GERIATRICS
A Study of Maturity

Fifth Edition

Barbara R. Hegner, MSN, RN
Esther Caldwell, MA, PhD

Contributor: *Carol Ann Mitchell, RN, MA, EdD*

Professor and Chair, Department of Adult Health Nursing
School of Nursing, Health Science Center
State University of New York at Stony Brook

Delmar Publishers Inc.®

Delmar staff:
Executive Editor: Barbara E. Norwitz
Associate Editor: Adrianne C. Williams
Developmental Editor: Marjorie A. Bruce
Project Editor: Judith Boyd Nelson
Production Coordinator: Helen Yackel
Design Supervisor: Susan Mathews
Art Coordinator: Michael J. Nelson
Art Supervisor: John Lent

Cover photos by Comstock, Positive Images, Skjold Photography

For information, address Delmar Publishers Inc.
2 Computer Drive, West, Box 15-015
Albany, NY 12212-9985

Printed in the United States of America
Published simultaneously in Canada
by Nelson Canada,
a division of The Thomson Corporation

10 9 8 7 6 5 4 3 2

Library of Congress Cataloging-in-Publication Data

Hegner, Barbara R.
    Geriatrics : a study of maturity / Barbara R. Hegner, Esther
Caldwell ; contributor, Carol Ann Mitchell.—5th ed.
        p.   cm.
    Caldwell's name appears first on the previous edition.
    Includes index.
    ISBN 0-8273-4531-3
    1. Geriatrics.   I. Caldwell, Esther.   II. Mitchell, Carol Ann.
III. Title.
    [DNLM: 1. Aging.   2. Geriatrics.   WT 100 H464g]
RC952.C353   1991
618.97—dc20
DNLM/DLC   90-139-05
for Library of Congress   CIP

Contents

Procedures

Preface

The first edition of *Geriatrics—A Study of Maturity* was published in 1972. This was long before the field of geriatric nursing became an independent discipline. However, the authors recognized at that time that there was a growing need for the specialized care required by an increasing population of older persons.

Each edition of the text has addressed changes in health-care delivery for the elderly, nursing care, and the economics of aging. Each edition has also devoted more attention to the multidisciplinary approach to the care of the elderly. The fifth edition continues this commitment to give health-care providers the latest information available on providing quality care to the elderly.

The authors welcome Dr. Carol Ann Mitchell as a contributor to the fifth edition. Dr. Mitchell is a noted authority in the field of gerontological nursing. Her insights help strengthen the base from which geriatric health-care providers learn to provide quality care and to enhance their skills.

The daily challenges that health-care providers face have never been more exciting or, at times, more frustrating. The potential for satisfaction in meeting these challenges has never been greater. The challenges that *Geriatrics—A Study of Maturity* helps prepare health-care providers to meet include the following:

- A growing population of young-old and old-old people
- The trend toward home care of the elderly and others within the community, and the support services that make this type of care possible
- The increasing cost of in-hospital care, which results in the release of sicker people to home care or to the care of other facilities
- The many health problems that affect an aging population
- The ethical questions associated with the use of technology to save and prolong life
- The rapid growth of geriatric care principles into a special discipline
- The effect of changing social programs that alter the way in which health care is paid
- The dramatic rise in the number of health-care facilities offering care for the elderly and long-term resident
- The shortage of professional nurses, especially those specializing in gerontology
- The growing need for health-care providers to assist professionals in giving care
- The changing mores of the society as a whole, which allow and encourage changing and diverse patterns of living arrangements
- A trend toward promoting wellness and self-care

Changes For the Fifth Edition

Throughout the text the authors promote the concept that the elderly in our society deserve care that will ensure the highest quality of life possible. To achieve this goal, the text has been expanded with new content, new photos and illustrations, and more detailed reviews. The new and revised content for the fifth edition include the following:

- NEW units
    - 11 The nursing team—members and roles, nursing process, nursing care plans, responsibilities of nursing assistants
    - 13 Legal responsibilities and residents' rights
    - 21 Mental and behavioral alterations in the aged, such as depression, delirium, and dementia, with guidelines for care by nursing assistants
    - 22 Sensory alterations in the aged, with guidelines for the nursing assistants' responsibilities for sight-impaired residents, blind residents, hearing-impaired residents, and deaf residents
- NEW Major topics
    Socioeconomic trends affecting the elderly
    Maslow's and Erickson's theories of needs and tasks
    Human sexuality and sexual expression, including bisexuality and homosexuality
    Multidisciplinary approach to care for the elderly
    Ethical standards in the care of the elderly
    Safety considerations for the elderly
    Infection control, including universal blood and body fluid precautions
    Alternative nutritional therapies such as nasogastric feeding, nasoenteric feeding, and hyperalimentation
    Durable power of attorney, no code orders
    Glucose monitoring
    Arterial and venous obstruction
    Sexually transmitted diseases
- Revised order of units to present content from general to more specific topics
- Vocabulary listing following objectives to identify terms for learners
- Summary in list form at the end of each unit for quick review
- Expanded reviews with more vocabulary activities
- Nursing diagnostic categories provided in selected units to provide a basis for understanding the development of nursing care plans
- Emphasis on the responsibilities of the nursing assistant in providing care for the elderly
- Updated statistics relating to the elderly—economics, health, community services and resources, insurance, care facilities and nursing care
- Updated information on aging theories and therapies
- More information on disease conditions commonly affecting the elderly, by body systems, and the nursing assistant's responsibilities for care
- Updated information on drug therapies; new content on the effects of "polypharmacy" on the elderly

The basic care procedures have been kept in the fifth edition. A listing of the procedures following the table of contents makes it easier to locate them in the text. Competency checklists for the procedures are provided in the Instructor's Guide as a teaching and evaluation tool.

The expanded Instructor's Guide also includes instructor objectives, review outlines, vocabulary lists, suggested activities, answers to unit reviews, section review questions and answers, comprehensive evaluation questions and answers, a list of text procedures, procedure evaluation forms, competency checklists, transparency masters, and a listing of instructional aids.

NOTICE TO THE READER

Acknowledgments

The authors wish to express their appreciation to the following instructors for their in-depth reviews. Their recommendations provided significant help to the authors in preparing the final manuscript.

Susan Kidd, RN
Massanutten Vocational Technical Center
Harrisonburg, VA

Barbara Gill, RN
Director of Nursing
Broward Convalescent Home
Fort Lauderdale, FL

Dianna Dee Mackey, RN, MA
Allied Health Department
Mission College
Santa Clara, CA

Elaine Polan, BS, RNC
Vocational Education and Extension Board
School of Practical Nursing
Uniondale, NY

Peggy K. Carr
Curriculum Specialist, Health Occupations
Vocational Curriculum Development & Research Center
Natchitoches, LA

Katherine Kucinkas, RN, BA, MA
Mansfield Business School
Nursing Assistant Program
San Antonio, TX

We gratefully acknowledge the Spanish translations of the glossary terms from Stuart Gedal, Maroli Licardie and Francisco Astorga of World Education, Inc., Boston, MA.

Section 1
Introduction to Aging

Unit 1
The Aging Population: Stereotypes

Objectives
After studying this unit, you should be able to:
- Define the aging process.
- Describe the demographics of the aged population.
- Explain the difference between a myth and a stereotype.
- Identify organizations concerned with problems of the aging.
- Define and spell vocabulary terms.

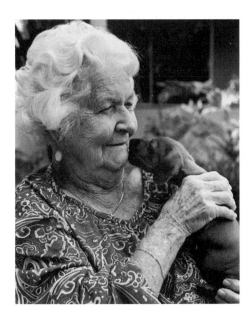

Vocabulary
Learn the meaning and spelling of the following words or phrases.

aged	myths
aging	old-old
demographics	senescence
geriatrics	senile
gerontology	stereotypes

Aging is a natural, progressive process beginning at birth, figure 1-1. It is an inevitable, universally shared experience. Advanced age is reached only by those who have proven themselves capable of survival. Physical signs of the aging process are easily recognized in the faces and hands of the elderly. Character and experience are etched in each.

Advancing from infancy to old age, an individual accumulates a wealth of impressions, skills, and knowledge and develops a particular life-style. By the time old age is reached, life has fashioned a unique and very special person. That person has exceeding value and worth and distinct characteristics and idiosyncracies, possesses human dignity, and deserves respect and support.

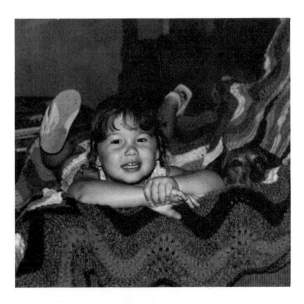
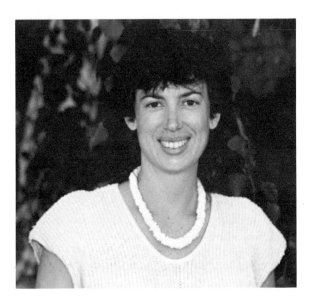
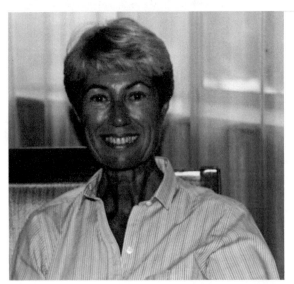
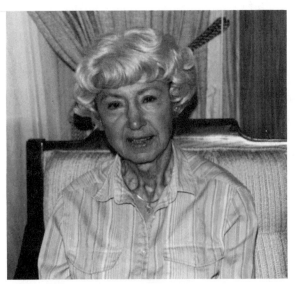

Figure 1-1   Aging is a progressive process from infancy to old age.

Terminology

Those who study old people and the aging process will come across some new words. *Geriatrics* is a word of Greek origin. It means care of the elderly. It is the branch of medicine and nursing that deals with old age and its diseases. Research into the aging process itself is called *gerontology*. *Senile* is a term that has become distorted in general usage. It properly means being affected with the infirmities of age. It has popularly come to mean mental deterioration. *Senescence* also means growing old. It refers to that period in a person's life when the changes characteristic of age have taken place. The term *aged* means old and usually refers to those over seventy-five. *Old-old* or fragile aged is a fairly new term meaning those older than eighty-five years.

Life Span

In the past two thousand years, the human life span has lengthened from twenty-two years to seventy years and more. Before 1900, children and young adults accounted for most of the deaths. The majority of the population died before age forty-five, with only 24 percent living beyond sixty-five. Since then, however, great strides have been made in the control of communicable diseases. Infant mortality rates and child care have improved. Today, old age has replaced youth as the time to die. Women tend to outlive men. In 1989, the average life span for women was 77.6 years and for men, 70.2 years. There are now four women for every three men aged sixty-five or older. It is thought that by the year 2000, older women will outnumber men by a margin of two to one.

The periods of life are pictured in figure 1-2. The chart shows that old age is now used to describe those over seventy-five. The age of later maturity begins at sixty-five. This is probably a much more realistic division. The majority of people are relatively healthy and vigorous at that age and still actively participating in life. About

Period of Life	Age Group
Neonatal	Birth to 1 month
Infancy	1 month to 1 year
Preschool	1 year to 6 years
School Age	6 years to 12 years
Preadolescent	12 years to 14 years
Early Adolescence	14 years to 16 years
Middle Adolescence	16 years to 18 years
Late Adolescence	18 years to 20 years
Early Adulthood	20 years to 40 years
Middle Adulthood	40 years to 65 years
Late Adulthood	65 years to 75 years
Old Age	75 years to 85 years
Old-Old Age	85 years and over

Figure 1-2   The periods of life

one-third of the sixty-five-year-old men are still in the labor force. In addition, the civic leaders of many communities are those of advancing years. Most older people are honored as valuable members of society.

The general attitude of Western society, however, is far different from the respectful attitude of Eastern cultures. In the past, Western society has often seen the elderly person as a source of embarrassment—someone to be tolerated, rejected, or simply ignored. Even the names chosen to speak of the aged—"senior citizen," "oldster," and "elderly"—reveal this feeling. Young people call themselves teenagers with great pride. However, people find it very difficult to call themselves or others "old" with the same pride. They often express preference for euphemisms like "senior citizen," "mature American," or "retired person." They are less amenable to "old person," "aged person," or "golden ager."

The twilight years, the golden years, and the sunset years are phrases used to describe the later years. Such terms make this phase of living seem like the end, not the peak years of life. This is probably why these terms are less acceptable.

In the last few years, education seems to have been improving attitudes toward the older population. What does being "old" really mean? To be old means that a person has successfully met and survived life's challenges. It means an individual has reached a state of maturity, endowed with certain wisdom derived from first-hand experience. It means someone has a storehouse of skills and knowledge that can be of great value to society.

In the past thirty-five years, society has been taking a closer look at the elderly people in its midst. More recognition is being given to the aging process and the needs of the aged. There are more than twenty-nine million persons over sixty-five years of age today, representing 12.3 percent of our total population. This number is growing constantly. We are an aging population. The twenty-first century will see, in its first quarter, 50 percent of the population over forty-five years of age. In fact, between 1900 and 1989, the total U.S. population tripled. The age group sixty-five or older increased eight times. It is estimated that at this same rate of growth, there will be more than fifty-eight million people over sixty-five by the year 2025. The implications of the statistics in terms of promoting satisfying lives are enormous.

These older Americans are most heavily concentrated in California, New York, and Florida. Most older Americans, 95%, live independent lives, together with spouses, or with other family members. A small percentage (3 percent of elderly men and 2 percent of the elderly women) live in the community with nonrelatives. Only 5 percent of the elderly require the supportive care of institutional living.

Organizations and Social Legislation

The Social Security Act of 1935 created for the first time a national system of retirement benefits for those over sixty-five. Two of the earliest groups to be concerned with the aged and their problems were the American Geriatrics Society (1942) and the Gerontological Society, Inc. (1944). The American Geriatrics Society is concerned with medical care. It publishes the *Journal of the American Geriatrics Society.* The Gerontological Society is concerned with all aspects of aging and publishes the *Journal of Gerontology.*

The first national conference on aging was called in Washington in 1950. From this initial conference, a federal committee was created, known as the Committee on Aging. This same year, the National Social Welfare Assembly, a large voluntary agency working for social reform, formed its Committee on Aging. It began immediately to work in the areas of employment and health care. This voluntary committee on aging evolved into an independent organization that in 1961 became known as the National Council on Aging (N.C.O.A.). The N.C.O.A. is an active and diversified organization offering counseling services, developing programs for the elderly, and publishing important information about aging.

The American Medical Association organized its Committee on Aging in 1955. Other state, local, and philanthropic organizations were formed in the early 1950s in response to the need. The Senior Citizens of America was organized in 1954, and The American Society for the Aged, Inc. in 1955, both voluntary agencies. To coordinate all the efforts, the American Federal Council on Aging was created by presidential appointment in 1956.

Efforts on behalf of the elderly gained momentum after the second White House Conference on Aging, held in 1961. Out of this conference emerged a document called the Senior Citizen's Charter or Bill of Rights, figure 1-3. Following this conference, the President's Council on Aging was established by executive order in 1962. The council conducts studies and makes direct reports to the President on matters of concern to the elderly. The American Nurses' Association also established its Geriatric Nursing Section in 1962.

THE SENIOR CITIZEN'S CHARTER

At the 1961 White House Conference on Aging, one group discussed the social and economic implication of population trends. This group also set up a statement of rights and obligations of senior citizens.

"Each of our Senior Citizens, regardless of race, color or creed, is entitled to:

"The **right** to be useful.

"The **right** to obtain employment, based on merit.

"The **right** to freedom from want in old age.

"The **right** to a fair share of the community's recreational, educational, and medical resources.

"The **right** to obtain decent housing suited to needs of later years.

"The **right** to the moral and financial support of one's family so far as is consistent with the best interest of the family.

"The **right** to live independently, as one chooses.

"The **right** to live and die with dignity.

"The **right** of access to all knowledge as available on how to improve the later years of life."

Balancing these rights are:

"The **obligation** of each citizen to prepare himself to become and resolve to remain active, alert, capable, self-supporting and useful so long as health and circumstances permit and to plan for ultimate retirement.

"The **obligation** to learn and apply sound principles of physical and mental health.

"The **obligation** to seek and develop potential avenues of service in the years after retirement.

"The **obligation** to make available the benefits of his experience and knowledge.

"The **obligation** to endeavor to make himself adaptable to the changes added years will bring.

"The **obligation** to attempt to maintain such relationships with family, neighbors and friends as will make him a respected and valued counselor throughout his later years."

This group also said that, with health and adequate income, and freed of physical compulsions, the need to conform, compete, or seek education for utilitarian value only, older citizens can be free to adopt new roles and status and develop unusual potentials.

Figure 1-3   The Senior Citizen's Charter is also known as the Senior Citizen's Bill of Rights. (Copyright 1965, the American Journal of Nursing Company. Reprinted from *Nursing Outlook,* November 1964.)

During this same period, the American Nurses Association recommended that a geriatric nurses specialty group be formed. This group received full recognition as a nursing specialty by 1966 as the division on geriatric nursing.

The 1960s saw much legislation and many programs develop on behalf of the elderly. In 1965, Social Security amendments brought Medicare and Medicaid into being. The Older Americans Act produced a wide variety of services and programs for the aged. The Administration on Aging was created with the signing of the Older Americans Act.

In 1967, the Administration on Aging became part of the new Social and Rehabilitation Service within the Department of Health, Education and Welfare. In that same year, the President recommended new legislation to further improve benefits for the aged. The recommendations were called "The Messsage on Older

Americans." The President's message stressed, "Our goal is not merely to prolong our citizens' lives but to enrich them." Six months later, the 1967 Amendments to the Older Americans Act were signed into law. Shortly thereafter, in 1969, the division on geriatric nursing developed and published the standards for geriatric nursing practice.

The third National Conference on Aging, held in 1971, revealed the effectiveness of the current programs. The 1970s showed rapid growth in the field of gerontological nursing, with the first certification in the field. In 1976 the name of the geriatric nursing division was changed. The new name reflects the broad involvement of nursing in working with both the healthy and ill aging person.

The 1981 White House Conference on Aging

The fourth White House Conference on Aging was held in the nation's capitol in 1981. There was a clear conflict between administration attempts to cut the national budget for social programs and the ever-growing needs of the elderly minority population. Social Security cuts were threatened. Out of this conference came a plank of eight recommendations labeled "Eight for the Eighties." Despite intercommittee hassles, there was agreement on the need to:

1. safeguard Social Security. The package of proposed cuts was only withdrawn after public outcry.
2. broaden opportunities for older workers to remain active voluntarily in the labor force.
3. assure income sufficient to maintain a minimum level of dignity and comfort. Supplementary Security Income payments were to be raised to the official poverty line immediately, with gradual increases over the decade.
4. enact a comprehensive national health plan for all Americans.

5. take interim steps to improve health care for older persons. Medicare and Medicaid services were to be expanded to include health maintenance costs such as prescription drugs and dental care. Also included were institutional care and community-based and in-home services.
6. develop 200,000 publicly financed housing units for the elderly each year throughout the 1980s.
7. complete a comprehensive service delivery system for older people. It would build on the foundation established by the Older Americans Act through partnership between various levels of government.
8. strengthen the federal commitment to the elderly by fostering research, education, and training.

Much has been accomplished since the 1981 White House Conference. Much is still left to be done.

Throughout the 1980s, the voices of advocates for the elderly have been heard in their attempts to prevent cutbacks in service and increases in health care supplementary costs. The movement has made a major effort to fight changes in Medicare and Medicaid provisions. The voice of the older population and its supporters has never been stronger.

Stereotypes and Myths

Stereotypes of people are rigid, biased ideas about people as a group. Stereotypes about aging and the elderly picture all members of the group as having the same characteristics.

Some stereotypes or fixed ideas about aging and the elderly are based in fact. For example, the belief that aging causes a loss in visual acuity is essentially correct. Beliefs about groups of people that are not even partly true are *myths*, figure 1-4.

Stereotyping is dangerous. It tends to assign characteristics to entire groups of people who may only have a single characteristic in common.

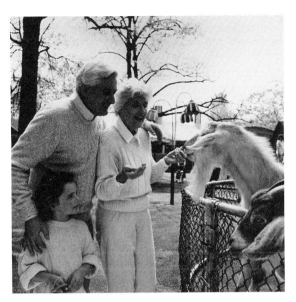

Figure 1-4 It is a myth that retirement means boredom and unhappiness for all those experiencing it. (Compliments of Squibb Pharmaceuticals—USA.)

Stereotypes do not consider the uniqueness of the individual. Stereotyping tends to harden attitudes and concepts, which then become self-fulfilling prophecies. In other words, if the elderly are treated as if these stereotypes are true, they will tend to see themselves in the same way. Seeing themselves in a particular way will prompt behaviors that authenticate the self-image. For example, a health care provider may take control of certain patient activities in the belief that patients are unable to care for themselves. If that action is persistent, it won't be long before the patients begin to believe they are not capable and will cease to try. In more practical terms, it might be quicker to feed stroke patients than to allow them to feed themselves. However, if feeding is continued, there is little incentive or encouragement for the patient to become self-sufficient.

The common stereotypes assigned to the aged are as easily believed by the elderly as by the young. The two age groups differ. The young apply the stereotypes to the elderly in general, while the elderly apply them to older people other than themselves. The older person considers himself or herself an exception to the rule.

The general stereotype of the elderly is one of weakness and vulnerability, with little hope, of little value to society, shunned by a society that is uncaring and unwilling to help or support. Resisting the temptation to stereotype all older people can best be achieved by accepting each older person as an individual. Each older person should be allowed to have as much personal control over life and activities as possible. Your role as a health care provider should be directed to supporting the elderly to remain as independent as possible. Remember that there really is no such thing as a typical older person. Each person is special and unique.

The following paragraphs describe some of the more common views (stereotypes) and misconceptions (myths) about aging and the aged.

Old Age

The first stereotype is that being old is determined by the number of years lived. This stereotype would have us believe that everyone is old at the arbitrary age of sixty-five. At this special moment, the person becomes old, retires from work, and gives up participating in life.

Studies show that most of those under sixty-four consider the median age of old people as sixty-six for men and sixty-five for women. This reflects a trend toward considering people old at a slightly later age than was previously the case. Interestingly, a sizable group who have already reached age sixty-five put less stress on chronological age. They emphasize other factors such as health and social involvement when describing the concept of "old." The active person projects a much younger image than one who is sedentary. Image also seems to be important when making such a value judgment.

The truth is that the world "old" is a nebulous term at best and must be applied on a highly individual basis. Being old is more related to how one feels and acts than to number of years lived.

Actually, the period of old age can be divided into progressive stages of increasing maturity. Chronological age is only one measure of age. It is important to recognize that the majority of people remain active and productive into their seventies and eighties. The elderly, however, are often limited by physical problems or severe and chronic illnesses that keep them homebound or institutionalized.

Work and Retirement

Another common stereotype relates to work and retirement. This stereotype says that work becomes less important as retirement age is reached and passed. It pictures the older person as gradually losing interest and satisfaction in work as retirement nears. The older worker is viewed as becoming more rigid and dogmatic in approach and missing an increasing number of work days due to illness and accident. Once retired, the myth continues, the elderly person dislikes being retired and is bored, with nothing to fill the time.

Statistics show that older workers have less absenteeism, fewer on-job accidents, and are no less efficient than younger workers. Older workers express more satisfaction with their jobs and are just as willing to learn new skills to increase their productivity.

It is a fact that mandatory retirement may remove workers from the work force while they are still highly productive and may not yet have reached their full potential. In 1989, about 18 percent of men over sixty-five were employed in some kind of work. About 8 percent of the women over sixty-five were employed. Both men and women often do household chores until they are in their eighties and nineties. Many older people enjoy active retirement as long as their health and finances permit. Travel and community and family involvement seem to be satisfying and fulfilling.

Shortening work hours is only one of the ways that workers can reduce their load and still continue to make a valuable contribution. The elderly do have more difficulty finding work af-

ter retirement or a layoff. However, the concept of massive intergenerational competition for jobs simply does not fit the facts.

More and more often today, older workers retired from employment in one field seek work opportunities and second careers in a related or unrelated field. For example, a 55-year-old postal clerk retiring from full-time employment after 30 years of service seeks and obtains employment as a structural mechanic in a local aircraft industry. Still in good health, he becomes vested for retirement benefits after 10 years of full-time employment. He also has the option of flexible, part-time employment after age 65.

Older women whose families are grown enter the work force. They continue working until their husbands retire or they reach their own retirement age.

Mental Processes

Some people believe that aging brings about deterioration of mental processes and an inability to make sound judgments. It is another stereotype that says that, as the individual ages, mental processes deteriorate and emotional adjustments become fragile. The elderly are seen as less intelligent, more forgetful, less adaptable, and more rigidly conservative. They are pictured as senile and depressed, seeing little hope or joy in their future.

Studies show, however, that older people continue to be able to concentrate, learn, and remember and to think and behave in logical ways, figure 1-5. They share the concerns of the young about health and the future. Older people do not perceive themselves as being less able to manage their own affairs. They are just as eager to be productive members of society. Of the very small percentage whose emotional stability is threatened, many can be helped with appropriate therapy. Keep in mind that, although external economic pressures are currently very high, the life satisfaction expressed by those over sixty-five is almost as strong as it is for those under sixty-five. It is true that as the years progress beyond eighty, less satisfaction is expressed. But

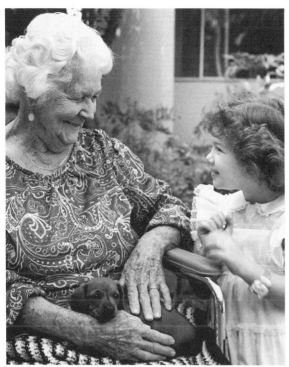

Figure 1-5 The majority of older people remain emotionally stable and mentally competent.

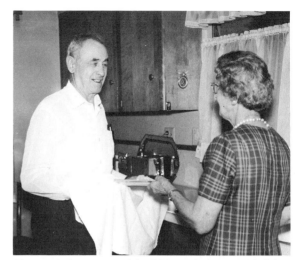

Figure 1-6 Many elderly people have satisfying interpersonal relationships with family and friends.

depression, withdrawal, and forgetfulness are not unique to old age. Satisfaction seems to be more related to economic circumstances and health than to chronological age.

Abandonment and Loneliness

Another stereotype is that society has abandoned the elderly, leaving them isolated and lonely. Society believes that they are a drain on its limited resources.

Studies show that, on the contrary, society has not turned a deaf ear to the needs of the elderly. It has supported legislation to benefit the older age group. Other studies show that 80 percent of the elderly live with someone, so loneliness is not a major problem. Many of those living alone have satisfying interpersonal relationships with a social network of family and friends, figure 1-6. Although most of the elderly maintain their own households, there is frequent interaction with

family members. The elderly provide numerous services to younger family members that would otherwise be costly not only to the family, but to society as a whole.

A growing trend in two-working-parent families is to call the older retired members into service to provide child care, figure 1-7. Younger

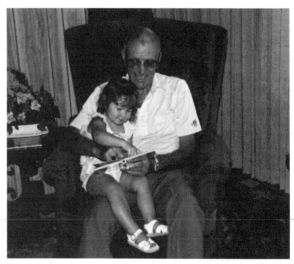

Figure 1-7 The elderly can be a positive influence on the lives of the young.

people in general treat older people with respect, and they desire only the same treatment in return.

Financial Security

A final myth involves the financial status of the elderly. This myth says that the financial picture of all elderly persons is bleak. This is an untrue misconception. Certainly, no one would deny that inflation and the threat of inflation, coupled with the enormous federal deficit and efforts to bring it under control, have affected the financial security of everyone. The elderly generally live on fixed incomes and have limited resources. They are more threatened than most. Still, overall financial requirements are not as great for the elderly, whose families have already been raised. Savings, pensions, Social Security, health assistance, and investments leave a marginal majority feeling that they are better off than they were. There are still millions living in poverty, but by no means is everyone in this situation.

The Minority

You might wonder why the myths and stereotypes persist in the face of such studies and statistics. There are several reasons. Obviously, some older people do not belong to the majority that has been described. Women and minorities are heavily overrepresented among the aged poor. They may well experience financial problems, illness, and social exclusion. In refuting the stereotype, remember that, although the percentages may be small, the actual numbers of people represented are not. To say that 5 percent of the elderly are institutionalized is to say that more than seven million people will become our patients and clients. The population over sixty-five is increasing, providing greater and greater opportunities for your service.

Those older people who are able to take care of themselves and can continue to live an in-volved, independent life will do so. However, even they will continue to need some degree of support. Society needs to work to increase opportunities for them. It must emphasize developing a safety net of care and support for those who are ill and infirm, are not financially secure, and must be cared for in various agencies.

Most textbooks on the aged center on the care of this minority population and its attendant problems and concerns. News media also focus on the unusual. In calling attention to the plight of the minority, the capabilities of the majority are frequently overlooked.

There is more than one way to describe a single circumstance. For example, if a glass of water needs to be emptied, it may be viewed as being three-quarters full. But if the need is to fill

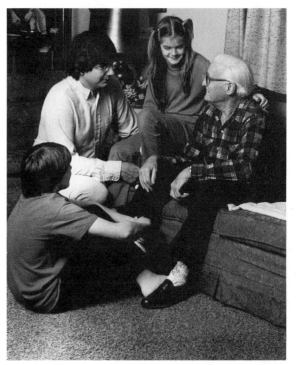

Figure 1-8 Living within a family unit affords the elderly a continuing sense of security.

the same glass, it may be viewed as one-quarter empty. Since our role as health care providers is to provide help, we must focus on the areas of need. In doing so, we must always bear in mind that, numerous as our patients or clients may be, they represent only a small fraction of people in their age group.

Needs of the Elderly

The basic needs of the elderly do not differ from the basic needs of other age groups. A sense of security is essential for peace of mind at any age, and the elderly are no exception, figure 1-8. They need to share love and affection and have adequate income, food, and shelter. Health needs are a paramount concern, because four out of five elderly persons have one or more chronic illnesses. Beyond this, the elderly need a sense of purpose and direction to their lives. There is no age limit on the creative portion of life.

Summary

- Aging is a natural process—an inevitable part of living. Those reaching advanced years do so because they have been able to adjust to life's challenges with success.
- The numbers of those reaching age sixty-five and beyond is growing rapidly, creating an increasing need for services.
- The basic needs of the elderly are the same as those of all human beings. Fundamentally, the elderly need to be treated as valued members of society.
- Beyond the basic needs, two areas of greatest concern are diminishing health and limited finances.
- In the past two decades, organizations dedicated to aiding the elderly have been formed at all levels of government.
- Social legislation has been passed that is beginning to bring a measure of security to the aged in our society.

Review Outline

I. Behavioral Objectives

II. Vocabulary

III. Terminology

    A. Geriatrics
    B. Gerontology
    C. Senile
    D. Senescence
    E. Aged

IV. Demographics

    A. Life span
    B. Periods of life
    C. Population concentrations
    D. Living arrangements
    E. Societal attitudes

    V. Organizations and Social Legislation

        A. Social Security Act of 1935
        B. American Geriatrics Society
        C. Gerontological Society
        D. National Council on Aging
        E. President's Council on Aging
        F. White House Conference on Aging

  VI. Stereotypes and Myths

        A. Definitions
        B. Dangers
        C. Specific stereotypes and myths

Review

    I. Vocabulary

Write the definition of each of the following.

      1. Aging _____
      2. Gerontology _____
      3. Stereotype _____
      4. Myth _____
      5. Senile _____

   II. True or False

      1. The majority of the elderly are living in poverty.
      2. Old age begins at sixty-five years of age.
      3. *Senile* is a term that has become distorted in general usage.
      4. The term *old-old* refers to people over eighty-five years of age.
      5. The current (1989) life span for women is approximately seventy-seven years.
      6. At age sixty-five, all men and women are ready for retirement.
      7. Many older Americans prefer to call themselves *oldsters*.
      8. The Social Security Act was first created in 1945.
      9. Chronological age is only one measure of age.
    10. More than one-half of the elderly population has one or more chronic ailments.

  III. Short Answers

      1. List four chronic ailments among the elderly.
      2. The demographics of the elderly show that
          a. at age sixty-five, _____ percent of men are still in the work force.
          b. by the year 2025, the number of people in the United States over sixty-five will be _____.
          c. the highest concentration of those over sixty-five years of age live in three states: _____, _____, _____.
          d. only _____ percent of those over sixty-five years of age require institutional care.

3. What conclusion would you draw from the statistics?
4. Describe the characteristics of the older worker.
5. How can stereotyping groups of people lead to false interpretations of the facts?

Unit 2
Developmental Tasks of the Older Person

Objectives
After studying this unit, you should be able to:
- Identify Abraham Maslow and Erick Erickson and explain how each has contributed to the understanding of human physical and psychological needs.
- List the psychological developmental tasks that must be met by the older person.
- Name four common periods of stress and major adjustment that people face in the later years of life.
- Describe the mechanisms to reduce stress.

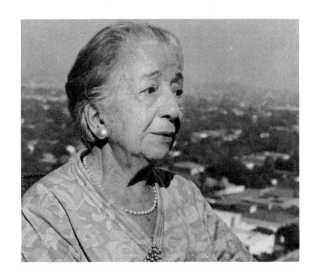

Vocabulary
Learn the meaning and spelling of the following words or phrases.

developmental tasks	mortality	personality
morbidity	partner	spouse

Socioeconomic Trends

Over the past forty years, many changes in society have altered previously established patterns. Women particularly have seen a change in their adult role. In the 1940s women were called into service for the war effort. Many remained in the work force after the war. Later, the women's liberation movement convinced many women that true fulfillment could come also by participating as a worker outside the home. The rising divorce rate has left many women as single parents supporting growing families. Inflation and the growing appetite for consumer goods have

also influenced the primary role of women as homemakers.

Today more than 50 percent of women with children under age six are in the work force. Many women who have remained in the home during the early years seek gainful employment when their children reach school age.

Another trend is for older retired persons to be asked to help two-working-parent families with child care. More and more grandparents who have raised their own children face retirement years raising their grandchildren.

Still another trend finds many women delaying pregnancy until their careers are well established. This often occurs just before their own "biologic time clocks" run out. This means that children are being born to older women who will be reaching their late middle adult years as the youngsters themselves reach maturity.

Women who are now entering their own retirement years, or later maturity, have lived through those turbulent times. The trends established in the 1950s and 1960s will continue to influence women's role expectations in the coming years.

Men, too, have experienced changes in society's expectations of them. Evidence seems to indicate that although men do help more with home and child responsibilities than they did previously, their role expectations have changed less dramatically than women's.

Physical and Emotional Development

As a person reaches each new phase of life, he or she accepts specific responsibilities and undertakes new roles. Throughout each of these developmental periods, the individual must make both physical and psychological adjustments. Two leaders in the field of human behavior are Abraham Maslow and Erick Erickson. Each has made valuable contributions to our understanding of the pattern of basic human needs and how people meet and handle the stresses and challenges that they face.

Maslow described the three broad groups of basic needs as physical, psychological, and sociological. He described these needs on five levels, figure 2-1.

Maslow found initially that the physical needs are the most important. The psychological or sociological needs can be fulfilled after the physical needs are met. His later writings indicate that physical and some psychological needs can be paramount simultaneously.

The most basic human concerns are those related to the physical functioning of our bodies. They include nutrition, rest, oxygen, elimination, activity, and sexuality. Illness and age create

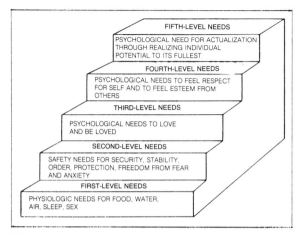

Figure 2-1   Maslow's hierarchy of needs (From Caldwell & Hegner, *Nursing Assistant—A Nursing Process Approach,* copyright 1989 by Delmar Publishers Inc.)

stresses that make meeting these needs a challenge for both the patient and the health care provider. For example, poorly fitting dentures and small appetites must be considered if adequate nutrition levels are to be maintained. Once basic physical needs are met, attention can be given to the next level of needs—psychological (emotional) needs. Many people can and do attempt to meet physical and psychological needs at the same time.

Maslow also found that the basic emotional needs of the elderly are the same as those at any age. There is a need to love and to be loved, with respect and dignity. Health care providers meet this need when they provide care promptly and gently. When health care providers treat people as respected individuals capable of making choices and decisions, people feel respected and their self esteem rises. When people make those in their care feel safe and secure, the social needs of the care receiver can be met by interacting with others in the society.

Personality

Exactly how each person goes about satisfying psychological needs depends upon one's personality. *Personality* is the sum of the ways we react to the events in our lives. Personality is gradually formed through experience. This creates a unique individual.

Erickson suggests that as we mature from infancy to old age, our personalities are formed. We pass through eight growing stages of self-identity. During each stage there are choices to be made and tasks to be accomplished. Erickson calls these the tasks of personality development, or *developmental tasks*. For example, the task of old age is to review life's challenges and accomplishments and to find final contentment. The tasks of various growth periods are summarized in figure 2-2.

Adult Role Establishment

For most people, the new responsibilities of adulthood begin when they finish school. Today, formal schooling is extending beyond the teen years, which in some cases postpones adulthood. Because the length of schooling varies, this discussion centers on the adult period between the ages of twenty-five and fifty. During these years, roles and responsibilities are fairly well defined as families are raised and careers are established.

Between twenty-five and fifty years of age mates are chosen, families established, and careers developed. These are busy years when,

for most people, health and energy are optimum. Toward the later part of this period, children mature and leave home for school and to establish their own families and careers.

Most men devote their lives to their careers and the support of their families. As long as physical health remains and they can continue in this role, they experience a feeling of independence and productivity. In the adult years, men often fulfill the authoritative and important role of father and provider.

The roles assumed by both men and women in their adult years may bring periods of frustration and indecision. However, they hold within them the potential for great satisfaction. The nature of the responsibilities provides opportunities for self-direction and fulfillment. Both men and women feel important as they successfully meet their responsibilities to their families and careers. Theirs is a full, productive life.

Middle Age
Final career advancement is achieved during middle age. After a time, this is followed by retirement. Children leave home and enter their own adult period. Health is usually still good, but some deterioration may be seen. Futures are less certain, and more time can usually be devoted to leisure activities. There can be years of financial pressure for those who are still responsible for their own aging parents, as well as for their own

TASKS OF PERSONALITY DEVELOPMENT	
Growing Stage	**Task**
Infancy	Learning to trust
Early childhood years	Recognizing identity as part of a family unit
School years	Skill development; constructive activities
Adolescent years	Developing identity as an individual
Young Adulthood	Forming intimate relationships, raising a family
Middle years	Carrying out one's chosen work
Old age	Integrating life's experiences

Figure 2-2 Tasks of personality development as summarized by Erickson. (From Hegner & Caldwell, *Assisting in Long-Term Care,* copyright 1988 by Delmar Publishers Inc.)

children. Financial needs often complicate planning an individual's own retirement.

The middle years are a time to develop and strengthen important relationships within the family and with friends. This is especially true for relationships between husband and wife.

Some people are able to prepare during their middle years for the changes to come. They make the effort to strengthen bonds with their husbands and wives and mature relationships with their children. They develop interests that can be enjoyed throughout life. Those with foresight and money begin to plan financially for their years after retirement. Others become so involved with current role expectations that they fail to recognize the changing nature of the role. When they come, the changes seem sudden, and coping is difficult. If a husband and wife can meet and expand their mutual needs as adults, they lay a foundation for their adjustment to later, postworking years.

Later Maturity

The period of later maturity is marked by gradual losses. There is a gradual loss of vitality and stamina and, for some, self-esteem. Physical changes signal the aging process. Sight and hearing diminish and hair turns gray. Chronic conditions develop and persist. This period is marked by the need to cope with the loss of a partner and friends.

It is no wonder that later maturity is a time when depression and introspection are more common. Support groups established in the adult and middle years can provide valuable assistance and social contacts. Persons in later maturity can function as important role models for younger age groups. The longer independence can be maintained, the more positive the changes are during this period.

Old Age

Old age is characterized frequently by decreased physical abilities and growing dependency. The need to deal with illness, loneliness, and loss of friends and loved ones, and the realization

of personal mortality, become important concerns.

Success in this final period depends upon the mechanisms of coping that the elderly have developed over the years. It also depends on the degree to which emotional and physical support systems are available. By the time old age has been reached, a person has experienced and somehow survived several major crises and multiple smaller ones. These are challenges that help develop the individual's personality.

During the later maturity years, a person must adjust to the loss of the parental role and the work role, and to retirement. In the old age period there may be the loss of a partner, living with illness and infirmities, and, finally, dealing with the loss of independence. In the lives of the elderly, several of these events may occur in close succession. The stress can be overwhelming.

Developmental Tasks of the Elderly

Meeting these challenges and making appropriate adjustments are the developmental tasks that the elderly must fulfill. Failure to adjust successfully to the changes can lead to depression, disengagement from society, and despair. Success brings with it a feeling of hope and wholeness from a challenge met and conquered.

Each of these changes is stressful for the older person. Techniques of stress reduction, tactfully applied, can ease the adjustments and allow the older person to enter more fully and completely into the final phase of life.

Empty Nest

When children mature and leave home, there is a definite period of adjustment. This is especially true for the mother. A woman's life can be very full when she is managing a home, with children dependent upon her for their basic needs. Many of her outside activities revolve around the children and their lives. If, during this period, she fails to develop some of her own personal interests, her life will seem empty when the children leave home to begin lives of their own. There is a sense of loss not only of the children, but also of the life purpose of motherhood. Hours can seem long. Apathy, stress, and a loss of direction may result. It is at this time that both husband and wife can do much to strengthen their own relationship. They can build common interests in preparation for the second adjustment period: retirement.

Retirement

Retirement means a tremendous adjustment for most people. No longer are they filling the family decision-maker roles of earlier years. Gainful employment is ended and, along with it, a measure of self-esteem may be lost. Personal opinions may not hold their former authority. Opinions are not as eagerly sought. This is particularly true because work is often intertwined with self-identity. Ask most Americans the question "Who are you?" and, besides offering their names, they will most often identify themselves by occupation. Jobs confer a sense of identity. When a job ceases, that person experiences stress and, sometimes, disintegration. This stress is easily projected to others, creating a strain on interpersonal relationships. Therefore, it is important to develop all aspects of personality throughout life, recognizing the many facets of identity.

Loss of a Partner

The loss of a *partner* requires major adjustments, figure 2-3. A partner is a significant other, male or female. A partner can be a housemate, a spouse, or a friend. This is sometimes a sudden, dramatic event, with little time for preparation. Even when death comes after a prolonged illness, a person is never fully prepared for its reality. The adjustment period is filled with grief and uncertainty. It does not matter that the partner may have been a close friend, a lover, or a spouse. The grief and uncertainty are still there.

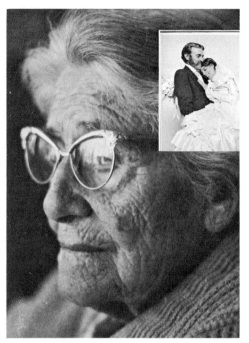

Figure 2-3   Death of a mate creates an empty space in the life of the remaining partner.

When a partner dies, decisions must be made about the future. Many factors, of course, influence the final decision. Age, personal health, personal wants, and financial security must all be considered. For a period of time, older persons may feel bewildered and alone trying to grapple with these momentous decisions, decisions that will have a great impact on their final years. Feelings of desperation, despair, and even anger and guilt may be so pervasive that major decisions are made poorly.

Because women outlive men by approximately seven years, the average woman will live those years, and in many cases more, as a widow, alone. Men, on the other hand, usually experience widowerhood at later ages. Still, both men and women or the partners in any life relationship experience the same emotional turmoil: anger, guilt, depression, and loneliness. The financial resources of the average widow are far more limited than those of the average widower. This in turn limits the available life-style options. The financial resources of the single elder of a homosexual relationship are even more constrained because most revenue laws favor legally married heterosexual couples.

The responsibility for social interaction is excused for a period of time. Society makes temporary allowances for the grieving period. After the grieving period, though, widows and widowers are expected to pull their lives together and resume some role in society. The need for intimacy that all humans share seems to be more readily met by men through remarriage. Twice as many widowers exercise this option as do widows.

For a woman who has been closely tied to her partner's identity (for example, "the minister's wife"), the loss of her mate may severely affect her own identity. Depending on the closeness and interaction with the partner's childhood family, the remaining partner may maintain some contacts with in-laws. But these become increasingly curtailed.

In some ways, men have more difficulty socializing than do widows, but loss of identity is not as great. Many men leave the instigation and promotion of social activities to their partners. The loss of a partner then cuts the lines of social involvement. The woman who has lost her partner still has those contacts. However, many social situations that involved couples are now closed to her.

The family usually makes decisions in the early bereavement period. This further reduces the older person's feeling of independence and self-confidence. Quite often, the death of one parent precipitates a major crisis in the homes and lives of the offspring as well. In addition to adjusting herself to the void left by her husband's death, a woman may have to make the additional adjustments needed when moving into the home of a daughter or daughter-in-law. Widowers may also be invited into the homes of children. Both

men and women, however, seem quite able and willing to maintain independent living quarters.

In many relationships, the partners may not be married. This doesn't diminish the magnitude of the loss, but may intensify the situation. Legal responsibilities may be more tenuous. For example, unmarried partners may not enjoy the same legal protection of property, or of survivor's insurance as husband and wife.

Family and friends play a tremendous role during the bereavement period. A close confidant, one who can listen, can make a real difference, figure 2-4. The bereaved are often obsessed with thoughts about the lost loved one. Opportunities to talk about the lost partner, to review and put into perspective his or her character—with good attributes and faults—help the person who is left to work through the grief. Adequate expression of thoughts ultimately

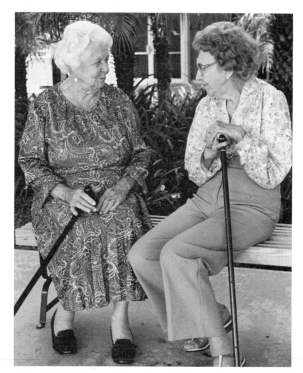

Figure 2-4 Having a confidant fulfills an important emotional need.

tends to make the negative characteristics unimportant. This leaves only an idealized memory with which to live. Men are less likely than women to have a close confidant, so opportunities to purify the lost partner's memory may be limited to family members.

Morbidity and Mortality

Morbidity (illness) and *mortality* (death) are the final adjustments that inevitably must be faced in the aging process. Older people have more illnesses. Although these illnesses may not require inpatient care, their chronic nature puts additional strain on changing body systems.

Poor health is not necessarily associated with aging. However, certain conditions such as hypertension, diabetes, heart disease, and arthritis, and impairments such as deafness, loss of teeth, and paralysis, grow more common with age. The longer the chronic condition persists, the more aware the older person becomes of its limiting effect. Initial anger and denial gradually give way to accommodating changes in activity and life-style. Individuals become aware that normal scnescent (aging) changes increase their own vulnerability.

The elderly person must make a major adjustment when it is necessary to give up independent living and become a resident in an extended care facility. Before they are admitted, many individuals undergo a series of emotional stresses. Making this decision is never easy for the family or for the person involved. Personal treasures may have to be given up, beloved pets put into new homes, and an entire life-style changed. A person's sense of independence is threatened just by knowing that there is a need for care and support in a facility.

After they are admitted, the elderly's new surroundings and people can raise the levels of anxiety and stress to such a point that a new resident becomes confused and disoriented. A health care provider's calm consistency and patience are vital factors in helping the new resident to adjust successfully and to complete this developmental task, figure 2-5.

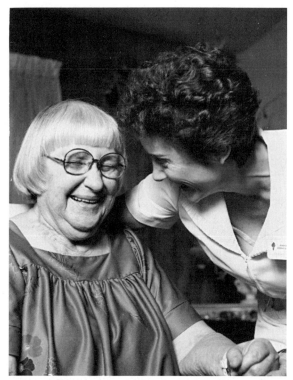

Figure 2-5 Loss of independence is a major adjustment for a person. The staff must be supportive as they take over responsibility for care.

Selections are made individually between the available options. The individual eventually begins to learn to separate from the usual patterns and activities of living, cope with the changes, and adapt by developing new patterns of living. Older people gradually redistribute their time and energies in ways that are most productive for them. The concept that we are mortal and must someday die requires a major adjustment in attitude. It is difficult enough to deal with the loss of a partner. Death is such a final act, but life does go on. It is far more difficult to deal with the idea that personal life eventually does not go on, that one's own death is an impending event.

Some people deny the need to adjust and throw themselves into activities to deny the future. Inevitably, though, for most the aging process, terminating in death, is accepted as a reality. Adaptive strategies are undertaken by most people. Older people redefine their physical and social interactions, taking on less and substituting alternate sources of satisfaction as the readjustment process continues. Values and goals are reviewed and coherence is sought at this stage of life.

Strategies for Reducing the Stress of Aging

The stresses just described are experienced by everyone at some time in life's journey. Strategies or techniques to cope successfully can be developed early in life. They need to be in place when the stress occurs.

Self-Confidence

The first stress reducer is confidence in oneself. Remember that only survivors prevail. Surviving should be a source of pride. Review the aspects of your life to date and try to identify difficult situations that you have worked through and solved. Take pride in these successes. Having confidence in your innate worth as a human being is the springboard from which all your other actions will come. As a health care provider, you must view those in your care with the same vision and build their positive self-image in the same way.

A Confidant

All tasks and problems seem more difficult when tackled alone. Sharing your thoughts and ideas with a special friend can help you gain a clearer perspective. Indiscriminately broadcasting your feelings and plans may tend to dilute them. But intimate sharing with a trusted person can solidify and enhance them. Feelings you could not express to a group can be dealt with in an intimate exchange. Having a friend is one of the best gifts you can give yourself. You may fulfill this role of confidant for your patients. This is especially true if you are working in an extended care facility. You may be selected as the one person with whom this special exchange can be made. Recognize the exchange as being very special. Give it the courtesy, support, and attention it deserves.

Support Networks

Beyond an intimate confidant, try to develop a support network of friends who share common backgrounds, goals, or experiences. Do not limit interaction to those with a similar background and experience. Each new relationship can enrich your life.

Try to develop a support network that, in time of crisis, will be there for you. This, of course, means that you must be a supporting part of the network when another member is in crisis. Older people who are moved out of their communities and into a residential setting lose their accustomed social support systems. You and the other residents or patients must fill the void.

The social network within an institution differs from the community network. Although you are part of the support, you cannot use the network for your own support.

Energy Conservation

When a crisis occurs, the event saps energy. Many things may need attention at one time. Important decisions may have to be made. Emotional stress drains energy.

First learn to set priorities. Everything cannot be accomplished at once. Often, if you put your energies into primary concerns, others automatically fall into place. As you plan your care assignments, you learn to set priorities. You organize your work so that all your tasks can be completed, but in descending order of importance.

Older people sometimes fret about minor things and forget to focus on really important activities. This can result from a habit begun early in life. Or it may be a delaying tactic to avoid facing a specific problem or task. Try to be sensitive to both possibilities as you help the elderly set priorities in stressful situations.

Family Relationships

At the same time that stresses are being felt and new roles are evolving, family relationships are also undergoing change. As children mature and gain independence, they become immersed in their own new roles and concerns. Some families remain close, maintaining frequent contact between parents and siblings. Other families, perhaps never close, become even more distant as time passes. The need for satisfying family relationships continues to be important, however, regardless of age. Recent studies show that most older persons do remain in frequent contact with younger family members.

Though husbands and wives can now spend more time with one another, figure 2-6, with fewer pressures and outside demands, younger family members seem to have less time to devote to their elders. Contact with youthful family members can be a source of tremendous pride

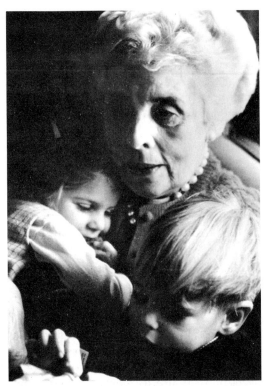

Figure 2-7   Contact with young family members can be a source of enjoyment for seniors.

and enjoyment for grandparents, figure 2-7. Is there anyone more thrilled than a grandfather watching his grandson up at bat or a grandmother holding grandchildren she seldom sees? Through relationships with younger people, older people experience a sense of continuing purpose in life. Seeing life being renewed and pursued through warm family relationships that span the generations can deeply enrich the lives of all.

The family is involved to some extent in each of the adjustment periods that have been described. When illness strikes or home care is no longer feasible, the health care team becomes involved and plays a vital role. Older people find the move to a strange new environment threatening. Families and partners may experience a

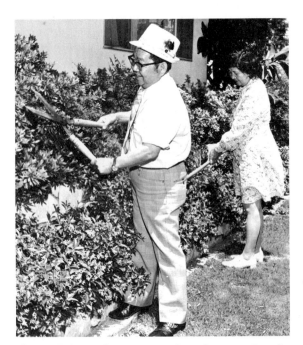

Figure 2-6   In later years, there is more time for husbands and wives to spend together.

sense of failure and guilt because the elderly person could not remain at home. The health care provider can help the patient achieve a sense of security with the staff and facility. He or she can help the family or partners work out their feelings about the move.

Family Reaction to Illness

Reaction to the onset of an acute illness or the prolongation of a chronic one varies in different families. Confronted with the health problem of an elderly member, some families may experience ambivalent feelings. They may demonstrate anger and other hostile feelings while they inwardly struggle with fears that they are inadequate for the tasks ahead. Some may feel guilt or shame because they did not provide more help and attention earlier. Others may resent the additional burden that illness imposes. They may feel so resentful that they reject the older person when love and support are most needed.

If the decision is made to place the older person in an extended care facility, family relationships may be placed under a tremendous strain. Once the move is made, some families demonstrate their rejection of the situation and the elderly person. They do so either by not visiting or by making routine visits with little loving warmth. However, family relationships must not be judged too casually or too quickly. Sometimes families do not visit older members because they do not know how to handle their own feelings. The conflict makes them uncomfortable. Other family members may not visit because the elderly person doesn't remember who they are. This is very painful. It may be difficult to understand the basic motivations, but the health care provider must try to maintain a nonjudgmental attitude while working with both family and patient.

Older patients in extended care facilities are there because there is no other place for them to receive care. Some receive regular visitors and have an opportunity to participate, at a distance, in family affairs. The restriction on child visitors made in general hospitals is not usually made in extended care facilities. Visits by youthful family members are often encouraged. The health care provider can help by assuring the family of the importance of their visits.

A large number of patients have few, if any, visitors. The health care providers and other patients gradually take the place of a family for those patients without visitors. In this case, the personnel's relationship with the elderly person needs to be a warm, receptive, but not mothering one built upon respect for the individual. This respect can be demonstrated by using the patient's proper name. Calling patients by general terms of endearment denotes familiarity, not respect. As the staff gets to know and understand individual patients and their backgrounds, realistic nursing care plans can be formulated that will enable the patients to reach their highest potential.

Health Team Relationships

Honest relationships have the best chance of being successful. Successful relationships are fundamental to effective nursing care. Before helping the elderly and their families work out their interpersonal relationships, health care providers must first come to grips with their own feelings about growing old and about old people.

True feelings are hard to conceal. They are revealed in the choice of words, the tone of voice, and the way patients are handled physically. Patients know whether a health care provider sincerely cares about them and the problems they face. They will be very aware of any reservations you may have about caring for them because they are elderly. It is important for staff members to resolve these feelings. Sometimes, talking honestly to others who are faced with the same situation can help clarify thinking. A discussion with an instructor and classmates may help the geriatric nursing assistant student.

Summary

- As people grow older, their responsibilities change and their life roles are altered.
- Maslow and Erickson have contributed greatly to our understanding of basic human needs and personality development.
- The characteristic roles of adulthood are essentially authoritative. They yield satisfaction and build identity and self-esteem.
- Roles are altered when crises force people to make adjustments in later maturity and older age.
- Major adjustment periods are the maturing of the young, retirement, loss of a partner, and major illness and the recognition of one's own mortality.
- Meeting and successfully coping with the multiple challenges of the later years are the developmental tasks of personality development.
- Stress reduction techniques should be learned early in life and be in place to provide maximum help.
- Healthy family relationships provide a sense of security for those undergoing a role change.
- When family support is lacking, as often occurs in extended care facilities, health care providers may function as a substitute.
- The health care provider who is mature, sincere, and sympathetic, and who is flexible in approaching individual residents, can become an important resource as a confidant and a part of the resident's social support system.

Review Outline

I. Behavioral Objectives

II. Vocabulary

III. Adult Role Establishment

    A. Socioeconomic trends
        1. More women in workforce
        2. Delayed parenthood
        3. Two-working-parent families
        4. Greater male participation in home responsibilities

    B. Physical and emotional development
        1. Maslow's hierarchy of needs
        2. Erickson's stages of personality development
        3. Adjustments at different life stages
        4. Special adjustments faced by the elderly
            a. Decreased physical ability
            b. Retirement
            c. Loss of a partner
            d. Loss of independence
            e. Acceptance of mortality

Review

I. Vocabulary

Write the definition of each of the following.

1. Morbidity _____
2. Mortality _____
3. Personality _____
4. Partner _____

II. Identify the following.

1. Abraham Maslow
2. Erick Erickson
3. Five trends that have influenced the traditional adult roles of women since 1940
4. Financial pressures for people in the late middle age period
5. Two major adjustments that usually must be faced in the later maturity years
6. Three major situations with which the person in the old age period must cope

III. Place the listed needs in order of Maslow's hierarchy.

	Need		Level
1.	To love	a.	First
2.	To be respected	b.	Second
3.	To be free from fear	c.	Third
4.	Food	d.	Fourth
5.	Security	e.	Fifth
6.	Need to love		
7.	Need for self-actualization		
8.	Water		
9.	Self-esteem		
10.	Sleep		

IV.   Clinical Situations

1.   One of the residents says that she can't join the community singing in the social room because she wants to clean out a drawer. What do you do?

2.   A member of the senior center begins to talk about her husband who recently died. What do you do?

3.   Another health care provider says she can't understand why Mrs. Rodan never receives visitors. How might you respond?

4.   You have been feeling very stressed for the past month. How might you go about reducing your stress?

5.   Mr. Ferber is very upset because his partner of 15 years fell and fractured his hip and has been hospitalized. What can you do?

Unit 3
Normal Psychosocial Changes

Objectives
After studying this unit, you should be able to:
- Describe the demographics of the aging population.
- List characteristics associated with the aged in some minority groups.
- Discuss age-related changes in intelligence, memory, and learning.
- Relate personality traits of the elderly to the problems of adjusting emotionally to aging.
- Describe reactions of the elderly to increased stress and defense mechanisms that may be employed.

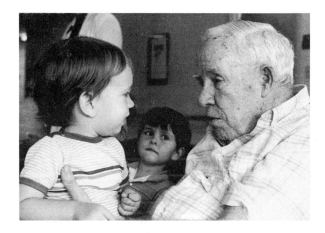

Vocabulary
Learn the meaning and spelling of the following words or phrases.

ambivalent	masochism	psychosocial
census	minority	rationalize
compensation	perceptual processes	society
defense mechanisms	phenomenon	substance abuse
denial	projection	withdrawal
displacing		

A *society* is any structured group of people with common interests and goals that functions within an accepted framework of cultural mores and customs. Members of the society interact in expected ways, following, to some extent, predetermined rules.

A society may be made up of a relatively small number of people who share a single, common interest. For example, the Audubon Society members all have an interest in birds. A society may involve an entire population, such as the culture or society established by the Mayan Indians. It may also be a city, a community, or the residents and staff of a large or small extended care facility. All societies have structure, set standards for their members, and expect their mem-

bers to carry out specific responsibilities and fulfill certain roles.

Society, as we know it, does not have the same expectations for each member all the time. Children fill one role in society, while adults fill another. Even within these large age groups, children, at different ages, are expected to behave differently, as are adults. Nevertheless, the expectations of society lead to the establishment of generally accepted characteristics for each level of development.

Society allows individuals to determine their own life-styles, within certain parameters. Society also establishes the process by which individuals become and remain members of cohesive groups. The outlaw fails to live up to society's rules and becomes an outcast. The person who reaches age sixty-five often becomes a member of a senior citizen group.

In the United States, many people have certain expectations for different age groups. Stereotypes and rules, or "norms," for behaving appropriately have evolved from these expectations. These norms, however, may not be very acceptable to those who have been labeled "old." As people grow older and experience changes related to age, their relationships with others may also change. Because the number of older people is increasing, society and its expectations may also change, figure 3-1. For example, as older people speak out more about what they

believe is appropriate behavior for themselves, younger people in society will begin to change their notions about what the rules should be.

Various aspects of many groups in society have been studied. However, there have been few studies of older people and the effects of cultural influences on them. Social scientists are the people who study the way in which personality interacts with societal expectations and restrictions.

Studies about self-concept, or attitude about oneself—what a person thinks, feels, and does—have shed light on some aspects of the elder person's personality. For the most part, self-concept is very stable and is not affected very much by aging. When there are changes, they are likely to be in autonomy, self-confidence, caring about others, and morale. Some studies have shown that life's events are more likely to affect self-concept and, in turn, a person's personality and how he or she adapts to changes. However, much still needs to be learned about the aging process and the effects of values, beliefs, rituals, attitudes, personality, and changes brought about by technology, war, and population explosions, and by changes in the family.

Characteristics of the Aging Population

What is the status of the members of our society who are part of the aged group? What role does society expect them to carry out?

Every ten years the government makes an extensive examination of the society as *census* takers gather information about the population. Statistics are compiled. Descriptions of living habits, age distribution, population concentrations, and public needs are generated. Using census information, public policy is formulated and funds are allocated to better meet current needs and projections of future requirements.

Although the last national census was taken in 1990, other governmental agencies, for example, the National Institute for Aging, also collect

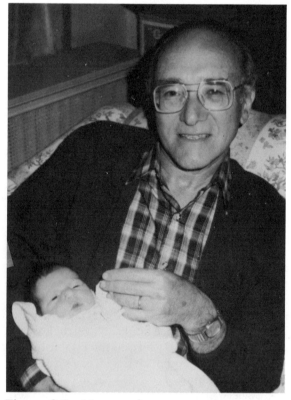

Figure 3-1   More and more grandparents are assuming care for their grandchildren as mothers increasingly go out to work. (From Morrison, *The World of Child Development,* copyright 1990 by Delmar Publishers Inc.)

census information. These studies revealed some interesting statistics about the older members of our society. Some students ignore statistics. They say that numbers are boring and charts are difficult to understand. Try to read this chapter carefully, thinking not just about the numbers but also about the human individuals that the numbers represent.

In 1987, those over sixty-five represented more than 12 percent of the population. Twenty-nine million people were either beginning or well advanced into the older years. In fifteen years, this number is expected to rise to over forty million. By the year 2025, 20 percent of the population is expected to be in this age group. One rapidly growing segment of the group consists of those in their eighties. The over-eighty-five group is expected to be about 25% of the population in the year 2020.

This massive increase in numbers will require careful planning if current and projected needs for assistance and services are to be met. Society must look at the projections and set priorities for public expenditures and programs. Health care providers must also examine the statistics carefully. To be successful, we need to learn about the characteristics of this group of people. Who are they? Where are they? What are their life-styles? These are questions that statistics can help answer.

Old-Age Subgroups

So many people are living into their eighth and ninth decades that the old-age group is divided into subgroups. Those who are sixty-five to seventy-four are considered the young-old. Those who are seventy-five to eighty-four are the old or middle-old and those eighty-four and older are considered the old-old. The role expectations for this latter group are far different than those for the sixty-five- to seventy-five-year-olds. Those over age eighty-four are considered to be frail, dependent, and needing the most services and care.

Looking at statistics help us to realize that the clients in our care will be largely women over eighty-five. Other statistics taken from various agencies, including the National Center for Health Statistics, reveal a great deal about our elders. For example:

- About 25 percent of noninstitutionalized Americans sixty-five and older are functionally limited with their basic activities of daily living (BADL) and independent activities of daily living (IADL). Of that, 25% need some assistance with their IADL.
- For those sixty years and older, 21 percent had no health problems, 30 percent had one health problem, and 49 percent had two or more health problems. Sixty-five percent of the latter group also had difficulty performing their activities of daily living.
- The major health problems of the elderly include arthritis, hypertension, heart disease, cataracts, diabetes, and strokes.
- The median income of the elderly increased by a greater percentage over the last two decades than did the median income of the younger adult population. Despite this improvement, about one of every seven Americans over the age of sixty-five lives in poverty.
- Elderly women are almost twice as likely as elderly men to be poor. Half of elderly, widowed, black women live in poverty.
- About eight of ten people sixty-five and over now describe their health as good or excellent compared with others their own age.
- Elderly men are more likely to be married and living with their wives. Elderly women are more likely to be widowed and living alone, with their children's families, or in institutions.
- The number of elderly women living alone has doubled in the last fifteen years.
- During the last decade, the number of elderly people living in central cities has declined. Meanwhile, the number living in suburbs and small towns has increased. Those suffering deepest poverty are in the inner cities or in rural areas.

- Half of those sixty-five and over who work do so on a part-time basis, compared with only one-third twenty years ago.
- In the 1988 election, 27 percent of those 65 and over voted.
- The major causes of death among the elderly include heart disease, cancer, stroke, and Alzheimer's disease.

The implications are clear. Many of those over sixty-five will need financial assistance and support services. In that group, women and minorities, especially those who fall into both categories, will be particularly needy.

The generally improved health status of those over sixty-five means that increasingly more people will live into their eighties and nineties and beyond. Perhaps the greatest emphasis should be placed on providing services for those over seventy-five, because they will have the greatest needs. Unless trends reverse themselves, increasing numbers of elderly women will be living alone or within residential care settings.

The elderly will most likely be found in suburban areas, away from major medical centers and health facilities. Greater numbers will be in the work force at least part-time. Chronic health problems will be common. In addition, at least a portion will be limited in their ability to care for themselves.

Active participation in politics means that, as a group, those over sixty-five will increasingly be in a position to determine public policy and to direct the expenditure of public funds, figure 3-2. More details about the aging population will be given in other units to which the statistics are particularly relevant.

Cultural Differences

By the year 2000, the number of aged minorities will exceed five million. A *minority* is a group of a limited number of people from the total population. Studies of disadvantaged minorities have greatly increased in recent years. The research findings have helped to identify characteristics that mark minority groups as different from the majority. Findings show that each group studied has its own special history. Usually, the histories are associated with negative stereotypes.

One study examined four minority groups: American Indian/Alaskan native, black (Afro-American), Hispanic American, and Pacific/Asian.[1] An attempt was made to examine how belonging to these groups affects the well-being and life-style of their elderly members.

1. J. Cuellar, E. Stanford, D. Miller-Soulé, *Understanding Minority Aging: Perspectives and Sources 1982.* University Center on Aging, College of Human Services, San Diego State University.

VOTING-AGE POPULATION: NOVEMBER 1984 AND 1980

Age Group	1984 Number of Persons (Thousands)	Percent Registered	Percent Who Voted	1980 Number of Persons (Thousands)	Percent Registered	Percent Who Voted
18 to 24 years	27,976	51.3	40.8	28,138	49.2	39.9
25 to 44 years	71,023	66.6	58.5	61,285	65.6	58.7
45 to 64 years	44,307	76.6	69.8	43,560	75.8	69.3
65 years and over	26,658	76.9	67.7	24,094	74.6	65.1

Figure 3-2   Older people have growing political power. (U.S. Bureau of Census)

American Indian/Alaskan Native

Statistical data about this heterogeneous group are extremely difficult to collect. Some live on reservations, some in inner cities, and some in other areas. Differences in culture, language, and historical experience compound the problem of assessing the situation accurately.

There are 293 federally recognized tribes and 58 tribes without legal status. More than one-third (36 percent) of American Indian elders speak only native languages. Studies have shown that the following statements can be made about this very diverse group.

- Cultural influences and tribal customs are strong. Services not under their control will be resisted. This is probably one reason that available services do not seem to meet their needs.
- Life expectancy is extremely short. It averages forty-seven years, compared to sixty-seven for white men.
- There is a higher incidence of some serious chronic illnesses among this group. Alcoholism and cirrhosis of the liver are 5 times higher than they are in other groups. Diabetes mellitus is 2.5 times higher, tuberculosis is 8 times higher, and influenza and pneumonia are 2.5 times higher. There is a lower incidence of heart disease and stroke, however. The leading cause of death is accidents, which directly relates to the hazards of this group's life-style.
- It is difficult to estimate the numbers of elderly because samplings differ. However, estimates range from less than 5 percent to more than 11 percent.
- Impairment levels of American Indians and Alaskan natives are comparable to those of non-Indian populations that are ten years older.
- Native Americans living in cities have experiences similar to those of poor, inner-city blacks. Their per-capita income is one-third the national average. The American Indian population tends to be less upwardly mobile than the black population, however.

Black (Afro-American)

In 1970, the number of older black Americans was 1.6 million. In 1981 the number had risen to over 2 million, or 7 percent of the population. Of this number, more than 59 percent were female.

As a group, blacks have a shorter life expectancy than whites, averaging 60 years for men and 68.3 years for women. But if a member of this group lives to age seventy-five, life expectancy is greater than it is for whites. This fact is referred to as the "crossover" phenomenon. In the over-seventy-five group, women make up 62.4 percent of the population. Note that many black men die before reaching the age of Social Security eligibility.

This minority group has been strongly stereotyped. Racism has restricted opportunities for middle-class jobs and education. Nevertheless, many blacks have raised their families to strive for middle-class values.

In all respects, aged blacks are worse off then their white counterparts. There is less money to live on, fewer sources of income, and greater dependency on Supplemental Security Income (S.S.I.) and public assistance. Of older blacks, 90 percent have Social Security pensions and 25 percent have S.S.I. benefits. Because Social Security benefits are tied to earned wages, the allotments may be small. Families who want to provide support for their elders are struggling against poverty themselves. One-third of elderly blacks live alone.

Fear and distrust of the bureaucracy inhibit use of available services. In general, elderly blacks live in substandard housing and are more apt to be renters than owners. Unemployment rates are higher than they are for whites. There are also fewer opportunities to prepare for retirement. Many are frightened and isolated in the inner city, where they are the victims of crime.

Chronic illness is a serious threat. The black elderly view their health as poor. However, they have less medical coverage and therefore receive less medical care and attention.

The elderly black woman is in a particularly serious predicament. She has four problems— she is old, black, a woman, and poor, figure 3-3. She may still play a significant role in her family. But high unemployment over her lifetime, menial jobs when employed, and poor education have most often led to low income, poor housing, and inadequate health care.

There is evidence that the situation is improving for younger generations of blacks. Much still needs to be done to achieve parity with other groups, however.

Hispanic American

Hispanics in America have their language as a common bond, but the language has also contributed to discrimination against them. They are of Mexican, Puerto Rican, and Cuban heritage. They usually live in metropolitan communities. The Mexican-American population is concentrated on the West Coast, especially in southern California. Cuban-Americans are concentrated in the Southeast and Puerto Ricans in the Northeast.

Some generalizations can be made about Hispanic Americans. First, this is one of the fastest growing minority groups. In 1970, they represented 2 percent of the population. In 1980, they represented 5 percent. Occupational history and income are generally higher than for other minorities. Unemployment is high, however, especially just before retirement. Educational background tends to be limited. Of Hispanic Americans, 25.7 percent live in poverty.

Occupations prior to this generation were largely agricultural. Only 55 percent were eligible for Social Security as compared to 76 percent of the white population. Few other retirement programs were available. Their lower socioeconomic status has led to a shorter life expectancy.

Hispanic Americans have a patriarchal society that tries to maintain support of the elderly

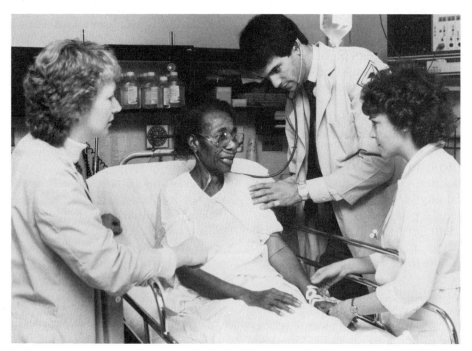

Figure 3-3   The single, elderly black woman is in the most serious need. (Courtesy Mercy Hospital and Medical Center, Chicago, IL)

through an extended family network. This type of support has become increasingly difficult as distances separate families. Hispanic Americans are a proud people and have a strong sense of dignity. This may partly explain why, as a group, they generally do not use available social service programs, figure 3-4. Some consider the need for help from a source outside the family a humiliation. There is little representation in state agencies for this group, and the language barrier places them at a disadvantage.

Even less information is available on aging among illegal aliens, although many thousands of Hispanic origin are living in the United States. Considering the difficulty of gathering data about this group, they will undoubtedly continue to be a subculture within the subculture of Hispanic minorities.

Pacific/Asian

This group of minority elders represents 6.5 percent of the U.S. population. The increase in Chinese, Japanese, and Filipino elders between 1960 and 1970 was three to five times greater than it was for white elders. This was partly because of the influx of immigrants, whose tenden-

cy is to move as families. The years between 1980 and 1990 have seen an influx in Vietnamese, Cambodian, and Laotian immigrants. This group is heterogeneous, representing many different subgroups. One-third of the population resides in California and one-fourth in Hawaii, figure 3-5. A great percentage (90 percent) lives in large urban areas and has difficulty meeting basic needs. This group is financially disadvantaged. Yet it underutilizes services, perhaps because it is unaware of them, unable to reach them, or feels a stigma attached to receiving them. Lack of bilingual/bicultural staff adds to problems between agency and client. Interestingly, Chinese American and Filipino American elder men outnumber elder women.

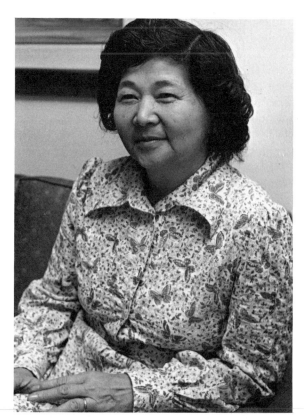

Figure 3-5 One-third of the Pacific/Asian population living in the United States lives in California.

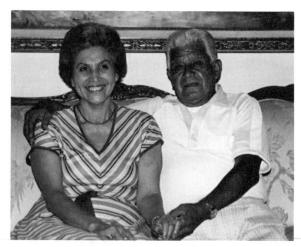

Figure 3-4 Hispanics have a great sense of pride and personal dignity. They often do not make use of available social service programs.

The members of this group will use services only if the following criteria are met:

• Services are local, within the neighborhood.
• The atmosphere is informal.
• The staff is bilingual, knowledgeable about the services that are available, and sensitive to the individual client's needs.

Psychosocial Adjustment to Aging

Psychosocial adjustments are both psychological and social adjustments. Self-concept, thinking, and morale tend to be very stable as a person ages. Contrary to stereotypes of ageism, most elders remain intelligent, thinking, adapting, and learning individuals. Older persons are confronted with many changes, such as loss of family, relatives, and friends through death or relocation. In addition, they experience changes in their role, their work, and even leisure activities. They may even confront discrimination. Possible socioeconomic changes may occur, because Social Security benefits account for only 38 percent of an elderly person's total income. This is a complex area involving sensory processes, perceptual processes, mental abilities, and emotions.

Senses and Perception

The senses are the major avenue for bringing reality to our awareness. Sensory losses, described in Unit 23, are common with advancing age. This means that the elderly may experience an imperfect awareness of reality. For example, hearing loss may mean that only part of a conversation reaches an aged person. Consequently, older people's reactions may not always seem appropriate to those who are communicating with them.

Perceptual processes are required to interpret sensory information. There is no serious decline until after seventy years. After this time, many elderly need more time to process sensory information and to respond. For example, you might ask a resident how she would like her hair fixed and find the response slow in coming. Be patient, understanding that it takes the older person more time to receive the information, process it, and then respond.

The majority of elderly people are mentally alert and competent. These people make up over 90 percent of the elderly population. They are active in the community and live independently or make their homes with their families. Many others with keen minds are in homes or other facilities that provide them with the necessary physical support. One cannot assume that because a person is no longer able to live alone, he or she is no longer mentally competent. A well-trained intellect and memory do not decline with age alone.

Many older people take advantage of educational opportunities in the community, as long as they are physically able, figure 3-6. Many colleges and universities allow older adults to attend classes without paying tuition or paying decreased tuition, or to audit classes. The more education an individual attains in the early years, the more apt he or she is to pursue intellectual activities in the later years. Unless pathology is present, there is no reason for intellect to decline with age. However, a sense of personal worth

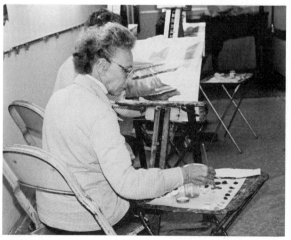

Figure 3-6 Many elderly persons take advantage of educational opportunities within the community.

and value is essential to a continuation of mental health and stability.

Custodial care is required for those who are no longer alert. Because health care providers give that care, they see a larger number of patients who do suffer from some degree of mental incompetence. Remember that only 5 percent of the total elderly population need custodial care and only 1 percent are found in mental hospitals.

Emotional Adjustment

Emotional adjustments in old age are extensions of the adjustments made earlier in life to many changes in circumstances. Personality characteristics and ways of reacting to stress are developed fairly early. By old age, personality patterns are firmly established. However, some traits may have been concealed. For example, less desirable traits such as envy, jealousy, and insecurity, which might hinder the individual in social and business interactions, are kept veiled in the younger years. At this age, making a good impression is socially and economically advantageous. In old age, the individual may feel that it is no longer necessary to hide these traits. Having less to lose, he or she can more openly reveal them.

As a person ages, personality traits become more pronounced. The stress produced by the circumstances and illnesses that accompany old age do not drastically alter the individual's personality. But they may disguise some traits while emphasizing others. The roles the elderly assume and the roles expected by society sometimes conflict. For example, an older resident sees himself as slowing down but still capable of dressing himself. The younger health care provider gives more assistance than is needed or desired. Conflict arises. When conflict develops, anxiety and frustration hamper successful adjustment. Decreased physical stamina only increases the difficulties experienced.

Old people have the same emotional needs and require the same supports for good mental health as young people do. They need to love and be loved, to feel a sense of achievement and recognition, and to have a degree of economic security. These needs are common to all human beings, regardless of age. The avenues for fulfilling these needs narrow greatly with age, however. For example, opportunities for social exchange and sexual expression, major sources of gratification, are generally reduced as the years advance. They are practically nonexistent for those confined to extended care facilities.

Defense Mechanisms   The Western world tends to relegate old people to a position of lesser significance. People who are now in their late maturity have participated in formulating and promulgating this attitude. It is no wonder, then, that the older these people become, the more their self-image declines. They, in fact, reject themselves. They expect only to be tolerated, as they previously tolerated their elders. Self-esteem is greatly threatened, and self-protective defense mechanisms are employed. *Defense mechanisms* are ways people respond that will protect their self-esteem. Some defense mechanisms that you will recognize in your patients are projection, displacement, rationalization, compensation, denial, and withdrawal. You may also recognize some of these defense mechanisms operating in your co-workers and in yourself at various times in your life.

A resident may claim that someone else joggled his arm so that his water spilled, rather than admit that the trembling of his own hands caused the accident. He is employing a defense mechanism called *projection*. Projection is a technique that places responsibility for one's action, thought, or feeling in someone other than oneself.

The resident who complains loudly that the staff ignores her just might be *displacing* the anger she is feeling about the infrequent visits of her family. Another resident might handle his disappointment over the same neglect differently. He might explain to anyone who will listen that his daughter cannot visit because she is such an important executive that she hardly has any free time. This resident has chosen to *rationalize* away his predicament, giving a logical explanation to cover his feelings of abandonment.

Someone who excels in one field to make up for a deficiency (real or imagined) in another is using the defense mechanism called *compensation*. One resident might spend hours each day crocheting to compensate for her inability to walk. Her handmade creations bring compliments, which enhance her sense of value and direct attention away from her disability.

When stress and anxiety become too great, some people simply refuse to face reality. This refusal is another defensive mechanism known as *denial*. An older person may simply refuse to admit that his hearing is not as acute as ever. He may complain that "those young assistants all mumble when they talk." There is certainly an element of projection in his assertion, but he is essentially denying the reality of his hearing loss.

Each of these defense mechanisms helps to keep the individual functioning while protecting self-esteem. When anxiety and stress become overwhelming, however, the only recourse for some is to absent themselves mentally and/or physically from the situation. This is known as *withdrawal*, figure 3-7. For example, a patient in a wheelchair might return to her room because the confusion of the day room is too stressful. She withdraws physically. But what about patients who lack the mobility to remove themselves physically from unhappy, uncomfortable, or stressful situations? These patients may escape into their own minds, fantasizing and daydreaming. Sometimes they carry on conversations with fantasy companions.

Self-Image Physical changes contribute to the loss of self-esteem with age. Wrinkles, graying hair, and the need for glasses or a hearing aid are difficult to deny, although many people attempt to do just that. This may be explained partly by our culture that values youth, attractiveness, strength, and slenderness. Some older people, however, emphasize inner qualities rather than physical attractiveness, and they are at peace with their aging.

Circumstances also contribute to loss of self-esteem and changes in self-image. Old age brings a series of losses, each influencing the way people

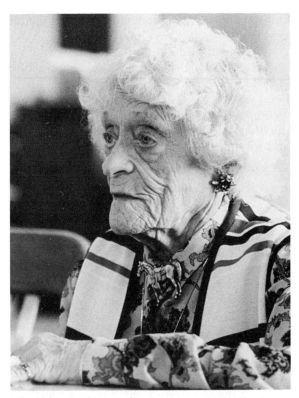

Figure 3-7   Emotional withdrawal eases stress that seems overwhelming. (Courtesy Long Beach Memorial Medical Center)

perceive themselves and their value to society. Perhaps one of the greatest losses is a change in roles. People have a wide variety of roles. Essential roles include being a parent, partner, homemaker, or worker. Social roles include friend, club member, or volunteer. Cultural expectations and health problems can decrease the numbers of roles that elders have and their ability to fulfill those that remain. For many, work is intimately linked with one's view of the self. A person may think of the self as a watchmaker, a plumber, a nurse, or a typist. When the work role is altered by retirement, a measure of one's self is lost as well. To the individual, a watchmaker, plumber, nurse, and typist all have social value. An ex-watchmaker or any ex-worker has lost equivalent social value. Retirement may also substantially reduce financial security. In a world of materialistic goals that are achieved through the expenditure of money, the older person is often denied this source of gratification.

Physical ailments, far more common in the elderly, are superimposed upon the transformation brought about by the natural aging process. Loss of the vigor and vitality of former years further alters the self-image.

The self-image is probably distorted most strongly by any circumstance that causes loss of self-esteem, status, or independence. Some of these circumstances have already been mentioned, for example, elimination from the work force. Independence and status are also affected when a person relinquishes a home to move in with a son or daughter or when a person is admitted to an extended care facility.

The role one assumes as an invited member of someone else's household is far different from the role one plays as head of one's own home. An ever greater role change takes place when one is admitted to a care facility. From a posture of independence or at least partial autonomy, the individual is cast into the role of "patient." Being a "patient" implies losing one's independence and individuality. Too often the environment of both situations fosters dependence and compromises the self-image.

Not all elderly people undergo drastic changes in self-image. Activities in the postretirement years bring a real sense of achievement to most, with a strengthening of the self-image. Participation in activities of social value, such as volunteer work or other forms of community service, can maintain or strengthen an individual's self-confidence, figure 3-8.

Many older people contribute to the community through their volunteer services. A Louis Harris survey in 1981 put the figure at 5.8 million or 23 percent of those sixty-five or older. The most active participants are volunteers who are white, retired, enjoy relatively good health, and have their own transportation. The value of these services in 1981 was estimated at $10.6 billion. Most of the older volunteers worked with their peers, but some worked with younger people. The majority of older volunteers provided

Age Group	Percent Who Did Volunteer Work (1981)
18 to 24	29
25 to 39	32
40 to 54	36
55 to 64	31
65 and over	23

Figure 3-8 Volunteer participation rates by age groups for 1981. These rates have remained fairly constant to the present. (A study for the National Council on the Aging, by Louis Harris and Associates, Inc., 1981.)

direct services that were often related to health or religious work. Some elderly said that they were not involved because of illness or poor health, lack of transportation, not enough time, and lack of opportunities. Without question, the elderly can and do continue to be a valuable resource for society.

Positive Adjustment

The most healthy emotional responses are guided by philosophies that accept aging as a natural, progressive step in life. Healthy attitudes recognize the strengths of wisdom as well as the limitations of the body. Healthy behaviors demonstrate an interest in living here and now. Healthy psychological adjustments are based on a realistic appraisal of the present circumstance. They build on positive aspects while coming to terms with negative ones. For example, an elderly person who loses a mate must adjust to the loss. Grieving is natural and healthy. Successful psychological adjustment is gradually made when the individual once more takes pleasure in the company of family, friends, children, and grandchildren (a positive aspect of the elderly person's life). At the same time, the person must recognize that memories are all that is left of the former relationship. This is a realistic appraisal and adjustment.

The elderly can best serve the young by acting as role models for them to follow in their own advanced years. The generation now in late maturity is living much longer than previous ones did, and the absence of role models creates anxiety and tension. Remembering the positive behavior of a grandfather or great-grandmother can help the younger individual adjust to the problems of aging.

The people most likely to make successful psychological adjustments are those who possess strong, positive personalities and inner strengths. People with less stable personalities who have not developed inner strengths tend to deny or fear the future, find no pleasure in the present, and gradually take their only comfort in memories of the past. Not all of the elderly have the same way of reacting to stress. However, the majority of them learned early in life the techniques of emotional survival that enabled them to reach their present advanced years. Remember that only 5 percent of the elderly require institutional care.

People continue to react and interact in the ways that they have found to be effective throughout life, following their own basic personality patterns. Those who have the most difficulty adjusting emotionally to aging are those who have deep, unmet emotional needs, those who have found social pressures and relationships difficult to handle all their lives. Now that they are older and their stamina is reduced, it takes less stress to produce an adverse response. Traits that may be encountered in these people include hostility, anxiety, self-punishment (*masochism*), defensive reactions, sensitiveness, and aggressiveness. Remember, defensive reactions are employed in an effort to protect self-esteem and reduce stress and anxiety. Sometimes people express these traits overtly. They may complain frequently, become involved in disputes with other patients, or be hurt or angered by minor incidents. At other times, personality traits are expressed more subtly. They may exhibit such regressive behavior as incontinence, rejection of fluids, or neglect of personal hygiene.

Sexuality

The chance for sexual expression is greatly hampered by the loss of a partner, limited opportunities, and the prevailing attitude of society that sex is the prerogative of the young. How the older person deals with sexual needs depends, in part, on previous sexual adjustment. The more active and satisfying the sexual experience has been, the more an individual will want to continue this activity into the later years. For those whose sexual interactions have been unsatisfying and even threatening, the later years offer a socially and personally acceptable reason for nonparticipation. Additional information about sexuality and aging is presented in Unit 5.

Reactions to Stress

Initially, when faced with stress, aging, or illness, people universally react with anxiety and fear. The level of emotional maturity determines the final response and behavior. It is common for older people to experience uncertainty and panic when first recognizing failing capabilities. They become greatly concerned about the unknown elements of the future. They wonder how their needs will be met when they can no longer care for themselves.

Fear is the dominant emotional response of this period. Fears are centered around the loss of independence and rejection by loved ones. Death becomes a more prominent concern. The overt behavioral pattern is one of chronic complaint. These complaints make the situation increasingly difficult for family or staff, who are sorely tried. Fears and anxieties, accompanied by feelings of frustration, cause agitation, restlessness, and nocturnal disturbances. The frustration experienced by the elderly is characterized by *ambivalence*, that is, being emotionally torn by *ambivalent* (opposing or conflicting) feelings—the desire for freedom and independence versus the desire for security and dependence.

Anxiety and fears are expressed in periods of depression and withdrawal. Crying, self-pity, and whining represent ways that patients overtly respond to their anxieties and fears. Withdrawal shows in lack of communication, temporary confusion, hallucinatory states, and general disorientation in time and place. As health care providers, it is important to report any observations that might indicate that these behaviors might be the result of *substance abuse* (inappropriate use of drugs). Patients having difficulty coping may resort to using alcohol or drugs. Elderly persons are more susceptible to having their cognitive and functional abilities seriously affected by alcohol and drugs. Often, when alcohol use is discovered, a person becomes hostile. These patients need to be reassured of two things. First, they have the ability to cope with their problems. Second, they will not be abandoned when they are no longer able to care for themselves. When they have withdrawn from the pressures of their problems, they need help in reestablishing contact with reality and support as they grapple with the solutions to their dilemmas. These patients are expressing a deep need for love and security.

The frustration experienced by the elderly is also revealed by aggressive behavior such as anger, hostility, and demands, figure 3-9. Some resort to bullying families, staff, or other patients in an attempt to relieve their feelings of helplessness. In periods of frustration, patients need help in expressing their frustrations in socially acceptable ways. At the same time, they need help in finding solutions to their problems and adjusting to those aspects of the situation that cannot be altered.

Some patients remain in a dependent role in an extended care facility because they believe this is the role the staff expects of them. They are afraid that any show of independence will result in retaliation from the staff. The elderly are very sensitive to the attitude of the staff. Health care providers must resist the temptation to promote dependence in their patients and be receptive to attempts at independent functioning. Supplying motivation is a primary nursing task. Nursing diagnostic categories related to psychosocial alterations are found in figure 3-10.

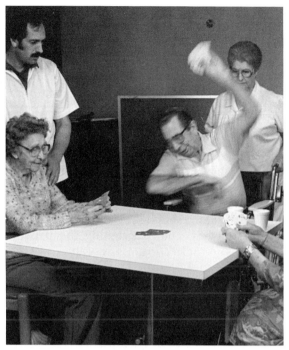

Figure 3-9   Aggressive behavior may result from the frustration felt by many elderly.

Actual or Potential
Alteration in family processes
Anticipatory grieving
Anxiety
Disturbance in self-concept: body image, self
Dysfunctional grieving
Esteem, role performance
Fear
Ineffective family coping
Ineffective individual coping
Knowledge deficit
Potential for violence
Powerlessness
Social isolation
Spiritual distress

Figure 3-10   Nursing diagnostic categories related to psychosocial alterations

The Health Care Provider's Role

The health care provider plays a vital role in the emotional adjustment of the elderly. In some instances, the staff provides their only stable relationships. It is with the health care providers' assistance that patients work through their fears, anxieties, and frustrations. The staff needs to apply the basic principles of caring and psychology to interactions with geriatric patients and their families. The staff must also be sensitive to the sociological aspects of these interactions.

Within the care setting, the health care provider can begin to build the patient's self-esteem and security by calmly accepting the patient's behavior and redirecting less desirable traits into positive channels, figure 3-11. The health care team can also work with the family and the community to encourage their support and acceptance of the elderly patient. Amazing changes in behavior are brought about when a patient ceases to fear rejection and feels that someone really cares.

Touch is a simple method of communicating intimacy, human warmth, and affection to patients, figure 3-12. Children accept physical contact as a natural part of their interpersonal relationships. As people grow older, touch tends to be restricted to spouse or lover, family, and friends. Yet the need for physical contact as a means of communication remains. So intense is this need that patients will sometimes engage in regressive behavior. They may become incontinent or physically aggressive, simply to engage in or prolong physical contact with the staff. Not all patients have this need to the same degree. The hostile patient may resent physical contact. Physical contact is desirable for many patients, however. It can easily be given through backrubs, touching a hand, or stroking a forehead. Quite often an elderly patient will reach out timidly to touch the hand of a staff member. This

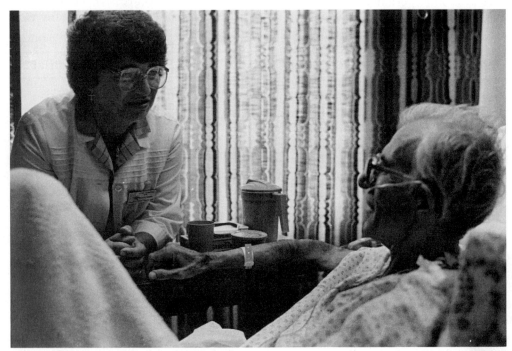

Figure 3-11   Positive interactions help the older person maintain healthy self-esteem. (Courtesy Long Beach Memorial Medical Center)

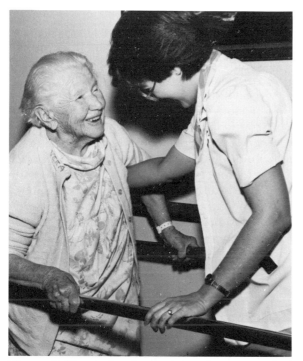

Figure 3-12   A simple touch can become an important moment of sharing.

moment of human sharing may be the beginning of an important supportive relationship.

The health care staff can stimulate social interaction by involving the patient with several staff members and patients. Good nutrition can be combined with social interchange at mealtime by having patients eat in a common dining room, with several people at each table, figure 3-13. Carefully chosen activities can help patients find satisfaction, fill the hours, and develop a sense of purpose. Attention to the physical needs of the patient is basic to the overall program of therapy and support.

The most significant part of therapy is the warm, nonjudgmental relationship the health care provider establishes with individual patients. Though the health care team must control the level of involvement to remain effective, sincere empathy establishes the therapeutic milieu. Almost no phase of geriatric care is as significant to the overall success of the regime as the health team-patient relationship. No type of health care offers greater rewards than the care of elderly patients.

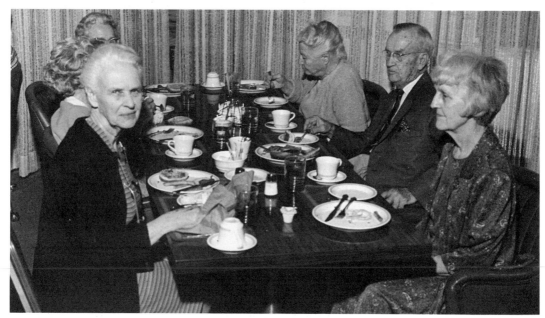

Figure 3-13   Eating in a common dining room permits positive social exchange.

Summary

- Throughout life, members of society interact. They make necessary adjustments so that personal values and behavior will conform with societal norms. These norms of expected behavior are applied by society to groups.
- The elderly as a group have certain characteristics and roles to fulfill. Adjustments to societal roles throughout life greatly influence the emotional adjustments of the later years. Each adjustment adds to or subtracts from the self-image.
- Healthful psychological adjustments make it possible to focus on positive aspects of life while realistically appraising negative aspects.
- Changes in body image and loss of self-esteem and independence hinder some elderly persons from making a healthful psychological adjustment to aging.

- Sexuality is an integral part of being human. It is an aspect of aging that health care providers often overlook or deny.
- Fears, anxieties, and frustrations of aged persons can be handled and the elderly person helped to find suitable solutions. This enhances personality integration. Failure to find solutions leads to personality disorganization.
- The health care team can help the patient/resident achieve a degree of security and emotional stability by organizing the environment, attending to emotional and physical needs, and providing social interactions.
- The health care team members can work with the family and the community to strengthen supportive bonds with the elderly.

Review Outline

   I. Behavioral Objectives

  II. Vocabulary

 III. Societal Expectations

 IV. Characteristics of the Aging Population
- A. General
- B. Cultural differences
   1. American Indian/Alaskan native
   2. Black (Afro-American)
   3. Hispanic American
   4. Pacific/Asian

  V. Emotional Adjustment
- A. Defense mechanisms
- B. Self-image
- C. Positive adjustments
- D. Reactions to stress

VI. The Health Care Provider Role

    A. Personal relationships
    B. Positive interactions
    C. Support of patient/resident and family
    D. Communication through touch

Review

  I. Vocabulary

Complete the crossword puzzle.

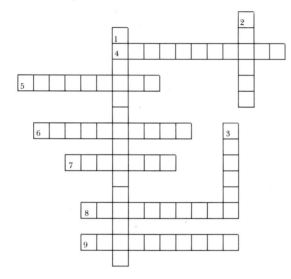

DOWN

1. Giving a logical but untrue reason to explain a circumstance
2. Government poll to gather information about the society
3. Refusing to recognize the reality of a situation

ACROSS

4. Having opposing feelings
5. Self-punishment
6. Directing anger against the wrong source
7. Structured group of people with common interests and goals
8. Absenting oneself mentally and physically
9. Placing responsibility for one's actions, thoughts, or feelings on someone other than oneself

  II. True or False

    1. Older people are generally unable to learn as well as younger people.
    2. More older men than older women are likely to be living with their spouse.
    3. Most people over sixty-five feel that their health is good or excellent.
    4. More elderly people live in inner cities than in suburbs.
    5. Less than one-third of those over sixty-five work at least part-time.
    6. One of every seven Americans over sixty-five lives in poverty.

7. Older people are politically inactive and seldom vote.
8. Elderly American Indians have a greater-than-average life expectancy.
9. Blacks are the fastest growing group of minority elderly.
10. A major number of elderly Pacific/Asian Americans live in California.

III. Short Answers

1. What are six defense mechanisms used to combat stress?
2. Why do many people feel they can more truly be themselves in old age?
3. What happens to basic personality traits as people age?
4. What is one reason an older individual may seem to react inappropriately?
5. In what way can the old best serve the young?
6. What are two characteristics of people most likely to make a successful psychological adjustment to old age?
7. If a positive emotional balance cannot be reached, what happens to a person's personality?
8. Providing there is no disease, how do the majority of elderly people function mentally?
9. What are three basic needs of people at all ages?
10. Why is the elderly's need for sexuality often unmet?

IV. Clinical Situations

1. A resident complains that he has been sitting in his wheelchair too long, when he has only been up for ten minutes. What defense mechanism might he be using?
2. A resident refuses to have her hair trimmed and insists that you spend time every morning arranging it. The resident who shares her room wants equal time spent cleaning and polishing her fingernails. What defense mechanisms might they be using?
3. A resident insists on bathing and dressing herself. Although she is capable, she is very slow. How should her independent nature be handled?

Unit 4
Normal Physical Changes

Objectives

After studying this unit, you should be able to:
- Define aging.
- Describe theories that explain the aging process.
- Describe the general physical changes that take place with aging.
- Differentiate between normal aging and the effects of illness.
- List some of the specific changes that take place in each body system.
- Identify therapeutic actions related to progressive changes that occur with aging.
- Differentiate between physical and chronological changes.

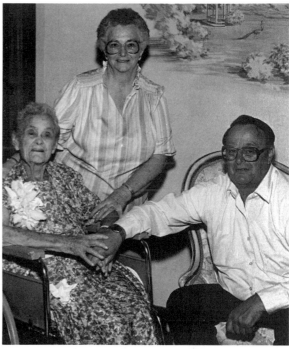

Vocabulary

Learn the meaning and spelling of the following words or phrases.

aging	insulin	
aldosterone	intertrigo	
aspiration	kyphosis	
autoimmune reactions	nocturia	theories
dermatitis	orthostatic hypotension	thyroxine
herniation	proprioception	vertigo
hypertrophy	pruritis	visual accommodation
hypochlorhydria	senescence	vital capacity
hypothermia	senile keratoses	

Aging is a natural process that brings about change in both physical appearance, figure 4-1, and functional efficiency. Physical aging is not simultaneous with chronological aging. There are many factors that influence the rate at which aging progresses. Senescence is different from aging. Aging is considered to be all the changes that occur normally with time. *Senescence* is the last stage of life in which aging occurs.

Theories of Aging

Over the centuries, people have tried to explain aging from scientific, philosophic, and religious viewpoints. They have also tried to find ways to postpone or prevent aging and to restore youth. You may remember from history that some European explorers came to the western hemisphere looking for the "fountain of youth."

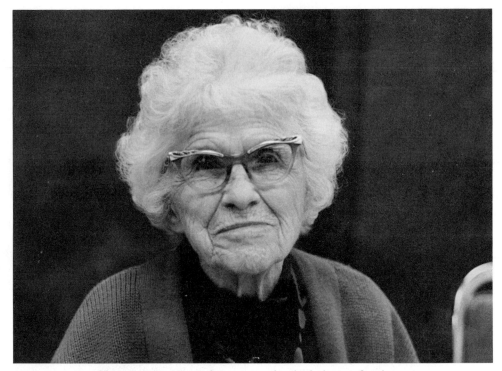

Figure 4-1   Note the many physical signs of aging.

Aging is still a topic under intensive research. Many theoretical explanations of aging exist. *Theories* are reasonable, logical attempts to explain events and processes that we do not understand. It is from theories and research, though, that we have been able to understand some of the mechanisms that guide and control the aging process. The rate of aging varies greatly from individual to individual, figure 4-2. All organ systems do not undergo changes at the same time. In order for a change to be considered a normal result of aging, it must occur in all individuals. It must not be seen just because certain disease states are more common among elders. For example, it cannot be assumed that heart disease is a result of aging just because it is prevalent among the elderly.

There are many theories of aging. Four of them are as follows.

- *Genetic Programming Theory.* This theory holds that life span is programmed at birth through the genes or is the result of changes in genetic material (D.N.A.) that occur with age.
- *Stress Theory.* This theory states that it is wear and tear on the body using up one's adaptive energy, not chronological age, that causes aging and eventual death. In other words, it likens the body to a complex machine that gradually wears out from use over the years. It holds that over time, body structures and the chemicals in the body change. This ultimately causes irreversible damage to the body's normal functioning.
- *Immunity Theory.* This theory is based on the unique ability of some body cells to identify abnormal changes in cells and to remove these cells from the body before they can form additional abnormal cells. It holds that this protective immune system becomes less efficient with age and that aging changes occur as more imperfect cells reproduce.

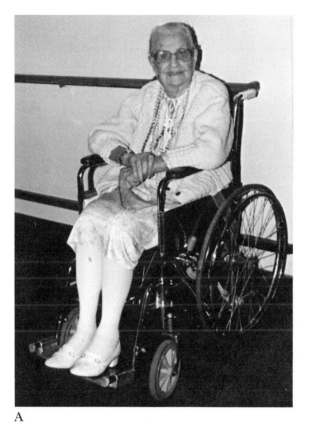

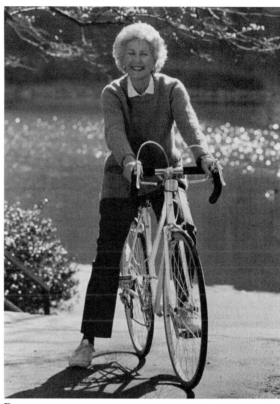

A   B

Figure 4-2A, B   The rate of aging varies greatly from individual to individual. (B—Courtesy of Squibb Pharmaceuticals—US)

• *Error Theory.* This theory is based on the notion that the nucleus, or the "brain" of the cell, releases inappropriate information that interferes with its normal function. As a result, the cell makes mistakes. Vital information is lost. As new cells develop, they are less able to perform their functions effectively. For example, the integration of complex body functions is controlled by the endocrine and nervous systems. With age, inadequate supplies of hormones produce a loss of function in this vital mechanism.

Aging is a complex, ever-changing process that occurs over time for all human beings. There is no one acceptable explanation for aging. Generally, it involves genetic programming, how the individual adapts to stressors, the physical environment, and emotional and social factors. Genetic and molecular studies promise to provide information that will have an effect on the aging process by the twenty-first century.

General Changes

Perhaps the most common complaints of the elderly are how much more easily they tire and how little vitality they seem to have. Less sleep seems to be needed, yet frequent rest periods are almost mandatory.

Physical changes are due to basic cell, tissue, and organ alterations. These cause all the body's functions to slow. The basic cellular metabolic rate decreases, cellular division and growth are limited, and newly forming replacement cells are less efficient. In some cases, cells replacing worn-out cells are not of the same type. For example, scar tissue cells cannot function in the same manner as the specialized cells they replace.

Disease increases the intensity and speed of the natural aging process. However, disease should not be confused with natural, progressive changes. Many of the signs of aging can be seen in older people. Younger people, however, may also be aware of some of these changes beginning within their own bodies. Aging does not begin at sixty or sixty-five years of age. It is a continuous process, beginning at birth, occurring in everyone.

Considerable emphasis today is placed on looking young. With the help of cosmetics, surgery, and artificial hairpieces, it is possible to disguise some signs of aging for a time. Sooner or later, however, each person must recognize that maturity has replaced youth.

There is probably no more beautiful person than one who accepts age and is content with life, one whose face mirrors the character that experience has fashioned. The aging process does not only involve loss. It also leads to a gain in emotional strength and coping abilities. The overall ability of the older body to respond to stress and to recover from injury, however, is greatly lessened, figure 4-3.

Systemic Changes

Senescent changes take place in each of the body systems, but not at any specific time or at any specific rate. A gradual process starting at birth, aging takes place at an individual rate. Throughout the body, tissues lose their elasticity. Redistribution and loss of subcutaneous fat change the usual body contours. Weight is usually gained in the fifties and sixties, reaches a plateau in the seventies, and begins to diminish thereafter. Fibrous changes decrease tone, mass, and strength of both skeletal and smooth muscles. There is general shrinkage in height, and postural changes, such as a slight flexion at the knees and hips, tend to further shorten stature.

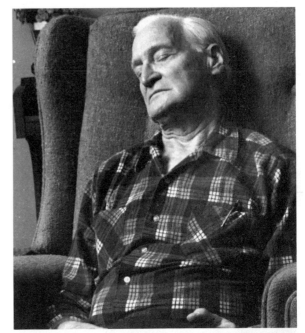

Figure 4-3 Frequent rest periods during the day help the elderly conserve energy.

Much of the shortening is attributable to changes in the vertebral column. During the seventh decade, a loss of 2 inches can be expected, figure 4-4. Secretory and endocrine cells become less functional, and nerve sensitivity is reduced. Changes in body chemistry also occur. The levels of potassium decline steadily, and demineralization of bone occurs.

Nervous System

Changes occur in the nervous system as a normal part of aging. These changes show themselves primarily by a "slowing down" in responding, thinking, reacting, integrating, and remembering. Some atrophy of brain tissue occurs. There is a thickening of the meninges, formation of senile plaques, and possibly interference with short-term memory. However, there is not necessarily an accompanying decrease in intellect. Studies have shown that elders can think and perform just as well as younger people if they are given enough time.

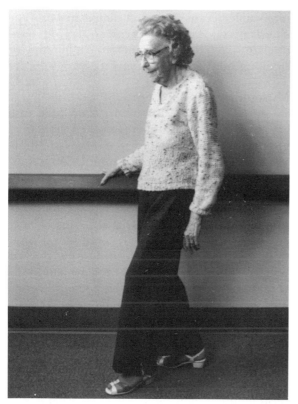

Figure 4-4   By the seventh decade, a loss of two inches in height can be expected. (From Caldwell & Hegner, *Nursing Assistant—A Nursing Process Approach,* copyright 1989 by Delmar Publishers Inc.)

Intellectual impairment and confusion are not always part of the aging process. Rather, they are signs that an elderly person has an acute illness or some other disability. Any recent change in behavior that involves confusion or changes in body functions should be reported to health care personnel, such as the supervising nurse or the physician. Appropriate examinations can be done to determine the cause of the change in behavior.

Nerve fibers degenerate. Nerve cells die and are not replaced as the body ages. Stronger sensory stimuli are needed to elicit a response, and reaction time greatly increases. Safe driving, which requires rapid response to stimuli, may

become a problem. There is a decrease in cerebral blood flow, brain size, and cerebral consumption of oxygen. Response to all sensory stimuli is slower and less accurate. This occurs because conduction of impulses along nerve pathways slows. Tactile receptors are less sensitive, so the older person does not perceive pain or injury with the same intensity as the young person. This is an important consideration, because injuries may go unnoticed and untreated. Pain itself may not be recognized or reported. Skin surfaces become thicker, drier, and less vascular. Sensory receptors are lost and it is difficult to stimulate the receptors. This can predispose the elderly not only to injury but also to falls and an uneven gait.

Elderly people often complain that food does not taste as it once did. In fact, as taste buds die, the sense of taste diminishes. About two-thirds of the taste buds are lost by the seventh decade, figure 4-5. The olfactory endings degenerate, and there is an increase in nostril hairs. This curtails the sense of smell. Loss of smell also

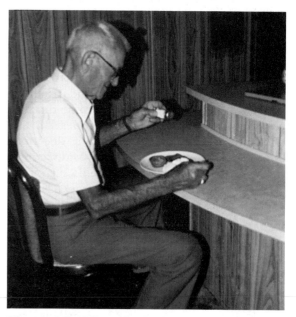

Figure 4-5   The elderly may tend to add more salt to their food in order to compensate for their diminished sense of taste.

alters the way food tastes, and appetites lag accordingly. Increased spices and more attention to how the food looks can help stimulate appetites. Care must be taken not to increase spices to the point that digestive disturbances occur.

Eyes and ears undergo gradual degeneration beginning quite early in life. Age has no monopoly on the need for corrective lenses to improve vision. In the elderly, peripheral vision is reduced, especially in dim light. *Accommodation* (adjusting) for vision at different distances is affected. In addition, the ability to adjust vision to differences in lighting is reduced. As the lens loses elasticity, the pupil becomes smaller and less responsive to light changes. Color perception diminishes, so bright colors are easier to see. Color blindness tends to increase, especially among men. Without glasses to correct these visual faults, the elderly person may become isolated and withdrawn. Glasses should be kept clean and close at hand. Lighting should be adequate, without glare. Bright colors can help residents more easily find their way.

Hearing, too, gradually diminishes. The ability to hear pure tone sound diminishes at all frequencies, especially high frequencies. But speech frequencies, which are relatively low, also seem to present difficulty. Not being able to hear all that is being said, the elderly are apt to feel left out. They may become frustrated and irritable as a result. Communication may become difficult. Not all the elderly can be helped by hearing aids, because much hearing loss is due to degeneration of the auditory nerve itself. Many elderly people resist the use of hearing aids even when they can be helped by them. To accept a hearing aid as a necessary means of continuing contact with others is to admit that aging has taken a toll. Some older people refuse to face this reality.

Proprioception (reception of internal stimuli) declines, joints become less flexible, and reflex reaction time increases. All three factors contribute to the falls suffered by elderly people. Older people often experience problems such as dizziness or *vertigo* that affect their balance and result in falls. Once a fall is started, recovery is almost impossible because reaction time is slowed. The elderly need to be taught to rise slowly from a bed or chair, from the toilet, and from a bending or stooping position.

Musculoskeletal System

Muscles lose strength, size, and tone with age. Intramuscular fat increases. Less storage of glycogen means that energy reserves are diminished. Response to nervous stimulation is slower, and the walls of organs become weaker. This predisposes the individual to *herniation* (protrusion of an organ out of its normal location) and problems of elimination. Hiatus hernia is more common after age sixty. Intervertebral disks thin, causing the individual to lose height and undergo postural changes. The spine bends, the chest falls forward, and the abdomen protrudes. *Kyphosis* (hunchback) is characteristic. The rib cage becomes more rigid and the costal (rib) cartilage somewhat more hardened. Joints are less flexible, and some osteoarthritis (simple wearing out of the joints) is fairly common. Bones become generally more porous and brittle, especially in postmenopausal women. Skeletal weight and flexibility diminish, and equilibrium is compromised. Care must be taken to protect the older person in any situation that challenges equilibrium. These include rapid turning, rapid rising, walking, or bending over. Grab bars and corridor railings can be important safety aids.

Respiratory System

Physical fitness through aerobic activities helps maintain cardiopulmonary functioning. Some losses are inevitable, such as the respiratory reserve required to respond to stress. These losses, however, do not usually interfere with normal activity unless the lungs are diseased.

Changes in the structure of the thoracic cavity influence respiratory function. *Vital capacity* (the amount of air that can be forced out of the lungs after the deepest inspiration) is decreased 25 to 30 percent, and breathing capacity drops by 50 percent. The alveoli enlarge and thin out, the bronchioles lose elasticity, and breathing becomes more rapid. The diaphragm becomes somewhat fibrotic and weakened. This lessens its efficiency. The rate of gaseous exchange is reduced, and shortness of breath is common. Changes in the larynx cause the voice to become weaker and higher pitched.

The elderly should be helped to maintain aerobic activity, such as walking, figure 4-6, or active arm exercise. They should be encouraged to eat nutritionally balanced meals and to avoid pollutants such as smoke. Encouraging these activities is an important responsibility of the health care provider.

The changes in the respiratory system due to aging make the elderly more susceptible to respiratory disease. The threat of serious respiratory infection increases with age.

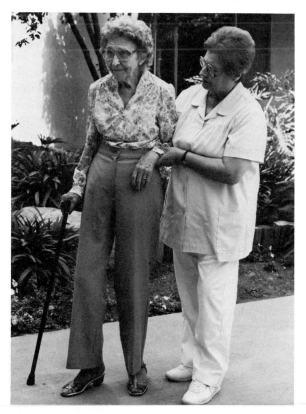

Figure 4-6 Helping elders maintain aerobic activity such as walking is an important factor for overall health.

Excretory System

Sweat glands diminish in activity, and changes are evident in the urinary tract. Kidneys decrease in size. Nephrons are lost as scars replace functional cells. Loss of smooth muscle tone and efficient vascular pathways may affect the amount of urine that is produced and eliminated. Production of urine is also hampered by decreased renal blood flow and reduced ability of the nephrons to filter urine. The kidneys of a seventy-year-old are only half as efficient as those of a thirty-year-old. Acid-base-electrolyte balance is adequate unless stressed by illness or fluid overload. Reduced bladder emptying makes infections more dangerous. *Nocturia* (nighttime urination) may become a problem when the urine-concentrating ability of the kidneys is diminished. Problems of emptying the urinary bladder are common because of the loss of pelvic muscular tone and the presence of such problems as prostatic *hypertrophy* (enlargement).

Changes in urinary function create problems for patients or residents and health care providers. The elderly often reduce their fluid intake and restrict their social activities for fear of being embarrassed by an "accident." These behaviors, however, can cause serious health problems. Health care providers can help elders by encouraging fluids, scheduling frequent bathroom breaks, helping elders dress in easily removed clothing, and by watching for changes in urinary or mental behavior that may indicate illness.

Cardiovascular System

Many experts in aging believe that exercising, maintaining normal body weight, and not smoking postpone age-related changes in this system. In fact, exercising at any age helps to delay further changes and can actually correct some problems.

Changes within the blood vessels are reflected throughout all systems. Fibrous changes in the smooth muscles of the vascular walls prevent them from expanding and recoiling normally. The walls become thickened and the lumens narrowed. Flow is diminished through the coronary arteries and even more to the kidneys and liver. Peripheral resistance to blood flow is increased, elevating the blood pressure. The uppermost limit of normal blood pressure in the person over sixty-five is 160/95 mmHg. Venous muscle tone decreases so that blood is returned less efficiently to the heart. Slowed blood return with position changes (*orthostatic hypotension*) can cause dizziness and contribute to falls. Edema may also occur in parts of the body that are located lower than the heart level. There are some fibrotic changes within the heart muscle and a degree of atrophy. Cardiac output decreases by 30 to 40 percent. The heart is slower in recovering its ability to contract. Chemical conversions are less efficient. Because functional ability is reduced, the heart frequently becomes enlarged (hypertrophied) with age.

Digestive System

The decrease in the number of taste buds has already been mentioned. The amounts of digestive enzymes, though still adequate, are also reduced. Decreased levels of hydrochloric acid (*hypochlorhydria*) are not uncommon, and dwindling secretion by intestinal mucosa reduces lubrication. Saliva becomes thicker, with less wetting ability. The tongue is less sensitive due to decreased circulation. Absorption may be limited because of changes in gastric secretions, decreased motility of the tract, and reduced blood flow to the intestinal tract. The decrease in absorption of iron can lead to anemia. Peristalsis is not as efficient because of changes in the smooth muscle, and elimination problems are often encountered. Decrease in anal sphincter reflexes can cause fecal incontinence. Altered activity patterns and soft diets adversely affect solid elimination.

The gag reflex is less active, and *aspiration* (drawing materials into the lungs) is a greater likelihood. The weight of the liver decreases. Although liver function studies may fall within normal ranges, many older people show evidence of hepatic insufficiency. This may include indigestion associated with intolerance to fatty foods, deficiency of fat-soluble vitamins, increased flatulence (gas), and poor ability to break down drugs.

Digestive complaints and problems should be minimized. Therapeutic interventions might include good mouth care, a high-fiber diet, increased fluids, and careful use of seasonings. A relaxing atmosphere in the dining room and an exercise program might also be emphasized.

Integumentary System

The skin reveals age as much as any part of the body. Loss of elasticity, adipose (fatty connective) tissue, and water undermine the skin foundation. The loss of fatty tissue makes the eyes appear sunken and the skin seem tight over the forehead, chin, and nose. This causes characteristic sagging and wrinkling, figure 4-7. Gravitational pull tends, over the years, to make the eyelids droop. Often the skin in the neck shrinks, leading to so-called age rings. Sebaceous glands in the skin are less active. With less lubricating secretions, the skin in general becomes dry and scaly, with a tendency to thin. Exposure to the sun further intensifies the tendency to wrinkle.

Skin that is covered shows very little change. This is quite evident when the skin of the face or neck is compared to the skin of an area that has not been exposed to the sun, such as the buttocks. Fair-skinned people seem to be more susceptible to damage from the sun than darker-skinned people. Sweat glands decrease in function and the elderly have difficulty responding to temperature changes and maintaining a balanced body temperature. *Hypothermia,* very low body temperature, is a dangerous problem. It is potentially life threatening for the elderly. Layered clothing, adequate nutrition, and adequate heat control are necessary to prevent this problem.

Finger- and toenails become thickened and brittle. They frequently split because of decreased peripheral circulation. Peripheral blood vessels are more fragile and more easily seen under the thinned epidermis. Small hemorrhages can occur due to the fragility of the blood

thought to result from environmental wear by weather and sun. *Senile keratoses* are roughened, scaly, slightly elevated, wartlike lesions thought to be related to sunburn damage in fair-skinned individuals. They must be watched carefully because they may undergo malignant changes.

The amount and color of hair undergo changes that are indicative of the normal aging process. Graying or loss of pigmentation is usual. Some graying is evident as early as the second or third decade. Genetics probably plays an important role in affecting the rate of change. As more and more pigment is lost, the hair becomes white. The loss of pigment is probably due to decreased circulation. Decreased oil makes the hair dull and lifeless. The amount of hair is reduced in some men, and the texture becomes coarser in other areas such as the eyebrows and face. Balding is an aging characteristic that first appears at widely varying ages. Again, genetics has a strong influence.

Endocrine System

In addition to changes in hormonal balance following menopause and those occurring with disease, other endocrine changes occur with aging. For example, there are higher levels of parathormone and the pituitary secretion, thyroid stimulating hormone (T.S.H.).

Thyroid The secretion of *thyroxine* (a hormone) doesn't seem to diminish. However, radioactive uptake of iodine by the thyroid, which it needs to produce thyroxine, is slowed. Oxygen utilization by the cells diminishes with age. Therefore, basal metabolic rate, which is under thyroid control, generally goes down. The older individual may seem less active and alert and complain of feeling cold as a result.

Thymus The immune response (the ability to resist effects of infectious agents) is less effective. Furthermore, instead of protecting itself against abnormal or foreign cells, the body increasingly loses its ability to recognize its own healthy cells and begins destructive processes called *autoimmune reactions*. Thymosin, a thymus secretion, is

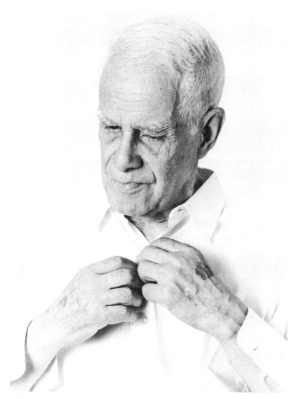

Figure 4-7 Skin changes reveal the aging process. Note the thinning and wrinkling of the skin and the presence of senile lentigines.

vessels. Peripheral circulation to the skin decreases, so that general skin nutrition is less satisfactory. Skin injuries are slower to heal. Too-frequent bathing and the use of some soaps can remove what little oil is present. Cleanliness is, however, essential in preventing many common skin problems such as *monilia* (infection), *pruritis* (itching), *dermatitis* (skin inflammations), and *intertrigo*. Intertrigo is an erythematous irritation of opposing skin surfaces due to friction.

Areas of skin pigmentation seem more pronounced with advancing years. Sometimes referred to as "liver spots," senile lentigines are not related to the liver at all. They are elevated yellowish or brownish spots or patches that occur on exposed skin surfaces such as the backs of the hands. Their cause is unknown, but they are

responsible for normal development of cells involved in the process. In early years, thymosin helps certain white blood cells to become programmed to the normal chemistry of the body cells and to reject that which is perceived as foreign.

Pancreas   *Insulin* is a hormone produced by the pancreas. The production of insulin and glucose utilization both diminish. Glucose tolerance decreases. The alpha cells of the pancreas produce glucagon, a hormone that raises blood sugar levels. Higher levels of glucagon also inhibit the use of glucose. This occurs because pancreatic alpha cells are not reduced as the insulin-producing beta cells are. Decreased exercise, unbalanced diets, and excess blood fat levels also contribute to glucose intolerance.

Adrenal Glands   *Aldosterone* is a hormone produced by the adrenal glands. Aldosterone levels are lower. However, there does not seem to be a loss in adrenal response to stress.

Gonads   In women, the decrease in estrogenic activity following menopause causes the vaginal wall to thin and vaginal secretions to diminish. Elderly women are thereby predisposed to vaginal inflammations. Fat redistribution causes the breasts to sag. Some degree of ovarian atrophy also takes place. Changes in hormone levels alone do not apparently alter sexual needs. Estrogens drop rather sharply between thirty and forty years of age, eventually reaching a lower plateau at about sixty years of age.

In men, response to sexual stimulation of the penis is slower and ejaculation may be restrained. Rather than posing a handicap, this enables the individual to engage in intercourse for a longer period of time before ejaculation. Blood levels of testosterone decrease gradually with age. The size and firmness of the testes diminish, and they do not elevate to the same degree during intercourse. There is a thickening of the seminiferous tubules and a beginning of degeneration. The production of sperm decreases. The seminal fluid becomes thinner and somewhat scanter. Ejaculation is not as forceful. Localized sexual sensations shift to a more generalized body response.

Genital response is directly related to the general health of the individual and to a positive self-image. It is also related to lifelong sexual patterns.

Figure 4-8 shows the nursing diagnoses related to the physiological changes due to normal aging.

ACTUAL OR POTENTIAL
    Activity intolerance
    Alteration in bowel elimination: constipation, diarrhea, incontinence
    Alteration in fluid volume: excess or deficit
    Alteration in respiratory function
    Alteration in tissue perfusion
    Alteration in urinary elimination: urgency, retention, incontinence
    Impaired physical mobility
    Impaired skin integrity
    Potential for infection
    Potential for injury
    Self-care deficits
    Sensory perceptual alterations

Figure 4-8 Nursing diagnostic categories related to physiological alterations.

Summary

- Though still adequate to maintain life, body functions generally slow down with advancing age.
- Basic changes in structure occur. There is a decrease in the number of functional cells, and they are replaced with scar or fat tissue.
- Atrophy and loss of muscle tone and mass alter the size and function of organs. Changes in circulatory patterns do the same.
- General efficiency of the body systems is reduced. Recovery from trauma and stress is delayed.
- Aging takes place in all body structures, beginning at birth. But the rate of aging varies with the individual.

Review Outline

   I. Behavioral Objectives

  II. Vocabulary

 III. Theories of Aging

       A.   Progressive stress
       B.   Genetic programming
       C.   Diminished immune response

 IV. Senescent Changes

       A.   General
       B.   Systemic
           1. Nervous system/intellect
           2. Musculoskeletal system
           3. Respiratory system
           4. Excretory system
           5. Cardiovascular system
           6. Digestive system
           7. Integumentary system
           8. Endocrine system

Review

   I. Vocabulary

Write the definition of each of the following.

     1. Aspiration _____
     2. Hypochlorhydria _____
     3. Nocturia _____
     4. Pruritis _____
     5. Senescence _____
     6. Vertigo _____
     7. Kyphosis _____
     8. Insulin _____
     9. Orthostatic hypotension _____
   10. Senile keratosis _____

  II. True or False

     1. Physical aging does not occur at the same rate as chronological aging.
     2. The mechanisms of aging are well understood.
     3. Loss of vitality is a common complaint of the elderly.
     4. As cells wear out, they are often replaced by scar tissue.
     5. The elderly body is less able to withstand stress and to over after injury than the young body is.
     6. The amount of digestive enzymes increases with age.

7. Adequate nutrition in the elderly may be hampered by their loss of taste buds.
8. Hearing may diminish greatly before the older person is willing to admit the loss.
9. Aging causes changes within the vascular system that are reflected throughout all systems.
10. Balding and graying of hair may occur at relatively early ages.

III. Short Answers

1. List three senescent changes you might expect in each of the following systems.
    a. integumentary
    b. nervous
    c. musculoskeletal
    d. cardiovascular
    e. endocrine
    f. gastrointestinal
2. Think about the oldest person you know in chronological age (number of years) and the oldest person you know in physical age (physical condition). Comment on each.

IV. Clinical Situations

1. A patient or resident tells you there is a reddened area on his foot but it doesn't hurt. What should you do?
2. A patient or resident sits in a semidarkened room and says she is afraid she will fall if she tries to walk. What should you do?
3. An obese resident has very dry skin, but the skin under her breasts and in the folds of her abdomen and axillae is inflamed, moist, and itching. What is the cause of this condition and how should it be treated?
4. Over the past week, a resident has become belligerent and incontinent. The resident also wanders at night and sleeps more during the day. What action should the health care provider take?

Unit 5
Human Sexuality

Objectives
After studying this unit, you should be able to:
- Compare sensuality and sexuality.
- Define terms related to human sexual expression.
- Identify different expressions of human sexuality.
- Discuss human sexuality in senescence.
- Identify therapeutic actions as they apply to expression of sexuality.

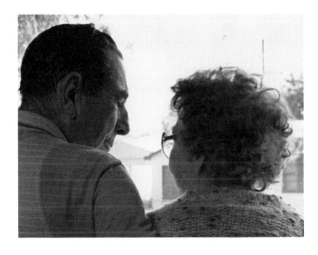

Vocabulary
Learn the meaning and spelling of the following words or phrases.

bisexuality	genitals	libido
celibate	heterosexuality	lover
climacteric	homophobia	masturbation
coitus	homosexuality	menopause
cunnilingus	incest	orgasm
dyspareunia	intercourse	potency
ejaculate	intimacy	procreation
fellatio	lesbians	sensual
gays		

Humans are complex, with physical, emotional, and spiritual facets. Each of these facets goes into creating special individuals, alike in some ways and unique in others. Each of these facets must be maintained, nourished, and used. Minds that are not used regularly become less functional. Feelings and desires that are unshared go unfulfilled. Bodies that are not exercised atrophy.

Sexuality is a special part of that wholeness. Sexual orientation begins long before birth when the genes of parents determine whether the new infant will have male or female reproductive organs and the nerves and chemicals that accom-

pany them. Sexuality and sensuality are part of human beings from birth to death.

Sexual expression is a basic human need like food, air, and rest. Many see older people and babies as being sexless because they are not capable of *procreation*. This is an inaccurate view. Babies are sensual beings—they love the feeling of someone holding, touching, and caressing them, figure 5-1. They respond with sounds and smiles when you speak to them. Penile erections on baby boys are often seen in the delivery room. Older people have not lost this basic response over the years. As they have matured, however, the need and ways of responding have also ma-

57

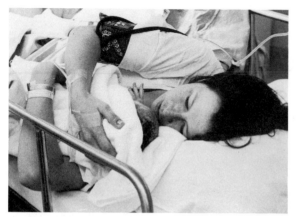

Figure 5-1 From the time of birth, humans need to be touched and to feel the love of other humans.

tured. Different ways of meeting the need have been investigated and measured against a developing moral code. Patterns of sexual behavior have been established. You may recognize your own sexuality and be aware of your sexual feelings. Yet you may find it difficult to accept those same sexual needs in others. This is particularly true when you consider the sexuality of those who are younger or older than yourself. This is true of most people.

In young adulthood, it is often difficult to believe that parents or grandparents or younger brothers and sisters have any sexual orientation. People in full maturity often find it difficult to appreciate the sexual behaviors of their children. This is natural and probably due to cultural training that places a taboo on *incest*. Incest is sexual relations between people too closely related to be married. Unfortunately, these restrictive feelings are often transferred to others outside the family, who are then seen as not being sensual or having sexual needs.

Sensuality and Intimacy

Feelings experienced by using the senses are described as sensual. Beautiful music is experienced through the ears, a sunset through the eyes. The soft, furry feel of a kitten is experi-

enced through the sense of touch, figure 5-2. The sweetness of candy is experienced through the sense of taste. Each sensation is pleasurable and its enjoyment leads to the desire to sample it again. That is the essence of the sensual side of our nature. When sensual experiences feel good, they raise the overall level of awareness and sense of being alive.

Sexual activities are highly sensual in nature. When pleasurable and satisfying, they impart a sense of well-being that is important to a happy life. Sexual behaviors involve the use and enjoyment of all the senses, not just those related to stimulation of the reproductive organs *(genitals)*. Nursing diagnostic categories that relate to sexual problems are *altered sexuality patterns* and *sex-*

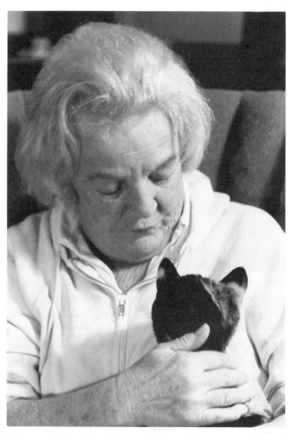

Figure 5-2 Stroking a kitten is a sensual (feeling) experience.

ual dysfunction. The first category includes problems with sexuality or sexual functions such as those occurring as a result of conflict or health problems. The second category describes dissatisfaction with sexual function.

Intimacy is a close relationship characterized by love and affection. Love and affection may or may not be expressed sexually. People can, and do, engage in sexual activity without intimacy. Some people also engage in sexual activity with another person for the feeling of intimacy and a need for touching. The other person may only be satisfying a sexual need, however. Intimacy is found between a mother feeding her baby, two children who are best friends, adults who are close friends, a husband and wife who are deliberately refraining from intercourse (celibate), and any couple expressing their love for one another sexually.

Human Sexual Expression

Since ancient times, celibacy, chastity, heterosexuality, homosexuality, and bisexuality have been both praised and condemned in many cultures and religions. It is not very different today, with perhaps a few exceptions. Homosexuality and bisexuality are no longer considered diseases by psychiatrists and psychologists, but rather part of the wide range of human sexual expressions. *Homophobia,* fear of homosexuality, still prevails to some degree. But this life-style is becoming more tolerated, if still not completely accepted.

Several Christian denominations now ordain nonheterosexual ministers, both men and women. Legislators are passing laws to establish and protect the rights of homosexuals, just as heterosexuals are protected. Homosexual couples are recognized as being just as committed to a relationship as are heterosexual couples.

Heterosexuality is the attraction the opposite sexes have for one another. Most dictionaries also define this term as the sexual relationship between the opposite sexes. Heterosexual relationships are the most common. Whether the partners are married or not, the relationship is characterized by intimacy and is frequently expressed in sexual activity. *Bisexuality* is defined as sexual attraction to members of both sexes. All people have the capacity to love and feel sexually attracted toward both men and women. Bisexuals choose not to have an exclusive heterosexual or homosexual relationship. *Homosexuality* is defined as sexual attraction toward a member of one's own sex, figure 5-3. Homosexual men and women tend to differ in their relationships. Thus, the definition is limited. *Gays* (this is the preferred term for male homosexuals) tend to have many sexual relationships. They are also capable of having long-term, loving relationships. Very few *lesbians* (this is the preferred term), on the other hand, think of themselves primarily in a sexual relationship. Rather, they think of themselves as women who love women in an intimate relationship. Celibacy may be the chosen preference not only for single men and women, but also for some married men and

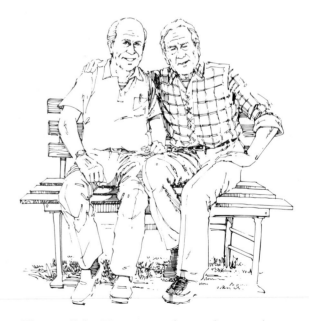

Figure 5-3 Homosexual couples are just as committed to a loving relationship as are heterosexual couples.

women. Celibacy used to mean single and abstaining from sexual activity. It did not necessarily mean chaste. Today people choose celibacy for various reasons. Being celibate does not mean being without love. It only means being without a sexual relationship with another person.

Sexual Expression and Morality

Human sexuality and its expression are tightly bound up with the attitudes and morality that an individual has been taught and accepted, figure 5-4. Religious beliefs and traditions play a major role in determining moral values. Each adult, you and those in your care, has developed a personal moral code that permits or disallows certain behaviors.

Your personal moral code might keep you from saying unkind things, and you would find these actions unacceptable in the behavior of others. Nevertheless, another's moral code might permit these behaviors. The same is true of sexual behaviors. Behaviors prohibited under one moral code may be perfectly acceptable under another. Sex between unmarried individuals, homosexuality, and masturbation are just a few examples of areas where different moral codes operate.

As a geriatric health care provider, you are ethically obliged not to force those in your care to accept your moral code. You must reserve judgment of others when they follow their own set of values instead of your own. You must also be careful not to let your verbal or body language reveal inner reservations and disapproval. For example, you may feel strongly that sexual release should only occur within the context of marriage with a loving partner. You may feel great dismay when you happen to notice an elderly resident relieving his sexual tension alone by masturbating. Remember, your negative feel-

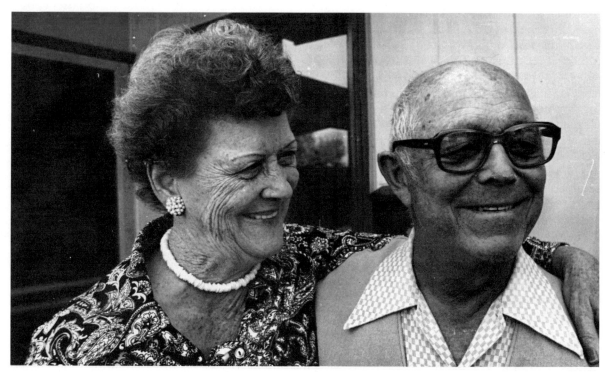

Figure 5-4 Sexual expression is a very personal reflection of attitude.

ings are influenced by *your* moral code. His moral code may place no prohibitions on his behavior. Make no judgment; shut the door and provide some privacy.

Just as you would not express disapproval of older couples making love, you must not encourage seniors into activities that they do not seek. Sexual attitudes influence sexual ideas. Men and women now in their sixties to eighties grew up in a restrictive era. They may feel guilty over their thoughts of sex. Few women were taught in that period to seek satisfaction of their sexual needs.

Human Sexuality and Aging

A slowing down of sexual activity in the late middle years is usually caused by boredom, lack of privacy, concern about loss of attractiveness, and fear of orgasmic failure. Relationships that have failed to grow and remain stimulating, those in which old hostilities and conflicts have not been resolved, are likely to transfer these problems to the sexual relationship with a loss of intimacy and sensuality.

In general, when opportunity is available, sexual patterns tend to remain stable throughout the adult and late adult years. Decreases in activity can be attributed to loss of opportunity, poor health, and the pressure of negative cultural attitudes.

Many older people continue to engage in pleasurable sexual activities. For heterosexual couples, this may or may not include *coitus. Coitus* refers to sexual relations or intercourse, figure 5-5. Older partners enjoy erotic (sexual) feelings derived from manual and oral-genital stimulation *(cunnilingus/fellatio). Cunnilingus* refers to oral-genital stimulation of the female and *fellatio* refers to oral-genital stimulation of the male. They sometimes seek more direct stimulation using a vibrator, alone or with a partner.

The need and desire to participate in sexual activity does not necessarily diminish with age. There is nothing in the aging process to prohibit sexual activity. As people grow older, however,

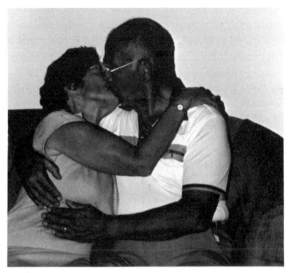

Figure 5-5   Sexual activity may or may not include coitus.

their physiological responses change. If understood, this can enhance the sexual experience.

Women in their middle years often report an improvement in their sexuality, figure 5-6. They feel more confident and self-assured. They are more willing to take the initiative. Menopause is not as dramatic an event as is often portrayed. It seems to be handled well by most women.

Hormonal Changes and Menopause

From age thirty onward, reproductive capacity decreases. The ovaries respond less effi-

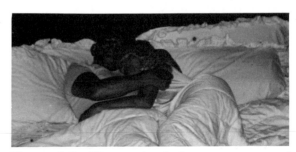

Figure 5-6   Women in their postmenopausal years often report an improvement in their sexuality.

ciently to hormones that are produced in the pituitary gland. After about age forty, ovulation becomes less frequent. From about forty-eight to fifty-two, menstrual cycles become irregular and finally cease. This period is known as the *menopause* or *climacteric*. Discomfort such as emotional tension and "hot flashes" may be experienced, but these can be controlled with hormone therapy. Hormone therapy also helps prevent a serious bone problem called osteoporosis, often seen in postmenopausal women.

The diminished level of hormones causes some changes in the reproductive organs. The vagina shrinks and becomes thin. The tissue loses some of its elasticity. There is less lubrication during arousal. The breasts and vulva lose fat and become thinner. Hormones also influence the mineral content of bones so with aging there is a loss of mineral content, and bones become more brittle.

There is no dramatic drop in sex drive *(libido)* nor any lessening in sensual pleasure or orgasmic response. The clitoris remains just as sexually sensitive. Although the sex flush diminishes, it bears no relationship to functional ability. Estrogen therapy improves bone maintenance and a mild lubricant such as K-Y jelly or vaginal cream can prevent vaginal discomfort during sexual activity or intercourse *(dyspareunia)*. Women continue to be capable of multiple *orgasms* (climaxes) well into their eighties.

Men have no definite end to their fertility. They usually do not go through a specific menopausal period as do women. After age forty, sperm production slows down. Between fifty-five and sixty, the level of male hormones diminishes somewhat, but not drastically. Men report that they do not feel as emotionally pressed to be dominant while making love and feel freer to be more tender.

About 5 percent of men reporting in one study experienced what might be described as a male climacteric. They characteristically felt weak, irritable, and tired. In addition, they had poor appetites and felt a decrease in sexual desire with a loss of *potency*. Potency refers to the ability of a man to engage in sexual intercourse (sexual union). This cannot be considered a common experience.

Male changes attributed directly to the aging process include the need for more direct penile stimulation and less physical need to ejaculate. There is also a decrease in seminal fluid, a lower and slower rise of the testes, and a less complete erection of the penis. None of these changes inhibit penetration. The older man is able to participate longer in coitus before the need to *ejaculate* (expulsion of semen) occurs.

In other words, as long as the individual is healthy, there is nothing in the aging process to interfere with good sexual function. The idea that sex is only for the young and attractive is a cultural myth that young and old alike have come to believe. Studies show that a key factor in maintaining sexual activity is the regularity established in younger years. In addition, sexual activity seems to slow the rate of normal aging changes.

Masturbating and fantasizing play a significant role in the sex lives of the elderly, figure 5-7. One recent study of people over ninety revealed that almost one-quarter (23 percent) masturbated to relieve sexual tension. The same study found that between 40 and 65 percent of active, healthy people aged sixty to seventy-one reported engaging in sexual intercourse frequently. This was also true for 10 to 20 percent of those seventy-eight and over. Opportunity and availability of willing and able partners were the determinants.

Every year, 35,000 couples in which one or both are sixty-five or older get married, figure 5-8. This is true despite frequent opposition to such marriages by children and other family members. There is a growing trend today for older couples to live together without benefit of marriage. This occurs because Social Security allotments are less for a married couple than they are for two singles living together. The economics make marriage a luxury these couples can ill afford. While in their working years gay and lesbian couples were denied the tax benefits of

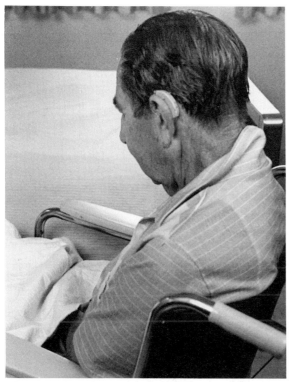

Figure 5-7 Masturbation offers sexual relief when a partner is not available.

married heterosexual couples, all couples may have a difficult time trying to live on Social Security benefits.

Impotence

True impotence in older men is usually more psychological than it is physiological. Some diseases such as diabetes can contribute to the inability of the male to achieve an erection. Certain surgical procedures and drugs such as tranquilizers, sedatives, and antihypertensives can have the same effect. There are implants that can help men achieve erections. These implants are soft, hollow tubes that can fill with fluid. The fluid is housed in the abdomen. When pressure is applied to the abdomen, fluid moves forward into the tube. This makes the penis firm and coitus easier.

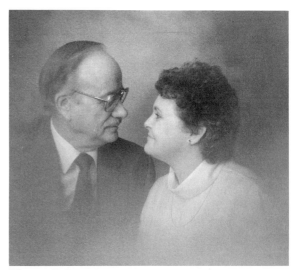

Figure 5-8 Thousands of older couples commit their love to one another every year.

Some men who have difficulty achieving erection are being helped with the use of prostaglandin therapy. Injected into the anterior penis just below the glans, either to the right or left of the midline, these local hormones can bring about an erection that can last several hours. The injections are not painful and can be self-administered.

Older men with erection problems, and their partners, can still enjoy manual and oral stimulation. This provides each partner with pleasure and satisfies the need for intimacy. The need for more direct stimulation can be helped with the use of a vibrator.

Sexual Expression in the Extended Care Facility

Only 8 percent of the elderly are hopelessly senile. This means that 92 percent of the elderly are still capable of some level of human loving.

In the privacy of their own homes, senior adults are free to carry out sexual activity any way they want. In an extended care facility, however, the situation is drastically different. Most extended care facilities and their residents are controlled by young and middle-aged people who believe the cultural myths about aging and sexuality. Many of the residents accept the cultural myths just as easily. The elderly may find it hard to believe that they could still be attractive. Those working in the facilities find that thoughts of sex in relation to the elderly make them uncomfortable.

There are more female residents in extended care facilities simply because women tend to outlive men. Many of the women may have been widowed for years. Failing to find another partner, they simply gave up hoping for heterosexual involvement. A few may have been separated from or have lost a lover to death (*lover* is the preferred term for a lesbian or gay partner). They may be reluctant to begin a new relationship. Some women find a partner, a person with whom they can have an intimate relationship, figure 5-9. They are able to express their sensuality once again in loving someone. This person may be a man or another woman. In either case, sensual or sexual expression should be respected and privacy provided.

There are some health problems that might interfere with sexual activity. These include cardiac illness, hypertension, atherosclerosis, arthritis, muscle and bone weakness, diabetes mellitus, hearing and sight problems, and depression. Even patients with these problems can be helped if they so desire and if there are willing, mature, knowledgeable health care providers to help.

Sex improves muscle tone and mildly stimulates the heart and respiration. Arthritis sufferers report several hours of relief from pain following sexual activity. This is thought to result from an increase in hormonal (cortisone) level. The elderly need to know that their desire for and participation in satisfying sexual activity is accepted. They need to know that health care providers will respect the opportunities available to them to engage in this recreational exercise. When opportunities for sexual interactions are limited, many men and women will derive satisfaction through self-stimulation (*masturbation*).

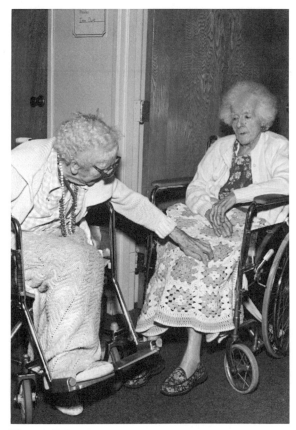

Figure 5-9   Some women residents find a partner with whom they can share a loving relationship.

This, too, should be accepted and respected, because it can bring pleasure and continued comfort to the later years.

Summary

- Elderly people are often viewed as sexless. To recognize sexuality in the elderly makes persons in other age groups uneasy.
- Greater awareness of the sexual needs of the elderly is beginning to be appreciated. Enlightened attitudes are leading health care providers to find ways of accommodating these as well as other needs.

Review Outline

   I. Objectives

  II. Vocabulary

 III. Sensuality/Sexuality

 IV. Sexual Expression and Morality

      A.   Societal attitudes
      B.   Personal attitudes
      C.   Health care provider attitudes
      D.   Modes of human expression
          1. Heterosexuality
          2. Homosexuality
          3. Bisexuality

  V. Physical Changes Affecting Sexual Response

      A.   Male
      B.   Female
      C.   Menopause

 VI. Sexual Expression in Extended Care Facilities

      A.   Opportunity
      B.   Support

Review

  I. Vocabulary

Match column I with column II.

Column I	Column II
1. Sexual desire	a. climacteric
2. Sexual intercourse	b. sensuality
3. Abstaining from sexual intercourse	c. dyspareunia
4. Pleasurable feelings experienced through the senses	d. libido
5. Oral sexual stimulation	e. celibacy
6. Sexual attraction by members of the opposite sex	f. heterosexuality
7. Another term for menopause	g. intimacy
8. Sexual self-stimulation	h. masturbation
9. Close relationship characterized by love and affection	i. coitus
10. Painful or uncomfortable sexual intercourse	j. cunnilingus

II. True or False

1. Sexuality is part of the essence of being a human being.
2. Sexuality is a basic human need.
3. Sensual feelings are those derived from stimulation of the senses.
4. Loss of potency is a frequent problem in most older men.
5. Seventy-year-old women are capable of multiple orgasms.
6. Older people do not like sexual activity.
7. Intimacy is sexual activity.
8. The term lover refers to any unmarried partner.
9. Commitment to a relationship is not as strong in a homosexual couple as it is in a heterosexual couple.
10. Some couples choose not to marry because single-person Social Security benefits are better.

III. Short Answers

1. List the ways that men and women change sexually as they age.
2. What percentage of the elderly are hopelessly senile, thus unable to be involved in a human loving relationship?
3. How do lesbians describe their relationships compared to gays?
4. What could an elderly woman use to reduce vaginal discomfort during sexual activity?
5. What is the benefit for a couple because an older man's need to ejaculate takes longer?

IV. Clinical Situations

1. You notice one of the elderly residents sitting in his wheelchair and you think he might be masturbating. What do you do?
2. Two elderly women are sitting on the bed with their arms about one another, stroking each other's face and hair. What do you do?
3. You walk into a room without knocking and find an elderly couple in bed, obviously undressed. They seem flustered. What do you do?

Unit 6
Living and Care Facilities

Objectives
After studying this unit, you should be able to:
- Name the government department that helps older people finance their homes.
- List various types of living facilities available to elderly people.
- Describe the services offered by a life-care community.

Vocabulary
Learn the meaning and spelling of the following words or phrases.

boardinghouse
condominiums
convalescent home
day center
D.R.G.s
extended care facility
home health services
H.U.D.
I.C.F.
intergenerational

life-care communities
metropolitan
mortgage insurance
multifunctional
multigenerational
N.C.O.A.
nursing home
rehabilitation
retirement community
rural communities

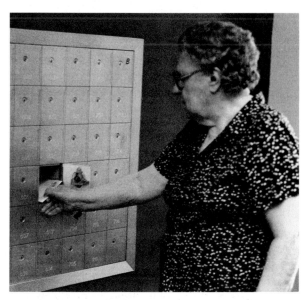

S.C.F.
sheltered/custodial care
    facility
subsidized

Housing for older people depends on individual preference, need, income, and availability. The choice is much the same for citizens of all ages. Most elderly persons prefer to live in familiar surroundings and to remain self-directed as long as possible. They wish to remain in their homes, with friends and neighbors nearby. Sometimes they want to move to living quarters closer to other family members. Institutionalization is a last resort. Some older people see their late mature years as an opportunity for self-fulfillment. They seek residences that will bring them into closer contact with their peers and away from the noise and stress of intergenerational living.

Geographic Distribution

Only a small percentage of those over sixty-five must live in institutions. About 95 percent of the elderly continue to make their home alone, with their spouse, or with a relative's family. Approximately 25 percent of those sixty-five and over live on farms or in rural communities with populations of less than 2,500. About one-third of the elderly live in large metropolitan areas. There is a trend among the more affluent elderly to live in the suburbs. More than one-half of the older population of metropolitan areas is now in the suburbs rather than the inner city. Almost one-quarter of the nation's elderly live in just three states—California, Florida, and New York. Large numbers also live in Illinois, Michigan, Ohio, Pennsylvania, and Texas. These eight states are home to almost half of the nation's elderly, figure 6-1.

Home Ownership

Because most women outlive their mates, three-quarters of the older men, but only about one-third of the older women, live together with their spouse. Four out of ten older women live alone. Almost four times as many older women as men live alone or with nonrelatives.

Home ownership is one of the elderly couple's principal assets, figure 6-2. As long as they are physically able to care for their home, most people enjoy the privacy and familiarity it provides. Approximately two-thirds of older couples own their own homes. Few of these are city dwellers. A large number of older couples still live in the house where they raised their families. However, houses that are large enough for a growing family are often too large and expensive for retired couples to maintain. Lack of mobility, money, and competition for available housing keeps many older people living in homes that are no longer appropriate for their needs. Entire neighborhoods may have changed around them. The fact the independent households are maintained does not mean that services are not needed. Much of the housing is old and in substandard condition. Many of those in independent households could benefit from health and social services.

Some community agencies sponsor senior work days during which young people fix up senior housing. These young people are paid by the agency or volunteer their time. They repair minor problems, paint, and do yard work.

In other communities, low-interest loan money is available. This money helps the elderly to employ reputable contractors to carry out more extensive repairs and renovations.

Church and synagogue groups also sponsor the activities of the young people of their congregations. These groups help seniors in similar ways.

Not enough housing is available at reasonable cost. In addition, much of what is available is not fit to live in. Moreover, the fixed incomes of the elderly make it difficult for those who rent to meet rising costs. National estimates find at least 30 percent of the nation's elderly in substandard housing. Almost one-half lack central heating. One-fifth have no toilet, bath, or shower. In recent years, more and more of the elderly have taken up residence in mobile home parks. Mobile homes for an individual or elderly couple are a convenient and economical source of private housing. In newer parks, recreational facilities are provided for the residents. Some homes are open to multigenerational living, while others are age restrictive.

PERSONS 65 + AS PERCENTAGE OF TOTAL POPULATION: 1988

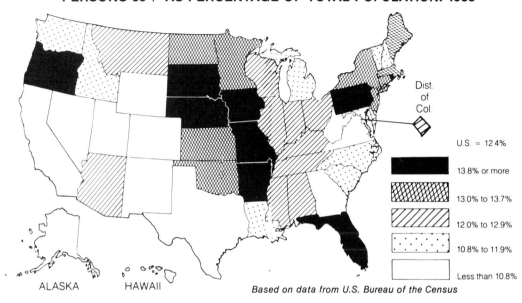

PERCENTAGE CHANGE IN 65 + POPULATION: 1980 TO 1988

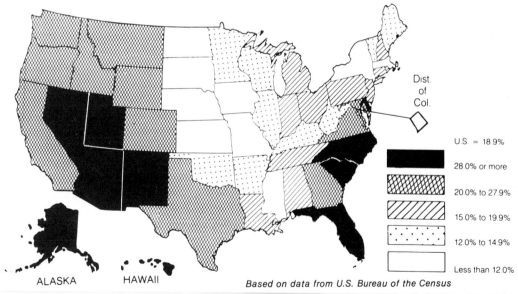

Figure 6-1 Population age sixty-five and older as a percentage of the total resident population. (From "A Profile of Older Americans: 1989," American Association of Retired Persons, 1909 K Street, NW, Washington, DC 20049)

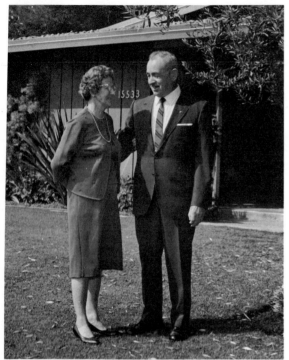

Figure 6-2 Home ownership is one of the elderly couple's principal equities.

Apartments and Rooming Houses

Apartment living offers convenience to the older couple who no longer wishes to be encumbered with the chores of home maintenance. *Condominiums* are privately owned apartments. All residents share the cost of maintaining communal areas such as halls and grounds. The condominium offers the elderly person the equity of home ownership without much of the personal effort needed to maintain a home. In addition, many condominiums offer greater protection against intruders. Some have special entry gates and, in more affluent areas, guarded gatekeepers.

Almost 33 percent of the women and 20 percent of the men live alone. Some elderly individuals living alone may find that rooming houses most nearly meet their needs. Simple meals can sometimes be prepared in the rooms.

Meals may also be included in the boardinghouse arrangement. Unfortunately, some elderly persons live in small, substandard rooms. They barely exist on their meager incomes. Old and alone, these people represent a poverty group only beginning to be recognized. They are likely to be found in the inner city, and a disproportionate number will be minorities.

Today, more and more elderly are joining the population of homeless who live, sleep, and exist on our streets. The homeless find food and shelter wherever they can, entering community shelters only when the weather becomes severe.

When the weather is very inclement, some communities open shelters for temporary care or give vouchers to low-cost private enterprises. Although some elderly prefer the freedom of street living, the majority would be relieved to know that shelter and food were consistently available to them.

Federal Assistance

The Department of Housing and Urban Development *(H.U.D.)* recognizes the relationship between home ownership and independent living. It provides mortgage insurance to help older people finance home purchases and loans and grants for home restoration. In addition, administration housing programs have sponsored low-cost loans to private and nonprofit sponsors to build low- or moderate-income housing for the elderly.

Some banks make reverse mortgages available to elderly homeowners. These mortgages use the property as collateral. The mortgage money provides for the current and future living expenses of the homeowner until the funds are all used up. This allows the elderly to continue to live in their own homes.

If the homeowner outlives the mortgage monies, the bank may take one of two steps. The bank may reappraise the property and, if it has increased in value, loan the homeowner additional money. The other step is that the bank may take possession of the property. The owner must then make other living arrangements.

The Department of Housing and Urban Development provides assistance to the elderly renter in two important ways. Through the rent supplement program, low-income elderly who are unable to pay full rent have a portion of their rent subsidized. Under another program, help is given to local housing authorities.. This enables them to construct low-rent public housing. Much of this new construction is designed specifically for the aged. Unfortunately, waiting lists for rentals are long, vacancies are few, and the housing may not meet an elderly person's needs. What is needed is a continuum of living arrangements within the same neighborhood to which the older person may move as circumstance and need dictate.

In spite of the growth and value of these programs, much still needs to be done to provide suitable and adequate housing at a reasonable cost for older citizens. The 1981 White House Conference on Aging pointed out that 200,000 homes needed to be constructed each year during the 1980s. Even today, this goal has not been met, leaving the housing needs of the nation sadly inadequate.

Medical Clinics

In some cities, medical clinics have been established in connection with low-cost housing projects. The medical clinic is staffed by nurses. It provides first aid and acts as a means of referral to other health services, figure 6-3. When a resident of such a housing project is admitted to one of the community agencies for health care, a nurse visits the hospital to maintain supporting contact. After the resident is discharged, follow-

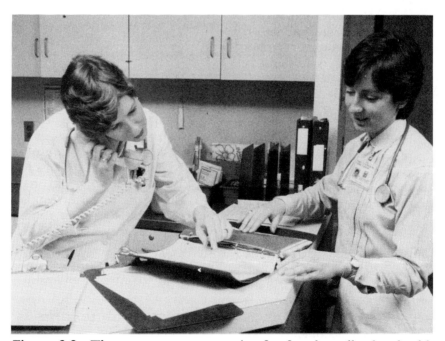

Figure 6-3 The nurse acts as an axis of referral to all other health services. (From Grippando & Mitchell, *Nursing Perspectives and Issues*, copyright 1989 by Delmar Publishers Inc. Courtesy The NYU Medical Center and Lou Manna)

up care is conducted in the home. The nurse usually maintains short health summaries. Working in this setting provides a unique opportunity to give service.

In the late 1980s, the approximately 600 nationwide community health care agencies recognized that the emphasis of care being offered was preventative in nature. It was more centered around maternal and child health.

Workshops were held to better coordinate activities of the Public Health Service and those services under the office of aging. The focus was on better utilization of senior centers as medical satellites for the community health centers. These centers included provisions for senior dental services, medical screening programs, and immunizations.

Home Health Services

Even when it becomes necessary because of illness, absence from one's own home causes great stress. The elderly strongly desire to return to their homes as quickly as possible. The application of DRG criteria also fosters discharge to home much earlier, often in a convalescent stage requiring considerable family support or assistance from community agencies. *Home health services* are available in some communities to help convalescing patients and the physically homebound in their own homes. These services provide help in many ways. For example, they can perform housekeeping chores, shop, or provide personal and professional care. The home health aide provides many of the direct services.

As early as the 1940s, hospitals showed an interest in providing some degree of care outside the hospital building. By 1955, fifty organized home health programs were scattered across the nation. These were all hospital based and served as an extended service. Home care was greatly expanded in 1965 under the amendments to the Social Security Act that instituted Medicare and Medicaid. Still, eligibility requirements are limiting. They require initial hospitalization or the ability to manage with intermittent care. Today,

there are over 2,500 home health programs certified for reimbursement under Medicare and Medicaid. Less than 20 percent of them are now hospital based, figure 6-4A and B.

Many important services needed to keep the elderly out of institutions are still not covered by home health programs. These include full-time housekeeping and heavy chore services. Home delivery of meals, errand running, and general companion services are also not covered. Some programs may include part-time nursing care, physical and occupational therapy, social service, speech therapy, some physician services, and the part-time services of a home health aide.

Some communities provide transportation and escort service, minor home repair and maintenance, telephone reassurance, visitors, and meal delivery. These are often sponsored by philanthropic and religious groups. The most successful home care programs allow for community and agency cooperation. This means including family members and friends as an important part of the team.

The Role of the Home Health Aide

The home health aide carries out personal care duties under the supervision of a doctor or registered nurse. Duties include food shopping, light meal preparation, light housekeeping, and personal care. Personal care includes helping the older person get to the bathroom or use a bedpan, bathe, ambulate, get in and out of bed, do prescribed exercises, and take medication, figure 6-5. Time spent with the client may be as little as one hour or as long as four. But the availability of these services can often make the difference between home living and institutionalization. This area of geriatric health care providers is one of the fastest growing of all health care services.

Retirement Communities

Retirement communities offer a life-style designed specifically for the older person. They are restrictive as to minimum age. Many require residents to be at least fifty-two. Recreational

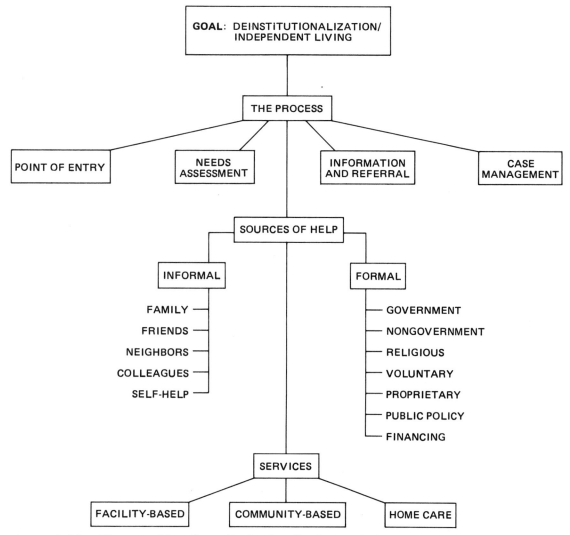

Figure 6-4A The transition from institutionalization to independent living is often made possible by in-home services made available through various sources.

facilities, health services, shopping centers, and churches are all conveniently located. Usually they are within the center itself. Different types of housing, from single homes to condominiums and apartments, are usually available at various prices. Electric cars and tricycles are common types of transportation within the community. Keeping active through recreational pursuits is stressed.

The elderly's response to retirement communities has ranged from enthusiasm to despondency. Some elderly people find renewed interest in life through community programs. They welcome the opportunity to make friends with their new neighbors. They are eager to enter into the activities and grateful to be away from the commotion of cities. They express pleasure at the convenience of facilities and relief at

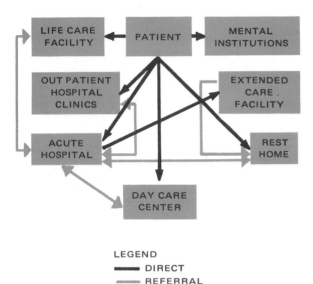

LEGEND
■■■ DIRECT
━━━ REFERRAL

Figure 6-4B   People may be moved to and from various health service areas according to need.

the absence of home maintenance chores. For others, the reaction is far different. Old friends are sorely missed. Adjustment to the new environment is difficult. Living in the community

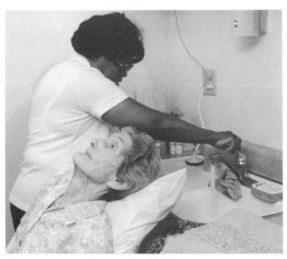

Figure 6-5   The home health aide assists the homebound person in many ways. (From Caldwell & Hegner, *Nursing Assistant—A Nursing Process Approach,* copyright 1989 by Delmar Publishers Inc.)

deprives them of companionship with other generations. They miss the security of knowing that family is nearby. As one disenchanted resident said, "Here we are, talking about our aches and pains, trying to fill the hours, waiting to see who will die next." The value of age-segregated living is still to be proven and is certainly not for everyone.

Life-Care Communities

Life-care communities represent still another type of housing specifically designed for the elderly. These apartment houses offer complete housing, health care, and recreational facilities.

An initial fee is charged when the person is admitted. A monthly fee covers all services including health care, meals, maid service, and linens. In some life-care residences, rental fees are scaled to accommodate lower income groups. All have variable accommodations and costs. Many are sponsored by local churches and other community groups, concerned over the inadequacy of housing for the elderly.

Some facilities are being designed specifically to meet the needs of handicapped residents. They are also being designed for those capable of self-care whose income is too high for rent subsidy but too low for complete self-maintenance. More and more elderly fall into this latter group.

Life-care facilities are built in areas that have easy access to public transportation and community activities. Residents are encouraged to participate in group activities within the residence, and to remain active in the community.

Life-care facilities include infirmaries that offer basic preventative services such as blood pressure checks and immunizations. Some infirmaries contain one or two beds for temporary care. A nurse coordinates the health care. He or she arranges for referral to other health facilities and provides follow-up care when a resident returns from a hospital or skilled nursing facility. The nurse is usually a resident of the facility and is on call for emergencies.

Health records are compiled on each resident and kept up to date. The nurse supervises the health practices of the residents and spends a large amount of time counseling them about their specific problems. Many people enter into life-care agreements when they are still healthy and independent. A life-care arrangement can offer security if an illness or infirmity occurs.

Many life-care communities are affiliated with an extended care facility (skilled or intermediate extended care facility SCR or ICF). Residents have top priority for placement in the facility if the need arises. These facilities provide further security for the older adult.

Living within the Family Unit

A small percentage of the elderly share the homes of younger family members. Three- and even four-generation families can be found sharing a single dwelling. This was once an accepted and expected form of life-style. It still is in many parts of the world.

It has become a less acceptable way of providing for older family members who may be made to feel they are intruding in the lives of younger family members, so the decision to move in with younger family members may be difficult for the older person. It may mean giving away, selling, or storing most of their personal possessions. Often it means being uprooted from familiar surroundings and friends.

Interpersonal relationships may be strained when an older person moves in. Even families that love the older person and accept the person's presence as the best arrangement may find the adjustment difficult. Stress is eased when the older person is made to feel needed. He or she should be allowed to share in the workload. Both the older person and the family unit should have opportunities to function independently. If possible, the older person should have a separate room that can be arranged to personal taste and where personal mementos can be kept. Unless tact is employed to protect dignity, the older person gradually loses self-esteem as the authoritative role is relinquished to younger family members.

Both the older person and younger family members should have the opportunity to participate in private social occasions and to entertain their individual friends. Occasional separations are sometimes wise. The older person may be able to visit other family members. This relieves the immediate family of total responsibility. Often a temporary foster home can be found for the older person, who may find relief from the emotional involvements of living with others for a while. Day care centers, which may be multifunctional, afford a safe haven while family members are at work or involved in their own responsibilities. If up and about, the older person should be encouraged to participate in activities that bring contact with other age groups, figure 6-6. As one older woman said, "Life can-

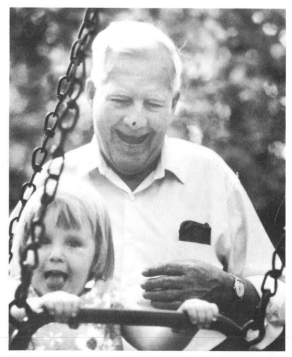

Figure 6-6   Elderly persons should be encouraged to engage in activities with other age groups.

not be dull when I see it renewed and made fresh with each new flower and child." Many older people get older, their level of income becomes lower, table 7-1. Many factors influence the their own age. Even a short daily break from one another can keep home relationships harmonious.

Day Centers

Throughout the country, multipurpose *day centers* have been established for the geriatric population. Most have been organized since 1965, when the Older Americans Act created the Administration on Aging, an agency of the Department of Health and Human Services. The last Harris survey revealed a high interest and participation rate in day centers. Some of these centers are funded by government agencies. Others are funded by churches and local benevo-

lent organizations. Some operations are under combined auspices. A church may provide the meeting place and other agencies may provide the actual services.

The health services offered are not the same at all centers. Some centers are strictly social and offer no health support. They simply provide a place where the older person can meet others with similar interests and problems to talk, to play checkers, chess, or cards, or to watch television, figure 6-7. Some centers offer exercise, dance, or craft classes, figure 6-8. The participants determine and plan the programs. Nutritionally balanced lunches may be provided at nominal cost or members may bring their lunches. In some cities, mobile canteen units, which take food to shut-ins, operate out of day centers.

Other day centers incorporate health benefits. Health examinations and health screening are routinely carried out. Through agencies such as the local health department, doctors, nurses, dietitians, and social workers visit the day center.

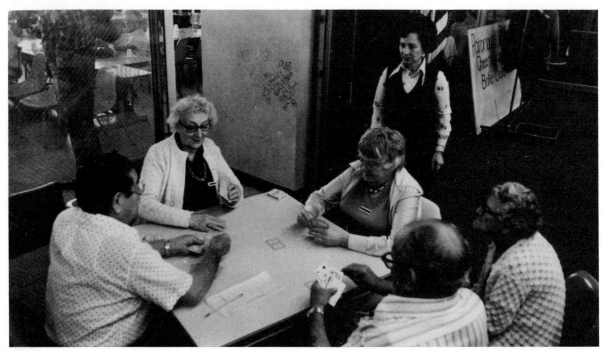

Figure 6-7   Day centers vary in services offered, but all provide an opportunity for social interchange.

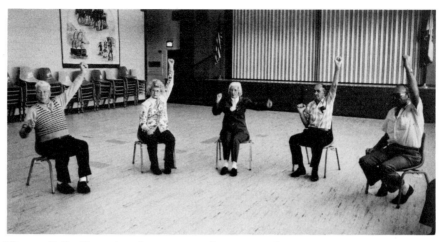

Figure 6-8 Exercise classes are often part of senior citizen programs.

Doctors and nurses use their visits to do health screening. They make referrals to the proper facilities for further care or study. General hygiene, with emphasis on proper foot care, is stressed. In some centers, mass immunizations are carried out by nursing personnel, figure 6-9. Special programs on nutrition and general preventative health measures may be offered each week or each month, with guest speakers from the community. Dietitians may speak to the group about general nutrition. They may also spend time prescribing special low-salt, diabetic, or bland diets that members need. Dietitians may also provide information to help people who live alone plan their nutrition more economically. Social workers can make members aware of other services that have been organized to help them. They can coordinate all available services to the best advantage of the elderly person. A professional team approach such as this is ideal. It leads to the best utilization of services. However, a nurse or social worker alone may have to provide all professional services. This one person examines, makes referrals, counsels, and even makes home visits to homebound members.

Besides decreasing the need for hospitalization, day centers provide a place for the elderly to spend their daytime hours pleasantly and safely.

When tensions are high at home, both the older person and the other family members need temporary separation. Senior centers are also becoming a source of continuing education for older people. Here older citizens can gain a sense of self-worth as they learn skills, engage in satisfying activities of self-expression, and come to realize the influence they can exert through the political process.

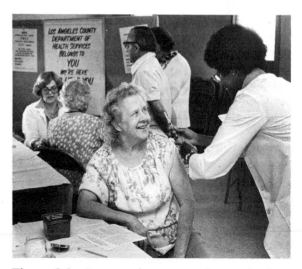

Figure 6-9 In some day centers, immunizations are carried out by nursing personnel.

Acute Care Hospitals

Persons in need of professional care may be admitted to a hospital or medical center in the community directly from their home or from another care facility. A fractured hip, pneumonia, a stroke, or a heart attack may require immediate professional attention. Acute care hospitals are not designed to provide long-term care. Therefore, as soon as the patient's condition warrants it, he or she is sent home or transferred to another care facility. Cost containment practices, such as the institution of D.R.G.s as a basis of reimbursement, have made early hospital discharge financially advantageous to acute care facilities. The availability of home care services and day centers also helps make earlier discharge possible.

Skilled Extended Care Facilities

Skilled extended care facilities (S.C.F.) offer progressive care. For those over sixty-five, most of the cost is covered by Medicare. The patient in this type of unit does not require acute nursing care. Here the focus is on *rehabilitation* (those efforts that aid people in achieving ways to improve their functional capacity so that they are able to be as independent as possible and have a satisfying life) and the greatest possible degree of independence, figure 6-10. New skills for carrying out the activities of daily living, such as self-feeding or walking after a cerebrovascular accident or an amputation, can be learned in this setting. Cases are reviewed periodically. The patient's progress is evaluated in light of established goals.

Patients are admitted to skilled extended care facilities from the hospital when they no longer need intensive nursing care but are not yet ready to assume responsibility for their own care. The criterion for admission to an extended care facility is potential for rehabilitation.

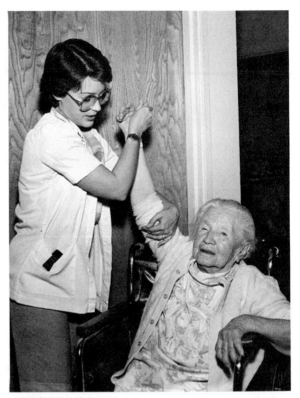

Figure 6-10   Rehabilitation is stressed in skilled extended care facilities.

Intermediate Care Facilities

If, following care in other facilities, there is no possibility that a patient can return to his or her former, independent life-style, care may best be provided in an intermediate care facility. Some homes provide "sheltered care" for ambulatory patients and are restrictive in their admission policy. They may accept only ambulatory patients and permit them to stay only as long as they are ambulatory. The majority of these facilities are not restrictive, however. They accept patients with varying degrees of dependence.

The major portion of direct patient care in this facility is given by nursing assistants working under the supervision of a professional or licensed vocational or practical nurse. Medications and treatments are professional responsibilities. But these functions may be placed in the hands of ancillary personnel, with the nurse giving somewhat remote supervision. In this situation, the responsibility for safe nursing care rests ultimately with the professional nurse. As a geriatric health care provider, make sure that you perform only those duties authorized by your job description.

Sheltered care patients require assistance in activities of daily living such as dressing, toileting, and eating. However, they do not need a great deal of physical nursing care. If the need arises for more acute nursing care, these patients are transferred to the acute care beds of a hospital. Ideally, movement to and from different health care facilities should be made without difficulty. There should also be a continuous record of the services provided.

Intermediate care facilities are one of the nation's rapid growth industries. The need for good, safe homes is evident. Although most facilities provide good care, conditions in some are substandard. The cost of others is prohibitive. A study by the Senate Committee on Aging identified such problems as abuse of seniors, fire danger, improper drug administration, and financial exploitation. The study also found a need for more qualified nurses and better enforcement of Health and Human Services (H.H.S.) standards.

Extended care facilities, many funded by Medicare, house close to one million residents. The move to an extended care facility, which are sometimes called *rest homes (nursing homes)*, is never an easy one. It usually is accepted only after a series of attempts to solve the problem of independent living.

Residents who are over eighty-five make up a large percentage of the nursing home population. In years to come, that percentage will double. Admission to a rest home may follow previous admissions to an acute care facility or extended care facility. Or it may result from an inability to care for the patient at home. Often

widowhood or loss of a home are precipitating factors.

Family tensions may develop when illness or infirmity increases the burden of care and decreases the flexibility of personality. When the burden becomes so great that the family unity is threatened, the older person will have to be moved to a different setting. The move will be easier if the older person is made to feel that his or her welfare is the principal reason for the move. Visits from the family then become extremely important. The health care provider can often act as a bond between patient and family. He or she can reassure the patient of the family's concern and encourage family members to visit and maintain contact with the patient.

Even when community-based services are available, Medicare eligibility policies create financial incentives to use nursing homes. In addition, the lack of community coordination acts as a barrier to continuum service. Some homes make provisions for husband and wife to remain together. Some homes, where sexual expression is recognized as a basic human need, provide areas where a couple can have privacy. But this is uncommon.

Care in sheltered facilities and skilled nursing facilities is largely supplied by non-professional personnel. As a geriatric health care provider, you are in a position to present an enlightened attitude. As a member of the nursing staff working in *homes for the aged*, you can greatly influence the quality of care. Mature, knowledgeable health care providers can do much to help hospital administrators and other personnel realize that, at times, everyone young or old needs privacy. A concerted effort is needed to overcome the prevailing negative attitude of some nursing home personnel regarding the sexuality of patients in their care.

Finding the right housing for the elderly is not always easy. The family health care provider can often provide sources of referral. The National Council on Aging (N.C.O.A.), a nonprofit, nongovernmental agency concerned with all problems of aging, publishes a national directory of nonprofit homes. Other listings can be obtained through local health and welfare agencies and through the local housing authority or community council. Homes should be visited and carefully inspected before placement is made. It is important to remember that only 5 percent of the elderly population is cared for in intermediate care facilities.

New Approaches

New, innovative approaches to providing safe, suitable housing for the elderly have been made. One such approach is the share-a-home concept. This places older people who need housing in touch with one another. Each newly formed household hires a cook and housekeeper. Another approach is to house the elderly together with students of college age. Certain facilities such as shops, restaurants, and libraries are common and allow for intergenerational mingling. Pilot programs seem to offer advantages to all concerned.

Mental Institutions

A number of elderly patients are found in institutions for the mentally ill. They represent only 1 percent of the total elderly population, however. Many of these patients have emotional problems that require professional psychiatric help. Other patients are confined because of temporary or transient confusion, organic cerebral changes, or because there is nowhere else for them to go. Alone, with no family and no financial resources, their only solution seems to be admission to a public institution. Loneliness, physical illness, and despair make them unable to manage for themselves. More information on mental breakdown is given in Unit 22.

Some long-term care facilities are designated as mental health facilities. They provide most of the same services as other long-term care facilities. However, the grounds of these facilities are enclosed, which allows residents with limited mental acuity (such as that associated with Alzheimer's disease) to be freely mobile.

Hospices

Hospices provide living arrangements for those with a limited life expectancy. Hospice care may be provided in the individual's own home or in a hospice building. Hospices and the hospice philosophy are covered more fully in Unit 18.

Referrals

If the health care provider is asked about the selection of a residence, he or she should remember that the elderly usually prefer to remain within their own communities. They need to be close to transportation, health services, and their place of worship. The best housing is simple in design. Cost and safety features are important. No one type of housing is suitable for all older people. Individual preference is important and should be the final determining factor.

There is a definite need for clear communication among the many different agencies that offer health care and housing for the elderly. This will ensure that these services can be coordinated to the best advantage. The health care provider in the community, whether specially appointed by an interested group, part of the visiting nurse association, or employed by the health department, is a logical person to function in this way. This person can act as a liaison between the patient and possible sources of help.

To fulfill this function, the health care provider must have access to the patient's medical history and the records of care and progress. The health care provider must be informed about special diets and treatments the patient needs in order to help the patient adapt the home situation to best advantage. Both long- and short-term goals need to be explicit. The patient's understanding of his or her condition must be carefully described. The nurse must devise ways to convey all this pertinent information to the appropriate agencies.

A basic referral form can be valuable in accurately transmitting patient information. A simple but complete referral form should become part of the patient's permanent record. It should move with the patient from agency to agency, making repetition and duplication of information unnecessary. No referral form is of value, of course, unless nurses understand its significance and recognize the importance of keeping it up to date. Unless this is done, essential information will be lost and real coordination will not be achieved.

Summary

- Most elderly people continue to live in the homes where they raised their families.
- The elderly prefer to remain in familiar neighborhoods, close to friends and younger family members. Home health care and day centers make this possible.
- Over the last twenty years, different types of housing accommodations have been developed specifically for the elderly.
- Rent subsidies, low-rent housing, and special loans for home purchase and improvement help the elderly to remain independent within the community.
- Entire communities have been developed for retired people. There is a strong emphasis on remaining active.
- Life-care communities offer total care for life under contractual agreements.
- In spite of the resources available to the elderly, some live on the streets with minimal help and shelter.
- Other housing arrangements depend upon need for assistance and care. These include acute hospitals, skilled care facilities, and extended care facilities.
- The decision to transfer from one facility to another, whether on a temporary or full-time basis, is difficult for all concerned. A great deal of compassion, tact, and understanding is needed to make the arrangements succeed. Ideally, the community should provide a continuum of facilities and services with easy transfer processes and maximum choice.
- Extended care facilities are becoming more numerous. Careful selection of a facility is important for an elderly person to ensure that the facility best meets his or her needs.

Review Outline

   I. Behavioral Objectives

  II. Vocabulary

 III. Living Facilities

      A.   Geographic distribution
      B.   Home ownership
      C.   Apartments and boarding houses
      D.   Retirement communities
      E.   Rooms or apartments within homes of younger family members

  IV. Care Facilities

      A.   Day centers
      B.   Life-care communities
         1. Complete health care
         2. Housing
         3. Recreational facilities

      C.   Acute care hospitals
      D.   Skilled extended care
      E.   Sheltered care
      F.   Intermediate extended care
      G.   Mental institutions
      H.   Hospices

V. Community Services

      A.   Federal assistance
          1. Rent subsidies
          2. Homeless shelters
          3. Reverse mortgages
      B.   Community health care agencies
      C.   Home health services
      D.   Medical clinics

Review

I. Vocabulary

Write the word from the vocabulary list that best completes each of the following statements.

    1. The living arrangements for some elderly may be _____ _____ subsidized or assisted by governmental agency money.
    2. A family consisting of a husband, wife, children, aunt, and grandmother might be described as _____.
    3. The elderly couple moved from their large home that was difficult to keep up to a less stressful _____.
    4. An agency that provides mortgage insurance to help the elderly is called _____
    5. A life-style especially designed for the active older person may be found in a _____

II. Short Answers

    1. Which government department provides mortgage insurance to help older persons repair and purchase homes?
    2. What help is available to older people who cannot pay full rent?
    3. What are the advantages of a condominium to an older person?
    4. What services provide enough help to make it possible for elderly people to remain in their own homes?
    5. What are factors that will make it easier for older people to move in with younger family members?
    6. What is the main function of extended care facilities?
    7. What is a sheltered care facility?
    8. What is another name for a rest home that cares for the total needs of elderly patients?
    9. What is the value of referral records?

10. List the services offered by a life-care residence.
11. Describe the services of a geriatric day center.
12. List the positive and negative aspects of living in a retirement community.

III. Complete the chart on sources of help for keeping the elderly living independently.

Sources of Help

Informal	Formal
a. _____	a. _____
b. _____	b. _____
c. _____	c. _____
d. _____	d. _____
e. _____	e. _____
	f. _____
	g. _____

IV. Clinical Situations

1. A neighbor wants to ease the stress of having her elderly mother move in with them. What would you suggest?
2. A new multipurpose senior citizen center opens in your neighborhood. A friend asks you to explain what goes on there. What would you say?

Unit 7
Financial Considerations

Objectives

After studying this unit, you should be able to:
- Describe the general financial status of those over sixty-five.
- Name four ways that people can prepare financially for the later years of life.
- List four major public retirement plans.

Vocabulary

Learn the meaning and spelling of the following words or phrases.

C.O.L.A.	Medicare
data	pension
E.R.I.S.A.	Social Security
I.R.A.	S.S.I.
Keogh plans	vesting
Medicaid	

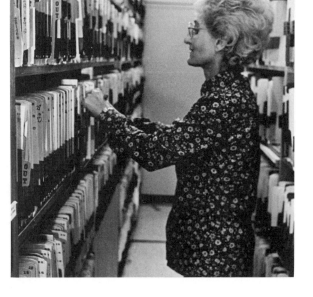

A Word About Statistical Data

Statistics provide important information (*data*) about populations and the relationship of the numbers of persons within those populations to the entire group. Statistics are just numbers and figures until they are organized and analyzed. The scope of the data and how the questions are worded may alter the final conclusions that are obtained. The analysis itself may group figures in such a way that important information is missed. For example, statistics tell us that in 1987 those aged sixty-five and over made up 12.2 percent of the population. The statistics also show that by the year 2000, this number will rise to 13 percent and continue to increase. What these statistics fail to reveal is that there is a rapidly growing segment of the elderly population over eighty years of age that is frail and requires supportive care.

Important as this information is, it becomes even more significant when it is combined with the birth statistics of the 1940s. This information tells us that the most rapid increase in the numbers of those in their eighties and nineties will be between the years 2010 and 2030.

These statistical data can be added to the fact that the Social Security system is financially funded only until the early part of the twenty-first century. Think what the large numbers of elderly, frail people who may not have the financial floor of Social Security could mean to each person individually and to the society as a whole.

New Data Gathering

The 1990 census should provide much information that is lacking in the current data about the elderly. It will break down groups of people into five-year age increments. This will provide information on how many elderly persons in each group are unable to carry out the activities of daily living without help, how much of their income comes from private pensions, and the numbers and types of people in the various care facilities. There are several important statistical-gathering groups who have already agreed to changes in data usage. These groups include the National Center for Health Statistics, the National Institute on Aging, and the Gerontological Society of America. The cost of information gathering and analysis is a drawback. Problems maintaining privacy and confidentiality also occur. Still, ways of learning more accurate information are essential if public policy is to be properly prepared and financed as we move through the 1990s to the twenty-first century.

Statistics may seem outdated when they represent findings of surveys more than five years old. In many cases, however, these statistics are the best that can be presented considering the restrictions on collecting and analyzing the data. As you read this unit, try to keep in mind the importance and limitations of statistical data.

Financial Planning

Plans for financial security in the later years must be made early in life. Preretirement planning, to be effective, should be started many years before retirement actually occurs. This is especially important for those of the "baby boomer" generation who are now reaching their forties. By the time they reach their own retirement years, there will be fewer people in the work force to contribute to their support. In addition, the current stabilized Social Security system may not be able to provide for them.

Of all the crises that must be managed in a lifetime, the crisis of retirement is one of the most

critical. For some, sixty-five is the age at which the crisis arrives. For others, it is much earlier. For a few, it never really comes. The problem of financial support in the postretirement years is an important aspect of the crisis that must be faced by nearly all of the elderly.

At the same time that income is sharply reduced, the elderly often feel the need for additional expenditures for health, figure 7-1. Four out of five elderly people suffer from one or more chronic conditions.

With retirement comes an increase in leisure time. There is more opportunity for recreational and entertainment activities than ever before. Unfortunately, these activities put additional burdens on the budget. The elderly must now spend money on fees, equipment, clothes, and transportation.

The vast majority of retirees have a fixed income that makes no provision for cost increases due to inflation or unexpected expenses. Social Security, a major source of income, is currently indexed to provide a cost of living adjustment *(C.O.L.A.)*. Even this assistance is threatened because of efforts to control the

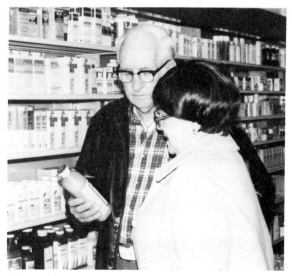

Figure 7-1 Personal health expenditures are greater for those persons over sixty-five.

federal deficit. So in reality, as costs of essential services rise, buying power dwindles. Simply providing for basic needs often becomes an awesome task. Special expenditures such as property upkeep have to be postponed or eliminated altogether. The financial situation of the postretirement years is such that many older people struggling with it often feel inadequate. They gradually lose confidence that they will be able to remain independent.

Financial Status of the Elderly

Few people are able to maintain a high level of income throughout their lives. In general, as people get older, their level of income becomes lower, table 7-1. Many factors influence the

financial picture. These include sex, race, health, marital status, and earning ability.

The current status of those in their retirement years has greatly improved over the last thirty years. This is particularly true for that segment of the elderly who are married, own their own homes, and have been regularly employed throughout their adult years. In fact, the older population generally has fared better than the population as a whole.

Since 1968, elderly incomes have grown in real terms. Those of the rest of the population have stabilized. In the years since 1968, there has been a 52.6 percent growth in the elderly income adjusted for inflation. The growth in real income for all households was 6 percent. In 1987, the median income among elderly households was $14,334 compared to $25,986 for all households, table 7-2.

The median net worth of older households in 1987 was $60,300. This figure placed it well above the U.S. average of $32,700. Nearly one-third of the elderly households have a net worth of $100,000.

Home Ownership

Home ownership is a major asset for the elderly. Nearly three-quarters of the elderly own their own homes. This makes home equity an important component of elderly wealth. Many older people were able to purchase homes when property and interest rates were relatively low. They now find themselves with property of greatly increased value. Moreover, after age fifty-five the government grants a one-time tax exemption on profits of up to $125,000 from the sale of a home, regardless of an owner's income. This makes home ownership have even greater value.

Banks are cashing in on this source of wealth. Under pressure from the Federal Housing Administration (*F.H.A.*), they are offering reverse mortgages that will allow the elderly to continue living in the home and receive a monthly income.

Unlike regular home equity loans, which pay the total loan amount up front, reverse mort-

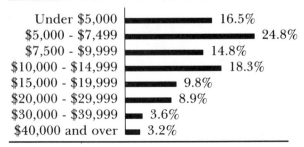

**PERCENT DISTRIBUTION
BY INCOME: 1988**

Family households with head 65 +

Income	Percent
Under $5,000	2.2%
$5,000 - $9,999	10.5%
$10,000 - $14,999	16.9%
$15,000 - $19,999	16.1%
$20,000 - $29,999	21.7%
$30,000 - $39,999	12.9%
$40,000 - $49,999	6.8%
$50,000 and over	12.9%

Nonfamily households with head 65 +

Income	Percent
Under $5,000	16.5%
$5,000 - $7,499	24.8%
$7,500 - $9,999	14.8%
$10,000 - $14,999	18.3%
$15,000 - $19,999	9.8%
$20,000 - $29,999	8.9%
$30,000 - $39,999	3.6%
$40,000 and over	3.2%

Table 7-1

| | ALL HOUSEHOLDS | | | OVER-65 HOUSEHOLDS | | |
| | Current | Constant 1987 Dollars | | Current | Constant 1987 Dollars | |
	$	1987 $	% Change	$	1987 $	% Change
1967	7,143	24,315		2,760	9,395	
1968	7,743	25,295	4.0	3,180	10,388	10.6
1969	8,389	26,007	2.8	3,329	10,321	−0.7
1970	8,735	25,567	−1.7	3,498	10,238	−0.8
1971	9,028	25,335	−0.9	3,813	10,700	4.5
1972	9,697	26,344	4.0	4,169	11,326	5.8
1973	10,512	26,884	2.1	4,583	11,721	3.5
1974	11,197	25,805	−4.0	5,292	12,196	4.1
1975	11,800	24,918	−3.4	5,919	12,499	2.5
1976	12,686	25,327	1.6	5,962	11,903	−4.8
1977	13,572	25,454	0.5	6,347	11,904	0.0
1978	15,064	26,243	3.1	7,081	12,336	3.6
1979	16,461	25,774	−1.8	7,879	12,337	0.0
1980	17,710	24,427	−5.2	8,781	12,111	−1.8
1981	19,074	23,835	−2.4	9,903	12,375	2.2
1982	20,171	23,750	−0.4	11,041	13,000	5.1
1983	21,018	23,976	1.0	11,972	13,657	5.1
1984	22,415	24,526	2.3	12,799	14,004	2.5
1985	23,618	24,952	1.7	13,254	14,003	0.0
1986	24,897	25,807	3.4	13,845	14,351	2.5
1987	25,986	25,986	0.7	14,334	14,334	−0.1

Source: U.S. Department of Commerce, Bureau of the Census; U.S. Department of Labor, Bureau of Labor Statistics, 1988.

Table 7-2 Median household income has shown an increase overall when compared with all household income 1967–1987.

gages advance the loan on a monthly basis. Under existing agreements, the principal, plus interest, is due either at the end of a specified term or when the house is sold or the homeowner dies.

There have been some problems with these mortgages. However, regulations instituted by the F.H.A. in 1988 sought to reduce some of the risks to the lenders if the homeowner refuses to sell at the agreed time and if the owner lives longer than expected and the loan is worth more than the property.

Banking institutions are also soliciting the savings of the elderly. They are offering, at no charge, services such as checking accounts, personalized checks, credit cards, income tax counseling, travelers checks, and photocopying. Many banks even sponsor clubs that present a variety of seminars or take members on short trips. Another factor influencing the financial well-being of this segment of the population is the fact that the elderly receive less of their income from wages and salaries. Therefore, they are less affected by changes in the labor market.

Looking only at the statistics given, one might be inclined to believe that reaching the golden years means prosperity and happiness for everyone. Another set of statistics reveals that although many elderly are enjoying greater financial security, there are still many who are not. Let's look at the financial situation of another set of the elderly. Remember that although they are a minority, this set of the elderly still represents millions of people.

Poverty

In 1984, for the first time, the poverty rate for the elderly dropped below the poverty rate for the nation as a whole. It was 12.2 percent as compared to a national average of 13.5 percent.

In the early 1960s, the Bureau of Labor Statistics developed a budget adequate to provide a modest standard of living for a theoretical couple. This couple was retired and over sixty-five, in good health, and lived in an urban area. Since that time, the budget has been regularly updated.

In 1987, the official poverty level for a single, elderly person over age sixty-five was $5,265. For a couple, it was $6,630.

About 3.5 million elderly persons were found with incomes below the poverty level. Eight million of the elderly take in less than twice that amount. Another 2.3 million, or 8 percent of the elderly, could be classified as "near poor." These people had incomes between the poverty level and 125 percent of this level. In 1987, nearly 40 percent of all the elderly were part of the poor or economically vulnerable group.

Elderly persons living alone or with nonrelatives were likely to have the lowest incomes, figure 7-2. Nearly 44 percent reported an income of $7,000 or less. Twenty-two percent reported incomes under $5,000. The median income also varied by race. Whites reported a median income of $8,098, blacks $4,974, and Hispanics $5,291. This means that one out of nine elderly white persons is poor, 31 percent of elderly blacks are poor, and about 25 percent of elderly Hispanics fall into this category.

Older women have the highest poverty rate (15 percent). This is especially true when the older woman lives alone. Many women over seventy-five are widows living alone. Most were not in poverty until their husbands died.

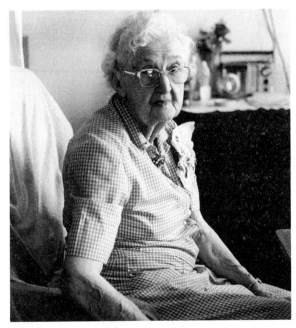

Figure 7-2   Elderly people living alone or with nonrelatives usually have the lowest income. (From Zins, *Aging in America,* copyright 1987 by Delmar Publishers Inc.)

Based on these figures, some elderly subgroups have a high incidence of poverty. These groups include women, the very old, those living alone, and minorities. Three times as many elderly blacks fall below the poverty line as elderly whites. Belonging to more than one of these subgroups, as by being old, black, and female, intensifies the poverty. Other subgroups with a high incidence of poverty are those who are not married, do not work, live on Social Security, and live in small towns and rural areas.

The southeastern states have the highest concentration of elderly poor. Mississippi, Alabama, Arkansas, and Louisiana have the greatest numbers. California, Connecticut, and Wisconsin have the fewest.

Poverty among aging minorities is increasing more sharply than ever before. Elderly minorities are two to three times more likely to be poor than are elderly whites. For aged blacks, approximately 50 percent live in poverty. Since 1979, the number of poor black women has increased by 20 percent. The number now stands at approximately 60 percent.

The elderly poor living in rural areas have an additional burden since they often do not have easy access to many of the services available in urban areas.

Most elderly people need almost all of their income for current expenditures. The biggest expenses are housing, food, energy, transportation, and health care. On an average, 57.5 percent of their income goes for food and 23.3 percent for energy, leaving only 19.2 percent for all other items. The latest Harris survey (1981) found that most people sixty-five and over regretted not having prepared better for the financial security of their later years.

Sources of Retirement Income

The major sources of income for the elderly include the government, current earnings from jobs, pensions, savings and investments, rents, inheritance, and money from relatives, figure 7-3.

Government Sources

The government provides four basic support systems for elderly income. They are Social Security, Supplemental Security Income *(S.S.I.)*, veterans' assistance, and other government pensions. The portion of the federal budget aimed at the elderly jumped from 16 percent in 1965 to 28 percent in 1988.

More older people receive Social Security benefits than any other type of public or private financial support, table 7-3. *Social Security* (Old Age, Survivors, and Disability Insurance) is a compulsory, federally sponsored insurance program that covers the vast majority of American workers. Payments to retirees depend on the amount they have paid into the plan during their working years. The amount they receive also depends on the age at which they begin receiving benefits. Current benefits are funded from current income rather than from past payments. Congress has passed legislation to increase income to the system over the next thirty years. This plus only moderate growth in the numbers

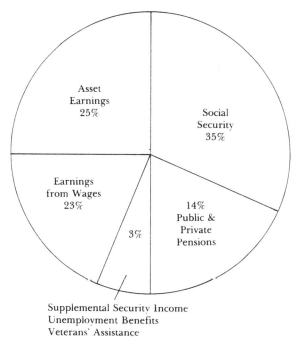

Supplemental Security Income
Unemployment Benefits
Veterans' Assistance

Figure 7-3 Sources of elderly income, 1988

SOCIAL SECURITY BENEFITS

If You Reach the Retirement Age in:	Average Earner: $21,410 in 1990	Maximum Earner: $49,800 in 1990
1990	6,713	$ 9,089
1995	7,091	9,826
2000	7,611	10,939
2005	8,175	12,174
2010	8,785	13,451
2015	9,436	14,720
2020	10,141	15,875
2025	10,892	17,057
2030	11,701	18,322

The normal age for full retirement benefits will rise in slow steps from 65 to 67 (in 2027) for people born between 1938 and 1960.

(Ramsden and Mullikin 1985, 63)

Table 7-3 Social Security benefits

of people receiving benefits should keep the Social Security fund solvent into the twenty-first century.

In 1988, it took 3.3 contributors to maintain one Social Security beneficiary. However, by the year 2035, the ratio of taxpayer to beneficiary will be 2 to 1. At that point, there may be another serious threat to this basic program.

Prior to Social Security, wages were the major source of support for the elderly. However, now more than nine out of ten elderly people receive Social Security benefits, and 65 percent depend on Social Security alone for income. For those whose income is less than $5,000, 80 percent have no other income but Social Security. One-fifth of the elderly living alone and two-fifths of the black elderly living alone receive 90 percent or more of their income from this source. Social Security, therefore, becomes the single largest source of income for the elderly. Current earnings from jobs of one or both spouses contribute far less to the incomes of elderly individuals living alone than they do to those who are members of households.

Recent amendments to the Social Security Act have increased the benefits and changed the amounts that can be earned without forfeiting benefits. Since 1979, employer and employee payments into Social Security funds have been gradually raised to help offset the enormous drains on the funds.

Some of the important changes in Social Security include those related to the eligibility for benefits and to Medicare. In the year 2009, full benefits will not be paid until the recipient reaches the age of sixty-six. The eligibility age will rise to sixty-seven in 2027. The Social Security rate, including Medicare, rose to 7.51 percent in 1989. The maximum Social Security Tax (FICA) wage base of $45,000 in 1988 increased to $48,000 in 1989. The maximum contribution also increased from $3,379.59 in 1988 to $3,604.80 in 1989.

From 1965 to 1988, the average retired Social Security entitlement rose from $1,015 to $5,341 a year. In 1989, a 4 percent C.O.L.A. (cost of living allowance) was granted. The allowance from S.S.I. in 1990 was $386 per month for an individual and $579 for a couple. Social Security now pays out $200 billion a year in benefits, mostly to the elderly.

Supplemental Security Income (S.S.I.) is a federal program with state supplements. It provides most of the public assistance for the disabled elderly.

Many elderly who might be eligible do not participate, however. A 1988 study revealed that about one-third of the elderly and disabled who could benefit from S.S.I. were not aware that the assistance is available. Others fail to participate because of the negative connotations of accepting "welfare," as well as an unwillingness to deal with the necessary bureaucracy.

Every state except Texas participates in S.S.I. either through supplemental checks or combined federal/state allotments. The aged disabled in Texas receive only federal payments.

The S.S.I. program enacted in 1974 provided $25 a month as a personal needs allowance for a person in long-term care. It provided $50 per month for a couple. In 1987, this amount was raised to $30 a month for an individual and $60 for a couple. In 1990 the allowance remained the same.

Veterans' assistance and government pensions are sent out to those elderly who have served the nation in either military or civil service positions. About 5 percent receive direct veterans' assistance, and 7 percent receive other governmental pensions.

Noncash Benefits

Any services for which the elderly make no direct payment add to their financial security. The Older Americans Act addresses needs that would either go unmet or those that would require the elderly to spend a considerable amount of their financial resources.

The 1965 Older Americans Act, figure 7-4, was created as a new federal program specifically designed to meet the social service needs of older people. It is a major vehicle for organizing and delivering social services to the elderly.

New appropriation legislation for the Older Americans Act was passed by the 100th Congress in 1987. This legislation authorized $1.2 billion to reauthorize the provisions of the Act through 1991. New rules under Title III provide for the needs of the frail elderly living at home. They also cover residents of long-term care facilities and persons at risk of abuse, neglect, or exploitation. Other amendments relate to outreach programs for the elderly who may be eligible for benefits under S.S.I., Medicare, and food stamp programs. Still other provisions are directed to the needs of the native American elderly and the disabled. In addition, other legislation has been enacted to assist with specific elderly problems, figure 7-5.

Title	Provision
I	Declaration of Objectives
II	Establishes the Administration on Aging
III	Grants for state and community programs on aging: for supportive services, nutrition services, nonmedical in-home services, long-term care ombudsman services, elder abuse prevention activities, health education, and special outreach programs for eligible persons
IV	Training and research program grants for demonstration projects on aging
V	Community service employment for older Americans supplies funds to subsidize part-time community service jobs (1987–1988 commitment supports 66,000 jobs)
VI	Grants to social and nutrition services for older Indians (native Americans) and native Hawaiians

Figure 7-4 Provisions of the Older Americans Act

OTHER PERTINENT LEGISLATION

S.S.I.

1. Increased personal needs allowance for nursing home residents under Supplemental Security Income programs.
2. Full benefits for S.S.I. recipients temporarily in institutions for three months for an additional three months when returning home.

Housing & Community Development Act of 1987

1. Authorizes monies ($621.7 million in 1988, $630 million in 1989) for federal housing programs.
2. Allows public housing authorities to give priority to families with a head of household at least fifty years old if there are vacancies.
3. H.U.D. required to conduct studies related to assisted housing for the elderly and to develop demonstration programs.

PL100-175

Legislation authorizing the President to call for a White House Conference on Aging in 1991 to recognize contributions of older Americans and to identify issues needing resolution and make recommendations for public action.

PLN100-203

Legislation relating to the funding of private pension plans, including:

1. imposing new minimum funding standards on single-employer defined benefit pension plans,

(continued)

2. increasing the annual per-participant premium charged for single-employer defined benefit plans by the Pension Benefit Guaranty Corporation,

3. increasing an employer's liability in the event a plan is terminated,

4. imposing certain restrictions on employers who wish to recapture assets in refunded pension plans.

Amended National School Lunch Programs

Permits adult day care programs to receive reimbursement under the child care food programs for meals and snacks for persons sixty years or older.

Figure 7-5 Summary of pertinent legislation affecting the elderly population.

In 1986, the Gramm-Rudman-Hollings legislation was passed in an effort to bring about a balanced budget in 1991. The impact of this bill has not been tested. Although the entitlement benefits such as Social Security are exempt, an increasing pressure to balance the budget could put restrictions on the administration of these programs.

Pensions

Most companies of any size today have retirement *(pension)* plans for their employees. This is especially true if the workers are union members. Although about 90 percent of older workers now have some form of retirement protection, only about 55 percent of workers in private industry are now covered. Only about one-half of that number actually receive a pension. In some companies, both employer and employee contribute to the retirement fund. In other companies, the employer makes all contributions. In the last thirty years, pensions have shown great improvement. Much of this gain has been due to union pressure. Unions have recently been losing membership. New high-technology companies do not unionize readily. Thus, gains may not advance further. They may even erode.

Company pensions vary greatly. They are often tied to expected benefits from Social Security. Some companies encourage employees to pay into savings plans by offering to match a percentage of the amount contributed. These savings may not be withdrawn until retirement time. After retirement, in addition to the savings, workers receive monthly pension checks based on their years of service.

In 1974, Congress passed the Employee Retirement Income Security Act *(E.R.I.S.A.)*. This law seeks to protect workers by regulating and overseeing the financing of private pension plans. It also offers some protection in case the company fails. E.R.I.S.A. makes no provision, however, for carrying retirement benefits from one company to another. Moving from one job to another can be costly to the individual in these terms.

The Tax Reform Act of 1986 requires vesting. This makes the worker eligible for pension benefits after five years of employment with a firm. Before 1986, most employees had to work ten years before becoming vested. *Vesting* means that an employee is entitled to part or all of an employer's contribution to his or her pension made after December 31, 1988. This is a particularly important provision for those older workers who enter second careers or move from job to job within a specific industry.

Further efforts are being made to safeguard pension funds. Companies that need financing have turned to so-called surplus pension monies. Surplus assets are those that exceed a company's current pension obligations to its employees and retirees. Legislation to impose an excise tax on fund usage may be enacted.

Many retired people who are not covered by Social Security are helped by railroad, teacher, or civil service retirement systems. Railroad retirement benefits are being paid to 930,000 retired workers and their families. Today there is one worker for every three retirees collecting benefits. The Railroad Retirement Board estimates that the number of retirees, which peaked at one million in the 1970s, has gradually declined. The number is expected to decline to 500,000 in the year 2010. Payroll tax increases enacted by Congress in 1983 and 1987 have kept the fund solvent. With the continuing decrease in recipients, the fund looks to be stable for the next twenty years. In 1989, the monthly benefits amounted to $730.

Public pensions for civil service workers and teachers often provide better benefits for participants than Social Security does. These pensions tend to relate returns to peak years of income and to contain cost of living clauses. They also involve high levels of participant contributions.

Private Savings

Since the early 1980s, great emphasis has been placed on developing personal saving strategies to assist in the retirement years. Tax incentives have been offered through I.R.A. and Keogh plans.

In 1981, the eligibility requirements for Individual Retirement Accounts were changed, making them available to almost all workers by 1982. These accounts allowed those currently employed to contribute up to $2,000 a year tax free to a special savings account called an Individual Retirement Account *(I.R.A.)*. These funds could be invested in a variety of nontaxable instruments. But they could not be withdrawn until the account owner reached fifty-nine years of age. At withdrawal, the funds and accumulated interest become taxable as income. Funds withdrawn prior to the eligible age are still subject to regular taxation and substantial loss of interest. This program was open to general participation until 1986. Restrictions were applied after 1986, making the tax deduction possible only for those who were not vested in another retirement program. *Keogh plans* still offer possibilities for the self-employed to save a specific percentage of their income for retirement.

Some effort needs to be made to protect the savings accounts of small savers who cannot util-

ize I.R.A. or Keogh plans. It is also necessary to find ways to include those unemployed through disability in a savings plan.

Only a small minority invest through insurance companies in annuities that mature when they retire, bringing in a small monthly income. Other people choose savings bonds plans and investments as ways of preparing a nest egg. Regular bank deposits lay a foundation of financial security for the later years. Few are able to use this system, however. Others invest in stocks and bonds. They develop a portfolio with retirement security as a goal. A small percentage supplement their incomes by renting property or space in their homes.

Fraternal organizations such as the Masons or Elks assist needy members. Some have established homes where aged members can receive care. But, in some cases, the older person must eventually turn to younger family members for financial assistance. Between 3 percent and 5 percent of the elderly report receiving cash gifts from younger family members. This situation poses its own set of problems. Working-age people are trapped between providing for their children, assisting their parents, and attempting to prepare for their own postretirement years.

The fact is that the majority of people regularly earn only enough to provide for their current needs. Little is left over. A large number of people have difficulty staying financially solvent throughout their working lives. Old age finds them in severely curtailed circumstances.

Public Assistance

State and local public assistance programs have greatly changed over the years, and the number of people requiring this type of help has decreased. This is probably a result of better coverage through Social Security. Changes in the requirements for assistance now make it possible for the elderly to earn some money and still receive benefits.

Many older people would rather be destitute than accept charity. Others are unaware that such benefits are available. In either case, social workers and others offering them help need to be sensitive in their approach. Older people must never be treated as second-class citizens or made to feel that they are a burden on society.

The potential for gainful employment is explored fully in Unit 8. This is another source of financial support as more workers take advantage of the opportunities promoted by changes in 1987 federal and state employment laws.

The Cost of Health Care

The chronic health problems of the elderly are a constant drain on their limited incomes, figure 7-6. Most of the elderly suffer from at least one chronic condition. Many have multiple conditions. Older persons over sixty-five average almost twice as many doctors' visits as younger persons. Hospital expenses account for the largest share of their health expenditures, followed by expenditures for physicians and nursing home care. An elderly American's second highest out-of-pocket expenditure is for prescription drugs. Only long-term care costs more. Many of the health needs of the elderly are now being met through the federally sponsored health insurance program called *Medicare*. They are also being met through various state-sponsored programs as well as through private insurance plans. State-supported services are called different names such as *Medicaid* or Medical. In 1987, Medicare spent $69 billion on hospital and doctors' fees on behalf of the elderly and disabled.

Despite cost containment efforts, expenditures for Medicare and Medicaid services rose so dramatically that both programs became threatened. One cost containment method instituted in the mid-1980s was D.R.G. reimbursement. *D.R.G.* stands for diagnosis-related groupings. Briefly, this means that disease conditions are classed into major groups. The government has established an expected length of hospitalization and specific rates of reimbursement under Medicare for each group. Other factors such as age, surgery, and complications are considered.

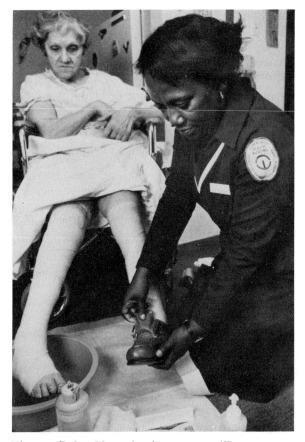

Figure 7-6   Chronic, long-term illnesses are among the leading health problems. (Courtesy Rush-Presbyterian-St. Luke's Medical Center, Chicago, IL)

But this method of reimbursement encourages hospitals to discharge patients as early as possible because they may keep funds for care if that care is not required. For example, if, under Medicare, payment can be made for seven days of hospitalization for a specific illness, and the patient is discharged after only five days, the hospital will still receive payment for seven days. If, on the other hand, the illness requires more than seven days in the hospital, the hospital must absorb the difference. This has resulted in many elderly people who still require nursing care being returned to the community or the extended care facility.

The Health Insurance of the Aged Act, Title XVIII of the Social Security Act, established Medicare to help those over sixty-five meet hospital and other medical costs. There are two parts to the Medicare program: hospital insurance and voluntary supplementary medical insurance. The first part is financed by contributions from employees. Employers pay an equal amount. It is also financed by the self-employed. Patients pay an initial amount, which is determined by the average daily cost of inpatient hospital care.

The majority of those benefitting from Medicare hospital insurance are over age sixty-five (29 million people in 1988). An additional 3 million disabled also receive benefits. The majority of beneficiaries have also purchased supplemental insurance (Medigap) to help pay for services not covered by insurance. This represents 8 million elderly. Premiums for the second part are financed in part by the federal government and in part by the individual. It is possible for those who have not worked long enough to be eligible for Social Security to purchase Medicare insurance by paying a monthly premium.

The Medicare Catastrophic Protection Act of 1987 and the Medicare Catastrophic Loss Prevention Act of 1987 were both passed by the 100th Congress and signed into law by the president. The new law took effect January 1, 1989. It was to be phased in completely over a period of four years. It limited out-of-pocket costs that Medicare beneficiaries would have to pay for hospital and doctor bills and for outpatient prescription bills that exceeded $600 per year.

The legislation required Medicare to pick up the cost of all covered hospital care after the payment of a single annual deductible. Starting in 1989, the annual deductible would be $564. In 1990, the maximum liability for beneficiaries under Part B would be $1,370 after an annual deductible of $75. Part B covered charges for participating physicians' fees and other outpatient services. About 98 percent of all beneficiaries would participate in both Part A and Part B of the plan. They would have had increasing amounts deducted from their Social Security

checks. After the limits had been met, Medicare would pay for 100 percent of the approved charges. Three other important provisions were also addressed in the bill: outpatient prescription drugs, mammography examination to detect breast cancer, and eighty hours per year for "respite" relief. The cost of respite care was provided to relieve unpaid family members from providing continual care.

The legislation was to be financed by increased costs to Medicare beneficiaries. Higher income people would pay a supplemental premium. Although the new laws were valuable, there was no provision for the cost of long-term care in an extended care facility or in the community.

Strong protests from the elderly about the additional costs to them prompted legislators to take another look at the plan in 1989. Subsequently, the legislation was repealed.

Title XIX of the Social Security Amendments of 1965 was a companion law to the original Medicare Act. It authorized grants to states to provide high-quality medical services to low-income elderly and other needy people. Title XIX established a single and separate medical program that replaced medical care cost provisions of Old Age Assistance and Medical Assistance to the Aged programs. This program offers benefits under varying names in different states. For example, it is known as Medicaid in New York and Medical in California. Over the years, the exact provisions of these acts have changed, and they continue to do so.

The Catastrophic Medicare Bill (HR 2470) altered Medicaid provisions. It required the joint federal/state program to pay all Medicare-required premiums, deductibles, and coinsurance amounts for beneficiaries whose incomes are too high to make them eligible for standard Medicaid, but who are still below the poverty level.

A major extension of the bill deals with the problem of spousal impoverishment. This situation develops when one member of a couple requires long-term care and the spouse must "spend down" all of their assets before the partner who needs care can qualify for Medicaid help in paying care facility costs. Under the new provision, the spouse remaining at home can keep an amount equal to 122 percent of the current poverty level (1989—$780 per month) for a couple, up to a maximum of $1,500 per month. The amount permitted would gradually increase until 1992. States would also have to permit the at-home spouse to retain at least $12,000 in assets or one-half of the couple's joint assets, up to $60,000.

The cost of these benefits come from savings to the program as Medicare picks up some previously paid benefits. They also come from the general treasury.

Medigap Insurance

About two-thirds of Medicare beneficiaries currently have private "Medigap" insurance policies. These policies offer coverage similar to that provided in the 1988 legislation. The Catastrophic Care Act gave Medigap insurers until January 31, 1989, to inform policyholders how the new act would affect existing policies and premiums. It also gave insurers until that date to explain any adjustments the company has made to eliminate problems with overlapping coverage. Medigap coverage is still needed to cover deductibles, the beneficiary's share of physician's fees, and some other expenses not covered by Medicare.

The Medicare system seems financially stable until sometime around 2005. There are fears that some of the program will need to be altered to help reduce the federal deficit and to keep the basic provisions solvent.

Long-Term Care

The third major influence on the financial status of the elderly is the cost of long-term care. Federal legislators have not faced this problem. This is an area that must be considered, because long-term care costs $40 billion each year. Some of this long-term care is provided in institutions and some in the community.

The older one gets, the greater the likelihood that institutional care will be needed. Approximately 5 percent of those over sixty-five are in nursing homes. However, 50 percent of those eighty-five and older require long-term care. Only 0.5 percent of those needing such care have insurance to help pay for it.

Medicare and private insurance cover less than 3 percent of nursing home costs. These costs averaged $24,000 to $25,000 per year in 1989.

More people are living today to become the frail elderly in their eighties and nineties. Long-term care will become increasingly costly as the population in care facilities grows. This population is currently growing by 1.5 million a year. To meet the projected demand for facility care, it is estimated that forty institutions must be built each month for the next eleven years. In addition, people must be prepared to provide the needed care. Home care supplied by paid health care providers ranges from $45 to $60 per visit.

It is estimated that 1 million families each year enter poverty because of the cost of long-term care. Medicare does cover some skilled care by a nurse or home health aide to eligible beneficiaries on a part-time basis. It is not enough to meet the need, however. It is estimated that 3.2 million elderly people need home nursing or other care to remain in their homes, table 7-4. Only three-fifths are receiving the help they need. Of that number, almost 2 million seem to be receiving help from relatives, friends, and paid visiting health care providers. And 1.1 million people need help in carrying out the activities of daily living. There is little doubt that long-term care and ways to provide it are major social issues.

Role of the Health Care Provider

Members of the health care staff have a rare opportunity and responsibility to help the elderly find and accept community programs. This is true whether the person in need is a patient or someone living in the same apartment or neigh-

PERCENT HAVING DIFFICULTY AND RECEIVING
HELP WITH SELECTED ACTIVITIES, BY AGE: 1984

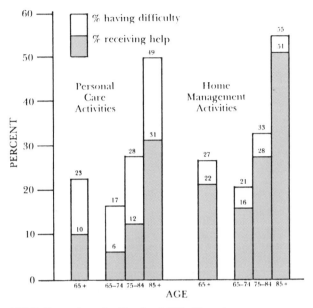

NOTE: Data refer to health-related difficulties only.
Based on data from U.S. Department of Health and Human Services

Table 7-4

borhood. To be able to help an older person with services they desperately need, you must first accept the older person with dignity and respect. If you are knowledgeable about available programs, you will be able to provide correct information. In addition, every cost containment measure you use as you carry out your duties will help to maintain the current levels of financial support.

Summary

- The financial status of the majority of elderly people has improved greatly over the last few years. However, there are still millions who live in poverty and do not enjoy financial security.
- Single women and minorities are the most vulnerable.
- Three factors determine the financial security of the elderly: retirement income, health care costs, and the cost of long-term care.
- The great majority of elderly people receive financial help through Social Security, civil service, and other public retirement plans, and through wages earned.
- Private-sector retirement programs, personal savings and investments, and financial help from relatives are also sources of income for this group.
- The Catastrophic Care Act of 1988 was a major move to help protect the elderly against the costs of catastrophic illness. But it failed to address the problem of long-term care and subsequently was abandoned.
- Efforts to control the federal budget deficit mean that Social Security benefits may not continue to grow as rapidly. Reduced deficits could lead to lowered interest rates. This could reduce a major source of income for the elderly.

Review Outline

I. Behavioral Objectives

II. Vocabulary

III. Interpretation of Statistical Data
    A. Importance
    B. Limitations

IV. Financial Status of Americans

V. Sources of Equity and Support

    A.   Home ownership
    B.   Individual savings
    C.   Employment
    D.   Pension plans
        1.   Private industrial
        2.   Governmental
    E.   Gifts from family members
    F.   Noncash benefits
        1.   Food stamps
        2.   Health care
           a. Medicare
           b. Medicaid
           c. Fraternal organizations

VI. Sources of Increased Costs

    A.   Health maintenance
    B.   Assistance with activities of daily living

Review

I. Vocabulary

Write the meaning of each of the following.

    1. D.R.G. _____
    2. C.O.L.A. _____
    3. S.S.I. _____
    4. I.R.A. _____
    5. Keogh plan _____

II. Short Answers

    1.   What precipitates the financial difficulties of old age for most people?
    2.   What is the major drawback to living on a fixed income?
    3.   What is the major asset of most older people?
    4.   On what is most of the income of elderly people spent?
    5.   What is the federally sponsored health insurance program for the aged?
    6.   Who finances the first part of the Medicare program?
    7.   Who finances the second part of Medicare?
    8.   What is the companion program to Medicare?
    9.   What has been the effect of D.R.G. on length of time spent in the hospital?
  10.   List four major public retirement plans.
  11.   Briefly describe the 1987 provisions of the appropriation legislation for the Older Americans Act.
  12.   What health care area was not covered for the elderly in the 1988 Catastrophic Health Care Bill and why was the act rescinded?

III. Clinical Situations

1. A neighbor who is blind and eligible for minimal Social Security benefits asks you if you know of any other program that could help. What do you say?
2. You are planning for your own financial future and reviewing ways to be financially secure after retirement. What are they?

Unit 8
Occupational Opportunities

Objectives

After studying this unit, you should be able to:

- Describe the characteristics of the older work force.
- Describe the psychological adjustments that follow retirement.
- Describe factors that contribute to retirement.
- List important sources of job placement for older workers.
- Describe possible opportunities for part-time employment after retirement.

Vocabulary

Learn the meaning and spelling of the following words or phrases.

A.A.R.P.	Operation R.E.A.S.O.N.
A.D.E.A.	retirement
ageism	R.S.V.P.
B.L.S.	S.C.O.R.E.
E.R.I.P.s	S.C.S.E.P.
Gray Panthers	V.I.S.T.A.
N.R.T.A.	

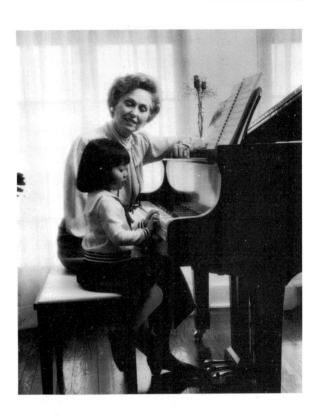

In the American culture, work is equated with personal value, both as an individual and as a contributing member of society. Working people reaching the age of fifty-five and beyond are faced with one of life's major decisions. The decision is when and how to retire from the paid work force.

Three major factors affect the exit of older workers from the paid labor pool. They are public policies regarding retirement, the person's physical ability to perform work-related activities, and the personal desires of the individual to either continue working or to engage in leisure activities.

Retirement Policies

The trend in recent years has been toward retiring at earlier and earlier ages. This trend has existed since the end of World War II.

Retirement programs in recent years have become increasingly liberal, allowing full benefits at earlier ages. Seventy-nine percent of the pension plans surveyed by the Bureau of Labor Statistics (*B.L.S.*) in 1983 had no minimum retirement age. Or they provided full benefits at age sixty-two or earlier. These facts were true of only 55 percent of the pension plans in 1974. In 1988, 37 percent of plans allowed for full-benefit retirement as early as age fifty-five, usually with thirty years of service.

Improvements in retirement income sources such as Social Security pensions and personal wealth contributed to early retirement ages. Early retirement (a term often used to describe retirement that occurs before the age of sixty-five) has become the norm. In fact, almost four of every five workers who obtained their initial awards for Social Security benefits in 1986 were between the ages of sixty-two and sixty-four. The vast majority were age sixty-two (Social Security Administration, 1987). Similarly, B.L.S. data show that, by age sixty-two, almost half of all men are completely out of the labor force (they are neither working nor looking for work). By age sixty-four, the B.L.S. definition applies to three-fifths of all men.

The average age of retirement for a male worker in 1989 was sixty-two years. The retirement age for women is complicated by a number of factors. Their choice of retirement age is closely related to the work history and pension resources of their mates. Many women who are at retirement age now had little work experience to allow them to build up pension benefits. Women who are divorced or never married need to depend upon their own resources. They tend to retire at ages comparable to their male counterparts.

Economic pressures, such as the two recessions in the early 1980s and foreign competition in the past decade, have prompted employers to seek ways to become more competitive and cost effective. One factor that has influenced employment and retirement patterns is automation, which has decreased the need for as many human workers. Another factor is the restructuring of companies, which results in the elimination of workers by layoffs or terminations. As part of this effort, some companies have instituted early retirement incentive plans *(E.R.I.P.s)* as a way to reduce costs and avoid laying off more workers.

The incentive programs reduce the number of forced layoffs, encourage early retirement, and reduce costs. This is achieved by replacing older, more highly paid workers with younger and lower paid, less experienced people. The national welfare is also influenced, as are changes in the work force and retirement planning. After decades of encouraging older workers to leave the work force early to make room for younger people, the trend is changing. Experts in industry and the government are anticipating a decline in the ratio of workers to retirees as the baby-boom generation reaches retirement age. They are beginning to institute measures to encourage the older worker to remain in the work force longer.

Moreover, in some areas people are beginning to look at the older worker as a national resource. They are being viewed as people, skilled and experienced, who can help fill the unfilled need for workers in the coming years.

Public policy is directed in part by laws. Two laws that have an impact on the retirement plans of older workers are the amendments to the Social Security Act (1983) and amendments to the Age Discrimination in Employment Act (A.D.E.A.) (1967). These amendments were approved in 1986.

The Social Security amendments raised the age of eligibility from sixty-five to sixty-seven for full-benefit retirement among persons born in 1960. The amendments to the Age Discrimination in Employment Act practically eliminated a mandatory retirement for most occupations.

Through these actions, the government seeks to encourage retirement at a later age. Government also wants to make it legally possible for all older workers to remain employed as long as they possess the physical ability and desire to do so.

As you can see, the private sector and government may be acting in opposition.

Physical Limitations to Work

Health is another factor in the participation of older persons in the labor force. A recent survey regarding ability to perform work-related activities found that the greatest problems existed when the work required stooping, crouching or kneeling, lifting, walking one-quarter of a mile, or climbing stairs.

Until the age of sixty-two, most men physically able to work do so. However, fewer than 80 percent to 90 percent of women age sixty and older are in the work force. The lower rate for women reflects not only age and physical ability, but also the large differences in work-life patterns of successive generations of women. It is only in the last two decades that socioeconomic changes have seen a rapid movement into the labor force of women of childbearing age. The women who are in their twenties, thirties, and forties today will approach retirement age with their own Social Security, investment, and pension plans. Because of a current greater emphasis on physical health, they should approach retirement age in better physical condition.

A similar survey found 58% of people ages 55-74 who had worked some time since their forty-fifth birthday had no difficulty in carrying out activities related to employment.

Many of the people who retired for other reasons could have remained in the work force. About two-thirds of those interviewed who had retired for other than health reasons indicated that they could work at a job or business if such an opportunity were available. But only 12 percent indicated a desire to do so. Among those who had retired for health reasons, only 28 percent said that they could work if a job were available. Of those people, only 10 percent really wanted to do so. Therefore, the majority of those who were retired for reasons other than health were not physically impaired. They could work, but few had a desire to do so. The majority who retired because of health said they could not work. It would appear that health, although a significant factor for some, is not the major reason that the older worker has elected to retire at an earlier age.

Personal Preferences

With current life expectancies, an individual may have between twelve and fifteen years of active living and as many as ten years of inactivity after retirement. Meaningful employment is essential to maintaining both emotional and physical health. Enforced idleness quickly produces loss of self-esteem and status. For most people, the years after retirement must be lived on a reduced, fixed income. Those who have derived fewer benefits from their work may still elect to retire early. This is especially true when low-paid work from which they gained little personal identity or pleasure is replaced by higher paying Social Security. It has been found that it does not take large amounts of pension income to induce workers to retire.

To many, the work ethic requires work for pay. This is then equated with personal value and worth. For most people, their work is an extension of themselves. Therefore, it is easy to understand how loss of regular employment can greatly reduce their view of themselves and the place they occupy in society. This is particularly true when an individual has enjoyed work, has been paid well for it, and has derived other satisfactions from it. Perhaps this is why more professional and white-collar workers exercise the option of deferring retirement beyond age sixty-five when there is a choice. For this second group of retirees, paid employment must be replaced by meaningful leisure occupations.

Conflicting social and economic policies make the future for retirement and employment unpredictable. Labor-force growth is expected to increase at only half the rate during the 1986–2000 period as it did in the previous fourteen years. More and more employers may follow the lead of those who have already developed programs designed to provide attractive, often innovative, work options for retirement-age workers.

In addition, with each successive generation of older workers, fewer will have worked in physically demanding jobs. More of them will have the educational background, particularly a college education, that will allow them more flexibility in the job market. Such profiles generally are associated with relatively high work participation rates and late retirement.

The Older Labor Force

In recent years, there has been a dramatic decline in labor-force participation by older workers. In 1985, 2.7 percent of men and 2.3 percent of women over age sixty-five were in the labor force. This represents fewer than 0.3 million of the postretirement-age workers still in the labor market. An estimated 32.3 million (84 percent) have worked some time since the age of forty-five. Almost all men and about three-quarters of the women have worked at some time.

Women leave the labor force primarily to rear children and to care for ailing family members. Some return for satisfactions, but many return for economic gain. They may also return to the work force because of widowhood, separation, divorce, or a husband's low earnings, disability, or unemployment.

In 1970, 6.1 percent of all women in their late thirties to forties who were out of the labor force the previous month reentered the following month. By 1987, this had risen to 10.4 percent. The same trend was seen among women in their forties and fifties, with a slight decline for those over age sixty.

Unless the trend toward early retirement changes, less and less time will be spent working and more and more time will be spent in retirement. A man born in 1988 can expect to live over seventy years, thirty-eight of which he could spend in the work force and fourteen or more in retirement.

For women, the picture is somewhat different. In 1983, 48.5 million women were in the work force. This represented a 52.9 percent participation rate. It reflected a slight increase over the 52.6 percent registered just a year before. There is a continuing trend toward more women entering the work force and remaining in it longer. Middle-aged women (from forty-five to fifty-four) have increased their participation from 38 percent in 1950 to the present high of over 62 percent. Once women reach sixty-five, there is a dramatic decline in the number of female workers, from a high of 11 percent in the 1960s to about 7 percent today. Participation rates for women between fifty-five and sixty-four have changed little over the last twenty years.

The changing economic climate and other social issues, such as a desire for greater income and the dramatically increasing divorce rate, have promoted a greater desire among women in their fifties and even sixties to seek employment. They bring with them little experience and limited skills. In the future, more of these women are likely to want to remain in the work force.

Sex and race are important determinants of occupations among the elderly who are employed. A study of the distribution of workers also reflects the move toward a more service-oriented society. A study by the National Council on Aging found that 63 percent of elderly workers were in clerical, sales, service, or professional jobs. At present, three-fifths of elderly white females are in white-collar occupations. About two-thirds of black females are in the service area, figure 8-1. About one-half of elderly white male workers are in white-collar occupations and one-quarter in blue-collar work. Over one-third of elderly black males are blue-collar workers. Nearly one-fourth are in white-collar occupations and one-fourth in service jobs.

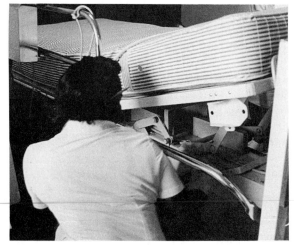

Figure 8-1   About two-thirds of black female workers are in the service area.

Farm occupations are more common among the oldest men. Nearly one-fifth of black and one-sixth of white working males age seventy and over are farm workers. This picture will probably change in the coming decades as more younger workers move off the farms and seek employment in urban areas.

Unemployment

In 1985, 13.2 percent of those age sixty-five and older participated in the labor force. That percentage is projected to continue to decrease, table 8-1. There is a slightly higher level of minorities employed after age sixty-five. This fact probably reflects their lower lifetime earnings and less financial security during retirement years.

Labor issues of unemployment, job displacement, and discouragement affect all workers or those seeking work. The older worker must also deal with age discrimination and forced retirement. Older workers, once unemployed, tend to stay unemployed longer, take lower paying jobs when they find work, and become discouraged and give up looking sooner. Over 300,000 older workers are no longer counted as unemployed because they have stopped looking for work.

High unemployment rates are generally related to education level. Those with the least education have the most difficulty finding new jobs. The jobs they do find are usually lower paying. One of the most common reasons given by older persons for not working is poor health. In many instances, they say they feel "too old" or are made to feel "too old." Job discrimination against the aged is a reality that cannot be denied. It is certainly a factor in the difficulty of finding suitable employment.

Many older workers who want to re-enter the work force are unable to do so after being laid off or forced to retire. Many workers, discouraged by an unsuccessful job search, simply end the search by permanently retiring.

The prevalence of age discrimination is difficult to understand in view of survey findings.

These findings indicate that older workers have much to offer society. They are viewed by themselves and employers as being mature, stable, reliable, responsible, and loyal. They need less supervision, are less distracted by personal concerns, and experience less absenteeism than younger workers.

Some of the myths that persist about older workers are that they are slow, frail, unadaptable, and often absent from work. Nothing could be further from the truth. Studies show there is no significant loss in productivity or performance and that older workers often exceed the output of younger workers. Labor-saving machines enable older workers to handle most jobs without difficulty. In fact, fewer than 14 percent of all jobs today require great physical strength and heavy lifting. Employer surveys prove that the attendance record of older workers is favorable when compared to younger workers. And young workers demonstrate as much resistance to change and inflexibility as older workers do. Despite government efforts and the regulations of the Age Discrimination in Employment Act, ageism persists as a subtle, if not overt, factor in job loss or failure to find employment.

In 1987, three-fourths of the unemployed men between fifty-five and fifty-nine were job losers. The probability of finding a new job tends to be lowest for the older worker. In a recent study, 43 percent of both unemployed men and women over age sixty-five had not reentered the labor force after being unemployed the previous month.

The older the individual gets, the poorer the prospects for reemployment after the job loss. After sixty-two, pensions and Social Security and/or savings help to cushion the financial need. About one-half of those unemployed who are fifty-five or older receive pension or Social Security benefits. Social Security payments also limit the amount of earnable income.

Currently, Social Security recipients younger than age sixty-five can earn as much as $6,120. After that, their benefit amount is re-

CIVILIAN LABOR FORCE AND PARTICIPATION RATES, BY RACE, SEX, AND AGE, 1970 TO 1985,
AND PROJECTIONS, 1990 AND 1995

[**For civilian noninstitutional population 16 years old and over.** Annual averages of monthly figures. Rates are based on annual average civilian noninstitutional population of each specified group and represent proportion of each specified group in the civilian labor force. Based on Current Population Survey; see text, section 1 and Appendix III. See also *Historical Statistics, Colonial Times to 1970,* series D 42–48]

RACE, SEX, AND AGE	CIVILIAN LABOR FORCE (millions)							PARTICIPATION RATE (percent)						
	1970	1975	1980	1984	1985	1990	1995	1970	1975	1980	1984	1985	1990	1995
Total[1]	82.8	93.8	106.9	113.5	115.5	122.7	129.2	60.4	61.2	63.8	64.4	64.8	65.7	66.6
White	73.6	82.8	93.6	98.5	99.9	105.5	110.1	60.2	61.5	64.1	64.6	65.0	65.9	66.8
Male	46.0	50.3	54.5	56.1	56.5	58.5	59.9	80.0	78.7	78.2	77.1	77.0	76.5	75.8
Female	27.5	32.5	39.1	42.4	43.5	46.9	50.2	42.6	45.9	51.2	53.3	54.1	56.2	58.4
Black[2]	9.2	9.3	10.9	12.0	12.4	13.6	14.8	61.8	58.8	61.0	62.2	62.9	64.1	65.3
Male	5.2	5.0	5.6	6.1	6.2	6.7	7.2	76.5	71.0	70.6	70.8	70.8	71.0	70.8
Female	4.0	4.2	5.3	5.9	6.1	6.9	7.6	49.5	48.9	53.2	55.2	56.5	58.6	60.8
Male	51.2	56.3	61.5	63.8	64.4	67.1	69.3	79.7	77.9	77.4	76.4	76.3	75.8	75.3
16–19 years	4.0	4.8	5.0	4.1	4.1	3.8	3.7	56.1	59.1	60.5	56.0	56.8	57.6	57.9
16 and 17 years	1.8	2.1	2.1	1.6	1.7	1.5	1.5	47.0	48.6	50.1	43.5	45.1	44.4	45.4
18 and 19 years	2.2	2.7	2.9	2.5	2.5	2.4	2.2	66.7	70.6	71.3	68.1	68.9	70.2	71.8
20–24 years	5.7	7.6	8.6	8.6	8.3	7.3	6.8	83.3	84.5	85.9	85.0	85.0	86.3	87.3
25–34 years	11.3	14.2	17.0	18.5	18.8	19.7	18.2	96.4	95.2	95.2	94.4	94.7	94.1	93.7
35–44 years	10.5	10.4	11.8	14.0	14.5	17.3	19.2	96.9	95.6	95.5	95.4	95.0	94.7	94.3
45–54 years	10.4	10.4	9.9	9.8	9.9	11.1	13.7	94.3	92.1	91.2	91.2	91.0	90.8	90.4
55–64 years	7.1	7.0	7.2	7.1	7.1	6.3	6.1	83.0	75.6	72.1	68.5	67.9	64.4	62.6
65 years and over	2.2	1.9	1.9	1.8	1.8	1.6	1.4	26.8	21.6	19.0	16.3	15.8	13.2	11.0
Female	31.5	37.5	45.5	49.7	51.1	55.5	59.9	43.3	46.3	51.5	53.6	54.5	56.6	58.9
16–19 years	3.2	4.1	4.4	3.8	3.8	3.4	3.3	44.0	49.1	52.9	51.8	52.1	51.8	51.2
16 and 17 years	1.3	1.7	1.8	1.5	1.5	1.3	1.4	34.9	40.2	43.6	41.2	42.1	41.4	41.5
18 and 19 years	1.9	2.4	2.6	2.4	2.3	2.1	1.9	53.5	58.1	61.9	61.8	61.7	61.3	61.2
20–24 years	4.9	6.2	7.3	7.5	7.4	6.6	6.3	57.7	64.1	68.9	70.4	71.8	73.8	76.3
25–34 years	5.7	8.7	12.3	14.2	14.7	16.4	16.2	45.0	54.9	65.5	69.8	70.9	76.2	81.1
35–44 years	6.0	6.5	8.6	10.9	11.6	14.5	16.9	51.1	55.8	65.5	70.1	71.8	75.9	80.5
45–54 years	6.5	6.7	7.0	7.2	7.5	8.8	11.4	54.4	54.6	59.9	62.9	64.4	67.8	71.3
55–64 years	4.2	4.3	4.7	4.9	4.9	4.6	4.7	43.0	40.9	41.3	41.7	42.0	41.9	42.7
65 years and over	1.1	1.0	1.2	1.2	1.2	1.1	1.0	9.7	8.2	8.1	7.5	7.3	6.4	5.5

[1]Beginning 1975, includes other races not shown separately.
[2]For 1970, Black and other.

Source: U.S. Bureau of Labor Statistics, *Employment and Earnings,* monthly; *Monthly Labor Review,* November 1985; and unpublished data.

Table 8-1   Participation in the labor force by those over age sixty-five is expected to decrease due to a variety of factors.

duced by $1 for every $2 earned. Workers between ages sixty-five and seventy can earn $8,400 before being subject to benefit reductions. After age seventy, the earnings test no longer applies.

Part-time Employment

The major reasons that persons over age sixty-five look for work are a need for greater financial security or a need for social and psychological interaction, or both. Part-time employment meets both needs. Over the last ten years, elderly men have made up 5 to 6 percent of all persons on voluntary part-time work schedules. Elderly women make up about 4 percent of the part-time work force. Although these are small percentages of the entire work force of all ages, they represent about one-half of those sixty-five and over. Part-time work for both men and women is becoming an increasingly important

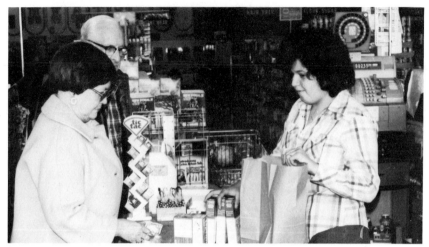

Figure 8-2   Money for food and necessities is the major reason those over sixty-five look for work.

means of supplementing income as fixed incomes fail to keep up with rising costs, figure 8-2.

Close to 50 percent of elderly men and 60 percent of elderly women are part-time employees. The older people get, the more they are apt to seek part-time rather than full-time employment.

Less is known about minority groups. Data specifically related to them is not available. In general, they are far more likely to experience labor market problems. They have higher rates of unemployment, experience greater levels of discouragement, have fewer financial resources, and ultimately reenter the work force at lower levels of pay. A report of the National Commission for Employment Policy (1985) found that labor market problems were four times higher for older blacks and three times higher for older Hispanics than they were among their white counterparts. The factor that will most strongly affect the job potential for all older workers is the overall pace of economic expansion.

Opportunities for part-time employment are greatest in the service sector. The service industries are less likely to have mandatory retirement ages. Pension coverage is also usually less than it is in other industries.

It is also possible to turn hobby skills acquired during the work years into part-time employment or self-employment, figure 8-3. Small appliance repair and teaching a craft such as knitting are two possibilities. There are many books at the library that suggest ways to turn avocational into vocational skills.

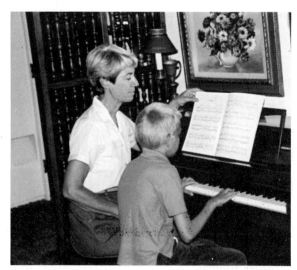

Figure 8-3   Older persons can often find part-time employment teaching their skills to others.

In one survey, more than one-third of older people in the preretirement years (fifty-five to sixty-four) indicated a willingness to undergo job training to acquire new skills. In addition, 17 percent of the men and 15 percent of the women over sixty-five indicated the same interest. New skills can be acquired free or inexpensively with a short-term investment. Most community colleges and state universities have adult education courses that are essentially free or require minimal registration fees. Learning ability doesn't diminish with age. In fact, intellectual functioning seems to be at its height between the ages of forty-five and eighty. Educational counseling at the school can often help people make the most appropriate plans for retraining. Job referrals and market analysis of job opportunities, available through the schools, help the older person make prudent, timesaving choices. Because high-technology jobs are not necessarily physically strenuous, many older people, after technical retraining, can qualify.

Older persons should be encouraged to review and list their current skills to see which can be adapted to current market needs. They should also be made aware of and put in contact with organizations that can assist them in their job search. One source of possible job ideas is the *Dictionary of Occupational Titles*. This directory lists occupations and occupational traits that can be transferred from one job to another.

Desire for paid employment, even on a part-time basis, is lower when workers have a higher level of education and a more secure financial status. It would seem that, surveys to the contrary, a desire for part-time work is based on a need for supplemental income.

Preparation for Retirement

Preparation for *retirement* (stopping regular work) should begin early (about ten years prior to expected retirement). This is especially true in terms of financial planning. During this early phase, the financial, physical, and social possibilities of the retirement period can be explored.

More and more progressive companies and unions recognize the psychological impact of retirement. They have programs to help employees prepare for it. Seminars, lectures, and group discussions focus on company and union pension plans, Social Security benefits, insurance, financial planning, and creative use of leisure time. Information is presented about community programs of special interest. These types of programs stimulate employees to do some long-range planning of their own, which helps employees adjust to retirement.

A sizable share of workers below retirement age indicate that they would prefer a phased retirement. They would like to work in their same line of work for the same employer. Unfortunately, many of those who would prefer to have a phased retirement do not have that opportunity. Unanticipated events, such as a disability or illness or a change in family responsibilities, or employers' preferences and pension rules that make such hour reductions impractical, eliminate this possibility.

Some companies are experimenting with shorter working hours for their older employees as a prelude to actual retirement. This trial retirement offers an opportunity to test retirement options for suitability. Unfortunately, such long-term planning is still the exception rather than the rule. For many, retirement is something that will happen some day, not something to think about today, no matter how close that day looms on the horizon.

Retirement

People are moved out of the labor force today in a variety of ways. Some firms adhere to regular retirement rules, especially in the upper echelons of management. Even in these instances, people may make the transition to retirement by retaining a consultant role. Other companies ease the transition by gradually extending the shorter work hours of the preretirement period. For example, older teachers are often permitted to teach fewer classes per semester.

Flexible work hours allow the spacing of activities for maximum benefits of energy expenditure. Jobs may also be redesigned to provide for more sitting or more daylight hours.

The retired person works less than full-time or year-round and receives a retirement pension. Before age sixty-two, retirement is due mainly to prolonged unemployment or disability. About 10 percent of the labor force leaves in their fifties. But at age sixty-five, there is a sharp drop in male employment. Women tend to withdraw from paid employment more gradually and earlier.

Loss of money and social contacts are cited as the major problems of retirement. Pensions are more generous in those medium- and large-size industries where unions have been long-term activists for their members. Smaller firms and service industries have lower pay and fewer pension benefits. Those with lower retirement benefits tend to remain in the work force longer. Therefore, they maintain income and social contacts in this way. Some firms maintain social contacts through newsletters and retiree get-togethers, figure 8-4.

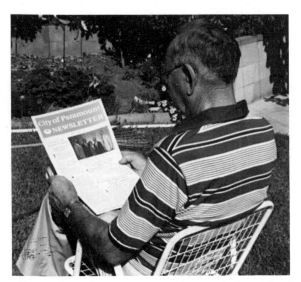

Figure 8-4 Company newsletters help retired workers keep in touch with former co-workers.

Age sixty-five has been the compulsory retirement age in many retirement programs since the late 1800s. In the 1960s, because of lengthening life spans, unions and companies began to take a more flexible approach toward retirement. Although no longer mandatory, age sixty-five is still the most common age of retirement if health is good.

Retirement still comes to many people when they are at the peak of their productivity. The average retirement age for men is now sixty-three. The occupations that seem most likely to retain older people are the professions, clerical work, farming, crafts, maintenance, housekeeping, and babysitting. Reactions to fixed retirement policies vary. They depend largely upon how effectively other company policies have paved the way and helped prepare the worker for the adjustments that must be made.

The majority of those over sixty-five give health as their main reason for withdrawing from the labor force. Sometimes specific health problems force early retirement. Many times, however, the older person just lacks energy to keep up the pace. Another factor that affects the timing of retirement is potential level of income. More and more people are taking advantage of early retirement prerogatives, even though they must accept a decrease in Social Security or company retirement benefits.

Companies use various incentives to ease older workers into retirement. In medium- and large-size firms, 90 percent of white-collar workers can retire by age fifty-five if they have worked the required number of years (usually about twenty). Some companies even supplement retirees' income until they become eligible for Social Security. Only 3 percent of private retirement plans have cost-of-living adjustments, however.

Early retirement is encouraged by those who feel that younger people should be given their place in the work force. Although it is true that technological change and automation are eliminating some jobs, other jobs are being created. The number of opportunities is increasing, not decreasing. To believe that the old must be sacrificed to the young is a grave mistake, both socially and economically.

Psychological Response to Retirement

Reactions to retirement differ. Initially, most feel a sense of relief. No longer must they be up at a certain hour, confined to a specific activity. Some feel the euphoria of vacation. This is sometimes called the honeymoon period. Previous fantasies about retirement are now measured against the reality. The thought, "Now I can do all those things I haven't had time for," prevails, figure 8-5. Others feel an immediate letdown and a sense of loss. These retirees face long, empty hours with no thought of how to fill them. The latter extreme is more often experienced when health and finance severely limit possibilities. Many women escape these extremes because, even when they are employed outside the home, they are more apt than men to have housekeeping activities to fill their time.

Following one of the two initial reactions, the retiree reaches a period of stability, which is either positively or negatively focused. Adjustment to retirement is one of the developmental tasks of aging. There is a definable retirement role based on social, physical, and financial independence. The retired person is aware of the expectations and begins to settle in. Negative self-images that are sometimes developed by retirees are more apt to result from poverty than from the vagueness of their new life-style. A gradual postretirement routine of activities is eventually developed, and the retiree completes a successful transition into this phase of life.

Retirement has been found to have few long-term effects on morale, life satisfaction, depression, or level of self-esteem. It might be concluded that most adults complete this developmental task with a minimum of upheaval. The key factors seem to be health, money, and a willingness to give up work routines.

Domestic problems sometimes arise for the couple when the husband retires. Quite frequently, the husband assumes a greater share of the household tasks than he did previously, with a subsequent loss of self-esteem, figure 8-6. In

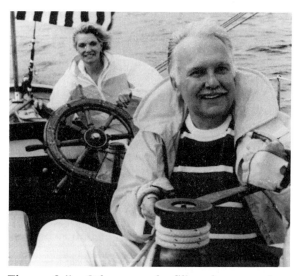

Figure 8-5 Other people fill retirement time with leisure activities. (Courtesy Marion Laboratories, Inc.)

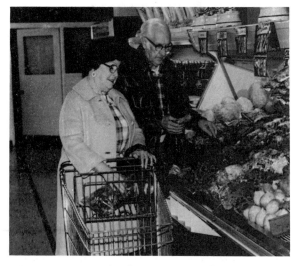

Figure 8-6 Retired men may take on a great share of household tasks.

future years, if the roles of men and women as provider and homemaker continue to merge, this transition may be easier. Stress can be eased if one or both members of the couple can get out of the house for part of the day. Even a brief separation can increase harmony in the home. Good sexual relationships can offer supportive warmth and enhance communications, helping to ease the adjustment.

Gradually a different reaction begins to take hold. As the days pass and the problems and potential of retirement come into closer focus, a more realistic appraisal may make anxieties and fears about the future press inward. Adjusting to a fixed income is not easy, especially in times of inflation and high prices. And with the loss of a job, there is a definite loss of social contact and routine. Unless new, socially satisfying avenues are pursued, the individual experiences a feeling of drifting with no purpose. Although health and finances determine adjustment to some degree, it may depend even more on the individual's personal philosophy and previous adjustment to life in general. If, over the years, the person has developed some skill in adjusting to change and overcoming hardships and retains a degree of optimism and flexibility, adjustment to retirement will be much easier.

Older people as a group find adjustments difficult. In some cases, they find it impossible to adjust. Retirees need help in seeing themselves in terms of the multiple skills they have acquired during their lives and not in terms of work classifications alone. They need to recognize that their skills have value that is not lost when their job title disappears. The vast majority of people retire and adjust rather quickly to their new life circumstances.

Occupational Opportunities

In general, older workers experience longer layoffs and have more difficulty than younger workers in finding new employment. Some steps have been taken to offer help.

Government Programs

One step has been to make arbitrary age discrimination in employment against the law. Another step has been to design programs of assistance. For those over seventy, job information centers have been established in many cities. The United States Department of Labor has developed guidelines to redesign jobs for older workers in an attempt to stimulate employment opportunities. Another program is the Senior Community Service Employment Program *(S.C.S.E.P.).* The U.S. Department of Labor also operates this program. It strives to find minimum-wage employment within the community for willing workers over fifty-five who are economically disadvantaged.

One of the most important sources of job placement for older workers is the state employment service, sponsored by the Bureau of Employment Security. There are more than 2,000 employment offices nationally, located in all the major cities. Some offer special counseling for older employees. Other services offered to the older worker by some of these units are group guidance, job-finding techniques, job placement, and referral to training.

In the 1960s, the Office of Economic Opportunity developed some programs for the elderly. These were limited projects or studies. Some have been taken over by community action groups.

One of these projects, the Foster Grandparent program, is jointly operated with the Administration on Aging. This program recruits, trains, and employs men and women over sixty to work with neglected, deprived, and mentally retarded children. Through the program, jobs are created for older people and a community need is met. The Foster Grandparents project has proven so successful that it has become an integral part of many community action programs over the last twenty years.

Another project that has been taken over by communities is *Operation R.E.A.S.O.N.* (Responding to Elderly's Abilities and Sickness Otherwise Neglected). This project was designed to help people over sixty find work if they were physically able to do so. It also helps elderly people meet their health needs through a referral service, figure 8-7.

The home health aide program was developed through cooperation by the Public Health Service, the Administration on Aging, and the Office of Economic Opportunity. It is another program designed to serve two purposes. The concept of home health aides recruited from older groups has spread nationally, and many older people are now finding employment. Many indigent, elderly, or handicapped people are able to remain in their own homes and avoid institutionalization.

Older people have been given employment as aides in other programs designed to reach and benefit the older population. For example, the Department of Health and Human Services has sponsored programs of social and rehabilitation service that are directed by state and local welfare agencies. However, they receive financial support from the federal government.

Although programs to provide training for employment are not designed solely for the benefit of the elderly, many healthy older people have benefited from them. Private organizations such as the Goodwill Industries offer rehabilitative vocational training to the disabled and elderly. Multipurpose geriatric centers and day centers sometimes offer counseling for employment. In some centers, an occupational therapist is available and provides interest-motivated therapy. The manual and creative skills taught can sometimes be turned to profit.

Some of the ambitious programs started in the mid-sixties to help the elderly find and keep gainful employment were cut back in the late sixties when the national economy slackened. The 1970s found readjustments in the programs. Changes in mandatory retirement age were a boon to many federal and state agencies, which opened offices to help older people find work. Once more, in the mid-eighties, there were cutbacks in both programs and services to the elderly as attention was directed toward controlling the federal deficit.

Private Opportunities

The private business sector in each community is a source of work opportunities for the older and retired worker. Individual businesses can sometimes be established through small business loans. For an enterprising older person, self-employment may be an intriguing challenge.

Older people should be encouraged to investigate job possibilities that they might not consider because of their sex. Men doing household or companion chores and women entering the more traditional male roles of salesmanship and management may be just the career changes that could bring the most money and satisfaction.

Other sources of employment referrals include professional trade associations, labor union employment services, and employment services for retired military officers. The National Retired Teachers Association (*N.R.T.A.*) and the American Association of Retired Persons (*A.A.R.P.*) sponsor Mature Tempo Inc. This is a temporary job placement service for retirees. Clubs and associations such as the Masons and Kiwanis are also good sources of job information. Most good jobs are filled through the recommendations of social or business contacts.

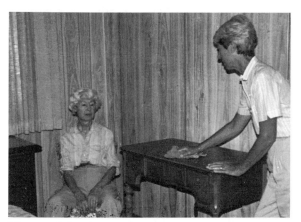

Figure 8-7 Operation R.E.A.S.O.N. matches the health needs of one person with the work needs of another.

Volunteer Work

The trend today is to become involved in some kind of meaningful work after retirement. Work need not be lucrative to be meaningful. Supplemental income is certainly welcome and often needed, however. When money is not a prime concern, many older people choose volunteer service as a way to remain active and useful.

Through volunteer work, many elderly people perform a valuable service for the community and reaffirm their own sense of importance, figure 8-8. Clerical skills are always in demand, such as folding circulars, addressing envelopes, and making telephone calls. None of these is a strenuous activity, figure 8-9, but all are vital to the operation of many civic and charitable organizations.

Retired executives can volunteer their services as consultants to young, struggling businesses. Organizations such as *S.C.O.R.E.* (Service Corps of Retired Executives), which was initiated by the Small Business Administration, channel these advisory services. The retired executive receives no compensation except reimbursement for out-of-pocket expenses. Both the small businesses and the executives seem to have

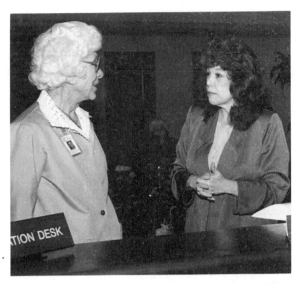

Figure 8-9   Older volunteers can perform much volunteer service if it is not too physically tiring.

derived great benefit and satisfaction from this arrangement.

Both the Peace Corps and *V.I.S.T.A.* (Volunteers in Service to America), the domestic counterpart of the Peace Corps, have welcomed the services of older people. Some retirees have been able to share their skills with people of many ages. Others have given service specially geared to other elderly people. Organizations such as the Scouts and the Y.M.C.A./Y.W.C.A. are always looking for people with time and talents that they are willing to share with young people. The problem is bringing the elderly and community opportunities together.

Three other volunteer programs provide opportunities for elder's service. The Retired Senior Volunteer Program *(R.S.V.P.)* serves in volunteer situations such as courts, libraries, nursing homes, Boy and Girl Scout offices, hospitals, and economic development agencies. The Senior Companion Program serves adults with special needs. The Action Cooperative Volunteers is a program in which older people volunteer one year of service to complete a community project.

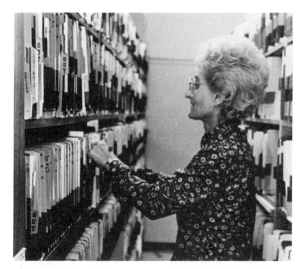

Figure 8-8   Volunteer work keeps this senior an active, productive member of society.

Political Involvement

Political involvement is an important way that older people can influence legislation that, in turn, directly affects them. Involvement can be local, regional, or national. By sheer numbers, a mobilized senior citizenry could bring about significant benefits. In the 1984 federal election, over thirty million voters were fifty-five or older. As a group, older people are more likely to vote than younger ones. The voice of the elderly is being heard more strongly. Ever-increasing numbers of older people, supported by other concerned citizens, strive to combat *ageism* (discrimination based on age) and improve life for the elderly.

The *Gray Panthers* is a movement begun in 1970 and still headed by its founder Maggie Kuhn, figure 8-10. It has become a means of national expression for the urgent reforms needed to protect the elderly. This loosely structured group of individuals is dedicated to working toward social justice and promoting involvement by all age groups in the social and political life of the nation. Areas of Gray Panthers' concern include increasing low- and middle-income housing and promoting in-home services and day centers as alternatives to institutionalization. Members of the group are committed to action rather than service. They are primarily supported by private donations. In 1973, the Retired Professional Action Group, supported by Ralph Nader's Public Citizen, Inc., joined the Gray Panthers to combined resources and talents. Today, the group is stronger than ever.

Role of the Geriatric Health Care Provider

At first glance, it may seem that retirement problems are primarily sociological and should be the concern of a social worker. But the health care provider often functions in a dual capacity as both nurse and social worker. Health care frequently brings health care providers into situations that expose retirement needs. For example, a public health nurse may be visiting other family members and meet the retired person. Home calls may be made on the retiree when either a temporary or chronic illness exists or when a retirement problem is recognized. Home health aides and geriatric-health care assistants often interact with family members, friends, and other health care providers. As a knowledgeable person, the health care provider can help the individual evaluate personal limitations, interests, and marketable skills. Referrals can be made to specific agencies operating in the community.

The Chamber of Commerce, libraries, and churches are good sources of information about local work programs for older people and areas where volunteer help would be welcome. Families may need help in assuming a supportive role for the postretirement employment of elderly

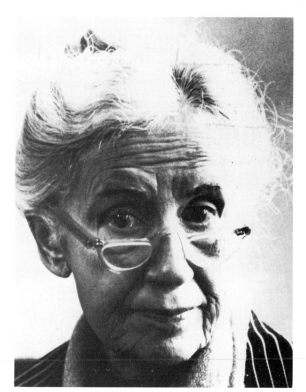

Figure 8-10 Maggie Kuhn, founder of the politically active Gray Panthers

members. Though the job the older person takes may not carry the same prestige as former employment, it is a worthy endeavor if it brings a measure of satisfaction to the individual. The health care provider who is familiar with local as well as national efforts to help retired people is a more valuable member of the nursing staff and the community.

Summary

• Retirement time is a period of major adjustment for the retiree and his or her family. The ease of adjustment depends in large measure on the reasons for retirement, the preparations made, the financial security, and the health of the retiree.

• Initial relief from the daily drudgery of a regular job may give way to feelings of anxiety, apathy, and withdrawal. A negative response is most common when ill health or inadequate personal finances make the future uncertain.

• Health care providers can do much to help retirees bring new meaning to their lives. They can direct retirees to sources for part-time employment or volunteer service.

• Developing trends have strong implications for the elderly. They include changes in the available labor force, early retirement, stress on federal expenditures for elderly needs, and movement to high-technology and service-oriented industries.

Review Outline

   I. Behavioral Objectives

  II. Vocabulary

 III. Retirement Policies

      A. Programs
      B. Age requirements
      C. Government policy versus private policy
      D. Age discrimination

 IV. Factors Influencing Retirement Decision

      A. Personal preference
      B. Physical limitations

  V. Characteristics of Older Labor Force

      A. Decline in numbers
      B. Increase in women
      C. Service oriented

 VI. Unemployment

      A. Trends
      B. Contributing factors

VII. Preparation for Retirement

      A. Personal planning
      B. Company programs

VIII.   Retirement

      A.   Definition
      B.   Associated problems
      C.   Psychological response

IX.   Occupational Opportunities

      A.   Government sponsored
      B.   Private (personal)
          1.   Self-employment
          2.   Volunteer work
          3.   Political involvement

X.   Role of the Health Care Provider

Review

I.   Vocabulary

In this unit, initials are used to designate a number of organizations, programs, or laws. Next to each set of initials, write the complete name.

    1.   A.A.R.P._____
    2.   A.D.E.A._____
    3.   N.R.T.A._____
    4.   R.S.V.P._____
    5.   V.I.S.T.A._____

II.   Short Answers

    1.   What two factors most affect the reaction to retirement?
    2.   What can companies do to help employees feel more secure about retirement?
    3.   When should retirement planning be started to be most effective?
    4.   What is the most common reason given for early retirement?
    5.   Give four examples of projects sponsored by the Office of Economic Opportunity to encourage employment for older people.
    6.   What are the aims of the Foster Grandparent programs?
    7.   What is the domestic counterpart of the Peace Corps?
    8.   Employment serves two primary functions. What are they?
    9.   What is the major reason for the trend toward more part-time work after retirement?
   10.   How can health care providers use an understanding of work opportunities in the retirement years?
   11.   Describe the goals of the Gray Panthers.

III.   Clinical Situations

    1.   A friend, age 55, asks if you think it is too early to plan for retirement. What is your response?
    2.   A friend who is retired wishes to supplement his income with part-time employment and asks you for suggestions. What is your response?

Unit 9
Recreational Opportunities

Objectives
After studying this unit, you should be able to:
- Name three factors influencing the choice of leisure time activities.
- List some activities that the elderly person can enjoy independently and that require little money.
- Describe types of recreational programs offered and types of recreational and care centers.

Vocabulary
Learn the meaning and spelling of the following words or phrases.

leisure
senior citizen center
social networks
volunteerism

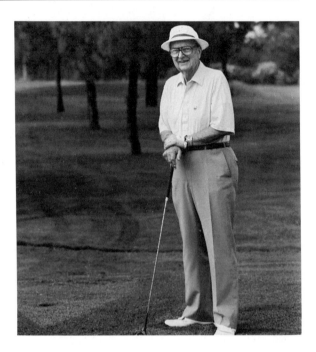

As the life span lengthens and people retire earlier, the postretirement years become longer—offering more time to be enjoyed or endured, figure 9-1. The value of these years depends on what activities are chosen to fill the hours. It also depends on to what extent these activities give the opportunity for creative self-expression and satisfaction. Today, the postretirement period averages about eight to fifteen years for men and fifteen to twenty-two years for women.

In the adult preretirement years, most people fulfill obligatory roles in the workplace and family setting. *Leisure* activity or recreation is balanced with purposeful work. Each brings a welcome change from the other. The later years offer a greater opportunity to participate in individually chosen, nonobligatory activities. To satisfyingly fill the hours, these activities must be more than just play, however. Studies show that both work and leisure activities can offer a sense of purpose and accomplishment. Both forms of activity provide pleasure and satisfaction, which may be inherent in the action, indirectly derived from the approval of others, or both. For example, you might feel creative enjoyment as you build a cabinet, extracting pleasure directly from the action. But you might also feel pride from knowing that your work is admired by family and friends.

Choice of Leisure Activities

Leisure time activities are individual choices. They meet highly personal needs. Those chosen in retirement will probably be similar to those chosen in the middle years.

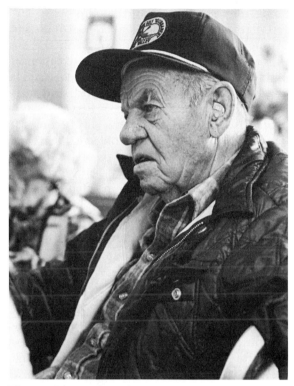

Figure 9-1 After the excitement of the final work day, a feeling of "let-down" comes to some retired people.

It is difficult to change a life's style of living. Leisure activities do not mean the same to everyone. A strong work ethic developed early in life and reinforced through a lifetime of practice may make it difficult to manage effectively the free leisure time that comes with retirement. Years of hard work, achievement, and delayed gratification can inhibit the relaxation that could come with less work, nonspecific goals, and the possibility of immediate reward. Some people may not be able to easily accept leisure as a legitimate way to spend their time. They experience feelings of guilt, depression, and anxiety when free time is unstructured. Not all older people may choose a leisurely life-style easily, even if it is available to them. They may need help in putting their work values into a different perspective, one that still maintains self-esteem. Those caring for them must be careful not to inflict their own personal work values on the elderly. For these people, activity that is productive leads to a positive self-image and a higher morale.

The more personal goals an individual has established, the more active he or she continues to be in pursuing them. If social participation has not been part of the individual's life-style before retirement, it will probably not figure largely in the life-style after retirement. If community involvement has been high in preretirement years, it will probably be sustained into the postretirement period.

In the early retirement years (sixty-five to seventy-five), activities tend to remain relatively unchanged from those pursued in younger years. This is true as long as physical health is maintained. There is, however, a gradual slowing down and greater participation in less strenuous activities. Beyond seventy-five, the person's activity decline is substantially greater. Physical health, financial security, availability of transportation, and established activity patterns are the critical factors in determining which activities will be chosen and the extent of social involvement.

Society today tends to view an increase in leisure activity as an earned right. Still, society expects the retired person to spend his or her time as an active, involved member of the community, engaged in constructive activities, figure 9-2. To the extent that the older person's activities are retiring and sedentary, he or she begins to be viewed as having less value. Studies indicate that the activities chosen by older people are not drastically different from those chosen by younger people. There are four exceptions. The younger person spends more time caring for other members of the family, in being gainfully employed, and participating in sports. The older person spends more time watching television. Otherwise, activities enjoyed by both groups are remarkably alike.

Although the general population may view older people as spending excessive time in private, isolated activity with not enough to do, old-

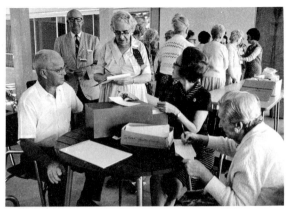

Figure 9-2 After retirement, there is greater opportunity for community activities such as voter registration.

er people don't view their own activities in this light. They also do not see themselves as without goals. It is wrong to assume that physical inactivity means no activity. Contemplation leads to a synthesis of experience, personality, and values. Well-being is difficult to evaluate. But if a person continues to have enthusiasm for life's experiences and to demonstrate happiness and contentment, it may be assumed that the individual finds life satisfying.

Most elderly people settle into a routine once they have adjusted to the end of paid employment. The routine is stabilizing and provides a degree of comfort. A person may choose to readjust in some ways, such as staying up later at night and sleeping later in the day, or eating at different times. However, some mental and physical activity must continue to be part of life.

One psychological theory is the activity theory. It implies that social activity is the essence of life for all people at all ages. It is through activities that mental and social well-being are established and maintained. Studies seem to bear out this theory. Activity is not the sole determinant of life's satisfactions, but it is an important factor.

Leisure is primarily a state of mind in which individuals feel free to choose activities from which they derive pleasure and satisfaction.

Some may continue gainful employment or volunteer service. People gain a sense of identity through these activities. Through interaction with others, they experience a sense of community and belonging. To have friends, to love and be loved, to have a place in the world, and to be recognized as a person of value are basic needs of people of all ages. Real idleness only becomes an important part of life in very old age. Even then, physical inactivity doesn't mean that important emotional adjustments are not being made.

One must also keep in mind that the activities of daily living require an output of energy, even when the person is assisted. These activities include dressing, eating, eliminating, and maintaining hygiene.

Social Networks

Social networks consist of those people and organizations that offer an individual the opportunity for support and socialization. It is through the individual's social network that psychological, social, and activity needs are expressed and met. Social networks may be limited to family and friends, or they may involve larger groups within structured organizations.

Family and Friends

Most older people continue to look to their families as the primary source of social relationships and activities. Older people living in their own homes spend much time caring for their personal needs and doing household chores. Over one-third of older Americans spend their leisure time at home in activities that can be done alone. These include watching television, reading, gardening, going on walks, and doing handwork, figure 9-3.

Maintaining and strengthening family ties takes a good deal of time. In addition, family responsibilities may continue to occupy early retirement years. Helping with household tasks, sewing, babysitting, visiting, and preparing for

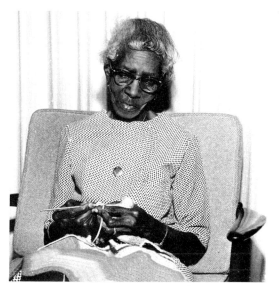

Figure 9-3 Sewing and handwork can be enjoyed independently.

family outings and gatherings can be enjoyable experiences for all concerned. Additional energy in the early retirement years is spent enhancing. relationships with a spouse. Activities in this period may also include greater participation with other couples who are also freed from rigid constraints of time and family. Traveling and entertaining friends increase accordingly.

Living alone without the support of family need not mean the end of socialization. Neighbors often take an interest in the elderly in their neighborhoods, dropping in for brief visits. Certainly there are some elderly who feel real social deprivation when living alone.

Pets

Pets can be a real source of pleasure to their owners. They help their owners overcome loneliness, offering an outlet for the expression of affection. We are only just beginning to understand the degree and value a pet offers to one who is elderly and alone.

Caring for a pet gives the owner a sense of purpose and helps him or her feel needed. Many

owners feel so strongly about their pets that they talk to them and treat them as part of the family.

Pets offer companionship, affection, and an assurance that their owners are needed and loved. Even having pets visit routinely lifts the spirits of the elderly.

Other Social Sources

When close family relationships are not available or fail to meet social needs, the older person may seek social relationships outside the home. A blending of activities from home and outside recreational sources offers the best opportunity for social fulfillment. For the millions of older people who live in large cities, anonymity and loneliness are major problems. Social relationships help elderly people overcome the loneliness of isolation.

When they have the opportunity to communicate with others with similar interests and to share these interests, older persons are able to find a degree of affection and greater security in self-identity. The meeting ground of common interests gives people an opportunity to maintain their status as individuals. This protects and enhances their self-esteem.

Visiting is an essential part of developing and maintaining social contacts. In fact, in a recent survey, almost half of those surveyed indicated that they spent "a lot of time" in this activity. Socializing with friends is an important activity throughout life, but especially in later years, figure 9-4. The lower the socioeconomic level, the more importance this activity assumes. The upper middle class elderly favor active participation in voluntary associations, sports, reading, and gardening, figure 9-5. Memberships in lodges and fraternal organizations are most common and increase in this group up to age seventy-five. The older people usually hold the positions of leadership. Becoming involved in church-related activities is another way or source of socializing. The middle socioeconomic group favors manipulative activities such as crocheting, woodworking, and baking, in addition to reading

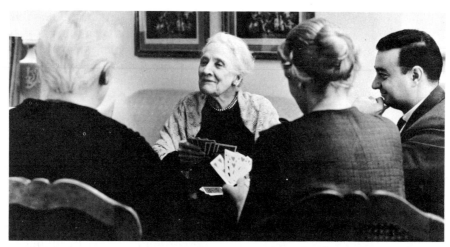

Figure 9-4   Playing cards with friends and family is a relaxing form of entertainment for the elderly. (Reproduced by permission of Knoll Pharmaceutical Company, Orange, NJ)

and watching television. Clearly, the availability of money and previous involvement influence choice of activities.

For the very old, even though more time is available for recreational pursuits, actual opportunities diminish. Decreasing energy is one deterring factor. Health problems and lack of

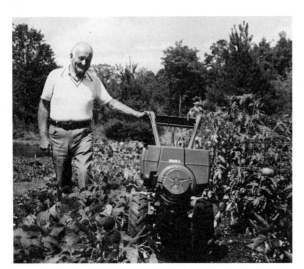

Figure 9-5   Gardening is a popular retirement activity. (Courtesy of Gardenway, Inc., Troy, NY)

transportation make getting to social outings a hardship. Some elderly people find that many of their old friends are gone, and the prospects for meeting new ones are limited. Some may even be frightened by the energy required to establish new relationships.

Circumstances may also have altered the elderly's living arrangements. Loss of a spouse may also lead to loss of the couple relationships both enjoyed. A move to a new neighborhood may mean loss of old friends and difficulty finding new ones. Under these circumstances, the older person who lives alone may become apathetic and seem to lack self-direction. Suddenly faced with hours to fill, he or she may not know how to begin. Insufficient money for transportation, proper clothing, and fees may also keep many people from taking the initial steps that would bring them into contact with outside social activities.

Individual Pursuits

Remember, individuals will not suddenly change interests greatly just because they have retired. If reading and gardening were primary interests in younger years, there is no reason to believe that square dancing and partying will become major interests of old age. Woodworking, sewing, and listening to the radio are also activities that can be enjoyed independently. They also require a minimal output of money. Art and craftwork can pleasantly fill the hours. At the same time, they can give a sense of artistic achievement, incentive, and purpose. Unfortunately, only a small percentage of the elderly occupy themselves with hobbies and crafts.

Many elderly people use their leisure time to contemplate their own lives and the meaning of life in general. Thoughts turn toward their religion, figure 9-6. A place of worship and its related activities may assume greater importance in the older person's life. If religious beliefs were important throughout their lives, they will remain important now. However, it should not automatically be assumed that all older persons become more religious. When attendance at religious services is desired but is not possible, every effort should be made to arrange for requested visits with the clergy and other members.

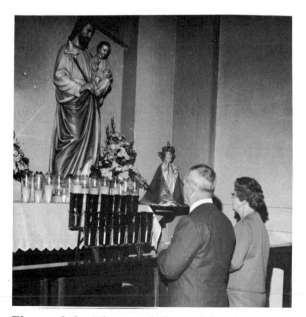

Figure 9-6 The need for spiritual comfort often assumes added significance for the older person.

When money is limited, public facilities such as libraries, adult education centers, and parks offer opportunities for low-cost entertainment. In some cities, libraries sponsor discussion groups, films, and travel lectures at no cost. Through adult education programs, more and more elderly people are proudly completing requirements for high school or college graduation.

The fact that many older people take advantage of cultural and educational opportunities points strongly to the need to recognize that leisure time activities for the elderly must contain intellectual stimulation.

Volunteerism

Many people over age 65 spend time freely giving their time and energy to benefit others. This is called *volunteerism*.

A large number of the country's older volunteers are between sixty-five and seventy years old. Some are in their eighties. In 1986, 43 percent of the sixty-five- to seventy-four-year-old group participated in volunteer activities. Twenty-six percent of the seventy-five and older population also donated time and energy to volunteer activities. The amount of volunteer time given ranged from less than seven to more than thirty-five hours a week. The average was just under five hours a week. In the past, women volunteered many more hours than men did. However, because women are now more actively involved in the work force, a greater proportion of volunteer work is being done by men. Fifty-one percent of women and 45 percent of men now volunteer their services.

Volunteer work is an important leisure time activity for 37 percent of the older age group. The highest proportion of volunteers are among the white middle and upper middle classes. More blacks and Hispanics are either joining the ranks of volunteers or indicating an interest in doing so.

Volunteer service is provided in a wide variety of ways, figure 9-7. Health-related and reli-

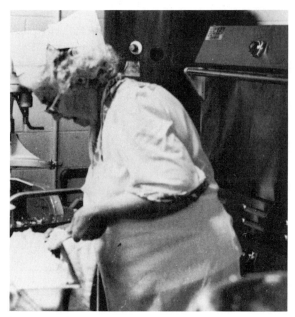

Figure 9-7 Almost one-quarter of the retired elderly spend at least part of their time in volunteer work. Here a senior helps prepare free meals for the needy.

gious activities are the most popular. Health-related activities include working in hospitals, health clinics, and extended care facilities. In these settings, volunteers sell in gift shops, deliver mail and flowers, or make visits. Others help community-based organizations such as the Red Cross and Y.M.C.A. or the March of Dimes. They work as receptionists and clerks or in care facilities for the elderly or very young. Church-related activities include singing in church choirs, teaching Sunday school, ushering, and serving on committees or in outreach programs.

Other volunteers provide transportation for the handicapped or elderly, register voters, lobby for passage of legislation, operate telephone hot-lines, and help publicize services within the community. Older volunteers also serve as sports coaches and as craft teachers. They counsel small businesses through *S.C.O.R.E.* (Service Corps of Retired Executives) and serve through *R.S.V.P.* (Retired Senior Volunteer Programs). They also participate in programs such as Meals on Wheels

and other shut-in services. They also participate in Foster Grandparent programs, figure 9-8, and work with organized youth groups such as the Girl Scouts and Boy Scouts. The reasons given for volunteering are a desire to help others, a sense of duty, and the satisfaction and enjoyment of the work.

Organizational Work

Many older people continue to be active in organizations that they joined in their youth. Fraternal organizations such as the Elks and Masons, civic and political groups, and special interest groups are well supported by their older members. Often, with retirement, older people cannot only attend meetings, but also become more active on committees. The expertise they bring is invaluable. Many of these organizational activities are independently pursued. Others become a group effort.

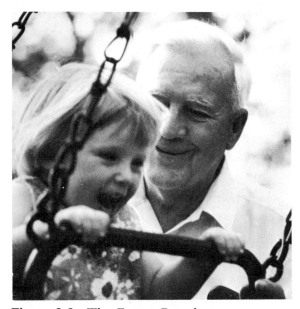

Figure 9-8 The Foster Grandparent program brings happiness to children and purpose to the lives of older people.

Adult Education

Adult education can meet a definite need, especially for that 10 percent of older people who are functionally illiterate. Many of these are older immigrants who never mastered English language skills. The number of older participants in continuing education is growing. Older adults make up nearly 50 percent of the higher education enrollment. These "gray students" appreciate the social contacts, the mental stimulation, and the opportunity to explore new topics.

Most older people who pursue additional education indicate that they do so for personal satisfaction and to meet new people. To meet the needs of those over sixty-five, there must be a wide variety of subjects from which to choose. There must also be innovative ways of presenting information in a nonthreatening manner.

Interest in formal education begins to lag when people reach thirty. It drops off sharply in the fifties. In preretirement years, education tends to center on skills and information useful on the job. After retirement, educational interests turn more to the arts and crafts and humanities. The more formal education an individual has achieved, the more he or she is likely to seek involvement in continuing education programs. There is every reason to believe that this trend will increase. It seems that there will be an increasingly higher level of education attained by the older population.

The general education attainment of the elderly population is about two years below that of the younger generations. Over the last thirty years, and especially in the last decade, the gap between the two groups has narrowed. In 1986, the median number of school years completed by those over fifty-five was 10.6, compared to a median of 12.2 for the entire population, table 9-1.

| | | PERCENT OF POPULATION COMPLETING— | | | | | | | Median School Years Completed |
| | | Elementary School | | | High School | | College | | |
RACE, SEX, AND AGE	Population (1,000)	0–4 years	5–7 years	8 years	1–3 years	4 years	1–3 years	4 years or more	
All races	146,606	2.7	4.7	6.0	11.9	38.4	16.9	19.4	12.6
Male	69,503	2.8	4.7	6.0	11.3	34.9	17.1	23.2	12.7
Female	77,102	2.5	4.6	6.0	12.5	41.6	16.7	16.1	12.6
25–29 years	21,619	.9	1.6	1.6	9.8	42.2	21.6	22.4	12.9
30–34 years	20,434	.9	1.7	1.6	8.2	40.1	21.7	25.7	12.9
35–44 years	32,508	1.2	2.5	2.6	9.0	38.9	20.5	25.5	12.9
45–54 years	22,662	2.3	4.0	4.7	12.6	42.0	15.2	19.1	12.6
55 years old and over	49,383	5.3	9.0	12.7	16.0	34.2	11.2	11.7	12.2
Black	**15,234**	**5.4**	**8.3**	**5.6**	**18.5**	**35.6**	**15.8**	**10.9**	**12.3**
25–29 years	2,684	.5	.8	1.2	14.1	47.0	24.5	11.8	12.7
30–34 years	2,417	.7	1.4	2.5	15.2	44.1	20.4	15.6	12.7
35–44 years	3,408	1.0	3.1	2.4	17.7	40.6	20.5	14.6	12.6
45–54 years	2,403	3.2	7.4	6.9	23.6	36.0	13.2	9.6	12.2
55 years old and over	4,323	15.6	21.2	11.9	20.7	19.5	5.5	5.6	9.2
Hispanic origin[1]	**9,030**	**12.9**	**15.9**	**8.1**	**14.7**	**28.4**	**11.6**	**8.4**	**11.7**
25–29 years	1,882	5.6	12.0	6.4	17.0	33.7	16.3	9.0	12.3
30–34 years	1,594	6.5	14.5	5.0	16.1	33.6	13.6	10.9	12.2
35–44 years	2,209	10.2	15.2	7.7	14.2	29.2	13.8	9.8	12.1
45–54 years	1,453	13.8	17.3	8.1	15.5	28.7	9.1	7.4	11.0
55 years old and over	1,891	27.8	20.6	13.0	11.2	17.7	4.8	4.9	8.1

[1]Hispanic persons may be of any race.

Table 9-1   Years of school completed, by race, sex, and age, 1986 (U.S. Bureau of the Census, unpublished data)

People who have not been in a formal school situation for years find it difficult to enter a classroom of people forty years younger. Those who are more self-assured already have an educated background. In addition, those who are motivated usually make the effort. A major reason for this increase in the number of older people continuing their education is that, following World War II, many people took advantage of educational opportunities offered under the G.I. Bill. Those who were in their twenties at that time (1941–1946) are in their sixties and early seventies now.

Universities, colleges, high schools, libraries, and senior citizen groups all offer courses, seminars, and discussion groups. These activities are mentally stimulating and allow older students to pursue academic status, increase their understanding of special interests, or open the door to new, unexplored fields.

Elder Hostels

The elder hostel program was first started in 1975. It has rapidly grown to meet educational and socialization needs of people age fifty and older. The elder hostel offers opportunities for seniors to visit educational institutions around the world. While there, they participate in short-term educational programs. In 1988 more than 160,000 hostlers enrolled in programs in all fifty states, Canada, and forty countries overseas. Participants stay in dormitories and have food available through the school cafeterias. There are no examinations. In addition, the costs of the entire program of housing, meals, and education are minimal. The program includes short study sessions in a wide variety of subjects and interest areas.

Although age alone does not limit learning ability, educational methods change. Older people were often taught to learn by rote rather than by the problem-solving methods used more commonly today. This may be one reason that older people often do not do as well on standardized tests as younger people do. Standardized tests also tend to be timed. They penalize the slower response time of older people. The more the intellect is used, the sharper it remains, however. Motivation is a key factor in successful learning. The great potential of adult education as a lifetime learning process is being developed to meet the needs of the older population.

Skilled Care Facilities

In some communities, adult education programs are made available to the residents in skilled care facilities. A teacher goes to the facility and, working with the activities director, plans short-term classes of interest and therapeutic value to the residents. The activities director is a designated person who spends at least twenty hours each week in the facility if there are fifty beds or more. This is a requirement for Medicare certification. Bedridden residents and those in wheelchairs should not be neglected. Each should be encouraged to participate in activities to the full extent of their abilities.

Geriatric health care providers can promote these activities by seeing that transportation to the activity area is available. They should also make sure that care is planned to leave time and energy to participate in activities. Structured activity, designed for individual residents to meet specific goals, is therapeutic recreation. Besides meeting specific self-image needs, these activities relieve boredom and add to the satisfaction of the individual's life. You may be asked to assist at the bedside for those unable to get to a communal area. You can bring a great measure of joy and stimulation by being patient and tactful.

Senior Citizen Centers

Since the Older Americans Act of 1965, many communities have undertaken to provide facilities and programs for the elderly. *Senior citizen centers*, where seniors can meet to enjoy programs and socializing, are springing up in both urban and rural areas. Senior centers, started as meeting places for the low-income elderly, are found in almost every community. They serve the needs of those with varying economic means. Through these centers, older people are offered discounts on commercial entertainment and reduced bus fares. Dial-a-Ride and similar programs provide transportation to and from shopping facilities and recreation centers.

Attendance at these centers has been rising since 1974, along with public awareness of them. Senior citizen centers are now available to more than 50 percent of the population over fifty-five. They are least accessible to those living in rural areas and in the South.

The National Senior Club directory listed three hundred senior citizen centers across the country in 1966. By 1986, this same volume listed three thousand senior centers and another three thousand clubs that meet at least once each week. Some of these centers are large, comprehensive units. Others are smaller clubs. The Golden Age and Over Sixty Clubs are examples of small clubs operating on limited budgets. Some of them are sponsored by local church groups that provide the meeting place. Others are self-sustaining through dues. Activities are usually planned by the members. They include cards, dancing, conversation, and games such as bingo and checkers. Some clubs have pool tables and shuffleboard and table tennis equipment. Sometimes coffee is made and members bring their lunches, spending the entire day together. Under the sponsorship of the club, arrangements are made for special events, sometimes at discount prices. These may be tours, plays, and other cultural events.

The larger recreation centers may be part of more comprehensive senior citizen centers. They may be tax-supported through city, county, or state agencies. Through the centers, older people can meet others of the same age with similar problems and interests. They often discover new avenues for service.

Parks are often the sites of these activities, with recreation departments handling the programming. Most outdoor activities such as camping and boating are undertaken by older persons under the sponsorship of the recreation department. Large, multipurpose centers are sometimes developed as community outreach by churches and other philanthropic groups. They provide recreational opportunities along with health, economic, and social services.

Some of the centers are classified as day centers and are open during the weekday hours. To be classified as a day care program, services must combine health and social activities. They are specifically designed to meet the needs of the elderly who live in the community and have some physical or mental limitations. Programs promote self-care and encourage members to be active to the extent of their personal limitations. Recreation activities are usually directed by a specially trained staff member. In addition, craft activities and even vocational training may be offered. Health and financial counseling are consistently part of the overall programming.

Recreation in Care Facilities

Patients in long-term care facilities need the stimulation of planned recreation, figure 9-9. But the type of activity must be carefully tailored to the needs, desires, and abilities of the patients. As a rule, institutionalization tends to limit activities and to sever community contacts. One of the few independent decisions left to residents is the choice of activities. This choice should not be denied to them. The health care provider in these facilities is often responsible for bringing some entertainment into residents' lives and providing some direction for their activities.

It is important for those who plan activities to keep in mind the age and possible physical limitations of the participants. To mention this may seem unnecessary. In one facility, however, beadwork, which requires coordination and good eyesight, was listed as a principal activity. Planning must take into consideration that older people have less coordination and are more apt to have hearing and vision deficiencies. The fact

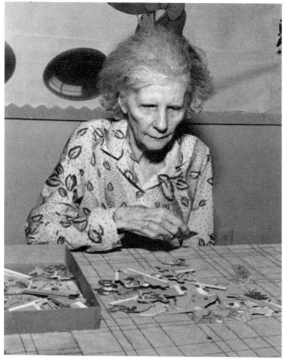

Figure 9-9 Residents in long-term care need the stimulus of planned recreation.

that recreation with a purpose is the most stimulating to mature people must also be considered. Finally, do not assume that lack of participation is necessarily bad. Older people like some time alone to contemplate. Activities that are planned by the participants are the most successful. Shows and skits call for many different talents. They are usually enjoyed by everyone. Planning exhibits and sales and making gifts for others are examples of activities that combine recreation with purpose.

Do not overlook the fact that older people enjoy television and an opportunity to converse with others and read. Areas should be available where these activities can be enjoyed. These are not costly activities, but they prove satisfying. With care, activities can be planned that meet special rehabilitation objectives. This is the therapeutic recreation mentioned earlier. The occupational therapist is a valuable consultant both in

care facilities and recreational centers. Singing, exercising, hand-clapping to music, simple hand crafts, and games can be enjoyed to some degree by bed patients, wheelchair patients, and even those who are mentally confused. For those patients capable of locomotion, marching and chair exercises can be stimulating as well as enjoyable. Most care facilities have a special room where out-of-bed patients can visit with one another. Recreation should be considered an important facet of overall therapy, figure 9-10.

Recreation in Life-Care Facilities

The operators of life-care facilities recognize the importance of recreation in the lives of the residents in several ways. All provide facilities for communal recreation with equipment similar to that in large centers. In addition, some have rooms where residents can entertain their personal friends. Information is posted about entertainment opportunities in the community.

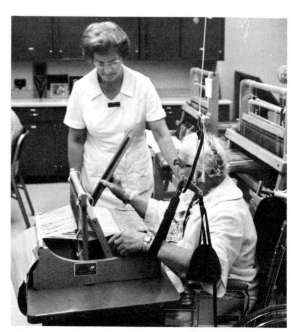

Figure 9-10 Activities provide a sense of achievement and meet rehabilitation needs.

Group arrangements are also made for tours and lectures.

Some facilities have an activities director on the staff. The programming in these facilities may be quite varied and extensive. Some residents make use of the volunteer services of community groups such as the Scouts. The most successful programs present varied activities from which residents can make personal choices.

Summary

- Leisure activities are an important part of healthful living.
- Recreation and opportunities for service need to be included among possible uses of leisure time.
- Since the Older Americans Act of 1965, emphasis has been placed on developing special centers for older persons. Many of these centers have stressed recreation and the productive, satisfying use of leisure time.

- Health care providers often play a vital role in providing health information and counseling, as well as recreational activities for the elderly in senior centers and extended care facilities.
- The freedom to choose whether and in what activities to participate is a vital element that must always be considered.
- Leisure activities help pass the time. But there must also be a balance between recreation and useful activity.
- More and more senior adults are taking advantage of opportunities to keep their minds stimulated in ways that contribute to their social, psychological, and physical well-being.
- Play loses its appeal when it becomes an everyday occurrence.
- Many elderly people lack the financial resources needed to meet their basic needs, let alone utilize recreational facilities. But many satisfying activities can be enjoyed at little or no cost.

Review Outline

   I.   Behavioral Objectives

  II.   Vocabulary

 III.   Choice of Leisure Activities

        A.   Life-style patterns
        B.   Current trends
        C.   Importance

  IV.   Specific Areas of Involvement

        A.   Family and friends
        B.   Social sources
        C.   Individual pursuits
             1.   Opportunities
             2.   Volunteerism
             3.   Organizational work
             4.   Adult education
        D.   Senior citizen centers

   V.   Recreation in Care Facilities

Review

I. Vocabulary

Word Puzzle—find and circle the words or initials defined.

```
A F S E N I O R J C E N T E R
M J O I K D Q B P C I A D J C
H R C O C H G L S G L K R E O
C G I A S P S C O R E H T K B
P I A J K B I F P L I N G O W
V O L U N T E E R I S M W M F
N S G B Z L C A S G U K C Q P
B D N M E I U Q V J R M L G H
U J E P A O K I P V E U H T W
G E T Q G L D N F Q C R R D U
S I W J R T P U A D I P A I U
A K O H I E W G L M K I O E R
L F R O R N T L J E Q B N T F
A M K U R P F C K U H I D O C
```

1. Free time
2. Participating in donated time and effort
3. Initials of a service organization of retired executives
4. A place where older people gather in the community
5. Initials of a service group offering programs for retired seniors
6. Group of people through which individuals can work to fulfill their recreational needs

II. Short Answers

1. What major factors hinder the elderly from participating in recreational activities?
2. What are the two elements needed in leisure activities?
3. Why is it important that the elderly choose their own leisure activities?
4. What are the major recreations of the elderly?
5. Name four recreational activities that cost little or no money.
6. Why do people often demonstrate greater interest in religion and religious matters as they age?
7. List five recreational or social activities in which a person who is chairbound might participate.
8. What is the relationship between physical activity and mental health or morale?
9. Who makes up the primary social network of the elderly?
10. When an elderly person lives alone, what role may a pet play?

III. Clinical Situations

1. An elderly resident expresses a desire to remain in her room one morning and read rather than participate in a group activity that you have planned. What is your response?
2. An elderly friend indicates an interest in learning a foreign language. But he is afraid that he is too old. What is your response?

CASE STUDY

Four people in their postretirement years have just moved into a new community. The community has active civic involvement in the problems of all age groups. There are programs of interest to youth, such as the Scouts and the Y.M.C.A., as well as to the aged. Cost-free programs are presented through the library and school systems. The community also maintains a geriatric day center. Band concerts and programs of general community interest are presented through the recreation department in the parks. Several churches in the area have programs designed for older people. There are, of course, the usual commercial entertainment facilities such as bowling and theater.

Mr. and Mrs. A are in their early sixties, enjoy relatively good health, are financially secure, and enjoy meeting people. They have traveled and have always been active in their church.

Mr. B is a vigorous man of sixty-eight who has always been interested in sports, has a fixed income, and until his move was a member of a bowling league. He has always worked with his hands and is interested in woodworking and tools. At one time he was a Scout leader.

Mrs. C is chairbound and, although her mind is keen, she tires easily. She is a former school teacher. She has recently moved in with her niece and husband.

Suggest leisure activities for each.

Section 3
The Geriatric Health Care Provider

Unit 10
The Health Care Team

Objectives

After studying this unit, you should be able to:
- Describe different kinds of long-term care facilities.
- Identify the roles and responsibilities of members of the health care team.
- Explain the need for different kinds of geriatric health care providers.
- Explain the role and functions of the geriatric health care provider.
- List the characteristics necessary for successful employment.
- Describe ethical standards that govern your employment and work with the elderly.

Vocabulary

Learn the meaning and spelling of the following words or phrases.

activities of daily living (A.D.L.)	geriatrics
	gerontology
aiding & abetting	hospice
ageism	intermediate care
client	facility (I.C.F.)
convalescent home	malpractice
ethical dilemma	negligence
ethics	patient
euthanasia	resident
extended care facility	rest home
geriatric health care technician	skilled care facility (S.C.F.)

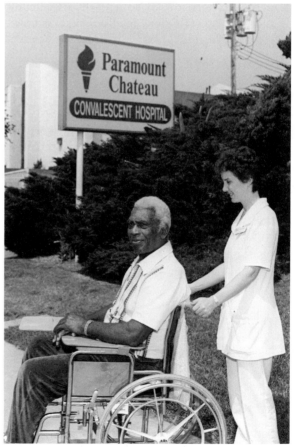

(From Hegner & Caldwell, *Assisting in Long-Term Care,* copyright 1988 by Delmar Publishers Inc.)

130

A geriatric health care provider employs special learned skills in the care of older persons who are ill or infirm. He or she may be a specialist in the field of *gerontology* (the study of aging) or the field of *geriatrics* (the study of illness in the elderly). He or she may be someone trained in basic nursing skills who applies these skills in the geriatric setting. The latter is called a *geriatric health care technician* or nursing assistant. This person gives care under the supervision and direction of a registered nurse (R.N.) or a licensed vocational/practical nurse (L.V.N./L.P.N.).

Registered nurses practice professional nursing, which includes many independent activities. Vocational or practical nurses practice technical nursing under the supervision of a professional nurse. Both are essential to good patient or resident care. In long-term care facilities, the L.P.N. often assumes "charge" responsibilities during the evening and night shifts.

Geriatric health care technicians may function as home health aides in a client's home. Or they may be employed in a nursing facility, figure 10-1, giving care to older patients who can no longer completely care for themselves.

In a health care facility, the technician may be called by various names. He or she may be known as a geriatric assistant or technician, nurse aide (N.A.), certified nursing assistant (C.N.A.), or geriatric nursing assistant or health assistant.

Care Facilities

"Long-term care facility" is a name applied to several different types of care providers. Other names given to long-term care facilities (L.T.C.s) include *skilled care facility (S.C.F.), intermediate care facility (I.C.F.), convalescent home, rest home, nursing home,* and *extended care facility.* The person being cared for in these facilities is usually called a *patient,* a *client,* or a *resident.*

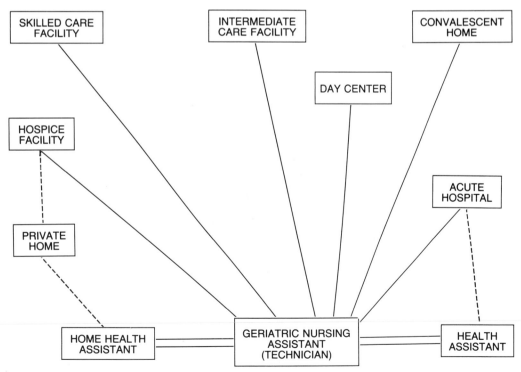

Figure 10-1   The geriatric nursing assistant functions in many different settings.

Although these agencies may provide care for more than one type of client, a large proportion of their clients are in the older age group.

Unlike patients in the usual hospital setting, who are acutely ill and need temporary, highly skilled care, residents of extended care facilities tend to be chronically ill and require long-term, often lifetime, care. Geriatric health care assistants also find employment in terminal settings such as a *hospice,* where people are cared for and supported during their final months or days of life.

Each facility that provides nursing service is authorized and regulated through state and federal guidelines. Federal, state, and local health agencies also inspect care facilities to make sure that the guidelines are being followed. The guidelines are translated into the policies or rules that govern the institution. Based on the policies, procedural manuals are written. These manuals describe the way that care will be given. The policies also help formulate job descriptions, which explain who will carry out the care. Through Medicare and Medicaid, federal and state revenues pay, in large measure, for the care of the patients or residents.

Multidisciplinary/Multidimensional Approach to Care

Caring for the elderly person is one of the greatest challenges in health care today. A small change in an older person's ability to perform self-care or household management activities, or receive help from a support person, can have a major impact on that person's life and health. Often a change affects not only the health of an older person, but almost all other dimensions of that person's life, including social and economic aspects. The elderly are especially vulnerable to disability from a variety of factors. These factors include disease, physical and emotional illnesses, and changes in their social and economic situations. Therefore, good care of older people requires a broad outlook, and a multidisciplinary or team approach to health care, figure 10-2.

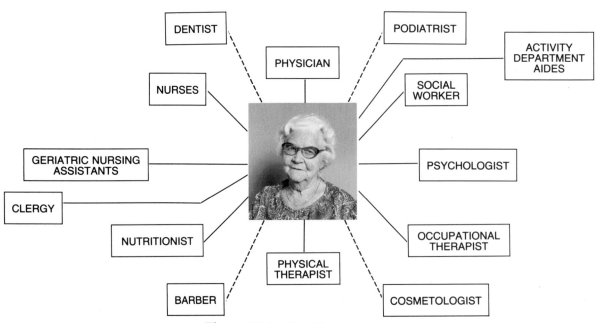

Figure 10-2   Health care team

Geriatric technicians or assistants are health care providers who are essential members of health care teams.

The health care team includes all those who directly participate in the care of the resident or patient. The resident or patient and family are always part of the team. Remember that total health care involves the emotional and social, as well as the physical, well-being of the resident or patient. Today, health care providers emphasize a holistic approach. This approach does not separate the physical from the emotional and social aspects of human life. Instead, it views the human being as a whole. It realizes that each area of a person's life influences the other areas. Residents or patients are treated as whole beings who are under stress from some physical, emotional, or social force.

The members of the health care team work cooperatively. Each contributes his or her expertise, figure 10-3, to develop care plans that work for the resident or patient. The care plan considers all aspects of the resident's or patient's current status, health, goals, and potential for rehabilitation.

Members of the Health Care Team

The exact makeup of the health care team varies. It depends on the type of care facility and the individual patient's or resident's needs. The basic team usually consists of the physician, the nurse who is responsible for the resident or patient, and the social worker. Other specialists join the team as need for their help arises. In the skilled care facility, patients or residents need more acute care and can benefit from a broad range of health team members, figure 10-4. Specific teams might include the physician; registered nurses, licensed practical/vocational nurses, and health assistants; the nutritionist; the pharmacist; and physical, occupational, and speech therapists, figure 10-5. They may also include specialists in the fields of audiology,

psychology, social work, and podiatry; the patient's/resident's priest, minister, or rabbi; and the patient/resident and family members.

In an intermediate care facility, residents require continuous monitoring, but less acute care. The physician, nurse, nutritionist, physical therapist, and social worker make up the basic team. Other specialists are included as needed. For example, the podiatrist might be included for consultation and a public health nurse might be included during discharge planning.

In an extended care facility or convalescent facility, residents are expected to stay for a long period of time, often for the rest of their lives. Here the primary team members include the physician, whose visits are not as frequent as would be in an acute care setting; the registered nurse, the licensed practical/vocational nurse, the geriatric nursing assistant, the nutritionist, physical and occupational therapists, the psychologist, and the social worker. Some therapists and specialists, such as a podiatrist and dentist, are not on-site team members. However, they make periodic visits to provide service. Other technicians such as barbers and cosmetologists may also make routine visits to provide service.

In a hospice facility, team members are available for personal care, pain control, emotional support, physical therapy, and spiritual support twenty-four hours a day. This same service can be provided in a patient's home or in a long-term care facility. The hospice team includes a physician, registered nurse, social worker, volunteers, home health aide, homemaker, physical therapist, and member of the clergy. The home health aide assists with personal care under the supervision of professional personnel in the home, just as the geriatric nursing technician does in care facilities.

Each health care team has a support group. Although it is not directly involved in patient or resident care, this group nevertheless contributes to the overall success of the program. It includes laboratory technicians and employees in the dietary, housekeeping, facility maintenance, and business departments.

Health Team Members	Role
Physician	Admits the patient, establishes the diagnosis, writes orders for medical care
Professional nurse (R.N.)	Evaluates the patient's needs, writes orders for nursing care, directs and supervises care, coordinates activities of other health team members
Technicians	
Practical or vocational nurse (L.P.N./L.V.N.)	Helps the R.N. evaluate the patient's/resident's needs and carry out the nursing care plan, supervises assistants
Geriatric nursing assistant	Gives direct personal care under supervision
Nutritionist	Supervises the meal planning
Pharmacist	Compounds and dispenses medicines
Physical therapist	Teaches and supervises activities that maintain optimum body functioning and mobility
Dentist	Treats dental and oral problems
Occupational therapist	Assists patients in activities that increase productive use of their time
Ophthalmologist	Cares for conditions of the eye
Recreational therapist	Directs patients in recreational activities in order to increase their enjoyment of life
Speech therapist	Tests speech communication skills and treats speech disorders
Podiatrist	Examines and corrects foot problems to increase comfort and mobility
Audiologist	Tests hearing and helps fit devices to improve hearing
Psychologist	Assists the patient and family in making emotional adjustments
Social worker	Assists patients and families in making social and economic adjustments to changes in their lives
Homemaker	Performs homemaking chores that enable people to remain in their own homes

Figure 10-3   Roles of various health team members

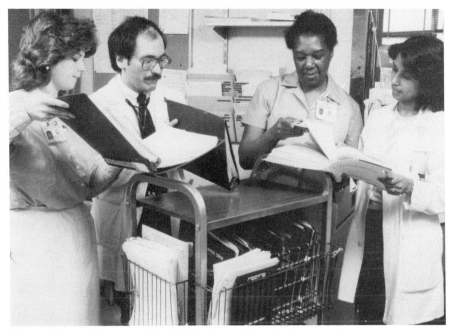

Figure 10-4   Many medical disciplines offer their expertise during the care conference. (Courtesy The NYU Medical Center and Lou Manna)

Characteristics of the Geriatric Health Care Provider

Not everyone is suited to work with the elderly. This field of nursing care requires a person who has a great deal of maturity, patience, sensitivity, empathy, and kindness. Dramatic recoveries are not the norm. Small gains must be satisfying.

In long-term care facilities, the residents are usually older and have multiple problems. The facility becomes a home as well as a source of physical care and emotional support. In this environment, geriatric health care providers not only provide for the physical needs of the resident but often assume the role of substitute family and friend. Close relationships develop between care giver and receiver. You will need to work closely and cooperatively with other staff members and help create an atmosphere of harmony and calm.

Personal Appearance

In large measure, you represent the facility to residents and their visitors. What you do and say and how you do it reflects not only on you, but also on the entire facility. You will be in close personal contact with your patients as you give care. In addition, your work, although rewarding, is not physically easy. Therefore it is particularly important that body odors be controlled, figure 10-6. A daily bath and the use of antiperspirants are essential. Thorough, frequent cleansing of your teeth should be routine. Many people object to strong perfume, after-shave lotion, and cigarette odors. They should be avoided. Hair and fingernails must be kept short and clean. If nail polish is used, it should be clear. Actually, nail polish should be avoided because germs collect under chipped polish. These germs are not easily removed, even with vigorous handwashing. Thus, infection is possible not only for residents/patients, but also for you and

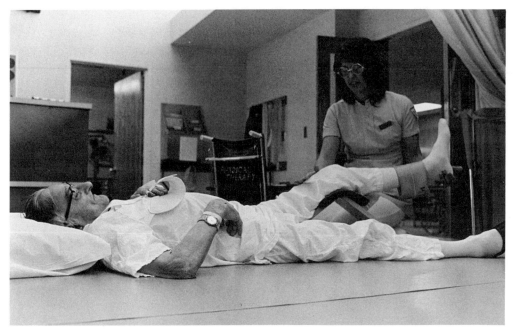

Figure 10-5A   The physical therapist is an important member of the geriatric health care team. (Courtesy Long Beach Memorial Medical Center)

others away from the work setting. Jewelry other than a watch, wedding ring, or professional pins is not part of your uniform. Stockings should be freshly laundered. Shoes and shoelaces should be cleaned daily. Fatigue will be lessened if the shoes give good support and fit the feet well.

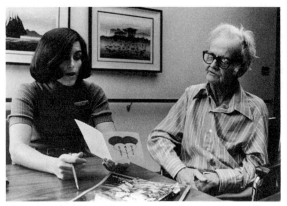

Figure 10-5B   The speech therapist works to improve verbal communication skills. (Courtesy Long Beach Memorial Medical Center)

Some facilities today allow assistants great leeway in selecting their uniforms. Other facilities have regulations governing the type and color of uniform to be worn. Know and abide by the rules of your facility. An identification badge worn on your uniform can help to dispel confusion as to your name, role, and responsibilities. Many state laws require that all types of health care providers wear name tags with print large enough even for those with sight problems to see your name and role.

Uniforms are to be worn in the facility and should not be worn elsewhere. They should not be worn when you shop or do errands. If your facility does not have an area for changing your uniform before and after you go on duty, wear a cover-up when you travel. Upon arriving home, remove your uniform, turn it inside out, and put it into the laundry. (Turning the uniform inside out lessens the possibility of germs brought from the health care facility spreading to the home.) Wearing a fresh uniform every day should become a habit.

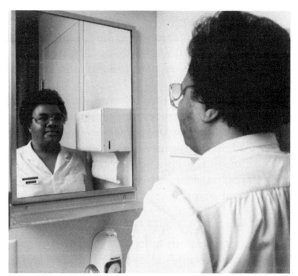

Figure 10-6 Good grooming begins with a clean body and hair (From Caldwell & Hegner, *Nursing Assistant—A Nursing Process Approach,* copyright 1989 by Delmar Publishers Inc.)

Being a health care provider requires enthusiasm and great energy. You will need a good diet and adequate rest, as well as recreation and stress reducing activities, to perform at your peak.

Personal Adjustment

You will have to make some personal adjustments in each new work situation. Facility policies (rules) are written for the protection and welfare of the residents. Facility rules need to be obeyed and orders from supervisors need to be carried out promptly, even if you do not agree with them. The ability to accept constructive criticism and profit by it is equally important. It means that you are willing to learn and grow. How well you are personally adjusted shows in many other ways. You demonstrate dependability and accuracy by reporting to work on time and completing your assignments carefully. If illness prevents you from reporting to work on time, it is essential that you notify your employer as early as possible. In this case, a substitute can be brought in to provide uninterrupted patient/resident care. You prove your reliability when

you follow procedures correctly and ask questions when in doubt.

Training and Education

Training programs for geriatric nursing assistants vary in length. Some are offered in public and private schools, and some are taught in the employing facility.

Since 1989, Medicare-Medicaid rulings have changed. They now require all nursing assistants working with Medicare/Medicaid patients/residents to complete a training program. They must pass state tests (written and skills performance) to become certified nursing assistants (C.N.A.). Many care facilities will only hire those people who have passed the tests and are certified.

You must learn and abide by the regulations of your own state. The basic training period is usually about six weeks. However, growth and learning will continue throughout your lifetime as a care giver.

Many facilities conduct ongoing classes to upgrade the skills of their employees, figure 10-7. These classes may be required or optional. You should take advantage of every opportunity

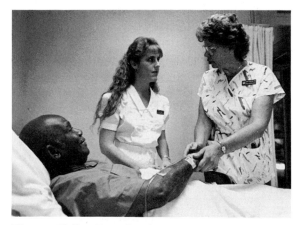

Figure 10-7 Ongoing in-service education and supervision helps employees upgrade their skills. (From Caldwell & Hegner, *Nursing Assistant—A Nursing Process Approach,* copyright 1989 by Delmar Publishers Inc.)

to increase your knowledge and sharpen your skills. The more proficient you become, the better care you will be able to give your patients.

Job Description

Your job description outlines the work for which you will be responsible, figure 10-8. For comparison, figure 10-9 gives a typical job description for a licensed practical/vocational nurse. In accordance with your job description, specific assignments for your daily work will be made.

As an employee, your direct assignment will usually be made by your charge nurse or team leader. When you accept responsibility for an assignment, you should fully understand the assignment and feel capable of handling it. If you have any doubt, discuss it with the charge nurse. Never hesitate to ask for clarification. Never be embarrassed to admit that you need help or instruction.

Remember, your assignment will be based on patient need and availability of staff. Sometimes your load may seem especially heavy. At other times, you may be able to offer assistance to another staff member. A cooperative attitude on

---

- Gather routine data about patients/residents to help in developing nursing care plans.
- Carry out assigned activities that help the patient/resident meet goals and contribute to the smooth functioning of the facility.
- Organize your own assignment and seek assistance as needed.
- Communicate observations and problems of patients/residents promptly to the appropriate team member.
- Participate in team conferences, sharing observations and making suggestions to help develop and revise care plans.
- Assume responsibility for your own actions.
- Participate in self-development programs.

Figure 10-8 Job description of a geriatric nursing assistant.

- Gather patient-/resident-related data to contribute to assessment and diagnosis.
- Carry out nursing activities prescribed in the nursing care plan to help patients/residents.
- Organize your own assignment and assist other team members as needed.
- Communicate observations of patients'/residents' responses and/or changes in condition to the appropriate team member.
- Participate in team conferences for developing and revising nursing care plans.
- Provide direction as a team leader or team member to geriatric nursing assistants.
- Assume responsibility for your own actions.
- Assume responsibility for continued learning.
- Administer medications and treatments as ordered.

Figure 10-9 Job description for a licensed practical/vocational nurse.

---

the part of all staff members tends to balance the responsibilities.

Many of your duties will involve helping patients carry out their *activities of daily living (A.D.L.).* These are activities that fulfill basic human needs. They include physical activities such as bathing, eating, eliminating, exercising, and resting. They also include psychosocial activities such as communication, interaction, and goal fulfillment. Goals provide a purpose for living. To be satisfying, goals must be personal and realistic. Residents with limited mobility may find satisfaction in reaching a recreation or day room to watch a favorite soap opera. Even a patient in bed can be helped to establish reachable goals that, once met, can afford a sense of achievement.

As a geriatric health care assistant, it will be part of your responsibility to maintain optimum client involvement, participation, and independence. You will adjust techniques to meet the individual needs and abilities of the people under your care. In addition, you may be assigned to carry out special procedures you have learned. These could include giving enemas or checking vital signs. You may be asked to keep the patient's room and other common rooms such as a day room tidy and to distribute water pitchers and food trays. Your assignment may also include participating in occupational and recreational therapy sessions. Participating in patient care planning is another important activity. Exact assignments will vary from facility to facility and from day to day.

Remember that each facility has a procedure book, figure 10-10. This book describes how each task should be carried out. Know where the book is kept and consult the book frequently until you are thoroughly familiar with the specific procedures at your facility. Look up any new procedure. Be sure you know your exact responsibilities for carrying it out. Always be prepared to accept your assignment and carry it out to the best of your ability, with a positive attitude.

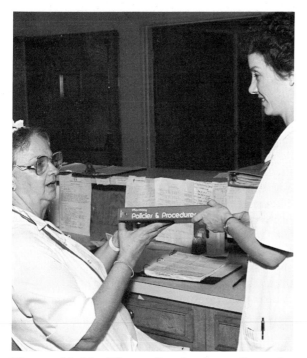

Figure 10-10   The policy book outlines the rules that govern the facility.

Responsibilities of the Geriatric Nursing Assistant

Geriatric nursing assistants are semiskilled workers. They can normally be expected to perform in certain ways, figure 10-11. An assistant who fails to give the care that is expected is guilty of *negligence*. For example, bedrails are to be up at night for many patients/residents. An assistant may prepare a patient for bed and forget to put up the bedrails. If the patient falls, the assistant is considered negligent. If a patient in postural supports is not checked regularly and circulation is impeded, there would be a case for negligence.

An assistant who gives care improperly or gives care in which he or she has not been instructed is guilty of *malpractice*. For example, an assistant may prepare an enema solution of a higher temperature than required. If it burns the patient, it would be considered malpractice. Turning a patient with an indwelling catheter so that the patient's position obstructed the flow of urine would also be considered malpractice.

Patients may not be forced to have care that they do not want. This means you may not threaten or use physical coercion. The patient's refusal, however, must be documented. Furthermore, you may not restrain a patient without a specific, written physician's order. To do so would constitute false imprisonment, which is illegal.

Because of the nature of their work, people employed in care facilities must have the highest degree of honesty and dependability. Despite careful screening of employees, dishonest acts may be observed. These range from the stealing of washcloths and patients' belongings to the stealing of drugs. If such an act is observed, it should be reported immediately to the charge nurse. Not reporting such an act is considered *aiding and abetting* the crime. As a geriatric assistant, you will find that opportunities for poor practice, illegal activities, and neglect are always present. Never be tempted. Honesty and integrity are the hallmark of the successful health care provider.

• Admit, transfer, and discharge patients	• Feed patients and pass trays
• Answer patient call lights	• Measure intake and output
• Ambulate and transport patients	• Assist with special procedures
• Bathe patients	• Carry messages
• Make beds	• Pass nourishments
• Assist patients with bedpans, urinals, and commodes	• Give oral hygiene
• Take blood pressure	• Care for patients with oxygen therapy
• Document patient's record	• Assist with physical examinations
• Clean patient unit and utility room	• Position patients
• Apply hot and cold compresses	• Provide postmortem care
• Change and pass drinking water	• Shave patients
• Give enemas	• Collect specimens
• Care for equipment	• Test urine and feces
	• Determine vital signs

Figure 10-11 Specific duties of geriatric nursing assistants

Patients may ask members of the staff to write a will for them. All matters of this nature should be reported promptly to the charge nurse. Writing a will is a legal matter for which you are not qualified. Signing a will as a witness can lead to legal complications and should also be avoided. There are legal aspects to everyday living as well as to every job. As a citizen, you will not have problems if you obey the law. As a geriatric health care provider, you will not have problems if you follow the policies and procedures outlined in the procedure book for your facility. Perform only those procedures that you have been taught. Know the lines of authority. That is, know to whom you are responsible. In all situations, remember that you are ultimately responsible for your own actions and their consequences.

Lines of Authority

Direct authority for the care that you provide comes to you through specific channels called lines of authority. Each facility has an organizational chart that explains the lines of authority, figure 10-12. Communication flows through the same channels.

The geriatric nursing assistant usually receives an assignment from the charge nurse or team leader. He or she reports to this same person upon completion of the assignment. This person is the assistant's immediate superior in the line of authority and communication.

If the facility is large, the assistant may function on a team whose leader is a registered nurse or a licensed practical nurse. In this case, the assistant's immediate superior is the team leader. The team leaders receive their assignments from the nurse in charge. This person is ultimately responsible for the total care of a certain number of patients/residents. This number may include all of the patients/residents on a wing, a unit, or a floor. In smaller facilities, the charge nurse may be responsible for all of the patients/residents in that facility. The charge nurse receives authority and direction from the supervisor (in larger facilities) and the director of nursing. The director of nursing works with the medical director and the facility administrator. The board of directors is responsible for the overall functioning and success of the facility. Physicians and other geriatric health care providers work with the director of nursing, administrator, supervisor, and charge nurse.

Facilities vary in the complexity of their staffing. You need to learn the lines of authority in your own work situation so that you function smoothly as a member of the health care team.

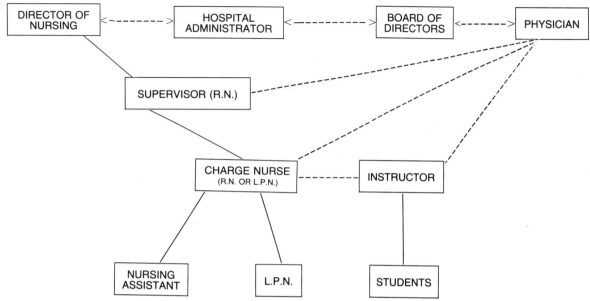

Figure 10-12   Lines of communication and authority in team nursing

Ethical Standards

The patient/resident is the most important person in any care setting. Elderly patients/residents often have many problems that pose ethical dilemmas for those who take care of them. The decisions made to solve individual, family, and societal problems of the elderly need to be based on professional, not personal, ethics. Professional ethics help health care providers to focus on the "ideal." They emphasize high-quality decision making and actions to carry out the decisions.

Personal and Professional Ethics

Ethics are basically the values or standards that guide behavior. Ethics are very similar to morals, rules, and principles. These morals, rules, and principles develop from custom. When a person acts according to these values, it can be said that this person is moral or principled.

Ethics, on the other hand, involve thought-

fully understanding and making decisions about human problems, even though these decisions may go against the care giver's custom. It is important to understand one's own values so that one can be sensitive to the values of others. These values may be very different. The geriatric health care provider should be able to accept that people have different value systems. He or she is then able to begin developing ethics that recognize that the patient/resident, or at times families or friends, is the ultimate authority in making decisions about care. This is extremely important when dealing with an ethical dilemma. An *ethical dilemma* is a choice that must be made between unsatisfactory or unacceptable solutions to a problem. In other words, because there is no one best answer to a problem, a person is said to be "caught between a rock and a hard place." Ethical dilemmas often arise in the care of elderly people. They include such issues as mental competency, confidentiality, death, mercy killing *(euthanasia)*, suicide, and the right to health care, or the right to refuse health care.

Critical Decisions in the Care of the Elderly

The belief that all patients/residents have legal and moral rights is the foundation for all ethical guidelines. The next unit describes these rights and the geriatric health care assistant's responsibilities concerning them.

Certain moral principles can help geriatric health care providers make ethical decisions in caring for older people. These include recognizing that all people deserve quality care, respect, and the privilege of making their own decisions. Quality care is determined by the unique situation of each older person. Older people expect and deserve respect and appreciation. They do not deserve to be treated as less than a person or as a joke. To do so is to be inhumane, amoral, and unethical. The name for this type of prejudice is *ageism*. All people, regardless of age, should be allowed to make their own decisions. People waive this right for a variety of reasons. In this case, decisions made by family, friends, or the geriatric health care provider should agree with the patient's/resident's values and past decisions.

Summary

- In different care settings, the person who receives care is referred to by different names. These names are frequently interchangeable. "Patient," "client," and "resident" are common terms.
- The geriatric health care provider is a specially trained person who cares for the older patient/resident/client. He or she works in a variety of health care settings, giving basic physical and emotional care. This person also helps patients/residents/clients in ways that allow them to fulfill their physical, emotional, and psychological needs.
- The geriatric health care provider has specific responsibilities that vary, depending upon the employing agency and the provider's level of preparation.
- Personal appearance and good grooming are important for successful employment.
- Lines of communication and authority must be clearly understood and followed.
- Medical and legal complications can be avoided if the procedure manual and facility policies are carefully followed and the rights of patients/residents/clients are assured and protected.
- Health care specialists with varied skills and training join to become members of the health care team.
- Each member brings to the team expertise in planning for the patient's/resident's/client's maintenance, well-being, and rehabilitation. The ultimate goal is to provide care and help the patient/resident/client reach optimum self-sufficiency.
- The composition of the team varies from facility to facility. But the geriatric health care provider always plays an important role, participating in the formulation, execution, and evaluation of a care plan.
- The highest quality of care is possible when health care providers use their special knowledge and skills, and ethical behavior, to help patients/residents/clients to achieve their goals.

Review Outline

    I. Behavioral Objectives

   II. Vocabulary

 III. Terminology Applied to Health Care Providers/Facilities

IV. The Health Care Team

    A. Members
    B. Functions

V. The Successful Health Care Provider

    A. Personality traits
    B. Personal grooming
    C. Identification
    D. Personal adjustments
    E. Training and education
    F. Job description
        1. Geriatric nursing assistant
        2. Licensed vocational nurse
    G. Lines of authority
    H. Personal and professional ethics

Review

I. Vocabulary

Write the definition of each of the following.

    1. Gerontology _____
    2. Ethics _____
    3. Ageism _____
    4. Health care provider _____
    5. Patient/resident/client _____

II. Short Answers

    1. What are two other names for a long-term care facility?
    2. When you report to work on time, what quality do you demonstrate?
    3. What are three essentials of good grooming?
    4. List four personal characteristics that enhance your ability to work with the elderly.
    5. What is the difference between moral and ethical behavior?
    6. Who has the ultimate authority to make decisions about care for an elderly person?
    7. Describe the responsibilities of each of the team members listed.
        a. Nutritionist
        b. Physical therapist
        c. Speech therapist
        d. Physician
        e. Social worker
    8. Explain how a convalescent home differs from a skilled nursing facility.
    9. Complete the lines of authority

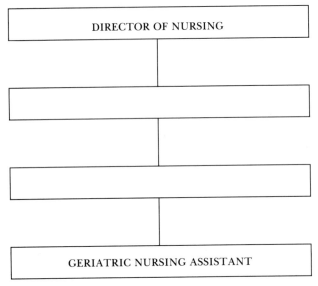

DIRECTOR OF NURSING

GERIATRIC NURSING ASSISTANT

   10.   Which three health care providers make up the basic health care team?

III. Clinical Situations

    1.   You notice that Mrs. Spencer seems very unsteady as she walks along the corridor. You want to report this fact to your immediate supervisor. Who is your supervisor?

    2.   Mr. Zweig tells you that if he has a "bad stroke," he doesn't want any lifesaving measures. His family tells you they want everything possible done to save his life. What kind of a situation is this? To whom do you report it?

    3.   You have been taught to carry out a nursing procedure in your training program. Another assistant tells you that, although the principles are the same, the procedure is done in a different way in this facility. What is your best course of action?

    4.   You hear a co-worker refer repeatedly to a patient/resident as a "silly old lady" or a "dirty old man." What kind of prejudice is this person showing? How should you handle it?

Unit 11
The Nursing Team: Roles, Responsibilities, and Functions

Objectives

After studying this unit, you should be able to:

- Define nursing and the aims of nursing.
- Identify all of the possible members of the nursing team.
- Describe the role, responsibilities, and functions of the various members of the nursing team.
- Explain the process used by the nursing team to deliver quality nursing care.

Vocabulary

Learn the meaning and spelling of the following words or phrases.

assessment
auscultation
B.A.D.L.
clinical nurse specialist
criterion
evaluation
geriatrician
hemiparesis
I.A.D.L.
implementation

inspection
intervention
gerontological clinical nurse
   specialist
geriatric nurse practitioner
nursing care plan

nursing diagnoses
nursing process
palpation
podiatrist
problem solving
psychiatrist
standards

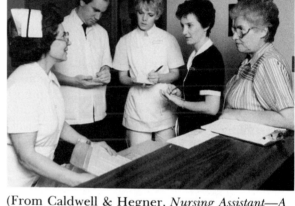

(From Caldwell & Hegner, *Nursing Assistant—A Nursing Process Approach,* copyright 1989 by Delmar Publishers Inc.)

Nursing is diagnosing and treating people's responses to actual or potential health problems. This diagnosis and treatment will maintain, restore, and promote health, or it will help people die with dignity. Nurses and the members of the nursing team achieve these aims by diagnosing patient problems and their causes. They treat these problems through physical and emotional caring, counseling, teaching, and coordinating all needed health-related treatments prescribed by various members of the health team. Nurses also teach, train, supervise, and coordinate the activities of the nursing team members. Professional nurses work both independently and together with other members of the health team in planning care with and for the patient/resident/client. The professional nurse is ultimately responsible for the nursing care and the coordination of all treatments for the patients/residents/clients in the facility.

Members of the Nursing Team

The nursing teams in most facilities are made up of registered nurses, licensed practical/vocational nurses, and nursing assistants, figure 11-1. The nursing team is responsible for giving care to a certain number of patients/residents/clients. *Nursing process* is the method used to determine the needs of the patient/resident/client and the nursing activities necessary to meet those needs and minimize the patient's/resident's/client's problems. Most problem-solving activities for patients/residents/clients take place during team conferences when all members of the team can be present. Because geriatric nursing assistants are the people who spend the most time with patients/residents/clients, their input is especially valuable. In addition to contributing observations and suggestions, the assistant will gain insight about the patient's/resident's/client's problems and the goals of therapies prescribed

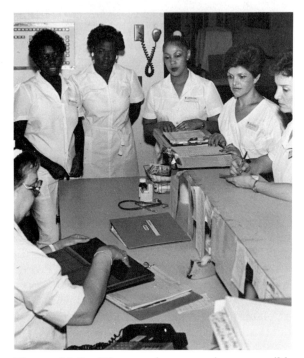

Figure 11-1   The nursing team is responsible for the care of a specific number of residents.

by nurses and other health team members. Team meetings may identify problems in attaining nursing goals and interpersonal conflicts or difficulties in carrying out assignments. Discussion then centers on solving the nursing problems. To that end, all members of the team make constructive suggestions.

At times there are patient/resident/client or nursing problems that the nursing team, under the leadership of the professional nurse, are unable to solve. These problems may be physical, emotional, or interpersonal. They may require the expertise of a nursing specialist. The *gerontological clinical nurse specialist* is an advanced nurse practitioner who has had further education and clinical preparation in the care of elders, sick and well, and in the management of personnel. The nurse may invite this specialist to provide consultation to the nursing team to help them solve a difficult problem. Another specialist with advanced preparation is the *geriatric nurse practitioner*. This individual has had further education and clinical preparation in the management of commonly occurring physical and emotional health problems of elderly people. The nurse practitioner is certified to provide advanced, expert nursing care. He or she can also perform certain acts such as diagnosing, prescribing medications and diagnostic tests, and managing commonly occurring acute and chronic diseases. Nurse practitioners generally work throughout the facility together with other nurses and physicians.

Nursing Process and Nursing Care of the Elderly

Nursing process is a systematic problem-solving activity that is similar to problem-solving methods used by other members of the health team. This problem-solving method, figure 11-2, is used to assess the patient/resident for the following reasons:

- To *identify problems*
- To *identify patient/resident goals* or outcomes

ASSESSMENT	DIAGNOSIS	PLANNING	INTERVENTION	EVALUATION
Inspection (visual observation)	Analyzing data	Goal setting	Caring	Standards
	Naming	Expected	Support	Outcomes
Palpation	Problem	outcomes	Teaching	Interventions
(examining by touch)	Identifying causes	Selecting activities	Helping with A.D.L.s	Revising care plans as needed
Auscultation (examining by listening)		Setting priorities		
Questioning				
Listening				

Figure 11-2 Components of the nursing process and related methods

- To *plan the activities* or interventions to help achieve the outcomes
- To *implement the plan*
- To *evaluate the plan of care* to determine how effective the interventions were in helping patients/residents achieve expected outcomes

Assessment

Assessment is the gathering of information. Assessment of older people is a very complex process. It requires knowledge of changes related to growing older and of all the dimensions of a person's life that may be affected by these changes. The process of collecting information from older people can be time consuming. In order to get accurate information, it is important not to rush older people. Instead, they should be helped to stay focused on the questions that need to be asked and should be given time to rest. Usually all the information needed to develop a plan of care cannot be obtained at one time, because elders fatigue easily. Also, a multidisciplinary and multidimensional approach requires more time for the various members of the team to collect the necessary information.

Nursing Diagnosis

Nursing diagnoses are statements of the problems or needs of a patient/resident/client and the probable causes or contributing factors. The nurse determines a nursing diagnosis after collecting and analyzing the information.

A nursing diagnosis should not be confused with a medical diagnosis. The physician, nurse practitioner, or physician assistant determines a medical diagnosis, which identifies the medical condition of the patient/resident/client. For example, the patient/resident/client has a medical diagnosis of "congestive heart failure." The medical diagnosis is different from the nursing diagnosis.

A nursing diagnosis consists of two basic parts. The first is a nursing diagnostic category (patient/resident/client problem) and the second is the contributing factor (influences on the problem). Nursing diagnoses are still in the developmental stage. Changes can be expected in the existing diagnoses and in the numbers of diagnoses yet to be developed. There are more than seventy-four nursing diagnostic categories. Of that number, there are certain categories that are especially seen with elderly people, figure 11-3. These diagnostic categories had to be approved by the special organization charged with this task, the North American Nursing Diagnosis Association (N.A.N.D.A.).

Planning

The treatment is written as a *nursing care plan* that focuses on nursing diagnoses rather than medical diagnoses. Each care plan includes nursing diagnoses, expected outcomes or goals, and the specific activities or interventions to bring about the outcomes. It also includes the standards (criteria) against which the plan is eval-

Activity Intolerance	Impaired Adjustment
Anxiety	Impaired Airway Clearance
Alteration in Body Temperature	Alteration in Bowel Elimination:
Alteration in Bowel Elimination: Diarrhea	Constipation
Decreased Cardiac Output	Ineffective Breathing Pattern
Altered Comfort: Acute Pain	Altered Comfort: Chronic Pain
Ineffective Coping	Impaired Communication
Diversional Activity Deficit	Ineffective Family Coping
Fatigue	Altered Family Processes
Fear	Excess Fluid Volume
Fluid Volume Deficit	Impaired Gas Exchange
Grieving	Altered Health Maintenance
Impaired Home Maintenance	Hopelessness
Hyperthermia	Hypothermia
Potential for Injury	Potential for Infection
Impaired Physical Mobility	Knowledge Deficit
Noncompliance	Unilateral Neglect
Altered Nutrition: More than body requirements	Altered Nutrition: Less than body requirements
Powerlessness	Altered Oral Mucous Membrane
Self-Concept Disturbance	Self-Care Deficit
Sexual Dysfunction	Sensory/Perceptual Alterations
Sleep Pattern Disturbance	Impaired Skin Integrity
Social Isolation	Impaired Social Interaction
Impaired Swallowing	Spiritual Distress
Impaired Tissue Integrity	Altered Thought Processes
Urinary Incontinence	Altered Tissue Perfusion
	Potential for Violence

Figure 11-3   Nursing diagnostic categories related to the elderly

dent's/client's progress. The nursing care plan provides for continuity of care. It is a written communication record that becomes part of the patient's/resident's/client's record. Nursing team members contribute to the development, implementation, and revisions of the care plan, figure 11-4. All team members should use the care plan to guide the care they give. The charge nurse or team leader works from these plans to assign team members to provide care to specific patients/residents/clients. Nursing care plans are revised frequently to reflect changes in the patient/resident/client. Therefore, it is important to consult the plan, noting any changes that may

have been made, before starting care with the assigned patients/residents/clients. If the patient or resident is transferred to another agency, the care plan is also transferred. Thus it provides the new staff with important information and promotes continuity of care.

Intervention

Intervention refers to tasks, activities, and actions to achieve a goal or outcome. Various nursing team members, based on their educational preparation and competencies, are responsible for planning interventions and *implementing* (putting in action) them. The plans are written

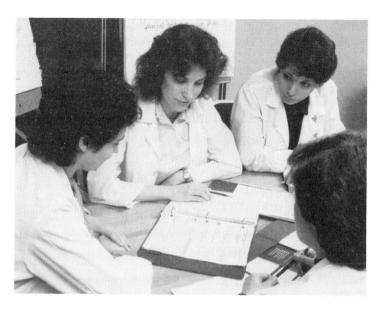

Figure 11-4A The team develops and follows the nursing care plan to meet the needs of the individual residents. (From Gippando & Mitchell, *Nursing Perspectives and Issues,* copyright 1989 by Delmar Publishers Inc.) (Courtesy the NYU Medical Center and Lou Manna)

on the nursing care plan for each patient, resident or client. The skills necessary to care for older people are no different from those needed for younger people.

How these skills are used, however, does differ from one older person to the next because their functional ability (ability to carry out A.D.L.s) varies so much. Generally, the elderly need more time to learn how to achieve their goals for activities of daily living. They also require more rehabilitation nursing techniques. They tend to do better when the same person works with them, because a trusting relationship can be developed.

Evaluation

Standards (measures of quality) are used to measure how effective the plan is in helping a patient achieve expected outcomes. *Criteria* (standards of judgment) for these standards are the specific evidence one would have that indicates that the goal has been met. Time periods during which outcomes should be attained are one type of criterion used. Generally, they are somewhat longer than they are for younger people. The procedure book is another standard used to evaluate care. Procedures and skills are

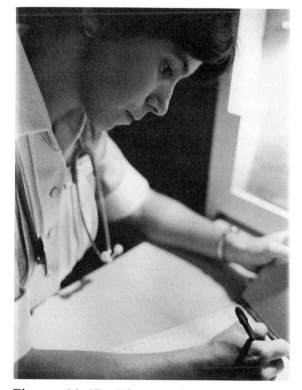

Figure 11-4B The nursing care plan is documented in the patient's record. (Courtesy Long Beach Memorial Medical Center)

developed based on the most up-to-date information. This ensures that patients/residents/clients can benefit from accurate, efficient skills. Geriatric nursing assistants have a great deal to contribute to the evaluation of care plans and patient/resident/client progress because of the amount of time they spend with patients/residents/clients and the trusting relationships they have with them.

How the Team Works: An Example

Phung Banh is a seventy-two-year-old Vietnamese widow recovering from a right cerebral vascular accident (stroke). She has been admitted to an extended care facility following hospitalization in a large medical center. She has been reluctant to get out of bed because she is afraid of falling and becoming more dependent. She has left-sided weakness (left *hemiparesis*). Although she drinks adequate amounts of tea and water, her appetite is poor because she does not like American food. She also has some difficulty swallowing as a result of the stroke. Her toenails are thickened and curling under. Her speech is clear but her vocabulary is limited. She has told the nursing assistant that she is worried about a granddaughter who has taken on "Western ways," and all of the family members are upset.

The charge nurse has assessed the patient and believes a multidisciplinary conference would be helpful. The physician, *podiatrist* (foot specialist), social worker, dietitian, physical therapist, public health nurse, and clinical nurse specialist are asked to join in the conference. They will help analyze the resident's nursing, medical, podiatric, nutritional, and physical problems. Thus, a realistic, quality plan of care can be developed. A family member is invited to help the team, especially the public health nurse, in planning for Mrs. Banh's recovery and eventual discharge to her home.

During the meeting, the resident's problems, needs, and areas of concern are analyzed. Suggestions are made. The geriatric nursing assistant's input is very valuable. The nursing assistant was the first person to observe some of the problems and report them to the charge nurse. The physician clarifies for the team the nature of Mrs. Banh's stroke and the kind of recovery that can be expected. The podiatrist is confident that once her toenails are cut and she has received foot care, she will have more physical stability and less pain in the nails. The physical therapist describes the kinds of range of motion (R.O.M.) exercises that would enhance the physical therapy program prescribed to increase Mrs. Banh's mobility. The dietitian agrees with the family member that Mrs. Banh's appetite would probably improve if Vietnamese food could be prepared for her. The public health nurse shares the home assessment with the team and suggests the kinds of activities that might prepare Mrs. Banh and her family for her return to home. The clinical nurse specialist assists the team in understanding the culture shock Mrs. Banh is undergoing with her first hospitalization and also how elders are treated in the Vietnamese culture. At the end of the conference, the charge nurse formulates the nursing care plan, figure 11-5. The nursing team members implement the plan and help revise it as Mrs. Banh progresses toward her goals. The primary expected outcome is that she will be independent in her basic (personal) activities of daily living (B.A.D.L.) and in most of her instrumental (social and household) activities of daily living (I.A.D.L.).

Summary

- Each member of the nursing team has a role to play in the health care of those for whom he or she is responsible.
- The nursing care is based on established nursing diagnoses.

Room 42A
    NAME: Banh, Phung   AGE: 72   MARITAL STATUS: Widow
    MEDICAL DIAGNOSIS: R. CVA
    NURSE: Eli Jacobi, RN
    PHYSICIAN: Dr. J. Nguyen

NURSING DIAGNOSIS	OUTCOME	INTERVENTIONS
Altered physical mobility related to left hemiparesis, fear of falling, long toenails	The patient will: • Use quad cane • Ambulate unassisted (by 4 weeks)	• Active ROM, QID, quad-setting exercises, BID • Ambulate 20 ft, increasing distance by 5 ft daily
Altered Nutrition: • Less than body requirements related to dislike of Western-world food • Dysphagia (difficulty swallowing) • Current Weight:	• Gain 1 lb/week until usual body weight of 102 lb achieved	• Have family bring in Vietnamese food for one meal a day • Have family encourage her to eat • Weigh weekly • Occupational consultation for Ms. Banh to prepare Vietnamese food in unit kitchen
Impaired communication related to language barrier (limited English)	• Communicate basic needs effectively • Increase vocabulary (daily)	• Arrange for translator • Post a list of basic Vietnamese words and English meanings • Add an English word a day related to B.A.D.L. and I.A.D.L.
Potential impaired coping related to Western cultural influences on life-style	• Express concerns and fears about Western ways (by discharge)	• Ask clinical/nurse/specialist for consultation to help identify ways to help family cope more effectively

Figure 11-5   Nursing care plan

• The professional nurse is responsible for making the nursing diagnosis. He or she will identify the nursing problems, plan the necessary interventions, evaluate the effectiveness of the plan, and supervise the care that is being provided by the nursing team.

• The plan of care is written on the nursing care plan, which is followed by the nursing team. The results are documented in the patient's/resident's record.

Review Outline

I. Behavioral Objectives

II. Vocabulary

III. The Role of Nursing in Health Care
- A. Diagnosing health problems
  1. Actual
  2. Potential
- B. Professional nurses
  1. Plan and direct patient/resident/client care
  2. Teach, train, and supervise other team members
  3. Give nursing care
- C. Licensed practical/vocational nurses
  1. Work under professional supervision
  2. Supervise work of nursing assistants
  3. Give nursing care
- D. Geriatric nursing assistants
  1. Work under supervision of R.N./L.V.N.
  2. Give direct nursing care

IV. Nursing Diagnosis
- A. Established by professional nurses
  1. Identifies problems
  2. Determines goals
  3. Plans interventions
  4. Implements the plan
  5. Evaluates the plan
- B. Guides patient/resident/client care

Review

I. Vocabulary

Match the words or phrases with their meanings.

1. The act of visually observing
2. Activities to help achieve the goals of the nursing plan
3. The act of listening to body sounds
4. Identifies the patient's/resident's/client's problems
5. Statement of the problems or needs of the patient/resident/client
6. Criterion
7. The act of feeling or touching with the hands
8. Instrumental activities of daily living
9. A physician who cares for the feet
10. Basic activities of daily living

a. Nursing diagnosis
b. Assessment
c. I.A.D.L.
d. Inspection
e. Implementation
f. Auscultation
g. B.A.D.L.
h. Standard
i. Podiatrist
j. Intervention
k. Palpation

II. Short Answers

1. What are the three major parts of a care plan?
2. List three ways that the geriatric nursing assistant is involved with the care plan.
3. What two purposes do care plans serve?
4. Which health care team member would have special expertise in the field of communication skills?
5. What does the charge nurse use to make individual assignments?
6. Which nursing team member has the ultimate authority to see that nursing care is given properly?
7. Who are the members of the nursing team?
8. What is meant by the nursing process?
9. Explain the difference between a medical diagnosis and a nursing diagnosis.
10. What are the two parts of a nursing diagnosis?

III. Clinical Situations

1. Your resident has had a stroke and is having difficulty walking with a walker. Which specialist might be called in as a consultant?
2. Your resident, who is terminally ill, has asked to die at home. What will your title be if you continue to care for the patient at home?
3. Your resident seems to be hard of hearing. Which member of the team would evaluate the hearing loss and assist in fitting a hearing device?
4. Everyone on the nursing team is "burned out" emotionally and physically caring for a confused, frightened, and combative resident. People on the team are irritable and there seems to be more daily interpersonal conflicts. What nursing expert could probably help the team a great deal?
5. A new staff member asks you to explain the nursing care plan. How would you respond?
6. You are having difficulty getting to work or class on time. Using the principles of the nursing process, show the problem-solving method to overcome the lateness.

    Assessment:
    Diagnosis:
    Planning:
    Intervention:
    Evaluation:

Unit 12
Communications

Objectives

After studying this unit, you should be able to:
- Describe factors that affect communication positively and negatively.
- Explain the difference between therapeutic communication and conversation.
- Describe ways that people communicate with each other.
- State the relationship between ethical behavior and communication.
- Use medical terminology appropriately in the communication process.
- Describe the communication process in oral reports and in charting on the resident's record.

Vocabulary

Learn the meaning and spelling of the following words or phrases.

chart	objective
communication	prefixes
confidentiality	subjective
empathy	suffixes
interpersonal	sympathy
relationships	tact
kardex	therapeutic communication
living will	

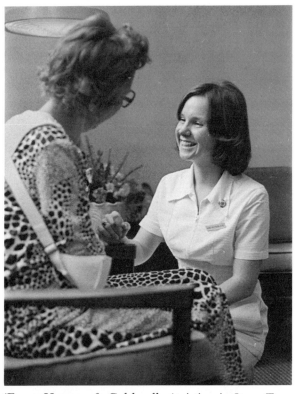

(From Hegner & Caldwell, *Assisting in Long-Term Care*, copyright 1988 by Delmar Publishers Inc.)

Communication is a dynamic interchange between two or more people. It involves verbal messages and nonverbal messages that are sent and received by all of the senses—seeing, hearing, smelling, touching, and tasting. In other words, all behavior is a form of communication. The purpose of communicating is to exchange ideas, beliefs, and opinions; and to give and request information. If both the person sending the message and the person receiving the message know the same information, then communication is successful. When the verbal message is blurred, confused, or interpreted incorrectly, it is usually the result of a contradictory nonverbal message.

One message may be communicated orally as people speak together. But other messages can be sent through the inflections in their voices and through their body language. You may have asked a co-worker to assist you in one of your tasks. The co-worker may have said, "Sure." The words conveyed a willingness to cooperate, but the co-worker's facial expression and voice inflection may have conveyed another meaning.

Some messages are easily transmitted without any words at all. The gentle touch of a hand, a smile, and attention as someone speaks all convey a message of respect and empathy, figure 12-1. Similarly, inattention, rough handling, and a closed facial expression all say "I don't care," regardless of the words being spoken.

Patients and co-workers send many messages. Some are verbal and some use body language. You need to be sensitive to all these messages. Remember that people are not always aware of the messages they are sending. The messages may be very subtle. For example, a patient who engages in bed-wetting may really be asking for the touch of another human being. The patient may not be aware of the reasons behind the bed-wetting, but the act may be based on this very real need. Skin contact, person to person, is extremely important in communicating a sense of caring and a recognition of the human essence of another individual.

When babies are little, they receive a great deal of skin contact. But as children grow, these intimate contacts become restricted to close family members. As adulthood is reached, skin contacts often become limited to friends, to a sexual partner, and to children and family. The elderly often suffer from sensory deprivation in this re-spect. They will, at times without self-awareness, create situations for skin touching. Through your personal touch, you can convey caring and concern.

Unlike conversation, *therapeutic communication* (communication with a purpose) within a health care facility is always a goal-oriented process. The geriatric health care provider uses communication to help patients make the changes necessary to achieve their goals. How a message is sent and interpreted depends upon many factors. People have different levels of maturity, backgrounds, experiences, cultures, intelligence, and ways of interacting with others. Communication is also affected by how free people feel to express themselves, how secure or anxious they feel, and how well their sensory organs function. Good communication skills and attitudes are extremely important for geriatric health care providers. Poor speech skills on the part of the sender and poor hearing on the part of the receiver can make communications very difficult. Your patient may speak a different language, may have impaired hearing, or may have lost language and comprehension skills because of a stroke. In each situation, communication can be hampered unless you are careful to speak slowly and distinctly. Choose your words carefully, face the person, and be patient and sensitive. Use gestures and, most of all, get the person's attention first so that he or she knows that you are talking to him or her.

Interpersonal Relationships

Communications are made easier by good *interpersonal relationships*. You develop interpersonal relationships with everyone you know, because to some degree you react to others and they react to you. Much of the satisfaction that you derive from your work is due to the relationship you develop with other staff members and those in your care. Good relationships with others begin with your own personality and attitudes. If you are a warm and accepting person with posi-

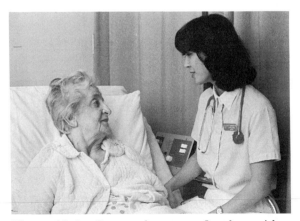

Figure 12-1 Care and concern for the resident are evident by this health care provider's body language. (Photo by B. Blair Brooks)

tive attitudes, others will most likely respond in the same way.

Every person entering a health care facility has his or her unique set of problems and concerns. All patients perceive their own problems and concerns as being of utmost importance. As you compare the conditions of many patients in your mind, it might seem that one has problems that are more serious than another, but *never forget that, to the patient, his or her own problems are the most important.*

Patients are composites of their life experiences, now complicated by illness, disability, and age. Social needs, spiritual needs, and physical needs must continue to be met. This is true even though the restrictions imposed by illness and age limit the ability to satisfy these needs through normal channels. This is naturally frustrating and puts great strain on the patient's ability to establish and maintain good interpersonal relations.

Loss of vitality, fear, pain, unrealistic perceptions of activities around them, worries about family, and lack of social support systems contribute to the patient's irritability and lack of cooperation. Some of these same factors—plus insecurity, fatigue, and personal conflict—influence relationships between co-workers as well. Finally, anxiety may also make visiting family members demanding and uncooperative. When one of their loved ones is no longer readily available to them, this adds stress to their lives. They are anxious to be reassured. It is in these situations that sensitivity and awareness of the needs of others, patience and *tact* (being non-offensive) are most essential, figure 12-2. Sometimes just quietly listening to another person or rephrasing the way you are communicating can change an entire interaction. Try to be aware not only of the words but also of the body language. Look for clues such as the tone of voice or the movement of hands. The health care provider who understands human behavior makes allowances for stress and realizes that older people, those who are sick, and their families need understanding.

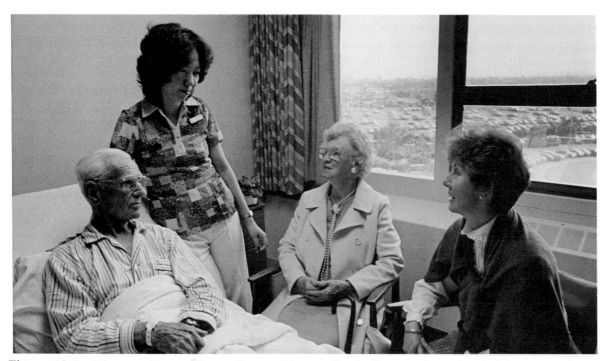

Figure 12-2   The nursing staff must be sensitive to the feelings and needs of visitors and family members.

Communication and Ethical Behavior

One influence on the way you relate to patients/residents and co-workers is the ethical code. Ethical standards guide the conduct of all those who care for the sick. When you assume responsibility for nursing care, you, too, voluntarily agree to live up to the ethical code. The ethical code addresses the most fundamental issues associated with interpersonal relationships between care giver and care receiver. One of the most basic rules of medical ethics is that life is precious. It is not always easy to keep this rule in mind when you are caring for a patient who is dying. This is especially true when you know that the patient is in pain or when there seems to be limited potential for prolonging a productive life.

Probably at no other time in history have the questions of ethics been under such scrutiny. When is life gone from a person on life support systems? How much heroic effort should be given in situations of terminal illness? Is a *"living will"* written by a terminally ill patient valid for those who wish no extraordinary means to be employed if their heart stops or their breathing ceases? These and many other questions are under consideration today. They will eventually be decided under the law.

Patients or residents will often tell you many personal things because of the *empathy* (ability to put oneself in another's position) and sensitivity you bring to the relationship. This encourages trust and security on the part of the resident, figure 12-3. What a resident tells you may be shared only with members of the health team. To maintain *confidentiality*, you may not tell even the patient's family anything. If family members ask you what has been said, you can politely tell them that the charge nurse should be able to help them with information.

Confidentiality of Information

This basic rule concerns what you see as well as what you hear as you work. Much of this information is of personal concern to the patient

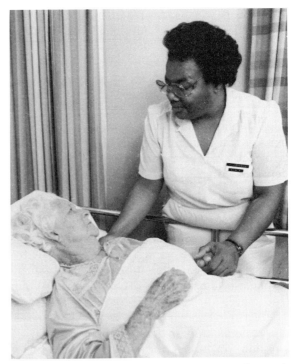

Figure 12-3   The geriatric nursing assistant is often in a position to learn private and confidential information. (From Caldwell & Hegner, *Nursing Assistant—A Nursing Process Approach*, copyright 1989 by Delmar Publishers Inc.)

and must be kept in strictest confidence. The pressure of age and illness may prompt patients to confide their deepest feelings and fears to you. Your close, daily contact with those in your care invites this type of intimacy. You also are in a position to observe the interactions between the patients and their visitors and to overhear personal conversations as you carry out your duties.

The ethical code forbids you from repeating this information or using it for personal gain. If you believe that the information is important to the welfare of the patient, you should promptly report the matter to your immediate supervisor. Only information that directly affects the patient's care and well-being may be repeated. Facts must be repeated only to your charge nurse and not within the hearing of visitors or other patients. Remember, your intent is not to gossip but to share information to benefit the patient. For example, if you have a patient who is worried about a husband with multiple sclerosis at home alone, you might well help by communicating this concern to the charge nurse. The charge nurse might then contact a social worker. A patient who is being harassed by a daughter to embrace the daughter's new religious beliefs might be helped by a visit from the facility chaplain. Arrangements can be made through an informed charge nurse. Note that although patients may discuss their personal problems with you, you must not add to their worries by discussing yours with them.

There is always a temptation to talk about work at lunch or during breaks. Discussing patients in this way is wrong, figure 12-4. The patient's chart is another source of personal information. The same rule of confidentiality holds true. Never discuss any patient information anywhere within earshot of visitors or other patients.

Patients, and sometimes their visitors, will question you about the patient's condition or treatment. Learn to evade these inquiries tactfully. Only the doctor or charge nurse can answer these questions properly. Refer these questions to your charge nurse. Treated with tact and courtesy and a smile, a refusal of this kind is rarely resented by patients or their visitors.

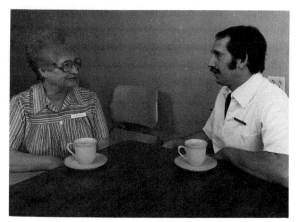

Figure 12-4 Information about patients or residents is confidential and must not be discussed casually with others.

Tipping

Patients are charged for the services they receive while in the care facility. The salary you are paid is included in that charge. The service you give depends on need, not on the patient's ability to pay. There is no place for tipping when service is based on need. If patients offer you "a little something," firm but courteous refusal is usually all that is necessary.

Keeping Promises

Trust is an important part of respect. It must be earned by consistent behavior. Never make promises that you do not intend to keep. If a promise must be broken, inform the patient/resident as soon as possible. Explain why you cannot keep the promise. For example, if you promise to carry out a special task for the patient/resident before lunch and you are too busy to complete it, let the patient/resident know as soon as possible.

Patients/residents feel more secure when they can have faith in the care giver. Keeping promises reflects your worthiness of that trust.

Co-Workers

So far the discussion has focused on ethical behavior in the interactions between the health care provider and the patient/resident. Ethics extend beyond this relationship into the interactions you have with your co-workers and employer.

Health care providers act as a team to provide the very best care. Therefore, they try to support one another, figure 12-5. If one health care provider has a particularly heavy assignment, offer to help as long as your own patients/residents are not neglected. Show your support by carrying out your own assignments so that someone else does not have to finish your work.

Be pleasant and do not gossip about your co-workers. If a new health care provider joins the staff, reach out to him or her by being friendly and cooperative. The manner of each team member helps to set the emotional tone of the entire facility. This does not mean, however, that if you see a patient/resident being mistreated or a

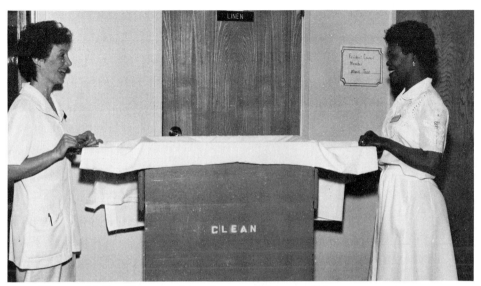

Figure 12-5 Teamwork makes working conditions more pleasant.

dishonest act being carried out, you should not take action. Loyalty to the patient/resident must come first.

Employer Relations

You also have ethical and legal responsibilities related to your employer. You should report to duty on time and be ready and willing to accept an assignment. Remember that you are paid to perform safely and responsibly. Notify your employer as soon as you know that you must be absent. To do otherwise puts not only the patient/resident and you in jeopardy, but your employer as well.

Supplies and equipment are costly. Each person must assume some responsibility in helping to contain the skyrocketing costs of health care. Do not open supplies unless you need them. Follow the policy about linen changes, unless there is a real need to do otherwise. Put equipment away safely. Report minor repair problems before they become major ones.

Speak only in positive terms about your supervisor and facility to others. If there is a problem or something is bothering you, seek clarification privately through the proper channels. If

you are not proud to be associated with your facility, you probably should not be working there.

Religious Expression

Adherence to the ethical code assures respect of personal religious beliefs, figure 12-6. People of all faiths or beliefs and those with no proclaimed faith are admitted for care. These differences must be respected. You show your respect when you inform the nurse of requests for clergy visits. You should be helpful and courteous, escort the clergy to the patient's/resident's bedside, draw the curtains or close the door for privacy, and leave the room. You should know correct information about the type of chaplain services available in your facility. You should also know whether a chapel is open for use by patients/residents and their families. Treat religious articles of the patient/resident—such as a Bible, crucifix, or Koran—with respect. Allow the patient/resident time alone to read, pray, or practice his or her religious beliefs.

Under no circumstances should you try to inflict your personal beliefs and value system on the patient/resident. If asked about your beliefs,

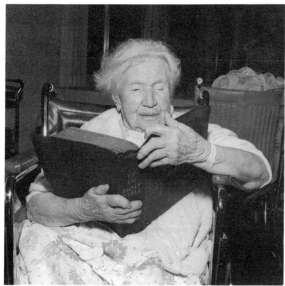

Figure 12-6 The personal religious beliefs of the residents must be respected.

it is better to try to redirect the inquiry to reflect the patient's/resident's own thoughts. For example, if the patient asks if you believe in life after death or in God, you might answer by saying, "You have been thinking about the meaning of life." Often this open-ended statement permits the patient/resident to reflect on his or her own thoughts and feelings.

Medical Terminology

In your role as a geriatric health care provider, you will need to communicate with other staff members in a professional way. Many of these communications will require the use of medical terms, abbreviations, and symbols. You will need to be familiar with each of these.

Many medical words have common endings (*suffixes*) or beginnings (*prefixes*). By learning some of the more common beginnings and endings, it is possible to understand the meaning of many new words. Learning the new words and

parts of words in this unit will make it easier for you to recognize the meanings of terms.

A combining form is part of a word that has a specific meaning. It may be a prefix, a suffix, or a root word. For example, "dys" is a prefix that means difficult. "Uria" is a root word that means urine. Your patient might tell you that she has a hard time passing her urine or urinating. You would report the problem to your charge nurse as "dysuria."

Shortened forms of words (often just letters) are called abbreviations. You will soon become familiar with abbreviations common to the world of health care. In addition, each facility uses its own special abbreviations. You will gradually learn the abbreviations used in your own facility.

The following commonly used abbreviations and combining forms are listed in groups to facilitate your learning. You will see and use these forms on medical records and assignment sheets. They may or may not be capitalized, depending on individual custom.

Time Abbreviations

a.c.–before meals
p.c.–after meals
A.M.–morning
P.M.–evening or afternoon
h.s.–hours of sleep (bedtime)
hr.–hour
b.i.d.–twice a day
t.i.d.–three times a day
q.i.d.–four times a day
q.2h.–every 2 hours

Patient/Resident Orders

A.D.L.–activities of daily living
ad. lib.–as desired
B.A.D.L.–basic activities of daily living
b.m.–bowel movement
c̄–with
C–Celsius
dc.–discontinue
Dr.–physician or doctor

Dx–diagnosis
F–Fahrenheit
ht.–height
I.A.D.L.–instrumental activities of daily
  living
lb.–pound
noct.–at night
n.p.o.–nothing by mouth
O$_2$–oxygen
per–by
p.o.–by mouth
p.r.n.–whenever necessary
q.s.–sufficient quantity
Rx–treatment (take)
s̄–without
spec.–specimen
stat—at once, immediately
tinct–tincture
ung. or oint.–ointment
wt.–weight

Diagnosis (Naming the Disease Process)

A.D.–Alzheimer's disease
A.S.H.D.–arteriosclerotic heart disease
C.H.F.–congestive heart failure
C.O.P.D.–chronic obstructive pulmonary
  disease
C.V.A.–cerebral vascular accident, also
  known as stroke
D.M.–diabetes mellitus
H.O.H.–hard of hearing
M.I.–myocardial infarction (heart attack)
M.S.–multiple sclerosis
P.V.D.–peripheral vascular disease
T.I.A.–transient ischemic attack (ministroke)
U.R.I.–upper respiratory infection
U.T.I.–urinary tract infection

Measurements and Volume

cc.–centimeter
L.–liter
ml.–milliliter
oz.–ounce
pt.–pint
qt.–quart

Weight/Height

in. or "–inch
kg.–kilogram
lb.–pound

Prefixes

a–from, without. *Example:* anemia–without
  adequate blood
ante–before. *Example:* antemortem–before
  death
contra–against, opposed. *Example:* contraindicated–against the usual treatment
dys–difficulty. *Example:* dysuria–difficult
  urination (also used to describe painful
  urination)
hyper-above, in excess of. *Example:*
  hypertension–high blood pressure
hypo–under, a deficiency of. *Example:*
  hypotension–low blood pressure
pneum–lung. *Example:* pneumonia–a
  condition involving the lungs

Suffixes

algia–pain. *Example:* neuralgia–pain in nerve
asis or osis–state, condition, or process.
  Example: arteriosclerosis–hardening of the
  arteries
ectomy–removal of. *Example:*
  laryngectomy–removal of the larynx or
  voice box
emia–blood. *Example:* glycemia–sugar in the
  blood
itis–inflammation. *Example:* gastritis–
  inflammation of the stomach
oma–tumor. *Example:* lipoma–fatty tumor
ostomy–creation of an opening. *Example:*
  colostomy–surgical opening into the large
  bowel (colon)

Combining Forms

cardi–pertaining to the heart. *Example:*
  cardialgia–pain in the heart

path–disease. *Example:* cardiopathy–disease of the heart

pneum–lung. *Example:* pneumonectomy–removal of a lung

Oral Communications

Telephone Etiquette

If it is necessary for you to answer the unit phone, your answer should be made courteously in the following manner:

1. Identify the unit or facility.
2. Identify yourself and your position.

For example, if you are in the west wing on the fifth floor of the facility and your name is Mrs. Brown, you might answer: "Five west, Mrs. Brown, geriatric assistant, speaking." This lets callers know immediately if they have reached the unit they want and if you are the person to answer their question. Facility phones should never be used for personal calls.

Oral Reports

The oral report is a special time of two-way communication between staff members. Report time is often used to make sure that all team members fully understand the nursing care that has been planned for the patients, figure 12-7. Reports are given from staff going off duty to the members of the oncoming shift. From the report you should learn the following information regarding each of your patients: name, location, medical diagnosis, doctor, nursing diagnosis, and special instructions in regard to care.

The staff member giving report will use the individual nursing care plan as each patient is

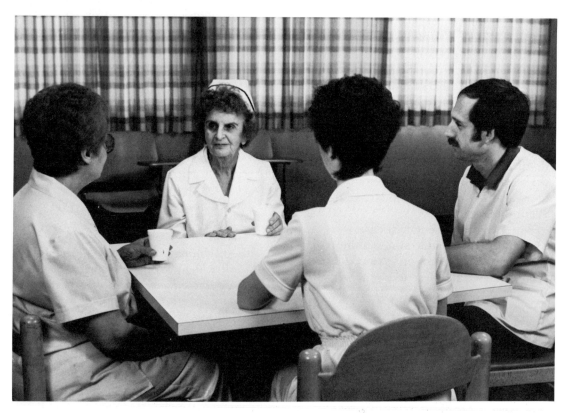

Figure 12-7   During report, patient/resident orders are discussed and assignments are made.

discussed. Nursing care plans are frequently kept in a special carrier called a *kardex*. Using the kardex as a guide, oral reports and assignments are passed on to other team members. Your charge nurse will review the kardex (nursing care plan) for each patient as you are given your assignment. If there is any doubt about your assignment, clarify it with your charge nurse or team leader before you start to work. Clear communication at this point can avert errors.

Usually, you will make a report about your patient to the charge nurse or the team leader just before the end of your shift. Be sure to include the identification and location of each patient as you give your report so there is no chance of misunderstanding. Discuss the care you gave and any special observations you made. Be brief but complete. If, for some reason, you were unable to complete your assignment, make sure your team leader knows exactly what is unfinished.

In summary, oral reports should be brief, complete, and contain information about only one patient at a time. Never leave the area without giving a report to your team leader.

Written Communications— The Chart

Written communication of patient information is made on the patient's *chart*. Charting is done by many members of the health team. In extended care facilities, the charge nurse may do the charting based on oral reports of the staff. Because sudden changes in a resident's condition are infrequent, charting is done less frequently than in the acute care setting. Charting is usually done a minimum of once each shift.

Part of the charting may be your responsibility, figure 12-8. All charting should be done legibly, in block printing. Block printing consists of making straight strokes and circles. Start by making large letters, then you can easily make them smaller. Some facilities permit charting in script, if it is legible. Most, however, prefer block print-

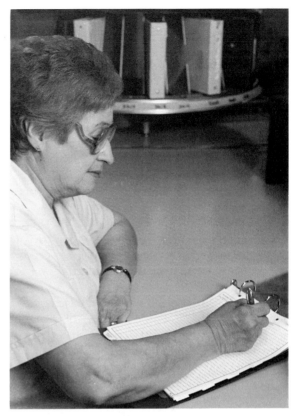

Figure 12-8 The geriatric nursing assistant adds her documentation to the resident's record. (From Hegner & Caldwell, *Assisting in Long-Term Care,* copyright 1988 by Delmar Publishers Inc.)

ing. Sign each entry you make with your first initial, last name, and title. Facilities usually use different colors of ink to identify each shift. Be sure to use the correct color for the time you are on duty. Everything charted relates to a particular patient. Therefore, the term *patient* is not used when charting. Notations should be short phrases, not sentences. The chart is a legal document. It may be called to court and read as evidence in case of lawsuit. Charting must be accurate and legible.

Every patient has a chart. The chart usually consists of different forms to be filled in with information concerning the patient. The following forms are usually included in the basic chart:

- A front sheet with information on sex, marital status, and admission diagnosis
- A physical examination and history record (maintained by the physician or advanced nurse practitioner)
- A progress chart (maintained by the physician or advanced nurse practitioner)
- A graphic chart for recording T.P.R. (temperature, pulse, and respiration)
- Nurses' notes of pertinent information about the patient/resident
- Flow sheets to record routine or frequent observations
- Reports of diagnostic studies
- Progress reports from other departments such as social services, dietary, restorative therapy, or activity department.

Other record forms are added based on the patient's condition. For example, the occupational therapist might add a consultant sheet. All records must be dated and identified with the patient's name, location, doctor, and hospital number. Many facilities now use addressograph cards that provide this information. If this is the policy at your facility, be sure that every sheet is individually stamped. The two records that will be most important to you are the graphic chart and the nursing notes.

The Graphic Chart

The graphic chart varies in form. But it always has two basic markings: the time in blocks across the top, and numbers relating to temperature, pulse, and respiratory (T.P.R.) rates along one side. Sometimes blood pressure, voiding, and defecation are also charted on this sheet. The T.P.R. rates are plotted by placing solid dots on the lines corresponding to the readings and the times the readings were taken.

Some facilities chart rectal temperatures in red. Others reserve red ink for all evening charting (7 P.M.–7 A.M.). An R should be placed above a rectal temperature reading and an AX above an axillary temperature reading.

Nursing Notes

How much routine care is to be charted depends on individual facility policy. Many facilities are using daily flow sheets, similar to the graphic sheet, to record routine care related to basic activities of daily living and treatments. Anything out of the ordinary should always be charted. A charting error should never be erased. A single red line should be drawn through it with the word *error* carefully printed and initialed. In other units of this text, attention is drawn to procedures and their effects that need charting.

Some health facilities are taking a new approach to charting. All health team members use the same record to chart observations and pertinent information about the patient. This record form is called a Problem-Oriented Record (P.O.R.). Recording is organized around specific problems of the patient.

For each problem, recording includes *Sub*jective information, or information given by the patient/resident. It also includes *O*bjective information, or information that is collected through the senses, such as seeing, hearing, or feeling. An *A*ssessment or judgment about the information related to the problem is also recorded. Finally, a *P*lan for meeting the patient's/resident's needs related to the problem is included. Some facilities also require that *I*nterventions, or what was actually done for the patient/resident, and *E*valuation of the effectiveness of the plan and interventions be recorded as well. These kinds of recordings are called SOAP or SOAPIE notes, based on the first initial of each section of the record, figure 12-9.

S = Subjective
O = Objective
A = Assessment
P = Plan
I = Intervention
E = Evaluation

Figure 12-9 The first letter of each aspect of documentation spells the word SOAPIE.

The geriatric health care provider is usually involved in charting on various parts of the patient's/resident's record. Charting is another form of verbal communication. Therefore, it is important to write legibly, using short phrases and correct abbreviations and spelling. The date, time, signature, and title of the person charting is always included. Each facility tends to modify forms and charting styles for its own purposes.

Observations

Observing patients is an important part of your responsibility in patient care. It is your observations that will be reported and charted, figure 12-10. Observing means more than just looking. To observe accurately, you must use all your senses. Note anything out of the ordinary and report these findings to your charge nurse. Experience and practice will enhance your skills in quickly recognizing unusual situations or changes in your patient's condition.

Your eyes and ears are your major senses for making patient observations. The more carefully and consistently you make observations, the more skill you will develop in quickly identifying unusual situations and responses. Do not, however, neglect the valuable information that reaches you through your other senses. You might note a change in skin color, a more rapid respiration, or slowing of a pulse. You might smell a strange odor, hear a moan, or feel an unusual lump in the skin.

Observations of the patient are of paramount importance. But you must also make observations of the environment and equipment pertaining to patient care and treatment. For example, drainage tubes have to be checked for flow. The drainage must be assessed for character, amount, and change. Equipment must be checked to be sure it is functioning properly and that power sources are intact.

Certain patient conditions make some

WHAT TO CHART	SAMPLE
Amount of assistance needed in ADL	Needs help dressing
Safety measures taken	Side rails up
Amount of food eaten	20% food eaten
Intake and output of fluids	1500 ml dark yellow urine
Procedures carried out	B.P. 148/98
Resident's physical and emotional responses	Face flushed, resists fluids, threw cup against wall
Complaints of discomfort	Difficulty breathing when lying down
Difficulties in communication	Does not respond to questions, repeats word "mama" over and over
Unusual odors	Greenish, foul drainage from area on left hip
Anything else unusual	Unable to move left arm, skin cyanotic

Figure 12-10 What to chart (From Hegner & Caldwell, *Assisting in Long-Term Care,* copyright 1988 by Delmar Publishers Inc.)

observations particularly significant. For example, attention to the skin color and respirations of a patient with pneumonia is particularly important. Attention to the condition of the patient's skin is particularly important if the patient is incontinent, because the urine enhances skin breakdown.

As you become more experienced, you will automatically make many observations when you enter any patient unit. You will quickly note equipment failure, drainage, body positions, and general appearance of both the patient and the room. You may be able to sense a problem or change even before you discover its nature. Remember, your observations must be promptly and accurately communicated to your charge nurse.

Time

Charting in international time is becoming increasingly common. With this system, time is not indicated by A.M. or P.M.. The day's twenty-four hours are identified by number. For example, midnight (12 A.M.) is recorded as 2400. The new day begins at 2400 hours, figure 12-11, and only the minutes are recorded for the first hour. For example, 12:10 A.M. is recorded as 0010. Noon is 1200 and 12:10 P.M. is 1210.

Summary

- Communication is a two-way exchange that carries messages between a sender and a receiver.
- Messages can be sent through verbal (oral and written) communication and nonverbal communication (the senses and body language).
- Geriatric health care providers need to be very sensitive and receptive to all forms of communication.
- The most successful communications occur when good interpersonal relationships are maintained and when the geriatric health care provider is committed to an ethical code of behavior.
- Formal patient records require the correct terms, abbreviations, and forms used in the facility.

A.M.	International Time	P.M.	International Time
12 midnight	2400	12 noon	1200
1	0100	1	1300
2	0200	2	1400
3	0300	3	1500
4	0400	4	1600
5	0500	5	1700
6	0600	6	1800
7	0700	7	1900
8	0800	8	2000
9	0900	9	2100
10	1000	10	2200
11	1100	11	2300

Figure 12-11   International time is becoming increasingly popular for charting. This figure shows A.M. and P.M. time converted to international time. (From Hegner & Caldwell, *Assisting in Long-Term Care,* copyright 1988 by Delmar Publishers Inc.)

Review Outline

    I. Behavioral Objectives

   II. Vocabulary

  III. Communication

        A.   Dynamic interchange
        B.   Verbal
        C.   Nonverbal

  IV. Therapeutic Communication

        A.   Goal oriented
        B.   Affected by many factors
             1. Level of maturity
             2. Background
             3. Experience
             4. Intelligence
             5. Functional sense organs
        C.   Requires freedom of participation

   V. Positive Interpersonal Relationships

        A.   Make communications easier
        B.   Enhance work satisfaction
        C.   Focus on patient/resident concerns

  VI. Communication and Ethical Behavior

        A.   Guide to behavior
        B.   Voluntary acceptance
        C.   Addresses fundamental issues between health care provider and recipient
             1. Sanctity of life
             2. Rules of confidentiality
             3. Impropriety of tipping
             4. Keeping promises
             5. Co-worker interactions
             6. Employer relations
             7. Freedom of religious expression

 VII. Communicating with Medical Terminology

        A.   Basis of staff communications
        B.   Combining forms
        C.   Abbreviations
             1. Time
             2. Patient/resident orders
             3. Diagnosis
             4. Measurements
        D.   Prefixes and suffixes

VIII.   Oral Communications

    A.   Telephone etiquette
    B.   Oral reports

IX.   Written Communications (Charting)

    A.   Nurses' observations
       1.   Descriptive notes
       2.   SOAPIE charting
    B.   Graphic charts
    C.   Flow sheets

Review

I.   Vocabulary

Match the word in column II with the meaning in column I.

Column I	Column II
1. Written information about the patient/resident	a. sympathy
2. Information collected through the senses	b. tact
3. Keeping information private	c. living will
4. Ways in which people interact with one another	d. empathy
5. A statement regarding a patient's/resident's desires about prolonging his or her life	e. confidentiality
6. Ability to place oneself in another's position	f. subjective
7. Information given by the patient/resident	g. objective
8. Relating in a manner that causes no offense	h. kardex
9. Summary of patient/resident orders	i. chart
10. Understanding of another's problems	j. interpersonal relationships

II.   Short Answers

    1.   What type of code guides the communication conduct of those who care for the sick and elderly?
    2.   To the patient or resident, whose problems are the most important?
    3.   What is a SOAPIE note?
    4.   Why is it wrong to talk about patient/resident concerns at lunchtime?
    5.   Explain each of the following steps of the nursing process and indicate how the geriatric nursing assistant participates.

STEP	NURSING ASSISTANT ROLE
Assessment	_____
Diagnosis	_____
Planning	_____
Intervention	_____
Evaluation	_____

III. Matching

Column I

1. a.c.
2. p.r.n.
3. p.o.
4. stat.
5. c̄

Column II

a. three times a day
b. whenever necessary
c. before meals
d. by mouth
e. after meals
f. at once
g. with

IV. Clinical Situations

1. You are taking Mr. Ramirez's blood pressure and hear him tell his daughter that he is worried about being able to pay his way in the facility. What is your responsibility?
2. The charge nurse has told you that Miss Berrenger must be assisted to ambulate. What does that mean?
3. The two residents in Room 418 offer to give you money for bringing fresh water. What is your responsibility?
4. The patient/resident tells you that she is changing her will to exclude her son. The son and daughter-in-law ask you whether "Mother has talked about wills?" What do you do?

Unit 13
Legal Relationships and Patient/Resident Rights

Objectives

After studying this unit, you should be able to:
- Describe the legal responsibilities of the health care provider.
- Recognize situations with ethical or legal implications.
- Explain the rights of people in your care.

Vocabulary

Learn the meaning and spelling of the following words or phrases.

abuse	gossip
aiding and abetting	informed consent
assault	laws
battery	liable
confidential	libel
defamation	negligence
ethical code	patients' rights
false imprisonment	slander

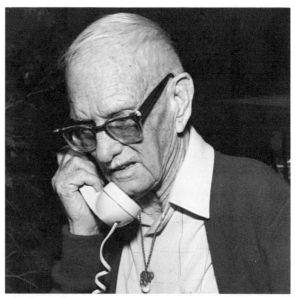

(From Hegner & Caldwell, *Assisting in Long-Term Care,* copyright 1988 by Delmar Publishers Inc.)

People who provide care to those who are ill or infirm agree to follow a specific standard of behavior. This standard is based on the ethical code and federal and state laws. The ethical code is a moral guide to behavior. The governmental guides are legal regulations.

Legal Standards

Standards are established by governing bodies on state and federal levels. For example, the joint commission on Accreditation of Hospitals has developed regulations for the services in various provider agencies. The nurse practice act of each state determines the types of activities that nurses may perform.

Standards are important because they state the expected level of care to be given. They also serve as a model against which practice and care can be measured.

Some rules and regulations set standards for the cleanliness and physical safety of the facility. Others concern the actual care and documentation of care given to the patients. Each plays a role in assuring that people receive the highest quality of safe, appropriate care and service.

Legal standards *(laws)* are guides to lawful behavior. They legally must be obeyed. When these laws are not obeyed, the care giver may be *liable* (held responsible) for legal prosecution. Legal guilt can result in the payment of fines or in imprisonment.

You need not fear breaking these laws if you are careful to do only those things that you have been taught and those that are within the scope of your training. You must keep your skills and knowledge up to date. You must act in ways that always keep the safety and well-being of the patient foremost in your mind. Make sure that you thoroughly understand directions for the care you are to give. You must perform your job according to facility policy. You must not harm the patients or their belongings.

If you follow these rules, you need not fear legal problems. But, if you fail to follow the rules, you may be held liable for any injury or loss suffered by the person for whom you are caring. You are more likely to avoid legal pitfalls if you are aware of their possibility. The following paragraphs describe some legal problems that you will wish to prevent.

Negligence

Health care providers are well trained. Normally they can be expected to perform in certain ways. When a care giver fails to give care that is expected or required by the job, that person is guilty of *negligence.*

You would be guilty of negligence if you injured a resident by not performing your work as you were taught. For example, you prepare an enema solution for a patient. That resident is burned because the enema solution is too hot. You would also be guilty of negligence if you did not carry out your job conscientiously. For example, your facility has a policy that bed rails must be up at night. In your hurry, you forget to secure the bed rails, and a resident falls out of bed and is injured.

Theft

Taking anything that doesn't belong to you makes you guilty of stealing. If you are caught, you will be liable according to the law. The article taken need not be expensive to be considered stolen. This applies to all articles that belong to the residents, to co-workers, or to the facility. If you see someone stealing something and do not report it, you are guilty of *aiding and abetting* the crime, figure 13-1.

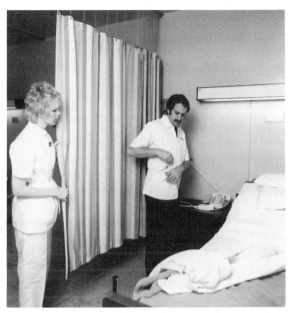

Figure 13-1 Taking anything that doesn't belong to you is stealing. (From Caldwell & Hegner, *Nursing Assistant—A Nursing Process Approach*, copyright 1989 by Delmar Publishers Inc.)

Because of the nature of their duties, people working in health care facilities must be honest and dependable. Despite careful screening, dishonest people are sometimes hired and things do begin to disappear. These range from washcloths and money to drugs and residents' personal belongings.

Sometimes workers are reluctant to report things that they see other people doing. Remember, however, that you are responsible for your own actions and must act properly. As a health care provider, the opportunities for poor practice, illegal activities, and neglect are always present. Always resist the temptation to lower your standards of practice. Honesty and integrity are characteristics of the sincere and conscientious health care provider.

Defamation

If you make false statements about another person to a third person and the character of the first person is injured, you are guilty of *defamation.* This is true whether you make the statement verbally *(slander)* or in writing *(libel)*. For example, if you inaccurately tell a co-worker that a resident has AIDS, you have slandered that individual. If you write the same untrue information in a note, you are guilty of libel.

False Imprisonment

Restraining a person's movements or actions without proper authorization is unlawful or *false imprisonment*. For example, residents have the right to leave the health care facility with or without the physician's permission. You may not interfere with this right. If you do interfere, you will be guilty of false imprisonment.

If you learn of a resident's intention to leave without permission, make sure that you inform the supervisor. The supervisor will handle the situation.

Using physical restraints or even threatening to do so in order to make a resident cooperate can also be false imprisonment. It is sometimes necessary to restrain the movement of residents to protect them or to protect others, figure 13-2. When used, a specific order by the physician is required *before* restraints can be applied. Nurse

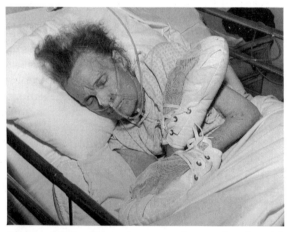

Figure 13-2   Restraints may be used only with the physician's order. (From Hegner & Caldwell, *Assisting in Long-Term Care*, copyright 1988 by Delmar Publishers Inc.)

practitioners or physician assistants can indicate the extent of restraint to be used and the reason for it. All restraints must be checked every half hour and must be completely removed every two hours. This is to ensure that the restraints are properly applied and are not interfering with the resident's circulation.

To avoid a charge of false imprisonment when using restraints, the care giver must be very careful never to apply or remove restraints on his or her own initiative. You must frequently observe and care for any patient who is restrained and document your actions and observations. Be sure to report any signs of irritation or circulatory impairment immediately.

Assault and Battery

Assault and battery are serious legal matters. *Assault* means intentionally attempting to touch the body of another against his or her will or even threatening to do so. *Battery* means actually touching another without that person's permission.

The care that is given is done with the patient's permission or *informed consent*. This means that the patient must know and agree to what you plan to do before you start. Consent may be withdrawn at any time. For example, you are assigned to give a patient a warm foot soak. Despite your explanation of the reasons for the order, the patient refuses. You may not force the patient to submit. To do so would make you guilty of battery. To threaten the resident by saying that you will get others to assist you if the resident refuses is to be guilty of assault. Either situation could make you liable for legal charges.

Always inform the resident of what you plan to do before beginning. Make certain that the resident understands. Don't rush into procedures, but allow time for the resident to ask questions. If the resident refuses the treatment, report the fact to the supervisor. Make sure you document the facts. Remember that you may not carry out a treatment against the resident's wishes.

Invasion of Privacy

Residents have a right to have their person and personal affairs kept confidential (private). To do otherwise is an invasion of privacy. Invading the privacy of another is against the law. The care giver should protect the resident's privacy at all times. When giving care, keep the resident's body covered as much as possible, with curtains drawn. Exposing the resident unnecessarily is an invasion of the resident's privacy. Common courtesy can often guide your actions. Knock before entering a room, figure 13-3. Do not eavesdrop when residents are with their visitors or when they are on the phone. Keep personal information about the residents and their activities private. Respect the residents' personal beliefs or views.

Abuse

Abuse of a resident makes you liable for legal prosecution. This means that you must report incidents of abuse by others or you can be held equally responsible for abusing the resident yourself.

Abuse can occur in several forms—physical, verbal, and psychological. Physical abuse does actual physical harm to the resident. This could occur if you handle a resident too roughly or perform the incorrect treatment on the resident. You must never hit or push or pinch the resident. The resident's need for food, water, and proper hygiene must not be neglected. To do so would make you guilty of physical abuse. Likewise, neglecting to turn the resident often or failing to carry out range-of-motion exercises would also be considered abuse. This is true because, in each situation, the resident is harmed in some physical way.

Verbal abuse may be directed toward the resident or may be expressed about the resident. If you use profanity or raise your voice in anger at the resident, if you call the resident unpleasant names, or if you tease the resident unkindly, you are verbally abusive. To call a person "pops" is degrading and abusive.

Psychological abuse occurs when you make the resident fearful of you. You do this when you threaten the resident with harm or threaten to tell something to others that the resident doesn't want known. It is psychologically abusive to make fun of or to belittle the resident in any way.

You must never abuse any resident. If you suspect that a person in your care is being abused by others, you should discuss the matter with your supervisor. Laws require that a health care provider who suspects abuse must report the situation so that the resident can be protected.

Anyone can be abused. But children and the very old are the most vulnerable. Usually, it is the health care provider or a family member who is responsible for the abuse.

It may be difficult to understand why anyone would abuse another who is weak or infirm. But it happens all too often. A few people may take satisfaction in feeling that they have control of others. Most abuse, however, probably arises out of feelings of frustration or fatigue.

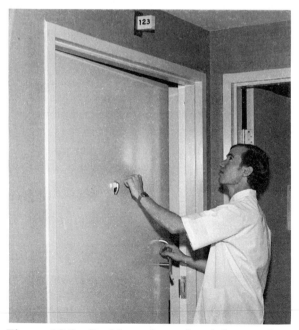

Figure 13-3 Residents have the right to privacy. Always knock before entering the room.

If you feel your tolerance level is being tested, you need to find ways to safeguard the resident and release your own stress. You might try to identify the exact cause of your irritation. You could talk to your supervisor about your feelings. Consider asking to be temporarily assigned to another resident. Try to reduce your overall stress and fatigue so you can bring a more positive, patient attitude to your job.

Legal Assistance

Sometimes residents wish to make a will or alter a current will. It is unwise for the health care provider to participate in this action in any way. Refer the matter to the supervisor who can make the appropriate arrangements for legal assistance.

Writing a will is a legal matter that you are not qualified to handle. Signing a will as a witness can lead to legal complications and should also be avoided.

There are legal aspects to everyday living as well as to every job. As a citizen, you do not have problems if you obey the law. As a geriatric health care provider, you will not have problems if you follow the policies and procedures outlined in the procedure manual for the facility in which you work. Perform only the procedures that you have been taught. Know the lines of authority. That is, know to whom you are responsible. Remember that in all situations, you are ultimately responsible for your own actions and their consequences.

Patient/Resident Rights

Each person being cared for has legal rights, called patient rights, based on laws that regulate the facility and the health care providers. The Patient's Bill of Rights is a document developed by the American Hospital Association. It spells out those rights that a patient can expect. It, or a similar document, figure 13-4, is given to and discussed with a prospective client before he or she is admitted to a facility. It is also posted clearly for all patients or residents to review.

Among these rights are the assurance that care will be given properly, privacy will be respected, and there will be no abuse. Residents will also be treated as respected individuals, capable of handling their own affairs and making their own decisions.

In addition, residents have the right to have their bill explained to them, even if the expenses are covered by a third party. They have the right to know the names of all the people who provide care. As long as residents are mentally competent, they have the right to refuse treatment.

In some states, following the Patient's Bill of Rights is mandated by law. In other states, the Patient's Bill of Rights must be followed before payment is made.

In addition to the Patient's Bill of Rights, each facility that is licensed for care is governed by specific policies and procedures designed to ensure a standard of care for each person. Following legal and ethical standards ensures the residents' rights and well-being.

Summary

- There are legal aspects to everyday living, as well as in carrying out every job.
- As a citizen, you do not have problems if you obey the law.
- As a geriatric health care provider, you will be legally secure if you follow the legal laws and facility policies.
- Patients have rights. Although they may not be legally binding in every state, they are generally accepted as being reasonable and right and should be kept in mind.
- Remember, in all situations, that you are ultimately responsible for your own actions.

87144. Personal Rights

(a) Each resident shall have personal rights which include, but are not limited to, the following:

(1) To be accorded dignity in his/her personal relationships with staff, residents, and other persons.

(2) To be accorded safe, healthful and comfortable accommodations, furnishings and equipment.

(3) To be free from corporal or unusual punishment, humiliation, intimidation, mental abuse, or other actions of a punitive nature, such as withholding of monetary allowances or interfering with daily living functions such as eating or sleeping patterns or elimination.

(4) To be informed by the licensee of the provisions of law regarding complaints and of procedures to confidentially register complaints, including, but not limited to, the address and telephone number of the complaint receiving unit of the licensing agency.

(5) To have the freedom of attending religious services or activities of his/her choice and to have visits from the spiritual advisor of his/her choice. Attendance at religious services, either in or outside the facility, shall be on a completely voluntary basis.

(6) To leave or depart the facility at any time and to not be locked into any room, building, or on facility premises by day or night. This does not prohibit the establishment of house rules, such as the locking of doors at night, for the protection of residents; nor does it prohibit, with permission of the licensing agency, the barring of windows against intruders.

(7) To visit the facility prior to residence along with his/her family and responsible persons.

(8) To have his/her family or responsible persons regularly informed by the facility of activities related to his care or services including ongoing evaluations, as appropriate to the resident's needs.

(9) To have communications to the facility from his/her family and responsible persons answered promptly and appropriately.

(10) To have his/her visitors, including ombudspersons and advocacy representatives, visit privately during reasonable hours but without prior notice, provided that the rights of other residents are not infringed upon.

(11) To wear his/her own clothes; to keep and use his/her own personal possessions, including his/her toilet articles; and to keep and be allowed to spend his/her own money.

(12) To have access to individual storage space for private use.

(13) To have reasonable access to telephones, to both make and receive confidential calls. The licensee may require reimbursements for long distance calls.

(14) To mail and receive unopened correspondence.

(15) To receive or reject medical care, or other services.

(16) To receive assistance in exercising the right to vote.

(17) To move from the facility.

(b) All persons accepted to facilities, or their responsible persons, shall be personally advised and given a copy of these rights at admission. The licensee shall have all residents or their responsible persons sign a copy of these rights and the signed copy shall be included in the resident's record.

(c) Facilities licensed for seven (7) or more shall prominently post, in areas accessible to the residents and their relatives, the following:

(1) Procedures for filing confidential complaints.

(2) A copy of these rights or, in lieu of a posted copy, instructions on how to obtain additional copies of these rights.

(d) The information in (c) above shall be posted in English, and in facilities where a significant portion of the residents cannot read English, in the language they can read.

NOTE: Authority cited: Section 1530, Health and Safety Code. Reference: Sections 1501, 1530, and 1531, Health and Safety Code.

Figure 13-4 Patient bill of rights (From Hegner & Caldwell, *Assisting in Long-Term Care*, copyright 1988 by Delmar Publishers Inc.)

Review Outline

   I. Behavioral Objectives

  II. Vocabulary

 III. Patient's Bill of Rights

   A. Developed by American Hospital Association
   B. Spells out patients' rights

 IV. Facility Policies to Protect Patients

  V. Health Care Provider Responsibilities

   A. Expected to perform in specific ways
   B. Failure can result in charges of
       1. Negligence
       2. Malpractice
       3. False imprisonment
       4. Defamation
       5. Assault and battery
       6. Invasion of privacy
       7. Abuse
   C. Honesty and integrity essential
   D. Does not provide legal assistance

Review

   I. Vocabulary

Match column I and column II

Column I	Column II
1. Abuse	a. Failure to give expected care
2. Liable	b. Injury to the reputation of another by making false statements
3. Aiding and abetting	c. Any action that harms others who cannot protect themselves
4. Laws	d. Legal rules
5. Negligence	e. Assisting others in illegal acts
6. Defamation	f. Legally responsible
7. Assault	g. Intentionally attempting to touch the body of another or threatening to do so
	h. Moral code of behavior

II. True or False

1. Patients/residents have the right to considerate care.
2. Patients/residents do not have the right to know their diagnosis because this might upset them.
3. Patients/residents must consent to all care given.
4. Patients/residents may refuse any treatment as long as they are mentally competent.
5. Patients/residents do not have the right to have their bills explained when a third party, such as an insurance company, is responsible for payment.
6. The patient/resident has the right to private communication.
7. The patient/resident has the right to know the names of all people involved in his or her care.
8. The patient/resident has the right to be treated with respect.
9. The patient's Bill of Rights is a standardized document that is legally mandated by all states.
10. The patient/resident has the right to know the facility rules and how they apply to him or her as a patient/resident.

III. Complete each statement.

1. When a person fails to carry out his or her job conscientiously and, as a result, a resident is injured, that person is guilty of _____.
2. Taking something that doesn't belong to you makes you guilty of _____.
3. Standards are important because they serve as _____ _____practice can be measured.
4. When laws are not obeyed, the person not following the law may be held _____.
5. If you prevent a resident from leaving the facility, without a physician's order, you may be guilty of _____.

IV. Clinical Situations

1. You notice another worker taking a patient's wallet. What should your response be?
2. A resident says that she has insurance coverage, but doesn't understand all of the charges that are being made. What should your response be?

Unit 14
Philosophy of Care and Rehabilitation

Objectives

After studying this unit, you should be able to:

- List ways to assist the elderly in rehabilitation.
- Assist a team in planning rehabilitation goals.
- Explain the rehabilitation philosophy.
- List special considerations for proper rehabilitation of the elderly.

Vocabulary

Learn the meaning and spelling of the following words or phrases.

ankylosing	occupational therapist
comatose	physiatrist
contractures	physical therapist
disability	prosthesis
hemiparalysis	recreational therapist
hemiparesis	rehabilitation
hemiplegia	

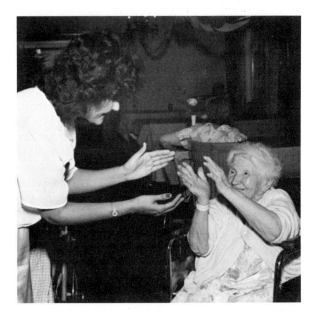

A philosophy is a system of guiding principles. The modern philosophy of *rehabilitation* holds that most patients have the potential for some degree of improved functioning. The conscientious health care provider looks for an increase in self-reliance in every patient seen. This is true whether the patient is in the hospital, a rehabilitation center, an extended care facility, or the home setting.

Rehabilitation must be viewed not as a separate activity but as part of everyday, basic health care, figure 14-1. There is no special time during the patient's illness when rehabilitation must begin or end. The earlier it can begin, the greater the chance of success. When rehabilitation is a routine consideration, preventative measures can be instituted early. These make restoration easier.

Sometimes the emphasis of rehabilitation is on physical improvement. But true rehabilitation also considers social and emotional adaptations and adjustments.

Preventative Measures

Progressive rehabilitation begins by preventing further deterioration of the patient's condition. Frequent position changes are essential to stimulate circulation and prevent pressure

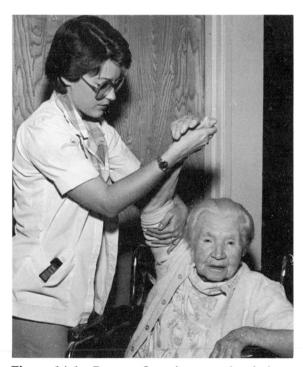

Figure 14-1   Range-of-motion exercises help to prevent further deterioration of the resident's overall condition.

areas. Maintaining proper alignment and applying appropriate range-of-motion exercises help prevent *contractures* (permanent shortening of muscles) and loss of joint activity from *ankylosing* (immobilization).

Encouraging the patient to be out of bed as much as possible and to carry on as many personal activities as possible builds self-confidence. It also lays the groundwork for specific rehabilitation. The longer that patients remain in bed and in a dependent state, the more they lose initiative and the harder it is to motivate them.

Rehabilitation Goals

The ultimate goals of any rehabilitation program are more independence in functional activities, a greater degree of personal usefulness, and increased social relatedness. For the elderly person crippled with arthritis, these goals may be expressed specifically in terms of learning to manage some personal activities of daily living, figure 14-2, and becoming a more cheerful person. Limited goals? Yes, perhaps, but they are important in the life of the individual. Even these are long-range goals for some. These goals can be reached only by slow, step-by-step movement toward such short-term goals as self-feeding or bathing.

Goals are highly individualized. They must take into account all of the patient's limitations, potential for rehabilitation, and readiness to participate. Realistic goals must be devised and frequently reevaluated. Basic goals are recovery of self-feeding and continence, independence in bathing and dressing, and some ability in transfer and mobility activities. In other words, they involve independence in carrying out the activities of daily living. Special rehabilitative needs and the planned therapy and care are details in the nursing care plan. Each staff member must be familiar with the plan for each individual patient and follow it consistently. Frequent consultation is needed to bring assessment of progress and adjustment in the plans in line with current status.

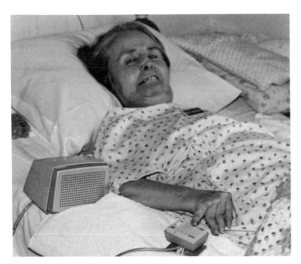

Figure 14-2 Equipment can sometimes be modified to meet unique patient needs, as in this case with the telephone and call bell.

Geriatric health care providers are in the unique position of working with the patient or resident daily. As a result, the geriatric health care provider can often make a valuable contribution to the process. The patient or resident may never have to leave the facility to benefit from rehabilitation efforts.

The elderly have complex health needs. Rehabilitation plans must be made accordingly, figure 14-3. For example, one goal for an elderly person might be to develop muscles that will permit greater wheelchair mobility. At the same time, staff members must consider that increased exercise might place too much stress on the patient's congestive heart condition.

Goals may first be perceived by the professional. But these goals cannot be met unless the patient perceives them as well and believes that they are worthwhile and achievable. Patients need to be actively involved, to the limit of their capabilities, in the selection of pertinent goals. Family members, too, may be asked to join the goal-setting team.

The patient's self-concept greatly affects the success or failure of a rehabilitative program. Many older people have gradually withdrawn

from social contacts and acts of independence. This is particularly true of the person who is institutionalized or lives alone. It is a sad fact that those who give care in institutions are largely responsible for this depersonalization. Often the staff believes it is quicker and easier to meet basic geriatric needs than it is to encourage self-care and self-expression. Dependence is fostered and independence discouraged. Unless patients see themselves as persons of value and worth, however, cooperative planning is not possible.

The first steps, then, in the rehabilitative process are to maintain or restore self-esteem and to determine how the patient views himself or herself and any specific disability. A *disability* (limitation) may be a challenge or a handicap, depending upon the patient's/resident's point of view. A positive relationship between health care provider and patient serves as the foundation from which inspiration, encouragement, and motivation arise. The nurse is in the best position to assess rehabilitation possibilities and to know when the patient is ready to participate in self-rehabilitation. The nurse will also benefit from information provided by other staff members who give care to the patient.

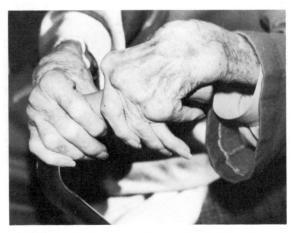

Figure 14-3 For a patient crippled by chronic arthritis, use of the hands becomes a frustrating experience.

Rehabilitation Centers and Teams

Rehabilitative services are offered through centers. Some of these centers specialize in specific types of rehabilitation. Such units are frequently part of large metropolitan hospitals or are associated with medical centers, figure 14-4. Others are operated by private, independent agencies. Skilled-nursing facilities emphasize rehabilitation services.

Rehabilitative services are directed by a team of professional people who work together to establish and reach realistic goals. At times, the team will consist of members from many disciplines. These may include medicine, recreational therapy, occupational therapy, psychotherapy, physiotherapy, social service, and nursing. The nurse often coordinates the combined effort. At other times, the nurse, doctor, and a few specialists make up the team. With a team approach, each team member sees the patient from a slightly different viewpoint. From the consensus, a specific rehabilitation plan is devised and recorded on the patient care plan.

Patients hospitalized in institutions with rehabilitation units can take advantage of these services. Many other patients utilize them on an outpatient basis. Outside of the centers, rehabilitative planning and services are provided by the physician, family, and public health nurse. The home health aide plays an important role in the rehabilitation of the home patient. He or she supplies encouragement and assists in therapy as directed. In all cases, patients/residents should be encouraged to demonstrate as much independence in self-care activities as is compatible with and safe for their specific conditions.

Special Geriatric Needs

Motivation is of prime importance in the rehabilitation process. Motivating the elderly patient may be especially difficult, however. Great skill, imagination, and ingenuity may be needed to help older people care enough about the future to make the necessary effort. Building their self-esteem is an obvious beginning, but it is only a beginning. Established goals need to be relevant, not remote. Patients need to experience success. They must be constantly encouraged and supported. They need to be led, not pushed, to greater independence. The elderly are less amenable to change than younger patients, and they will actively resist too much pressure. The young are inexperienced. They are more willing to take risks than are the elderly, whose experi-

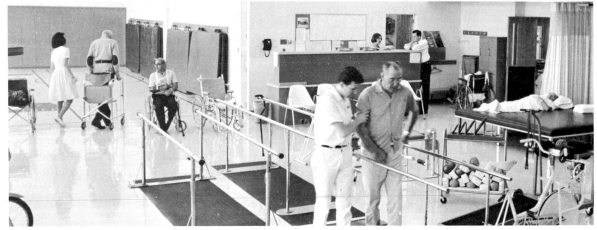

Figure 14-4 A rehabilitation unit associated with a large medical center offers a wide range of rehabilitation services.

ences warn them of possible consequences. The elderly also lack the energy to meet unrealistic expectations.

The health care provider's supportive role is essential. A positive, hopeful attitude can be the most important factor in motivating the patient to keep trying. Perhaps the most difficult task is knowing when to offer assistance and when to stand back, offering only moral support. Initial attempts at self-care are apt to be ineffectual and cause the patient embarrassment. The perceptive health care provider will ensure privacy, accept and minimize mishaps, and praise successes. The elderly have less self-confidence than do the young. Therefore, they need more encouragement. They need to be constantly reassured that the effort is worthwhile and that they are worth the effort. Family support is often negligible or missing altogether. The more consistent the staff is about sustaining the effort, the more the resident will cooperate and respond. Apathy, depression, and resignation keep some elderly people from making even a token response. The health care provider, in constant contact with them, can offer the continuous support and encouragement needed to stimulate a positive response. He or she can help them see tasks through to completion.

Patient fatigue is another important factor in geriatric rehabilitation. Aging in itself robs a person of stamina and energy. Chronic illness drains the remaining reserves. The elderly need time to learn or relearn and to practice rehabilitative skills. They must space their efforts with rest periods.

Any aids that can decrease the amount of energy the elderly patient must expend on a specific task should be used. For example, transfer activities are easier if the height of the bed can be adjusted and an overbed trapeze is in place. Overbed scales and mechanical lifts conserve the resident's energy. Moving from wheelchair to toilet is facilitated when grab bars and raised toilets are available. The patient feels a sense of security if a safety belt is in place as attempts are made to walk. Support equipment such as canes and walkers need to be readily available and in good repair. Safety belts can offer support and stability.

The goals of rehabilitation are, of necessity, limited. Setting goals for a level of rehabilitation that can be achieved only after years of effort is unrealistic for a person whose life expectancy is short. The more practical approach is to seek improvement in those areas that are likely to produce immediate benefits and satisfaction. It is difficult for the older person to see minor improvements or even to find value in some of the short-term goals. But any advance that is noticed and finds approval brings about a corresponding improvement in the patient's morale, emotional response, and willingness to keep trying.

Social Rehabilitation

Health care providers must treat all patients with respect and refuse to allow them to think of themselves as helpless and hopeless. This is the first step in social rehabilitation. The nursing staff can influence the social environment, encouraging the social contacts between patients. This will strengthen morale and a sense of identity, figure 14-5. The elderly need to interact with others even if participation must be limited. A person does not have to have full use of his or her arms and legs to enjoy music and conversation, to read, or to watch television with others. Even the way that beds or wheelchairs are arranged can increase opportunities for social rehabilitation, figure 14-6. Sometimes resocialization is the first step in the rehabilitation process. It gives the individual a reason to want to enter more fully into the entire rehabilitation program.

The Stroke Patient

Rehabilitation following a stroke (C.V.A.) may be a prolonged process. Strokes often leave patients both physically and intellectually impaired. Patients may have few usable communication skills. Motor loss may range from total *hemiparalysis* (paralysis of one side of the body) to partial loss of function in an arm or leg *(hemiparesis)*. Reflexes such as swallowing and bowel and bladder control may also be lost.

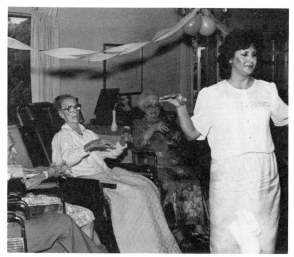

Figure 14-5 A day room offers a place for social exchange and rehabilitation.

When a patient is admitted to an acute care facility, he or she may be *comatose* (unconscious) and in danger of death. Even during this early critical phase, rehabilitative efforts can begin. Range-of-motion exercises are carried out and the staff attempts to establish a line of communication with the victim.

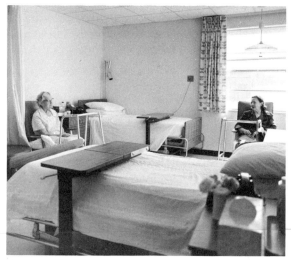

Figure 14-6 Bed arrangement encourages conversation.

Rehabilitation efforts increase in intensity as the patient begins to recover. Occupational therapy directed toward small muscle motor control, physical therapy planned to improve mobility, and speech therapy are introduced. All disciplines, with the continuous support of nursing care, begin to move the patient toward an optimum level of self-sufficiency.

When acute care is no longer needed, the patient may be transferred to a skilled-nursing facility. In this facility, rehabilitation is paramount and the patient is helped to reach optimum functional ability. Reaching this point, the patient may be discharged to home or transferred to an extended care facility. Whether at home or in an extended care facility, a patient's rehabilitative goals must continue to be pursued.

This process may have taken many months of effort. Understandably, patients and staff will both face moments of depression during this time. Some facilities provide sources of psychological support for both patients and health care providers. This is a valuable service that can mean the difference between success and failure. The staff must be alert to signs that the limit of physical capacity has been reached. They must not push patients beyond that limit. Dyspnea, dizziness, color or pulse changes, or complaints of pain should not go unheeded. Despite the devastating effects of stroke, many patients are able to regain a good measure of independence.

The Heart Attack Patient

After a heart attack, a patient is often fearful of undertaking any activity that is believed might provoke another attack. These patients tend to be depressed, believing that they will have to cut back their activities severely.

For a period of time activity will be limited, especially if cardiac bypass surgery was needed. Recuperation only takes a few weeks, however. During this time, the patient is put on a regime of gradually increased activity. Diet, weight, and blood clotting levels are controlled, and the patient is discharged to home.

Once home, fears do not automatically cease. An especially troublesome area is that of participation in sexual activity. Both partners may fear that coitus will precipitate another attack. Professional counseling can help to alleviate this concern. Studies show that sexual intercourse is no more demanding than climbing two flights of stairs. Furthermore, position during coitus plays a role in the amount of energy required. Adjustments in position can reduce the effort for the convalescing partner.

Activity in all areas is gradually increased. Most people return to something close to their former life-style. It is true that a number of patients succumb to a subsequent heart attack. But this is due more to the nature of the disease processes that led to the original heart attack than to a resumption of the activities of daily living.

The Prolonged Hospital Stay

Today, prolonged hospitalization results from a serious illness that requires acute care. Patients who are not acutely ill are transferred rapidly to other facilities. The very seriousness of a health problem such as cancer or the need to have a breast or limb amputated fosters a sense of dependency in the patient.

Rehabilitative efforts to promote independence must be started early. Three patient goals are sought. The first is to adjust to a change in body image. The second is to learn the use and care of supportive equipment. The last goal is to believe that independence in activities of daily living is both possible and preferable to being dependent on others. It is sometimes the most difficult goal to achieve.

Adjusting to an altered body image such as the loss of a breast or leg is difficult at any age. But it is particularly hard for the elderly, who may already be having trouble adjusting to the changes that age alone brings about. Great caring is needed to reassure older people that their essence has not been lost and is no less dear.

Learning to apply a *prosthesis* (artificial part), or use and care for equipment when eyesight is poor and hands tremble, is not an easy task. Some older people initially reject the whole idea. They refuse to look at the surgery or attempt self-care. A great deal of judgment is needed to know when and when not to intervene in the process, when to carry out the procedure and when to stand back and wait. This kind of judgment will come with experience.

Gradually, patients can be motivated to adopt a more independent state of mind. Patience, experience, and sincere caring are the key elements of success. In each special rehabilitation situation, the informed, empathetic geriatric health care provider plays a vital role. He or she offers support and encouragement, minimizes failures, and praises successes.

Summary

- Rehabilitation, as it relates to the older resident, recognizes special needs.
- Positive attitudes enable the health care provider to give the instruction and support needed to meet these needs.
- Rehabilitation goals must be established in cooperation with the resident. These goals must take into account individual handicaps and potential.
- Goals must be realistic.
- The older person can be encouraged, but never pushed toward their goals.
- Rehabilitation must consider the needs of the total individual although restoration of a specific function may be stressed.
- The success or failure of a rehabilitation program depends in large degree upon the health care provider's attitude. It also depends on the resident's self-confidence and his or her confidence in the health care provider.

- Most residents are capable of some degree of increased self-reliance, even when a specific program is not planned.
- Rehabilitation potential must be sought in all residents. Some rehabilitation goals must be incorporated in the resident's health care plan.
- Rehabilitation is most successful when there is opportunity for continuity of resident care.

Review Outline

    I.   Behavioral Objectives

   II.   Vocabulary

  III.   Philosophy of Rehabilitation

        A.   Increased self-reliance
        B.   Part of basic health care
        C.   Must begin early
        D.   Prevention of further loss
            1.   Maintain alignment
            2.   Remain mobile
        E.   Consideration of emotional and social factors

  IV.   Rehabilitation Goals

        A.   Part of large hospitals
        B.   Associated with medical centers
        C.   Programs planned by teams
            1.   Nurse coordinator
            2.   Recreational therapists
            3.   Occupational therapists
            4.   Psychotherapists
            5.   Physiotherapists
            6.   Social therapists
            7.   Medical therapists

  VI.   Special Geriatric Needs

        A.   Motivation
        B.   Immediate goals
        C.   Support
        D.   Energy conservation measures
        E.   Resocialization

 VII.   Major Conditions Requiring Rehabilitation

        A.   Cerebral vascular accidents
        B.   Heart attacks

Vocabulary

I. Vocabulary

Find as many words as you can from the vocabulary list. Circle each word in the puzzle below and write it and its definition.

I	L	C	M	E	P	H	G	R	L	C	O	E	M	J	S	S
A	E	N	V	L	D	Q	U	A	L	K	G	P	C	S	I	C
K	W	G	B	Q	U	C	I	O	I	B	F	O	N	S	H	A
P	N	N	K	J	R	N	U	D	N	X	N	J	Y	L	Y	O
P	R	O	S	T	H	E	S	I	S	T	H	L	G	S	E	W
M	N	E	I	B	M	J	D	P	R	G	A	P	C	K	I	H
D	O	Q	L	T	G	A	M	A	E	R	K	B	O	N	B	D
I	A	H	C	O	A	K	C	F	A	D	N	A	N	E	W	M
S	J	Q	F	L	H	T	C	P	C	O	M	A	T	O	S	E
A	N	K	Y	L	O	S	I	N	G	B	J	E	R	H	A	T
B	X	A	E	R	P	M	P	L	K	Z	N	L	A	W	O	I
I	D	V	C	G	E	F	A	Y	I	A	P	K	C	L	F	B
L	R	I	M	H	Q	U	I	E	N	B	Q	F	T	T	E	H
I	B	T	D	I	H	L	C	V	M	Q	A	X	U	P	W	G
T	M	Z	P	T	A	W	Z	L	D	H	X	N	R	R	Y	B
Y	O	A	I	K	O	E	P	X	T	Y	Q	U	E	Z	T	U
K	C	J	N	D	I	L	B	R	G	M	D	I	S	R	O	M

II. True or False

1. The philosophy of rehabilitation holds that all patients are capable of improved function.
2. Long-term goals are more readily accepted by the elderly than they are by younger persons.
3. One aspect of rehabilitation aims to prevent further deterioration of the patient's condition.
4. Patients must be ready both emotionally and physically if rehabilitation is to be successful.
5. The professional team establishes rehabilitation goals for the patient.
6. The resident's self-image has little influence on the success or failure of a rehabilitation program.
7. One of the health care providers most important contributions to the rehabilitative effort is to motivate the resident.
8. Rehabilitation centers are often associated with smaller hospitals in rural settings.
9. A feeling of self-worth is important to the rehabilitative process.
10. A disability may be a handicap or a challenge, depending upon the person's attitude.

III. Short Answers

1. List four ways that elderly residents differ from younger patients with rehabilitative needs.

2. Describe the health care provider's role in the rehabilitation of the elderly person.
3. List the three ultimate goals of rehabilitation.

IV. Clinical Situations

1. You find a resident struggling to put on her artificial leg. What do you do?
2. A resident complains of pain when you carry out range-of-motion exercises on his shoulder. What do you do?

Unit 15
Safety Considerations

Objectives

After studying this unit, you should be able to:

- List intrinsic and extrinsic factors that contribute to accidents.
- Describe health care provider actions that can contribute to or prevent accidents.
- Explain the principles of infection control.

Vocabulary

Learn the meaning and spelling of the following words or phrases.

asepsis	IV standards
antiseptic	medical asepsis
autoclave	nosocomial
concurrent cleaning	pathogenic organisms
contaminated	postural restraints
disinfection	proprioception
disposable	sharps
exudate	sterile
fomites	sterilization
incident	terminal cleaning
isolation technique	

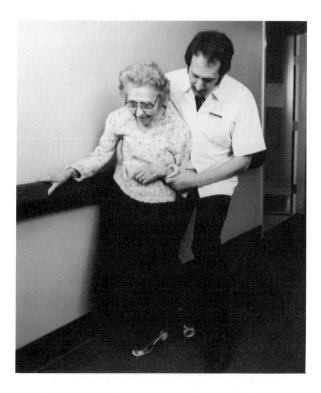

Safety is the concern both of the elderly person and of those responsible for that person's health care. Some older people neglect simple safety precautions because they do not understand their importance. Others more actively resist any suggestion that safety precautions are needed. For example, one seventy-eight-year-old woman became indignant when a nurse suggested that shoes with broad, low heels would give her better balance. The patient had always worn stylishly high-heeled shoes. She fully intended to continue wearing such shoes, even though she was recovering from a fractured hip. Some older people may deny the need for safety. To do otherwise would be to admit that they are no longer as independent and sure of themselves as they used to be.

Constant vigilance is needed to safeguard the elderly both at home and in patient care facilities. Responsible people must continually assess situations for potential hazards. They must then see that these threats are controlled or eliminated. As they carry on their work, geriatric health care providers must adopt safety practices that protect their own health as well as that of the patients.

Causes of Accidents

The facts of an accident do not necessarily explain the cause. Intrinsic or extrinsic factors may be at fault. Usually, it is a combination of factors that leads to an accident.

Intrinsic Factors

Intrinsic factors are those within the patient. Cerebral ischemia or temporary hypoglycemia, often found in the elderly, can cause momentary dizziness. Tremors may be present, resulting in loss of balance and a fall.

An older person may have difficulty maintaining equilibrium during postural changes. The person may bend over to pick something up and lose balance when quickly straightening up, figure 15-1. Changing too rapidly from a sitting to a standing position can also cause the older person to lose equilibrium. This sensitivity to rapid postural change can be seen when an elderly person who has been in a supine position on the examining table is raised too quickly to a sitting position. It also occurs when a resident who has been sleeping in a dorsal, recumbent position is raised too rapidly for morning care. Dizziness and momentary nausea are often experienced under these circumstances.

Position changes should always be made slowly. They should provide sufficient time for the older person to gain equilibrium. Elderly patients should not be left alone immediately following a postural change.

Decreased visual acuity is another intrinsic condition that affects safety. When a person sees well, objects such as slippers on the floor or loose electric cords are easy to avoid. For the elderly

person, such objects can be hazardous. Visual faults also interfere with depth perception. An elderly person is apt to misjudge distances. When bending over or leaning forward, he or she may topple and receive a head injury. Once a fall is started, reactions are often too slow to prevent it. Increased reflex time and decreased *proprioception* (reception of internal stimuli) are thus also intrinsic factors related to accidents.

For many, confusion and forgetfulness, which create hazardous conditions, are intrinsic factors. When confusion is present, the simplest activities can threaten safety. General confusion requires constant supervision. But temporary confused periods, such as those that occur on awakening or when there is a change in environment, are apt to go unnoticed until tragedy occurs. Untoward reaction to drugs or drug interactions can also lead to confusion. Gas burners turned on but not lit, food left to burn and start fires, and medication taken in error are only a few examples of the many possible accidents that can occur. In patient care facilities, a confused patient may attempt to come to the assistance of another and be met with impatience and irritability. Injury can result as a tug-of-war ensues. The geriatric health care provider must be aware of the possibility of this type of accident and be prepared to intervene when necessary.

Extrinsic Factors

Extrinsic factors, or outside influences, are responsible for a variety of accidents. Some examples are changes in furniture locations without warning, unlighted hallways, inadequately identified medicines, and accumulated trash. These may all contribute to serious accidents.

Types of Accidents

Persons aged sixty-five and over make up more than 11 percent of the population. But they account for 28 percent of all accidental deaths and 13 percent of all hospitalized accident victims. There can be no question that, when past sixty-five, a person is far more prone to accidents. As a result of accidents, the elderly often

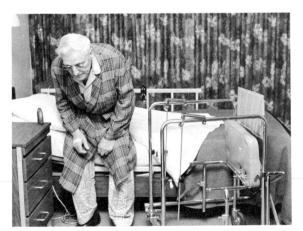

Figure 15-1 Loss of balance is a common cause of falls.

face long-term rehabilitation and even death. Falls are a major contributor to accidental injury.

Falls

Falls account for three-quarters of all accidental fatalities among people over sixty-five. Falls at home are usually the result of tripping, slipping, climbing, or reaching for inconveniently placed items.

Shoes are frequently the source of problems. Well-fitting shoes with broad, low heels offer the most support. Sore feet and foot problems cause many older people to resort to the immediate comfort of bedroom slippers. Unfortunately, most slippers have soft soles, fit loosely, and offer no support. Proper shoes are no solution unless they fit securely on the feet, the heels are not allowed to run down, and shoelaces are tied, figure 15-2. Bending down to adjust the

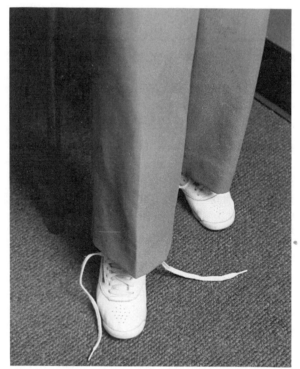

Figure 15-2 An untied shoelace is a threat to safe ambulation.

laces can be a difficult task. Nylon elastic shoelaces are convenient, but they cause problems for those suffering from peripheral vascular disease. Anything that constricts interferes with an already compromised circulation. Extra-long shoe horns make it easier to put on shoes.

Seniors may trip when clothing, such as a loose robe, is too long. This problem is easily solved by shortening the garment to ankle length. Toys or other items left in walk areas are often tripped over. Even doorsills can be perilous. Walk areas should be kept clear. Whenever possible, doorsills should be removed. Cords of any kind should be secured to baseboards, not left loose. Running them over doorframes rather than across rugs decreases the possibility of tripping.

Homes where the elderly must climb stairs are especially hazardous. Narrow or high steps are difficult for them to navigate. A toe can easily catch on loose carpeting, causing a nasty fall. Several things can be done to increase the safety of stairways. All carpeting can be secured. Any that is worn and threadbare should be replaced. The top and bottom steps can be painted to alert the elderly person to their presence. A railing can be provided and kept in good repair, figure 15-3, as many elderly people will lean heavily upon it. Lights that can be operated from both the top and bottom of the stairs are helpful. If possible, the light should shine at floor level. Stairways must be kept free of litter.

Handrails along corridors and grab bars near the toilet and bathtub, figure 15-4, are safety factors, if strategically placed. A variety of handrails and grab bars are produced commercially. Satisfactory ones can also be made by a home carpenter. The chief consideration is that they be securely fastened to the wall and be the right height. A dim light left on in passageways and in the room of the older person at all times is not expensive. It can prove of great benefit.

Falls are often the result of slipping. Floors can be made to shine with no-slip wax. Otherwise, highly polished waxed floors can be dangerous. Loose scatter rugs should be elimin-

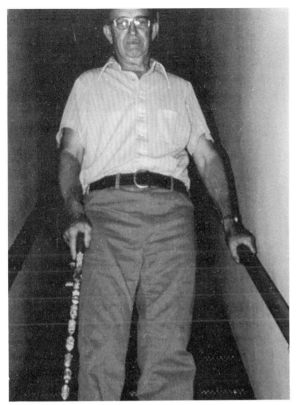

Figure 15-3 Handrails are helpful in maintaining balance when walking or going up or down stairs.

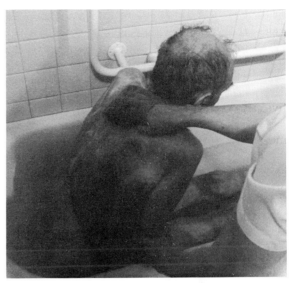

Figure 15-4 Grab bars can prevent serious injury.

ated. Spills of any kind should be wiped up immediately, figure 15-5. Even small spills can be dangerous. The tips of walkers, canes, and crutches should be rubber tipped for traction. Rubber tips are of little value when they become worn and uneven. They should be replaced before they become a danger.

Most falls take place in the bathroom. Place no-slip strips or a rubber mat in the tub or shower. The older person must be cautioned not to use bath oils, because they make the tub even more slippery. A good safe soap container is essential, because soap in a wet tub is a hazard. A shower or bathtub chair is an asset for those who have difficulty getting in and out of the tub, figure 15-6. Commercial shower chairs are avail-

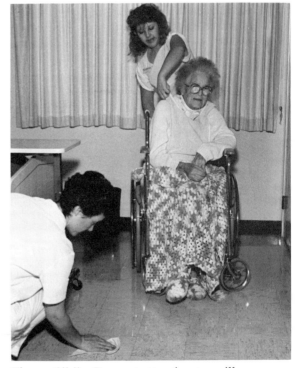

Figure 15-5 Prompt attention to spills can prevent accidents.

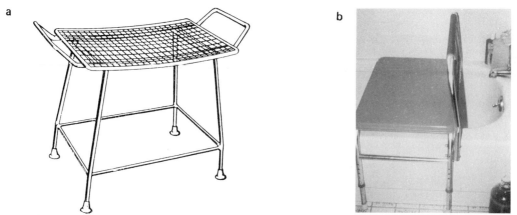

Figure 15-6   The shower bench and bathtub seat are safety items for the elderly.

able, but a regular chair can also be used. Showers with chairs are standard equipment in many patient care facilities. Patients can be easily transferred from a wheelchair to this kind of shower. Patients should never be left alone in a shower or tub without specific instruction to do so.

Raised toilet seats are convenient. They make toileting safer for the older person, figure 15-7. Getting on and off a low toilet can cause an

elderly person to lose balance and fall. Here again, handrails are both convenient and an important safety factor.

For the elderly individual at home who must venture out in bad weather, there are metal attachments for canes that cut into the snow and ice, providing better leverage, and tripod cane tips for better stability, figure 15-8. Walking in ice, rain, or snow is never wise for the elderly.

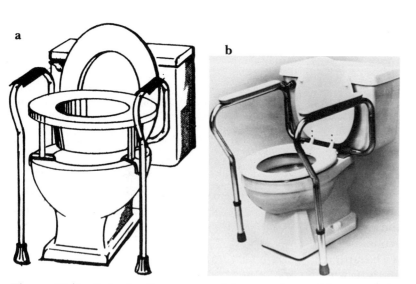

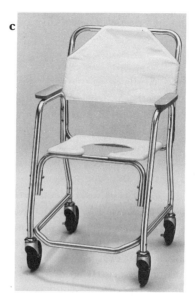

Figure 15-7   Raised toilet seats, grab bars, and portable commodes make toileting easier and safer for the elderly. (Photos courtesy Invacare Corporation)

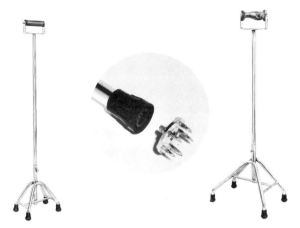

Figure 15-8 Quad canes and adaptable ice grippers are stability aids for the elderly.

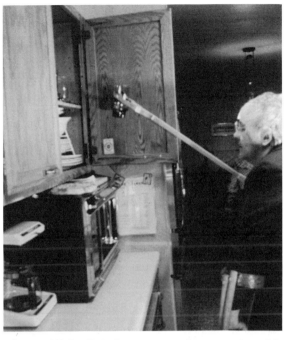

Figure 15-9   Reachers are an inexpensive aid.

When going out cannot be avoided, however, footwear such as rubbers and overshoes should be worn and should fit properly. Salt and gravel should be used on wet or icy walks to provide a better grip.

Beds, chairs, and couches of the proper heights are important if accidents are to be avoided. Furniture should be low enough so that the feet are flat when sitting. However, it should be high enough so that rising to stand is not difficult. Arms on chairs are helpful, and there should be enough room under the chair to put one foot back while rising.

Climbing is a dangerous activity for the older person, whether stepladders, footstools, or chairs are used. Articles should be arranged so that bending and climbing can be avoided. For hard-to-reach articles, the use of tong-like reachers should be encouraged, figure 15-9.

Almost 70 percent of patient-related accidents in care facilities are due to falls. Safety hazards exist in these facilities as well as in the home. Many of the same safety precautions can be applied. For example, lighted hallways, guard rails, and non-slip floors can help prevent injuries. But additional hazards exist in the care setting because of the greater frailty and feebleness of the residents and the types of equipment in use.

In many facilities a nurse will use an instrument called a fall risk factor indicator to assess a new resident. If a resident has a score that indicates the potential for a fall, staff can be more alert and implement more safety measures.

Falls can also be prevented if facility policies are followed exactly. For example, residents are often injured by falls that occur as they try to get out of bed. For this reason, facilities have a fairly uniform policy regarding the height at which beds may be left and the use of side rails.

Beds should be left in the lowest horizontal position when health care providers are not giving care. Side rails should be checked and left securely in place before the resident is left alone. Side rails should be lowered only when beds are in the lowest horizontal position. They should be up at night and whenever the condition of the resident requires their use for protection.

Side rails should never be used to attach tube or intravenous lines or catheters. Raising and lowering the side rails could squeeze or pinch off the tubing and injure the resident.

Equipment-related Injuries

Equipment-related accidents can be prevented by checking for and reporting needed repairs promptly. Used equipment should be disposed of in the proper containers or returned to storage.

Health care providers should check for frayed electrical wires. Electricity should not be misused by overloading electrical circuits, using ungrounded circuits, or using the wrong size electrical cords with equipment.

Most facilities dispose of *"sharps"* such as needles and blades in special containers. Broken glass should not be picked up with the hands. Larger pieces can be picked up with forceps. Smaller pieces can be picked up by moistening several thicknesses of paper towels and gently bringing the edges together so fingers do not touch the fragments.

Injuries sometimes result when the health care staff uses equipment improperly or fails to provide adequate protection and support during its use. There is no justification for this kind of neglect. Staff members must know how to operate equipment, such as resident lifts, gurneys, or wheelchairs, before they use the equipment with residents. Equipment must be kept in safe operating condition. Any malfunctions should be reported at once. In addition, a sign should be placed on the equipment so it will not be used. All facilities have procedures to follow when reporting dangerous conditions or unsafe equipment. Health care providers should learn what they are and follow them when they observe something amiss.

Signal Lights (Call Bells)

The health care provider should always check to see that the signal cord functions and is left within easy reach of the resident's hands. Remember that the signal light is the resident's means of letting others know that there is a problem or need. The health care provider also must ensure that the resident knows how to use the signal to summon help. Residents should be carefully instructed in the use of the signal cord and allowed to demonstrate its use. Residents should also be shown the location of the emergency buttons in each bathroom.

Safety Belts/Supports

Safety belts should be secure when in use. These should be used when the frail elderly are being transferred from bed to chair or commode. They should also be used when support is needed to sit in a chair or to assist in ambulation, figure 15-10.

Supports are used for resident protection. They are frequently used to support the posture while sitting and sometimes while the individual is in bed, figure 15-11. *Postural supports* can be jackets, belts, or straps that help the patient maintain proper body alignment. When used to protect the disoriented resident, there are guidelines that must be followed. A physician's order must be obtained before applying supports/restraints.

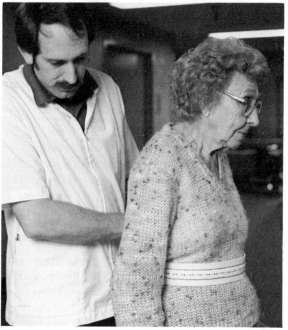

Figure 15-10 The gait belt offers support for the resident who is unsteady when walking.

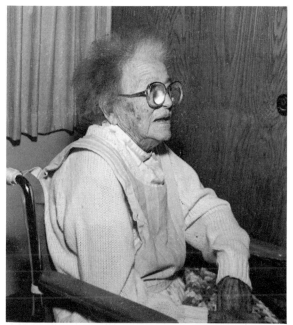

Figure 15-11   Soft restraints or postural supports should only be used to protect the residents or others from injury.

Supports/restraints should be used only after all other methods have been tried. For disoriented residents, having a family member sit with the resident may have a quieting effect and make the use of restraints unnecessary. More often than not, the use of supports/restraints increases the resident's agitation. Struggling against the restraints leads to exhaustion. Even the confused and disoriented resident interprets their use as punishment. Communication decreases as a result.

Because residents are immobilized by restraints, there is an increased risk of pneumonia, stasis of circulation, and skin breakdown. There are times, however, when restraints are the only way to keep a resident from dislodging intravenous injection needles and pulling out tubes. Soft restraints are best. They should be removed as soon as possible. Refer to the checklist in figure 15-12 for the use of supports/restraints. See the following procedure for applying supports/restraints.

Guidelines for Using Postural Supports/Restraints

1. A doctor's order for postural supports is always required. The reason for the order is given in the resident's record.
2. Always be sure there is a doctor's order for a postural support and that the reason is given before you put one on a resident.
3. Never apply a restraint that you have not been taught to use.
4. Even if a resident doesn't understand, always explain why you are putting a postural support on.
5. Check the resident frequently. When you do, talk with her and reassure her.
6. Check the circulation of the part restrained. Leave space for two fingers to slip between the restraint and the skin.
7. Check the resident every 15 minutes for comfort needs, fluids, toileting, eating.
8. Untie the support every two hours and check for irritation or poor circulation.
9. Reposition the resident every one to two hours to prevent skin breakdown.
10. Never tie a support to side rails; always attach it to the frame of the bed, wheelchair, or stretcher.
11. Never tie a support to a chair or bed without wheels. You could not move the resident quickly in an emergency.
12. Use half-bow knot/quick release knot and secure out of the resident's reach.
13. A call bell must always be in easy reach for the resident.
14. It may be necessary to pad the restraints for very thin residents.
15. In the case of an emergency, you may have to cut the restraints with scissors rather than taking the time to untie them.

Figure 15-12   Checklist for the use of supports/restraints. (From Badasch & Chesebro, *Essentials for the Nursing Assistant in Long-Term Care,* copyright 1990 by Delmar Publishers Inc.)

Also refer to figure 15-13 for a checklist of actions that the health care provider must perform at the beginning and end of each procedure involving direct care of the resident. These steps protect the safety and dignity of the resident. They also ensure that the resident knows what procedure is to be done and has the right to refuse treatment.

Beginning Procedure Actions

- Wash your hands.
- Assemble all necessary equipment.
- Knock on door and pause before entering resident's room.
- Politely ask visitors to leave. Tell them where they can wait.
- Identify the resident.
- Provide privacy by drawing curtains around bed and closing door.
- Explain what you will be doing and answer questions.
- Raise bed to comfortable working height.

Procedure Completion Actions

- Position resident comfortably.
- Leave signal cord, telephone, and fresh water where resident can reach them.
- Return bed to lowest horizontal position.
- Raise side rails, if required.
- Perform general safety check of resident and environment.
- Clean used equipment and return to proper storage, according to facility policy.
- Open privacy curtains.
- Wash your hands.
- Tell visitors that they may re-enter the room.
- Report completion of procedure.
- Document procedure following facility policy.

Figure 15-13 Beginning procedure actions and procedure completion actions.

PROCEDURE 1

Applying Postural Supports/Restraints

1. Wash hands.
2. Assemble the support/restraint you will need as specified in the physician's order.
3. Recheck that there is a written order from the physician for the support/restraint.
4. Make sure you have the correct resident by checking the wristband and asking the resident's name. If the resident is confused, verify identity by checking the wristband.
5. Tell the resident what you plan to do and why. Your attitude should be positive and gentle.
6. Remember that the support/restraint is to be used *only* when the resident is in a chair or bed with wheels.
7. If a vest support/restraint is used, make sure the opening is in the *front*.
8. Tie the restraint under the wheelchair out of the resident's reach, or tie it to the frame of the bed.
9. Check the resident for proper positioning. Maintain good body alignment.
10. Pad bony areas under the support/restraint to prevent friction. This is especially important for very thin residents.
11. Use a half-bow or quick release knot to tie the support/restraint to the wheelchair or bed.
12. Make sure that the call bell is within the resident's reach.
13. Check the resident frequently.
14. Remove the restraint at two-hour intervals. Check the skin for signs of irritation. Exercise the restrained limbs to ensure adequate circulation.
15. Report completion of procedure. Record:
    time support/restraint was applied
    type of support/restraint applied
    how resident tolerated procedure

any observations you made during the procedure

Staff Conduct

Your behavior can prevent or contribute to accidents. Remember to walk, never run, within the facility. Never engage in horseplay. Keep to the right of corridors when transporting residents. When transferring a resident in a wheelchair or on a stretcher, always back into rooms and elevators. Support chairs with your foot so they will not slide out from under residents. Always use wheelchair brakes when residents are transferring into and out of the chairs.

Carefully survey the environment for physical hazards such as protruding bed wheels or gatch handles. Put equipment away when no longer needed. Do not permit blankets used to cover residents to touch the floor. Wipe up spills immediately. Make sure there is adequate lighting, especially during evening and twilight hours.

Following procedures as taught and carrying out orders promptly and correctly help assure safe care. Frequent review of the resident care plan is important so that nursing care can be altered to safely provide for resident needs. For example, a resident may be on a soft diet when you go off duty. During the evening, a slight stroke may have left the resident unable to swallow. When you return the next morning, the order may have been changed to nothing by mouth. If you fail to check the updated care plan and attempt to feed the resident a soft diet, a serious choking accident may occur. Many accidents can be avoided if health care providers always follow orders and procedures.

Use proper body mechanics during each activity. Improper use of the body when moving equipment or lifting and transferring residents is another cause of accidental injuries to staff and to residents. The principles of good body mechanics must always be kept in mind when performing these actions. The procedures related to the use of proper body mechanics may be reviewed with your instructor. They are found in Unit 27.

Other Hazards

Fires and Burns

Every year there are news reports of tragic fires in extended care facilities where many lives are lost. Over one-fourth of all deaths from burns occur to those over sixty-five. Many of these fires could have been prevented.

It is the responsibility of all geriatric health care providers to know the fire plans for the agency in which they work. All licensed facilities must have fire control equipment, such as sprinklers and fire extinguishers. Federal and state regulations mandate written plans to be followed to safely evacuate residents in case of a fire. Fire escapes should be clearly marked. Routine fire drills should also be conducted. Fires spread rapidly, and the elderly can do little to help themselves in the confusion. It is up to staff members to execute the plan of action that provides for their escape. All staff members must take the initiative in learning the placement of fire extinguishers and how to use them, figure 15-14. Fire drill procedures should be regularly reviewed in staff meetings, figure 15-15.

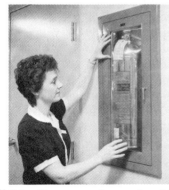

Figure 15-14 Every employee should know the location of fire extinguishers and how they are operated. (From Caldwell and Hegner, *Nursing Assistant, A Nursing Process Approach*, 5th edition, copyright 1989 by Delmar Publishers Inc.)

- Keep calm
- Follow fire policy of facility
- Move residents to safety
- Sound alarm
- Close windows and doors
- Shut off air conditioning
- Shut off other equipment as specified in facility policy
- Shut off oxygen
- Do not use elevators

Figure 15-15   Fire actions

The home, too, is often the scene of fires and burns. Sometimes gas is turned on but not lit. Oil burners may be turned on and, because the lighting is slow, there is a flare-up. Burns often occur from water or foods that are too hot. A mixer faucet on the washbowl and a governor on the shower or tub faucet to prevent the temperature from rising above 110°F can help prevent serious burns. In care facilities, temperature of bath and shower water and application of heat must be carefully controlled. Residents are generally not allowed in bathing areas alone. Checking the temperature of food before serving it is also important. Scalding can occur when hot fluids such as tea or coffee are spilled. Be sure trays are arranged in such a way as to prevent accidently knocking over hot liquids. Call the elderly's attention to the presence of hot containers and their placement on the table or tray.

A forgetful person may allow food to boil over on the stove and be burned trying to rescue it. Or, in boiling over, food may put out the flame, allowing gas to escape. Temperature positions on stoves and other appliances should be marked so that the elderly person can easily determine the proper setting. Raised or brightly painted figures help. The same method can be used to mark temperature settings on an iron. Home cooking and ironing may have to be supervised. But this must be done as inconspicu-

ously as possible to protect the self-esteem of the individual.

Severe burns may result from falling against open heaters that have been turned on to warm a bathroom. Recessed wall heaters are safer. Lights operated by wall switches eliminate the possibility of electrical shock, particularly near water. Still, many elderly people live in housing that provides chain pulls on lights over kitchen and bathroom sinks.

Trash is always a fire hazard. Elderly people tend to accumulate it either because they are saving various items or because they cannot manage trash disposal. Getting them to part with their saved treasures is sometimes quite a task.

For the elderly person who smokes, large deep ashtrays are safer than small ashtrays. Small ashtrays may be missed and fires may be started if the user is uncoordinated or has tremors. Smoking should be restricted to supervised areas in care facilities. Fire laws prohibit smoking in bed when patients or residents are unattended. A single uncontrolled spark may fall into an inaccessible area, smolder, and burst into flame hours later. Smoking restrictions apply to residents and staff alike. Those residents who are permitted to keep smoking materials at their bedside or on their person require extra vigilance. Residents without special permission who are observed with matches must be reported immediately.

Special situations within the care facility make the danger of fire greater. Whenever oxygen is in use, fires burn more rapidly. Special care must be taken when storing oxygen. While it is in use, no open flames (cigarettes, lighters, candles) or flammable liquids such as alcohol or nail polish are permitted. Use of electrical equipment such as razors or radios is also prohibited. Oxygen may be piped directly into the room through wall outlets. If oxygen cylinders are used, they must be secured to prevent falling. Visitors must be warned about oxygen precautions. They should not, under any circumstances, be permitted to smoke while they are visiting.

Electrical fires are common. They are caused by circuits overloaded with appliances, frayed wires, and loose connections. Ungrounded plugs should be reported and replaced by three-pronged ones. Sometimes heating equipment fails or flammable material is stored too close to heating elements. Be alert to all potential fire hazards and report them immediately.

In case of fire, always remember to first protect the safety of those in your care. Remove them from danger, shouting for assistance. Once your charges are safe, sound the alarm. Do not panic. Remember, only clear thinking can avert disaster. Once the alarm has been sounded, follow the evacuation plan as practiced. The patients will be frightened and confused. The staff must remain calm and controlled.

Poisoning

Accidental poisoning may occur unless precautions are observed. Perhaps the most important precaution is to have sufficient light at all times. The older person's medicines should be stored separately, away from the general family medicines. All medicines must be clearly labeled. A routine should be established for medications that must be taken regularly. Internal and external medications must be separated. "External only" medicines should be marked in some special way. This could mean placing a small piece of sandpaper on the bottle, marking it with a special color, or running a pin or tack into the cork top. Cleaning materials should always be stored separately to avoid a mix-up.

In the care facility, additional precautions will have to be taken. Confused residents may mistakenly pick up bottles of cleaning fluid or perfume and attempt to drink them. Visitors may bring in medications that are left at the bedside and then ingested by others.

Medications will normally be kept under lock and key, controlled by the nurse. The door to the medicine area should not be readily accessible to residents. It should be kept locked when not in use. Occasionally a medication such

as amyl nitrate or nitroglycerine will be allowed to be kept at the bedside for immediate use. These medications must be carefully monitored to prevent them from being overused or used by others. Be alert to behaviors that might indicate that medications are being hoarded. For example, patients may spit out and hide the pills after the medication nurse departs.

Choking

Food, saliva, or medications can cause a blockage of the respiratory tract. Improperly fitting or unused dentures can make chewing difficult. Large morsels of food can slip downward easily. Following a stroke, patients may have diminished gag and swallowing reflexes, which contribute to choking.

Feeding procedures should take these factors into account. If choking should occur, a quick response can be lifesaving. The Heimlich maneuver (see Procedure 2) and cardiopulmonary resuscitation (C.P.R.) should be employed. These techniques require special skill, which can be developed through practice. The Red Cross and American Heart Association conduct classes in these skills. Everyone should take the opportunity to learn. Many facilities require geriatric health care providers to be certified. These facilities provide classes with instructors from the American Red Cross or the American Heart Association. An instructor within the facility may also be certified by the American Red Cross to teach the C.P.R. technique.

PROCEDURE 2

Assisting the Conscious Choking Person (Heimlich Maneuver) (figure 15-16)

1. Stand behind and to one side of the victim.
2. Wait if the person starts to cough.

Note: If the person can cough, the obstruction usually is moved.

3. Clench fist, keeping thumb straight.
4. Place fist, thumb side in, against abdomen between navel and tip of sternum.
5. Grasp clenched fist with opposite hand.
6. Push forcefully with thumb side of the fist against midline of abdomen, inward and upward six to ten times.
7. If victim becomes unconscious:
    a. Place victim flat on floor on his or her back.
    b. Kneel and straddle victim.
    c. Place one hand flat on stomach between waist and sternum.
    d. Place other hand at right angles to the first.
    e. Push in and up in quick movements.
8. If the obstruction is still not dislodged, C.P.R. should be started by a person certified to do the procedure.

Whenever an emergency occurs, follow the guidelines shown in figure 15-17.

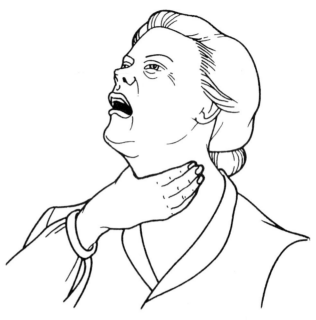

THE DISTRESS SIGNAL THAT THE RESIDENT IS CHOKING.

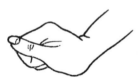

1. FORM A FIST

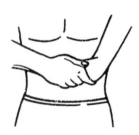

2. PLACE ARMS AROUND RESIDENT'S WAIST

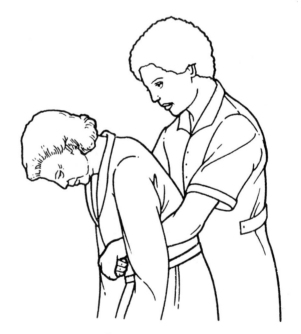

3. GIVE 6-10 UPWARD THRUSTS

Figure 15-16   Heimlich maneuver (From Hegner & Caldwell, *Assisting in Long-Term Care*, copyright 1988 by Delmar Publishers Inc.)

- Keep calm
- Assess situation
- Signal for help
- Never leave the resident alone
- Follow the directions of professionals

Figure 15-17 Actions in emergency situations

Infection Control

Hospital-acquired infections are called *nosocomial* infections. Elderly people are particularly vulnerable to infections of the respiratory and urinary tracts. Chronic illness, a less efficient immune system, and general frailty are all contributory factors. Germs may be spread easily from one resident to another while in common meeting areas such as day rooms or dining rooms. Visitors and the health care providers themselves can be the source of infectious organisms.

The Center for Disease Control (C.D.C.) located in Atlanta, Georgia issues guidelines to protect people and prevent the spread of infection. To safeguard the resident and yourself, you must understand the nature of infectious disease, how it is transmitted, and the steps you should take to prevent spreading it to others. Infections are caused by *pathogenic organisms* (germs). They can enter the body through the skin and the mucous membranes of the respiratory system and gastrointestinal tract and through the genitourinary tract. These organisms leave the body in similar ways. Coughing and sneezing are a major way that germs are passed from person to person. Germs may also be carried on the hands of health care providers or on equipment or articles (*fomites*) if they are not cleaned properly. Articles carrying infectious organisms are considered to be *contaminated*. Body secretions such as mucus, urine, saliva, feces, or discharge (*exudate*) from wounds can carry germs. *Medical asepsis* is the way in which germs are controlled within the care setting. Each person follows the same technique, thus

assuring the well-being of both staff and residents.

Hand Washing

Hand washing is extremely important. It is the basis of medical aseptic technique, figure 15-18. It should be done before and after toileting, handling a bedpan, handling food, feeding a resident, and caring for each resident. Warm water makes good lather and is less damaging to the skin than hot water.

CAUTION: Do not lean against the sink or allow the uniform to touch the sink.

It is essential that each person use the same technique, following it exactly.

Medical asepsis includes the use of *disposable* (not reusable) latex gloves whenever handling body secretions. This includes blood, saliva, sputum, feces, urine, or sexual secretions. This procedure is part of the Universal Precautions for protecting health care providers and patients/residents from infectious diseases, figure 15-19. Gloves should be used only once. Then they should be carefully removed so that the hands are not contaminated. The use of gloves during routine care may or may not be part of your facility policy. Gloves should never be a substitute for proper hand washing. Medical asepsis also includes thorough cleaning of articles, such as bedpans, that come into contact with residents.

PROCEDURE 3

Hand Washing

1. Assemble the equipment you will need:
   soap (a soap dispenser is usually mounted near the sink)
   paper towels
   waste can
2. Turn on faucet using a paper towel held between hand and faucet.
3. Drop towel in waste container.
4. Wet hands. Keep fingertips pointed downward.
5. Obtain soap from soap dispenser and lather.

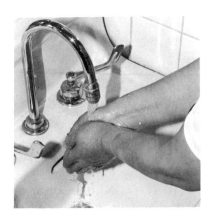
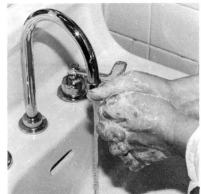
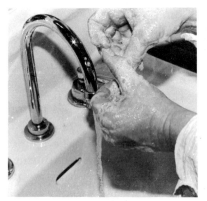
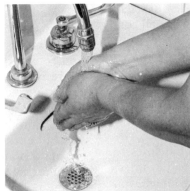
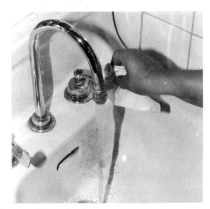

Figure 15-18   Proper handwashing is the foundation of the medical aseptic technique. (From Hegner & Caldwell, *Assisting in Long-Term Care*, copyright 1988 by Delmar Publishers Inc.)

6. Rub hands together in a circular motion and by interlacing fingers.
7. Rinse and repeat lathering. Continue rubbing hands for one minute.
8. Clean fingernails.
9. Rinse well. Keep fingers pointed downward.
10. Dry hands thoroughly.
11. Turn off faucet using another paper towel.
12. Drop paper towel in waste container.

Environmental Cleanliness

Attention must always be paid to the general cleanliness of the environment. This is known as *concurrent cleaning.* The daily or concurrent cleaning of equipment is an important job. Damp dusting will cut down on the amount of dust. This is important because germs can be spread in dust.

Stretchers and wheelchairs are usually made of materials that can be kept clean with soap and water. Bedside equipment, such as bedpans and urinals, wash basins, emesis basins, and IV *standards* (poles), can also be cleaned with soap and water. (IV standards are poles, usually made of stainless steel, that can be attached to the bed or stand on the floor. They are used to hang bags of fluids that are given to patients/residents through tubes in their veins.)

Concurrent cleaning may be included in the responsibility of the health care provider. However, it may be the responsibility of the housekeeping staff.

UNIVERSAL PRECAUTIONS

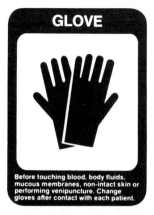

GLOVE

Before touching blood, body fluids, mucous membranes, non-intact skin or performing venipuncture. Change gloves after contact with each patient.

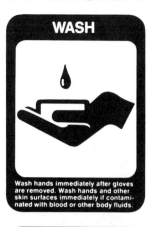

WASH

Wash hands immediately after gloves are removed. Wash hands and other skin surfaces immediately if contaminated with blood or other body fluids.

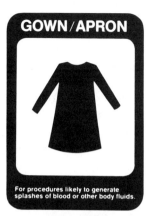

GOWN/APRON

For procedures likely to generate splashes of blood or other body fluids.

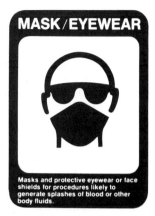

MASK/EYEWEAR

Masks and protective eyewear or face shields for procedures likely to generate splashes of blood or other body fluids.

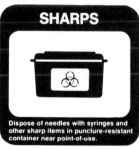

SHARPS

Dispose of needles with syringes and other sharp items in puncture-resistant container near point-of-use.

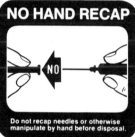

NO HAND RECAP

Do not recap needles or otherwise manipulate by hand before disposal.

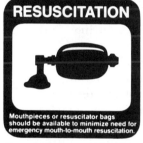

RESUSCITATION

Mouthpieces or resuscitator bags should be available to minimize need for emergency mouth-to-mouth resuscitation.

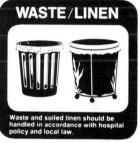

WASTE/LINEN

Waste and soiled linen should be handled in accordance with hospital policy and local law.

Figure 15-19   Universal precautions (From Caldwell and Hegner, *Nursing Assistant, A Nursing Process Approach,* 5th edition, copyright 1989 by Delmar Publishers Inc.)

When a patient/resident is discharged or moved to another part of the facility, the room must be thoroughly cleaned. This *terminal cleaning* may be part of the geriatric nursing assistant's responsibilities or it may be done by the housekeeping department. The following procedure provides the general steps for terminal cleaning.

PROCEDURE 4

Terminal Cleaning of Patient/Resident Unit

1. Assemble the equipment you will need:
   Basin of warm water   laundry hamper
   soap   newspaper for
   brush   waste
   cleaning cloths   scouring powder
   disinfectant   stretcher
     solution   radiator brush

2. Remove any special equipment. Be sure it is clean and returned to the proper storage area.
3. Remove all disposal material from bedside table and wrap it in newspaper to be disposed of according to facility policy.

Note: Do not dispose of anything that may be claimed by the resident or by family members.

4. Remove all basic equipment from bedside stand.
   a. Wash reusable equipment with hot water and detergent and/or sterilize it according to facility policy.
   b. If equipment is disposable, clean it and send the equipment home with resident or place in waste receptacle.
5. Strip bed and place linen in laundry hamper.

6. Place pillows on chair.
7. Take rubber drawsheet, if used, to utility room and wash it with soap and water. Rinse it with disinfectant solution. Allow to dry thoroughly. Some facilities put plastic drawsheets in the laundry.
8. Move stretcher beside the bed. With help, lift mattress from bed to stretcher.
9. Dry-dust coils of the bedsprings, using a long-handled radiator brush.
10. Using a cleaning cloth and disinfectant solution:
    a. Wash plastic cover on mattress with a damp cloth and damp-dust pillow surface.
    b. Wash bed frame, including the bedsprings. Remove parts for thorough cleaning, using scouring powder if needed.
    c. Wash bedside table inside and out. Leave drawers open to air.
    d. Wash bedside chair after placing pillows on mattress.
    e. Wash lamp and call bell cord.
11. Damp-dust all surfaces of mattress and pillows.
12. Place clean equipment in bedside stand and stock according to facility policy.
13. Wash hands.

Cleaning Contaminated Articles

Some contaminated articles such as tissues or dressing are disposable (not to be reused) and can be completely destroyed. Follow your facility policy for disposal. Many facilities have on-site incinerators to burn such disposables. Other, more expensive articles must be cleaned and reused. To be safe for reuse, they must be disinfected or sterilized.

Disinfection means to destroy pathogens. This is usually done with chemicals. All articles to be disinfected must be washed and dried. Then they must be left to soak the required length of time in the disinfectant solution. All parts of the article must come into contact with the disinfectant. Tubes being disinfected should be filled with the disinfectant. Instruments should be opened or taken apart and then submerged in the disinfectant.

Sterilization means the destruction of all microbes, even organisms that do not cause disease. Heat in some form is usually used to sterilize. Some articles may be boiled for twenty minutes or more. Others may be sterilized in steam under pressure in a machine called an *autoclave*, figure 15-20.

The autoclave works like a pressure cooker. Special tape is used to secure coverings on articles to be sterilized in the autoclave. The tape changes color during the process, giving evidence of sterilization. When the article could be harmed by heat, special gas autoclaves are used. Thermometers may be sterilized in this manner.

Opening Sterile Packages

You may be involved in a *sterile* (free from all microbes) dressing change. As a geriatric nursing assist, you may be asked to get sterile supplies

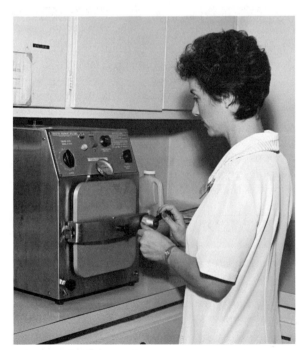

Figure 15-20 Sterilization is achieved by using an autoclave.

and perhaps assist the nurse by opening them. There is a procedure to be followed in opening sterile packages.

PROCEDURE 5

Opening a Sterile Package

Article Wrapped in Paper
1. Wash hands.
2. Check seal of package to be sure it is intact. If it is not intact, do not use the package.
3. Using both hands, grasp each side of the separated end of the package and gently pull package apart, figure 15-21.
4. Do not open package completely until physician or nurse is ready to use the contents.
5. When the physician or nurse is ready to use the contents of the package, open it only far enough to expose the end to be grasped.
6. Physician or nurse then withdraws article from package, being careful not to contaminate the article.

Article Double-wrapped in Cloth
1. Wash hands.
2. Check seal of package for color change. Color change indicates that the package has been sterilized.

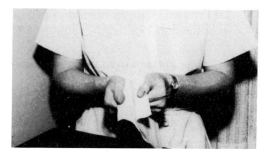

Figure 15-21 When opening a sterile package, never permit your fingers to touch the contents. (From Hegner & Caldwell, *Assisting in Long-Term Care,* copyright 1988 by Delmar Publishers Inc.)

3. Place package fold-side up on a flat surface.
4. Remove tape seal.
5. Unfold flap farthest from you by grasping outer surface only between thumb and forefinger.
6. Open left flap with left hand using the same technique as in step 5.
7. Open right flap with right hand using the same technique as in step 5.
8. Open final flap (the one nearest you).
9. Touch only the outside of the flap. Do not stand too close and do not let uniform touch flap as it is lifted free of package.
10. Pull flaps open completely so they do not fold back over the sterile field.

Residents or patients ill with infectious disease should be segregated. Sometimes isolation precautions must be followed.

Anything that comes into contact with a patient who has an easily transmitted disease is considered to be contaminated. It must be handled in a way to prevent spreading the disease to other patients and to staff. *Isolation technique* is the name given to the method of caring for patients with easily transmitted diseases. All staff members *must* use the same technique. Each facility has its own procedure for isolation technique. In many larger facilities, there is a staff member whose responsibility it is to ensure that all infection control and isolation technique procedures are followed by all employees.

The isolation area may be a unit or a single room. A room with adjoining sink and toilet facilities is best. Some facilities have special sections that are used only for the care of patients with infectious diseases.

Hand washing, wearing gloves, and using a covering gown are basic to isolation technique. The purpose of a gown is to prevent self-contamination and contamination of the uniform. At times, a mask is also required. Masks are effective for only thirty minutes. They must cover both nose and mouth. A clean gown or impervious apron must be put on before entering an isolation room. Discard the gown before leaving the room.

Frequently used equipment remains in the patient's unit. Special handling is required for all articles or specimens that leave isolation. Two people, one inside the isolation unit and the other outside the unit, are needed to carry out some procedures. Uncontaminated persons and objects are commonly called "clean." Contaminated persons and objects are commonly called "dirty."

Isolation procedures are exacting and may be reviewed with your instructor. Maintaining your own health is important in eliminating yourself as a source of infection.

PROCEDURE 6

Isolation Technique— Setting Up the Unit

1. Wash hands.
2. Assemble the equipment and supplies you will need:
   sign (universal precautions, isolation, or precaution)
   bedside table or cart
   isolation gowns
   masks
   disposable gloves
   paper bags
   plastic bags
   laundry hamper
   laundry bags marked "Isolation"
   antiseptic solution dispenser

Outside the Door to the Isolation Unit

3. Place the precaution or isolation sign on the door.
4. Place the bedside table or cart next to the door.
5. Stock the table with gowns, masks, and gloves, paper and plastic bags, and laundry bags.

Inside the Isolation Unit

6. Line waste container with plastic bag.
7. Place laundry bag marked "Isolation" in laundry hamper.
8. Put antiseptic solution dispenser over sink.
9. Check supply of paper towels and liquid soap in foot-operated dispenser.
10. Place basin of disinfectant solution for soaking contaminated articles near sink.

PROCEDURE 7

Putting On and Removing Gown and Mask

1. Outside the isolation unit, remove rings and secure inside a uniform pocket.
2. Remove watch and place in a plastic bag.
3. Wash hands.
4. Adjust mask over nose and mouth and tie securely.
5. Put on gown, slipping arms into sleeves.
6. Grasp ties at the back of the neck and tie.
7. Reach behind and overlap edges of gown to cover uniform completely. Tie waist ties.
8. Put on disposable gloves, with cuffs covering the cuffs of the gown.
9. Once work in isolation unit is completed, remove gloves using the procedure for removing contaminated gloves.
10. To remove gown in isolation unit, undo waist ties and loosen gown at waist, figure 15-22.
11. Holding a clean paper towel, turn on faucet.
12. Discard paper towel in waste basket.
13. Wash hands carefully and dry using paper towels.
14. Using paper towel to operate dispenser, wet hands with antiseptic solution and rub together. Air dry.
15. Using a dry paper towel, turn off faucet. Discard paper towel.

ISOLATION PRECAUTIONS

Room _____ Date _____

Isolation Type _____

☐ Private room necessary
☐ Door Must be Kept Closed
☐ **Mask** Necessary When:
　　☐ Entering Room
　　☐ _____
☐ **Gown** Necessary When:
　_____
☐ **Gloves** Necessary When:
　_____
☐ "NO" Red Bags
☐ Red Bag _____
☐ Sharps Container in room
☐ _____

INFECTION CONTROL DEPT.

Figure 15-22 Various means are used by the infection control department to inform health care providers about precautions to be followed for specific patients. (Courtesy Elizabeth Clark, RN, MPH)

16.　Undo mask. Holding by ties only, place it in laundry hamper.
17.　Undo neck ties of gown and loosen gown at shoulders.
18.　Slip fingers of right hand inside left cuff of gown. Do not touch outside of gown.
19.　Pull gown down and over left hand.
20.　Pull gown down over right hand with the gown-covered left hand.
21.　Fold gown with contaminated side inward. Roll and place in laundry hamper or waste container, if gown is disposable.
22.　Wash hands.
23.　Remove watch from plastic bag.
24.　Open door with clean paper towel. Prop door open with foot and drop towel in waste container.

PROCEDURE 8

Removing Contaminated Disposable Gloves

1.　Slip fingers of right hand under cuff of glove on left hand. Touch glove only.
2.　Pull left glove down to cover fingers and expose thumb.
3.　Slip uncovered thumb under cuff of glove on right hand.
4.　Pull right glove down until it is inside out over fingers.
5.　Touching only inside surfaces of gloves, remove gloves from both hands.
6.　Discard contaminated gloves according to facility policy.
7.　Wash hands.

Transferring Food and Disposable Items Outside the Isolation Unit

　　Two people assist in the transfer. One person is inside the unit and the other person stands outside the door of the unit. Leftover liquids and food from the resident's meal are discarded in the toilet (or according to facility policy). Be careful not to splash as the material is discarded.

　　For transfer of a disposable item, follow these guidelines:

1.　Door is opened by holding a paper towel. Door is propped open with foot.
2.　Person on the outside holds a cuffed plastic bag over hands to receive tray and other disposable items.
3.　Person on the outside secures top of plastic bag tightly.
4.　Disposable (throwaway) items such as dishes and plastic forks, knives, and spoons may be placed in waste container inside the unit.
5.　Dressings are sealed inside the room in a plastic bag. The person inside the room then places the plastic bag in the larger plastic bag held by the person outside the room.

6. The person outside the unit then secures the second bag. The bags are tagged with the appropriate destination: laundry, kitchen, central supply, or maintenance. The bags may be color coded for infectious waste. Tags may also be placed on them to indicate infectious waste. Once the bags arrive at the right location, the contents are disposal of according to facility or department procedures.

Note: In many facilities, gowns, gloves, and other items are all disposable.

Transferring Nondisposable Equipment Outside the Isolation Unit

Equipment that must be reused (nondisposable) may be double bagged in paper, labeled "isolation," and sent to central supply for sterilization. Some equipment may also be washed and soaked in a disinfectant solution in the room for a specified period of time before being sent for sterilization.

Collecting a Specimen in the Isolation Unit

To collect a specimen in the unit, follow these guidelines:

1. Place a clean specimen container and cover on a clean paper towel.
2. Place specimen in container without touching the container.
3. Properly dispose of the receptacle in which the specimen was collected.
4. Remove disposable gloves.
5. Wash hands, dry with paper towels, and put on a new pair of disposable gloves.
6. Cover specimen and label container.
7. Double-bag the specimen (using the same procedure as the one for equipment leaving the isolation unit).
8. Attach requisition slip to container and give it to person outside the unit.

9. The second person takes the specimen to the laboratory or notifies the laboratory for pickup. Follow facility policy.

Care of Laundry in the Isolation Unit (Double-Bagging)

Clean linen is brought to the unit as needed. Soiled linen is placed in a bag in the laundry hamper. When it is one-half to two-thirds full, the top is closed and the bag disposed of as follows:

1. The person outside the unit cuffs and holds a specially marked laundry bag and receives the soiled laundry bag.
2. The cover of the outside bag is securely tied. The linen is disposed of according to facility policy.

Transporting the Patient in Isolation

Notify the charge nurse or others in the department where you will be transferring the patient that a patient from isolation is on the way. Identify the patient, tell what is planned, and specify how the patient can be assisted. After reassuring the patient, you should:

1. Cover wheelchair or stretcher with clean sheets and wheel it in to the patient's room.
2. Put on a clean gown, following proper procedure, and assist patient into wheelchair or onto stretcher.
3. Mask the patient, if ordered.
4. Wrap sheet around the patient and instruct patient not to touch wheelchair or stretcher.
5. Remove gown just before leaving unit, following facility policy.

Geriatric health care providers can do much to limit the spread of infection. Keeping patients and their environment clean is a basic step in limiting the development of infections and the transfer of infectious material to others.

If a resident is placed in isolation, be sure you know the type of isolation and precautions to be followed. *Enteric* precautions are carried out when the infection is transmitted via the fecal-oral route; *respiratory* precautions, when the transmission is via respiratory secretions.

Incident Reports

Despite careful supervision and adherence to procedure and policy, injuries occur. After the emergency aspects of the situation have been handled and the victim is taken care of, a record of the *incident* (happening) must be made. This written statement is in addition to any oral report that might have been made. Staff members are often reluctant to make such reports, fearing that they are acknowledging responsibility for the incident. But the incident report is simply an objective documentation of the facts as they are known. The statement should contain no conclusions. It should indicate only what was seen or heard, the date and time of the incident, and any care given or action taken. The incident report becomes part of the patient's official record and is reported to the family and physician.

In legal actions, the incident report is considered separate from the patient's chart. Incident reports are considered to be the property of the facility. Because they are not part of the patient's chart, incident reports must be subpoenaed separately in a lawsuit.

Summary

- It is the responsibility of all health care providers to safeguard the in-hospital patient and to follow safety measures wherever the elderly are found.
- Serious consequences often result from falls, burns, poisoning, and nosocomial infections.
- Safety means constant vigilance. The entire staff must make safety rules and hazard prevention a growing part of their awareness.
- Although only one or two elderly people may be the concern of a single family, health care providers in a facility are responsible for the safety of a large number of elderly.
- The elderly in a care facility are more frail, sometimes confused, and generally less able to help themselves than are elderly in the community.
- Careful adherence to safety procedures and facility policies can prevent many accidents, both to residents and to staff.
- When incidents do occur, rapid intervention can contain the damage.
- A report regarding the incident must be made as soon as possible. Such a report becomes part of the legal record.

Review Outline

   I. Behavioral Objectives

  II. Vocabulary

 III. Elderly Accidents

     A. Intrinsic factors
       1. Physical disease
       2. Poor equilibrium
       3. Decreased visual acuity
       4. Confusion/forgetfulness

      B. Extrinsic factors
1. Dislocation of living quarters
2. Poorly lighted areas
3. Inadequately identified medications
4. Accumulated trash

IV. Types of Accidents

      A. Falls
1. Contributing factors
   a. Tripping
   b. Climbing
   c. Reaching
2. Safety measures
   a. Well-fitting clothing
   b. Clear walking areas
   c. Secure carpeting
   d. Adequate lighting
   e. Handrails/grab bars
   f. Special equipment

      B. Equipment-related
1. Contributing factors
   a. Poor condition
   b. Improper use
2. Safety measures
   a. Safe conditions
   b. Competent usage
   c. Proper staff conduct

      C. Fires and burns
1. Contributing factors
   a. Confusion
   b. Unsupervised smoking
   c. Presence of flammable materials
2. Safety measures
   a. Safe evacuation plans
   b. Supervised activities
   c. Prevention of trash accumulation

      D. Poisoning
1. Contributing factors
   a. Confusion
   b. Mistaken medications
2. Safety measures
   a. Supervision of residents
   b. Care of cleaning materials
   c. Proper labeling of medications

      E. Choking
1. Contributing factors
   a. Diminished gag reflex
   b. Poorly fitting dentures
   c. Large pieces of food or medications

2. Safety measures
    a. Careful feeding procedures
    b. Heimlich manuever

V. Infection Control

   A.   Universal Precautions

   B.   Hand washing

   C.   Gloving

   D.   Isolation procedures

VI. Incident Reports

Review

I. Vocabulary
Write the definition of each of the following.

1. Autoclave _____
2. Exudate _____
3. Fomites _____
4. Nosocomial _____
5. Medical asepsis _____

II. Short Answers

1.   What type of patient should not wear elastic shoelaces?
2.   What is the best means of preventing patients from tripping on loose garments?
3.   What is the best means of eliminating the hazard from doorsills?
4.   What can be used to make toileting safer and more convenient for the elderly?
5.   What can be used to decrease the hazard of wet or slippery walks?
6.   What is the safest type of heater?
7.   Why is accumulated trash a common source of fire in elderly households?
8.   Why is it a good idea to have a light burning at all times?
9.   Safety in a care facility means safety for two groups of people. Who are they?
10.   Why do many elderly people tend to ignore safety precautions?
11.   Why is it dangerous to change an elderly person's position rapidly?
12.   What is the primary cause of accidental injury to the elderly?
13.   What are the important safety features of shoes?
14.   List four ways that the safety of staircases can be improved.
15.   List three examples of accidents that can be caused by a confused patient.
16.   What are the health care provider's responsibilities in regard to fires?
17.   What is meant by terminal cleaning?
18.   What are pathogens and how many affect patient safety?
19.   What action is the foundation of medical asepsis?
20.   What is the special technique of segregating people with infectious diseases from others called?

III. Clinical Situations

1. You walk into a room and the elderly resident is lying on the floor. What do you do?
2. You see a visitor going into a resident's room with a lighted cigarette. What do you do?
3. You were present when an accident occurred. You now must document the incident. What will you include in the report?

Unit 16
Nutritional Aspects of Aging and Diet Therapy

Objectives

After studying this unit, you should be able to:
- Name the basic four food groups.
- Explain the reasons for malnutrition in the elderly person living alone.
- Describe the digestive changes that take place with age.
- Discuss the factors that must be considered in purchasing food for the elderly.
- Discuss means of providing nutrition for people who cannot provide for themselves.
- Recognize the signs of dehydration.

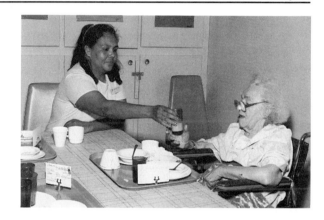

Vocabulary

Learn the meaning and spelling of the following words or phrases.

achlorhydria	gavage	nutrients
carbohydrates	hyperalimentation	nutrition
cellulose	hypochlorhydria	periodontitis
congregate	hypoproteinemia	protein
defecation	intravenous infusion (I.V.)	pyarrhea
fats	minerals	therapeutic
flow rate	nasoenteric tube	vitamins
force fluids (F.F.)	nasogastric tube	withholds
gastrostomy tube	nitrogen imbalance	

Nutrition is the process by which the body uses food for growth and repair and to maintain health. The signs of good nutrition include healthy hair, clear skin and eyes, a well-developed body, an alert expression, a pleasant disposition, healthy sleep, and a good appetite, figure 16-1. Malnutrition is evidenced in the elderly by anemia and decreased vitality. Other signs of poor nutrition are shown in figure 16-2. Malnutrition affects all body systems, making them less efficient.

Food is normally taken into the body through the mouth. The mouth is the beginning of the digestive tract. Digestion is the process of breaking down foods into simple substances that can be used by the body cells for nourishment.

Essential Nutrients

To be well nourished, the body must receive foods that supply heat and energy, build and repair body tissue, and regulate body functions.

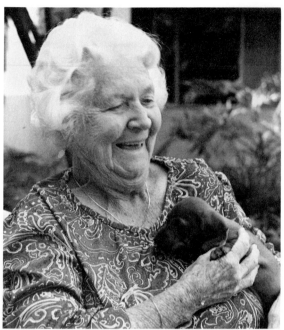

Figure 16-1 Proper nutrition contributes to vitality as shown in the face of this elderly woman.

These foods are called *nutrients*. The six nutrients essential to health are proteins, carbohydrates, fats, minerals, vitamins, and water.

Proteins

Protein is the basic material of every body cell. It is the only nutrient that can make new cells and rebuild tissue. The foods that contain the greatest amounts of protein come from animals.

- Hair loss
- Dull hair
- Dull eyes
- Smooth tongue
- Rashes
- Muscle wasting
- Tooth loss
- Scaling skin
- Nail ridges

Figure 16-2 Signs of poor nutrition

They include meat, fish, poultry, eggs, milk, and cheese. Other protein foods are beans, nuts, and lentils.

Carbohydrates and Fats

Carbohydrates and *fats* are called energy foods. The body uses them to produce heat and energy. When more food is eaten than needed, the body stores it as fat. Fats are also important in helping the body to use vitamins. Foods that contain the greatest amounts of carbohydrates come from plants. They include fruits and vegetables and foods made from fruits and vegetables. Examples are bread, cereals, and macaroni products. Carbohydrate foods also supply the body with roughage *(cellulose)*, which is important in maintaining regularity. Fats come from both plants and animals. Foods rich in fat include butter, pork, nuts, and egg yolks.

Vitamins and Minerals

Vitamins are substances that regulate body processes. They are designated by letter names: A, B-complex, C, D, E, and K. Vitamins help to build strong teeth and bones and promote growth. They also aid normal body functioning and strengthen resistance to disease. Vitamins B and C are water soluble. Vitamins A, D, K, and E are fat soluble. *Minerals* help to build body tissues, especially bones and teeth. They also regulate body fluids such as blood and digestive juices. The minerals needed in the daily diet include calcium, phosphorus, iodine, iron, copper, potassium, and sodium. Vitamins and minerals are present in a wide variety of foods.

Water

Water is also an essential nutrient. It is needed for all body processes. Approximately 2 ½ quarts (2½ liters or 2,500 milliliters) need to be replaced daily. Fluids are lost from the body through urine and feces, perspiration, and breathing. Older people are encouraged to keep fluid intake at about 3 quarts (3,000 milliliters) daily unless there is some special reason not to do so. Inadequate intake of fluids can predispose a

- Confusion
- Dry, inelastic skin (poor skin turgor)
- Dry, brown tongue
- Sunken cheeks
- Concentrated urine
- Poor fluid intake
- Lethargy

Figure 16-3   Be sure to report signs of dehydration.

person to infection, constipation, decreased bladder distensibility, fluid and electrolyte imbalance, confusion, and dehydration. Renal disease and cardiovascular disease may make it necessary to limit fluids. Dehydration can sometimes develop quite rapidly.

There are many causes of inadequate fluid intake. They include lack of access to water, altered mental states, fear of incontinence, lack of motivation, and inability to obtain liquids and drink without help. All health care providers must be alert to the elderly person's need for water. They must make sure that fresh water is available and is offered (unless counterindicated). An order for *force fluids* (F.F.) may be given. *Force fluids* means that the resident must be encouraged to take as much fluid as possible. The indications of dehydration that are listed in figure 16-3 should be noted and reported.

Nutritional Requirements

Nutritional requirements for the aged are essentially the same as those for other adults. However, the elderly have less of a need for calories, a greater need for vitamins and minerals, and a reduced tolerance for fats, sodium, and refined sugars. The rule should be to improve the nutrient quality while reducing quantity of food. Increased fiber and more reliance on whole grains and complex carbohydrates is beneficial. Fewer calories are needed because activity is decreased and the basal metabolic rate is lower. The average daily calorie intake for older women should be about 1,800 until age sixty-five. It should then be reduced to 1,600 calories per day. For older men, the average number of calories should be about 2,400 daily. The amount should be reduced to 2,050 after age seventy-five. Vitamin and mineral levels need to be increased in the elderly. These substances are not utilized as efficiently as a person ages.

Undernutrition is fairly common among people over fifty-five years and is not always evident with casual examination. The elderly are most often deficient in calcium and iron, folic acid, magnesium, vitamin B-6, and thiamin. This is especially true of those who live alone. However, a recent survey demonstrates that more than one-third of those living in extended care facilities who were included in the survey were not adequately nourished. Most often the problem is a protein/calorie deficiency (P.C.D.). This is very serious because it can become irreversible, and thus life threatening.

The four food groups should be included each day. These are fruits and vegetables, dairy products, breads and cereals, and meat and fish, figure 16-4. The consistency of foods and method of preparation may need to be altered. This will compensate for poorer chewing ability, less production of saliva, and decreased digestive power.

Nutritional assessment must become an integral part of every patient workup. In addition, an ongoing assessment should be included as part of each patient's nursing care.

Fruits and Vegetables

Four or more servings of fruits and vegetables should be included in the daily diet. Use leafy green and yellow vegetables—raw, cooked, frozen, or canned. These provide vitamin A, calcium, and iron. Leafy green vegetables also furnish riboflavin, niacin, and calcium. Citrus fruit, tomatoes, and raw cabbage provide vitamins C, A, and B-complex. When potatoes and other vegetables and fruits are eaten in fairly large amounts, they provide thiamine, vitamins A and C, calcium, and phosphorus. The fruit, vegetable, and grain groups should provide 48 percent of dietary carbohydrates.

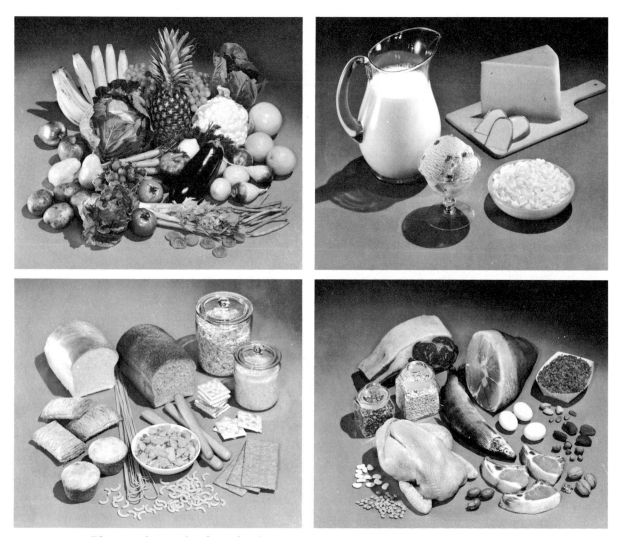

Figure 16-4   The four food groups should be included in the daily diet.

The elderly will find fruits and vegetables easier to manage if they are cooked and chopped or diced. Servings of vegetable and fruit juices are easily assimilated and provide vitamins and minerals. If a blender is available, many different drinks can be made from fresh fruits and vegetables to tempt lagging appetites. Commercially prepared baby foods can also be used to increase fruits and vegetables in the diet. These are especially good for those without teeth and for convalescents. The addition of spices can make these foods quite palatable. Be careful that they are not so spicy that they cause gastric distress.

Dairy Products

This group provides calcium, phosphorus, riboflavin, protein, vitamin A, and fat. The following dairy foods contain calcium equal to that in one cup of milk. They may be substituted for milk.

1 ounce hard cheese	12 ounces cottage
4 ounces creamy	cheese
cheese	2-3 dips ice cream

As few elderly people drink milk regularly, the daily requirement of the equivalent of two glasses often must be met in other ways. Cheese and other foods made from milk are a good substitute. Eggnogs and milk shakes provide a refreshing change of nourishing fluid intake. Soups, custards, puddings, and ice cream are other ways that milk can be introduced into the diet. They are often enjoyed by the older person because they are not too sweet and pose no problem in chewing. Skim milk and buttermilk are preferred to whole milk because of their lower fat and calorie content. They provide the essential nutrients without adding unnecessary weight. Besides being low in fat and calories, powdered skim milk is easy to mix and store. It is also economical for the person who lives alone. In case of lactose intolerance, sources of protein and calcium other than milk or milk products must be substituted.

Breads and Cereals

This group provides carbohydrates, thiamine, niacin, iron, and roughage. Four or more daily servings are advised. However, it is not uncommon to find carbohydrate foods forming the bulk of the elderly person's diet. The less expensive but higher calorie carbohydrates make up a high percentage of the diet because they are softer and easier to chew. They also require less preparation. Because enriched and whole grain foods offer the best source of vitamins and minerals, the elderly should be encouraged to include them in their diets. Roughage such as bran promotes peristalsis and elimination.

Meat and Fish

This group provides protein, some iron, phosphorus, and B-complex vitamins. Dried beans, peas, or nuts are an alternate source of incomplete proteins. The meat group is the most expensive food group. For this reason, it may be omitted by those on limited incomes. Two or more servings are the daily requirement (1 gram per kilogram of body weight). Many older people never achieve the requirement, however. They should be encouraged to buy variety meats such as sweetbreads and liver and other cuts that are

less expensive but equal in nutrition. Hamburger, a common choice, is graded for fat content. Sometimes the more expensive is a better buy because it has less fat. Eggs and beans, excellent sources of protein, can be incorporated with other foods if the elderly person objects to eating them alone. Eggs are good protein unless cholesterol is to be limited. Egg substitutes can then be used. In some parts of the country, fish is less expensive than red meat. It is better to broil meats than to fry them. Broiling meats at high temperatures is believed to create carcinogens. Since meat has a longer transit time through the intestines than many other foods it has been linked to cancer of the bowel. Overcooking tends to dry out meats, making them more difficult to chew.

Related Problems

The less active older person needs fewer calories. But keeping the calorie level under control is not easy. Obesity is a major problem in the younger and middle years. It is a real threat to longevity. Controlling calories is best accomplished by decreasing the amounts of fats and carbohydrates. The older person does not always tolerate large amounts of fat well. Flatulence and diarrhea can result from this intolerance and can be very uncomfortable.

One of the biggest dietary problems is to provide sufficient roughage to maintain regular, natural elimination. Stewed fruits, especially stewed prunes, whole grains, and adequate water can solve this problem if taken regularly.

If the diet is adequate, vitamin and mineral supplements are unnecessary. There is little problem if a wide selection of foods is available and if the elderly recognize their value. Unfortunately, their diet is often deficient in vitamins and minerals. Once a deficiency exists, it is difficult to correct.

Eating habits are established early in life. By the time a person reaches old age, likes and dislikes are deeply entrenched. Over the years, food preferences have been influenced by cultural patterns as well as economic status. Many times, former favorites become troublesome, causing indigestion, gas, or shortness of breath. Sometimes fad diets and so-called youth or health foods are tried in hopes of regaining vigor and vitality.

Foods are often chosen because they are filling rather than nourishing. Periodontal disease, neglected teeth, and changes in taste tend to deaden appetites. Dry mouth and burning of the tongue, common complaints, are probably caused by decreased circulation and decreased saliva production. Poor nutrition is particularly common among those who live alone. Sipping tea and nibbling toast stills hunger but does little to provide essential nutrients, figure 16-5. This type of diet is high in carbohydrates but low in proteins and vitamins.

The elderly are so seldom physically activity that any prolonged activity can lead to *hypoproteinemia* (abnormal decrease in the amount of protein in the blood). This is compounded when protein is deficient in the diet.

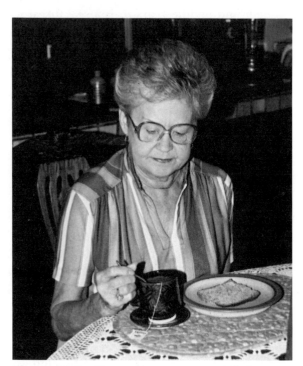

Figure 16-5   Tea and toast may satisfy hunger, but they do not provide essential nutrients.

Digestive Changes

Specific changes take place in the digestive tract with age. In the mouth, the number of functioning taste buds and the amount of saliva decrease to about half. The oral mucosa become thinner and lose some resiliency. Therefore, they are more easily injured when coarse foods are eaten. The amounts of digestive enzymes decrease, but they remain adequate for digestion. *Achlorhydria* (lack of hydrochloric acid) or *hypochlorhydria* (hydrochloric acid below 0.14 percent) is not uncommon. Intolerance to lactose is fairly common; thus elders often complain that they have indigestion after eating milk products. Aging brings about changes in absorption rates of nutrients such as calcium, iron, and vitamins. Loss of muscle tone throughout the alimentary tract slows the digestive process and causes irregularity of elimination.

Malnutrition

There have been limited studies on the food habits and dietary intake of the elderly. In general, it has been found that they take in less food and suffer from deficiencies in protein, calcium, iron, and the B vitamins. In addition, they frequently suffer from a *nitrogen imbalance*. A nitrogen imbalance results when the body takes in less protein, the source of nitrogen, than is required. At the same time, many older people suffer from obesity due to excessive calorie intake. Fluid intake is often inadequate. Older people may believe that by limiting their fluid intake, they can control incontinence. An elderly person can quickly become dehydrated, however. Dehydration can lead to serious consequences. If fluids are somewhat restricted in the evening hours, extra effort is necessary to assure adequate fluid intake during the day.

Some patient care facilities make fluid intake the responsibility of the medication or treatment nurse. This person makes special efforts to encourage fluid intake each time the patient is contact, figure 16-6. Every member of the nurs-

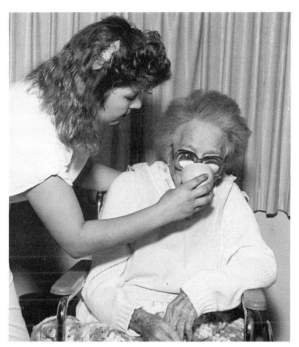

Figure 16-6 Fluid intake needs to be encouraged.

ing staff should take an active part in assuring proper fluid intake, even if not specifically assigned this duty.

Social Factors

Eating is in part a social activity. It is more enjoyable when there is company, and everyone eats better in congenial surroundings.

An elderly person living alone in a rooming house with limited cooking facilities has little recourse but to eat in restaurants. This can put an impossible strain on a retirement budget. Yet a diet of soup, coffee, and tea cannot provide adequate nourishment. When such people are also limited by physical disability, their situation can be particularly serious. A person living alone often loses interest in preparing and eating nutritional meals. Apathy and loneliness reduce the appetite even when cooking facilities are available.

Patient care facilities recognize the social aspect of eating. They provide communal eating areas where all ambulatory patients and those in wheelchairs gather for meals and between-meal snacks. However, it must not be assumed that all people will want to eat in such a communal setting. Some with disabilities may feel uncomfortable. Others may feel uncomfortable in the presence of disabilities. Communal eating should be encouraged, not forced.

Life-care facilities have restaurant service where the residents are served at regular tables. Friends look forward to meeting each other at mealtime. Some senior citizen centers have improved the nutrition of the elderly in a social setting by providing balanced, low-cost meals for their members.

Congregate (group) nutrition projects have been funded under Title VII of the Older Americans Act, figure 16-7. These government-supported programs are designed to encourage seniors to come out of their homes and meet in a social setting to eat and assure adequate nutrition. Some programs are held in conjunction with senior centers. Others are sponsored by churches or other civic groups. There are no financial means tests to qualify for these meals. A major purpose of these programs is to improve social interactions as well as to provide nourishment.

Chewing Problems

Mouth and dental problems are a common occurrence in the later years. Sores and odors, dental caries, lack of teeth, and poorly fitting dentures all plague the elderly. Over 90 percent of those persons between sixty-five and seventy-five years suffer some degree of periodontal disease. Denture statistics tell us that 50 percent of Americans over sixty-five have lost all their teeth. By the time Americans reach seventy-five, two-thirds are toothless. The statistics are frightening. What is really sad is that much tooth loss is needless.

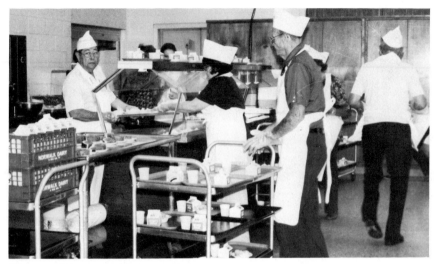

Figure 16-7   Nutrition projects have been established to provide one hot meal a day to people in need over the age of sixty.

Pyorrhea or *periodontitis* is a gum disease and is the chief cause of tooth loss. It is a condition in which pockets of pus form about the roots of teeth in the alveolar ridge. Preventative dentistry and proper tooth brushing and flossing in the early years are essential if pyorrhea is to be avoided.

Some people lose their teeth and manage to eat with the hardened gums. Chewing hard food is impossible. But it is little short of amazing how well many people actually do. Most, however, are fitted with and try to wear either partial or complete dentures. The presence of dentures influences the choice of foods. The lower plate is usually more stable. Therefore, people tend to bring food down upon these teeth when chewing, rather than biting down with the upper plate. Many foods such as raw fruits and vegetables and corn on the cob are avoided.

As a person ages, the alveolar ridges tend to be reabsorbed. This makes the fitting of artificial teeth difficult and unsatisfactory. Wobbly or ill-fitting dentures make the mouth sore and eating difficult.

Purchasing and Storing Food

Convenience foods—those that require little or no preparation—are found in increasing varieties in supermarkets. Their moderate servings are useful to the elderly person living alone. There is little waste, and each week there are new and tempting combinations. Expense is a factor that cannot be ignored, however. For many older people, it is the determining factor. Also, labels must be read. Some convenience foods contain additives such as sugar and salt that may need to be avoided.

The economy-minded homemaker saves by buying in bulk and at sales. There is no advantage to buying in bulk when items perish before they can be used, however. Buying in bulk also means many items to carry. Few elderly people can manage the heavy packages. Sale buying means that a large percentage of a limited budget must be allocated to a single type of food. Few older people can afford to do this. Upstairs apartments, shopping centers that are some distance from home, and the need to depend on buses and walking to transport parcels all influence the individual's choice of foods.

The kind of equipment that is available in the home for preparing and storing food also affects buying. Some of the elderly have only a hot plate or top burner. This prohibits the use of foods that require an oven. The size and temperature of cold food storage equipment must also be considered in making food selections. When only an icebox is available, frozen foods cannot be kept at all, and perishables cannot be kept for very long.

Older people can be helped to buy more efficiently. Always keeping their personal circumstances in mind, some suggestions that might be made include:

1. Make a list after checking current supplies; consider replenishing one staple at a time.
2. Plan meals based on the basic four food groups.
3. Buy only enough fresh fruits and vegetables to last a few days.
4. Remember that ground beef will keep refrigerated only one or two days. It should be frozen if it is to be kept longer.
5. Determine what container size is best. Buy the largest quantity compatible with personal needs. Unit pricing helps to determine the best buys.
6. Read labels for contents. Check dates for freshness.
7. Make sure that snacks are nourishing and not high in calories.
8. Steam vegetables minimal amounts of time to preserve vitamins.
9. Arrange eating times to meet individual preference.
10. Enjoy meals in a relaxed manner, with company if possible.

Feeding the older person who lives within the family unit requires some modification of the menu. But eating properly when one lives alone is much more difficult. In an effort to help meet the basic nutritional needs of the elderly person who is housebound, a unique program called "Meals on Wheels" was developed.

Meals on Wheels originated in England in 1939. It was first offered in the United States in 1954 in Philadelphia. Since then, many cities have established similar mobile canteen units. The service delivers directly to the shut-in one hot meal a day and enough cold food for two other meals. The daily cost is small. It is subsidized by both private and government sources. In addition to providing meals, the daily delivery is a small but important social contact.

To help meet the nutritional needs of low-income Americans, the Administration on Aging administers the National Program for Older Americans. This program is designed to provide inexpensive, nutritious meals to older Americans who have little money or those who have difficulty shopping and preparing well-balanced meals.

Through this program, nutrition projects have been established throughout the country. Their aim is to provide one hot meal a day, at least five days a week, to people in need who are over sixty and their spouse, whatever his or her age. Some of the meals are served through nutrition programs housed in churches, senior citizen centers, or public housing. The guidelines for meal planning under these programs require that the meal provide at least one-third of the recommended daily allowance of nutrients as established by the Food and Nutrition Board. Participants may pay for part or all of the meal. They may receive the meal free if they cannot afford to contribute. There is no means test to qualify. Hundreds of thousands of seniors receive one meal a day in this way. However, many eligible people do not participate because of ignorance or lack of interest.

Food stamps are available to low-income elderly through welfare services. The stamps extend buying power. They can be used to buy foods, to pay for food in service areas, or to pay for home-delivered meals.

Patients in Care Facilities

Diets in a hospital or extended care facility will be prepared by the dietary department and will include the essential nutrients. The way that the diet is prepared and its consistency will depend on the individual patient's condition and needs. Strict dietary control may be needed. Special *therapeutic* (treatment) diets, figure 16-8, include selection from the basic four food groups. The food may be altered in consistency or components to meet a personal need.

Institutions usually have four standard diets: liquid, soft, light, and regular-select or house. Labels on the trays will indicate the type. Sometimes color coding is used. Learn to recognize the types of food allowed in these diets to avoid mistakes. Always double-check the tray before it is served. The diet will be part of the patient care plan. Special instructions about feeding will also be listed on the care plan. Know the instructions for each of your patients.

Regular Diet

The regular-select or house diet is a normal diet based on the basic four food groups. It includes a great variety of foods. It excludes only the very rich, such as pastries, heavy cakes, fried foods, and highly seasoned foods, which might be difficult for inactive people to digest. Because an inactive person does not require as many calories as an active one, the calorie count of the regular diet may be somewhat lower than in the normal diet.

Clear Liquid Diet

The clear liquid diet consists of liquids that do not irritate, cause gas formation, or encourage bowel movements *(defecation)*. It replaces fluids that may have been lost by vomiting or diarrhea. It is a temporary diet because it is inadequate, composed mainly of water and carbohydrates for energy. Feedings are given every two, three, or four hours as prescribed by the physician. The foods allowed are:

tea
coffee with sugar but without cream
strained fruit or vegetable juice with gelatin
fat-free meat broths
ginger ale (occasionally)

Full Liquid Diet

The full liquid diet does supply nourishment. It may be used for longer periods of time than the clear liquid diet. It is given to patients who have acute infections, to patients who have difficulty chewing, and to those whose conditions involve the digestive tract. It includes all the foods allowed on the clear liquid diet in addition to the following:

strained cereal (gruel)	milk and cream
	plain ice cream
strained soups	strained vegetables
sherbet	and fruit juices
gelatin	junket
eggnog	malted milk

Six to eight ounces are usually given every two to three hours. A blender can convert many foods into liquids, adding variety to the diet.

Diabetic	Amounts of carbohydrates, fats, and proteins are balanced and prescribed. Concentrated sweets are restricted.
Low Sodium (sodium restricted)	Amounts of sodium are specifically prescribed, e.g. 500 mg sodium. Sodium-rich foods such as milk and bacon or salted nuts are excluded.
Low Fat	Foods with high fat content such as whole milk and eggs are restricted. Use of fats for preparation of food is avoided.
Calorie Restricted	Limits the number of calories while balancing nutrients.
High Protein	Amounts of high-protein foods such as meat, fish, eggs, and cheese are increased.

Figure 16-8   Special diets

Soft Diet

The soft diet includes liquids and semisolid foods that have a soft texture and are easily digested. It is given to patients who have infections and fevers, those who have difficulty chewing, those who are progressing from a liquid diet, and those whose conditions involve the digestive tract. The foods allowed on the soft diet are low residue, which means that they are almost completely used by the body. The foods are also mildly flavored, slightly seasoned or unseasoned, and prepared in a form that is easily digested. Although this diet nourishes the body, between-meal feedings are sometimes given to increase the calorie count. The following foods are usually allowed on the soft diet:

soup	angel or sponge cake
cream cheese	gelatin
cottage cheese	custard
fish	pudding
fruit juices	plain ice cream
cooked fruit	white meat of chicken
(sieved)	or turkey
tea, coffee	beef and lamb
butter	(scraped or finely
milk, cream	ground)
cooked cereals	cooked vegetables
eggs (not fried)	(mashed or sieved)
small amounts	
of sugar	

Foods to be avoided are:

coarse cereals	gas-forming foods
spices	(onions, cabbage)
fried foods	rich pastries and
raw fruits and	desserts
vegetables	foods high in
	roughage

Light Diet

The light or convalescent diet is an intermediate stage between the soft and regular diets. It is used for convalescent patients, for those with minor illnesses, sometimes for preoperative or postoperative patients, and for older people. It differs from the regular diet only in

the method of preparing the food. Because digestibility of food is of prime importance, foods should be baked, boiled, or broiled rather than fried. Rich, spicy, and coarse foods should be avoided. The following foods are allowed on the light diet:

refined cereals	broiled or baked lean
any bread except	meat
bran	fruits, except those
butter, cream	high in cellulose
bacon	vegetables, except
tea, coffee	those high in
small amounts of	cellulose
sweets	

Foods to be avoided are:

rich pastries	coarse cereals
heavy salad	pork (except bacon)
dressings	vegetables and fruits
fried foods	high in cellulose

Puree Diet

The pureed diet includes foods from each of the four food groups. This food has been placed through a blender.

Therapeutic Diets

There are many other types of special or therapeutic diets. These are designed to meet the dietary needs of patients with particular conditions. For example, the patient with a congestive heart problem would probably be on a sodium-restricted diet. You will become more familiar with components of special diets as you gain clinical experience. Some special diets that you will serve are the diabetic diet, the low-sodium diet, the low-fat diet, the calorie-restricted diet, and the high-protein diet.

Older patients to be discharged from the hospital or other facility should have the opportunity to discuss their food problems with someone who can give them nutritional information and suggestions. An understanding of basic nutrition enables the nurse to offer this kind of help. The nurse should try to learn about the patient's personal food preferences when the patient is admitted to the hospital. An understanding of the patient's nutritional needs should grow as health care is given. All members of the health staff can help to gain and share information about the patient's preferences. This can help the nurse in teaching the patient.

The morning care period is usually when the greatest amount of continuous time is spent with the patient. This is an ideal time for the casual conversations that reveal much about the patient's nutritional understandings and home situation. It is also one of the best times to correct false ideas and make positive suggestions.

Patients in Extended Care Facilities

Mealtime may be the highlight of the patient's day. It should be as pleasant as possible. The same basic diets as those prepared for the hospitalized patient will be served. In general, food servings are smaller to accommodate shrinking appetites, figure 16-9. The elderly can be almost overwhelmed if food servings are too large.

In many extended care facilities, several small meals rather than three large meals are served. The evening meal is usually light, since patients may find sleeping more difficult after a heavy meal. Often a small snack just before bed-

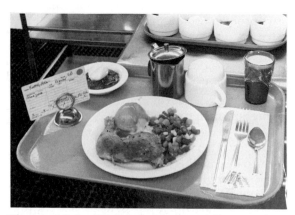

Figure 16-9 Well-balanced, smaller servings are more appealing to the elderly appetite.

time or during the night makes the use of sedatives unnecessary. Hunger can cause the patient to awaken and wander during the night. In these cases, try spending a few minutes with the resident and offer something light to eat or drink rather than seeking medication immediately. This technique often satisfies, enabling the resident to go back to sleep.

Care must be exercised in feeding weak, elderly residents. There is always the danger of aspiration. Coughing is the only clinical sign to tell the health care provider that a small amount of food may have been aspirated. Residents should be supported in a raised position while eating to decrease the change of aspiration. If the resident's condition does not warrant this, then feeding with a tube *(gavage)* is preferred. Feeding by gavage is a special technique and must only be carried out by those who have received special training.

The health care provider should take time feeding the resident, making the most of this opportunity for social contact. Being hurried when eating reduces the appetite. Foods may need to be rewarmed if they become too cool for enjoyment.

Responsibilities of the Geriatric Health Care Provider

Helping with meals is one of the major responsibilities of a geriatric health care provider. This includes serving the tray, assisting those who can feed themselves, and feeding those who are unable, figure 16-10. You may be assigned to serve supplementary nourishments and fresh water or to assist with tube feedings. Always note how much is taken of each serving. If the patient or resident is having intake and output monitored, be sure to measure and record accurately.

Supplementary Nourishments

Milk, juice, gelatin, or custard may be served to residents, usually in the midmorning, midafternoon, and before bedtime. Wash your hands

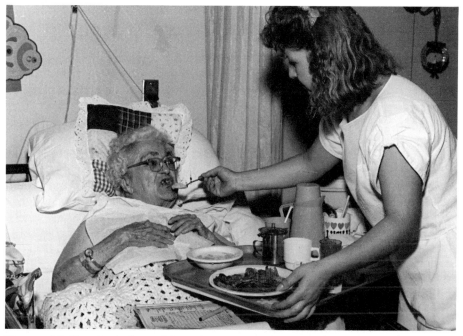

Figure 16-10   Assisting with a feeding should be a pleasurable experience.

before you start. Check the nourishment list for any *"withholds"* (patient is not to be served food) or special dietary instructions. Allow residents to choose from the available nourishments whenever possible. Assist those who are unable to take their nourishments alone. Pick up used glasses and dishes after the resident has finished and return them to the proper area. Record nourishments on the intake record if ordered.

Changing Water

It is important to provide fresh water for residents, since water is essential to life. Older people often do not drink enough water. Sometimes there will be a specific order for "force fluids." In some states, "force fluids" means that sufficient fluid must be provided to document 1,500–2,000 cc in twenty-four hours. Providing fresh water is one way to encourage the resident to increase the intake of fluids. The procedure for providing fresh water varies greatly. In some facilities, the water pitcher and glass are replaced with a new sterilized set each time water is pro-

vided. More often, the pitcher and glass are washed, refilled, and returned to the patient's bedside table. In all cases, be sure you know whether the resident is allowed ice or tap water and what the preference is.

Assisting with Feeding

Prepare in-bed seniors for their food trays by offering the bedpan and helping them to wash their hands and face. The head of the bed should be raised, if permitted. The position can also be adjusted with pillows. Sitting in a chair often will stimulate the resident's appetite. The overbed table should be cleared. Anything unpleasant, such as emesis basins or bedpans, should be removed from sight. Eating should be an enjoyable experience.

After you have washed your hands, assist the patient by cutting meat, pouring liquids, or buttering bread. Allow patients to do as much for themselves as their condition or orders permit. If a patient is blind, explain the arrangement of the tray as items relate to the face of a clock. At times, you will be responsible for the entire feeding procedure. It is important that you be pleasant and unhurried. The procedure for assisting those who can feed themselves and the procedure for feeding the individual who needs help may be reviewed with your instructor.

Alternate Ways to Provide Nutrition

When there is a disease of the digestive tract or other reasons that food cannot be taken in the normal way, it is necessary to introduce glucose and electrolytes to the patient's body through the veins. This is called an *intravenous infusion* or I.V. I.V. fluids do not have the essential nutrients necessary to build and repair tissue so they are used as a temporary measure only. The speed at which the I.V. solution enters the patient's body is called the *flow rate*. The rate is expressed in drops per minute. Report to the nurse if the drip chamber is full or the flow rate is different from

the one that was ordered. The nurse will also start and monitor intravenous infusions and change bottles when necessary. Be alert for bottles that are nearly empty. Call them to the attention of the nurse before the fluid runs out.

When patients are unable to take adequate nutrition by mouth and their nutritional needs are not able to be met with supplemental intravenous infusions, it may be necessary to provide nutrients through a tube leading into the gastrointestinal tract (gavage). There are several ways that this may be accomplished. For example, a *nasogastric tube* can be passed through the nose into the esophagus and into the stomach, figure 16-11. Nutrients are introduced into the patient through this tube. This is the most common technique used.

A *nasoenteric tube* is similar, but it is allowed to move further into the digestive tract until it comes to rest in the small intestine, figure 16-12. On occasion, a tube leading directly into the stomach through the abdominal wall (*gastrostomy tube*) is employed.

Tube feedings (gavage) require special

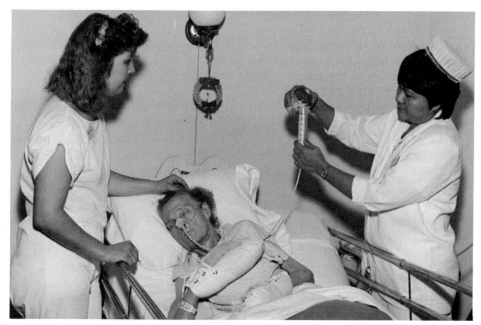

Figure 16-11 Gavage provides nutrients directly into the stomach through a tube.

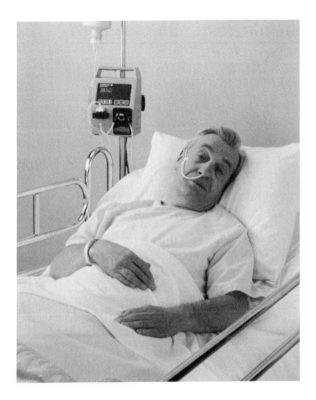
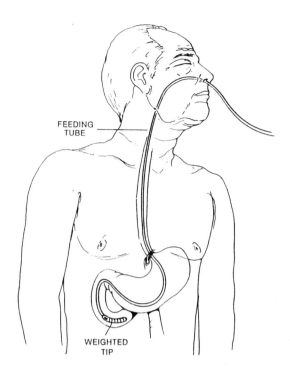

Figure 16-12   Nutrients supplied through a nasoenteric tube that leads directly into the small intestine (Reprinted with permission of Ross Laboratories, Columbus, OH 43216)

skills. Therefore, the nurse (R.N. or L.P.N./L.V.N.) will perform the procedures. The geriatric nursing assistant, however, may be asked to help by preparing the equipment and caring for the patient before, during, and after the feeding.

A nurse inserts the nasogastric tube. The tube is then clamped and taped in place. The free end of the tube is kept covered until it is used for feeding.

Patients must be positioned in a semi-Fowlers or high Fowlers position. Serious consequences can result if the gavage tube is not in the correct position. Make sure not to dislodge the tube when giving care. Do not allow secretions to build up around the external openings to the nose (nares). This could cause irritation and tissue breakdown.

The liquid formulas may be introduced by gravity drip or attached to a pump. The pump is attached to an I.V. standard by the patient's bed, figure 16-13. The pump delivers a set amount of the liquid at a predetermined rate.

Report any deviation of the rate to the nurse. Watch for signs of aspiration, such as excessive coughing, dyspnea, or cyanosis. Let the nurse know before the infusion is completed.

Some patients may even require *hyperalimentation*. In hyperalimentation, a catheter is placed in a large vein, usually the subclavian (under the collar bone). It is advanced to the superior vena cava near the heart. High-density nutrients are thus delivered directly into the bloodstream. This is a sterile procedure and will be performed by the professional staff. Once the tube has been inserted, the site will be covered with a dressing that must not be dislodged.

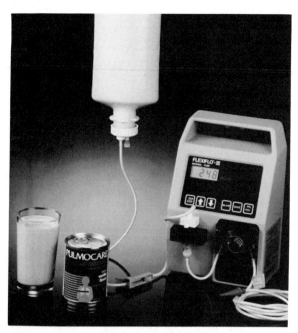

Figure 16-13 The enteric feeding pump controls the amount of nutrients administered and the rate of administration. (Reprinted with permission of Ross Laboratories, Columbus, OH 43216)

Summary

- The nutritional requirements for the elderly are essentially the same as those for the average adult. The older person's caloric needs, however, are lower and the need for vitamins and minerals is greater.
- Food preparation should be altered to allow for slower digestive processes and poorer chewing ability.
- Food habits are firmly established early in life. Great tact and skill are needed to bring about changes in eating patterns when age or physical conditions make changes necessary.
- Eating is a social as well as a nutritive process. Appetites are often improved when eating takes place in the company of others.
- The nursing staff assisting with feeding needs to make those occasions pleasant as well.
- The older person at home may need help in planning practical, nutritious meals that can be conveniently bought, stored, and prepared.

Review Outline

I. Nutrition

    A. Growth and repair
    B. Maintenance of health

II. Signs of Good Nutrition

    A. Healthy hair
    B. Clear skin and eyes
    C. Well-developed body
    D. Pleasant disposition
    E. Healthy sleep
    F. Good appetite

III. Essential Nutrients

    A. Proteins
        1. Growth and repair
        2. Sources

        a. Meat
        b. Fish
        c. Poultry
        d. Eggs
        e. Milk

  B. Carbohydrates
      1. Energy
      2. Roughage
        a. Plant sources
        b. Animal sources
      3. Vitamins and minerals

  C. Fats
      1. Energy
      2. Utilization of vitamins

  D. Vitamins and minerals
      1. Regular body processes
      2. Vitamins—letter designations

  E. Water
      1. 2½ liters needed daily
      2. Inadequate fluids can lead to dehydration
      3. Fluid limitations in specific health conditions

IV. Average Daily Calories

  A. Females up to sixty-five years—1,800
  B. Females over sixty-five years—1,600
  C. Males up to sixty-five years—2,400
  D. Males over sixty-five years—2,050

V. Nutritional Requirements of the Elderly

  A. Similar to other adults
  B. Fewer calories
  C. More vitamins and minerals
  D. Selections included from four food groups

VI. Undernutrition

  A. Common in elderly
  B. Common deficiencies
      1. Calcium
      2. Iron
      3. Folic acid
      4. Magnesium
      5. B vitamins
  C. Nutritional assessment essential

VII. Four Food Groups

  A. Fruits and vegetables
  B. Meat and fish
  C. Dairy products
  D. Breads and cereals

VIII.   Related Problems

    A.   Obesity
    B.   Irregular elimination
    C.   Eating and socialization
    D.   Chewing
    E.   Purchasing and storing foods

IX.   Standard Diets

    A.   Regular (house)
    B.   Clear liquid
    C.   Full liquid
    D.   Soft
    E.   Light
    F.   Pureed

X.   Nutrition in Care Facilities

    A.   Standard diets
    B.   Special diets
       1.   Diabetic
       2.   Low sodium
       3.   Low fat
       4.   Calorie restricted
       5.   High protein
    C.   Geriatric Health Care Provider Responsibilities
       1.   Serve diets
       2.   Feed patients
       3.   Provide supplemental nourishments
       4.   Change drinking water
    D.   Alternate Ways to Provide Nutrition
       1.   I.V.
       2.   Gavage
       3.   Hyperalimentation

Review

I.   Vocabulary

Complete the puzzle by filling in the missing letters of words found in this unit. Use the definitions to help you discover the words.

```
              N _ _ _ _ _ _ _
        _ _ _ _ U _ _ _ _
    _ _ _ _ _ _ T _ _ _
        _ _ _ R _ _ _ _ _ _ _
          _ I _ _ _ _ _
          _ _ T _
      _ _ _ _ _ I _
        _ _ _ _ O _ _ _ _ _ _
              N _ _ _ _ _ _ _ _ _
```

1. Substance essential to body growth
2. Roughage
3. Elimination of solid wastes
4. Related to treatment
5. Nutrient designated by letters
6. Storage form of energy
7. Nutrient that is a basic material of every cell
8. Nutrient used primarily for energy
9. Tube used to gavage

II. True or False

1. Eating patterns and preferences are usually established late in life.
2. Calorie requirements are usually less for the elderly than for the young.
3. When activity decreases, appetite usually increases.
4. Fruits and vegetables are easier to eat if they are cooked, chopped, or puréed.
5. The diets of elderly people are often high in carbohydrates because these foods are inexpensive and easier to chew.
6. The chief cause of tooth loss is periodontal disease.
7. Overcooking meats will make them tender and easy to chew.
8. Eating should be a pleasant experience.
9. The diet of the elderly is most often deficient in vitamins, minerals, and fats.
10. Controlling calories is best accomplished by decreasing the amounts of fats and carbohydrates.

III. Short Answers

1. Why is the elderly person living alone most apt to be malnourished?
2. What is the value of a program such as Meals on Wheels?
3. How does the presence of dentures influence the choice of foods?

IV. Clinical Situations

1. You serve a tray to a resident who is blind and unable to help himself. What do you do?
2. A resident is dehydrated and has an order for F.F. What does this mean?
3. The nurse asks you to assist with a nasogastric feeding. How will you position the patient?

Unit 17
Functional Abilities and Activities of Daily Living

Objectives
After studying this unit, you should be able to:
- Explain the difference between basic activities of daily living (B.A.D.L.) and instrumental activities of daily living (I.A.D.L.).
- List ways to assist elderly people in their B.A.D.L.s and I.A.D.L.s.
- Explain the importance of helping elders maintain independence in their A.D.L.s.

Vocabulary
Learn the meaning and spelling of the following words or phrases.

activities of daily living (A.D.L.)
anorexia
assessment
basic activities of daily living (B.A.D.L.)
contracture
crotch
decubitus
decubitus ulcers
dermal ulcer
elimination
functional status
gastatory
geri chair
hygiene
impaction
incontinence

instrumental activities of
daily living (I.A.D.L.)
pressure sores
range of motion (R.O.M.)

R.E.M.
toileting
transfers
ventilation

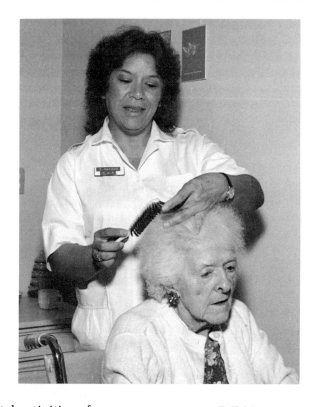

A healthy *functional status* means that the individual is able to take actions that ensure that basic human needs are fulfilled. It also means that the person is able to function within the framework of society.

A person's functional ability, or status, is assessed in the areas of physical and mental health, activities of daily living (A.D.L.), and social status. The need for a comprehensive functional assessment or evaluation was discussed earlier. Knowing only a person's illness provides little information about an elder's self-care ability and functional status. Problems of physical health, mental health, or social function can affect an elderly person's ability to perform A.D.L.s. These problems can eventually lead to loss of functional ability in all areas. *Basic activities of daily living (B.A.D.L.)* include bathing, dressing, *toileting* (taking care of elimination needs), *transfers* (moving from place to place), and feeding. *Instrumental activities of daily living (I.A.D.L.)* are more complex. They usually require interaction with others, to some degree. Included are housekeeping, shopping, doing the laundry, managing money, taking medicine, using transportation, cooking, and using the telephone. It is difficult to know exactly what the elderly are capable of doing without some form of accurate assessment.

There are instruments, or scales, that measure these abilities. They are often found in the resident's record. Two scales often used to measure basic A.D.L.s are the Katz Index of Activities of Daily Living and the Barthel Index. They are very similar although each measures these basic activities in slightly different ways. The Katz Index is scored by indicating whether the elderly person is independent or dependent. The Barthel Index adds a "needs assistance" score.

Knowing what an elderly person can do is important in planning care so that independence is not compromised. If a health care provider tries to save time by assisting or doing the activities of daily living for an elderly person often enough, the result is dependence. Activities of daily living are common to all people, young and old, at home or housed in institutions. Society expects senior adults to find ways to satisfy their basic needs in socially accepted ways. It is not always easy for the elderly to fulfill this expectation. Shopping for nourishing food may be difficult when money is scarce and transportation inconvenient. A decrease in activity and exercise may impair elimination. Physical ailments may limit normal social interactions.

The institutionalized elderly have much more difficulty in carrying out basic and in-strumental activities of daily living. The nursing staff must keep the human needs in mind and devise ways of helping the elderly in their care.

The elderly individual should have as much control as possible over how and when the activities of daily living will be carried out. Even if someone else actually does the task, the desires and input of the resident or patient must be considered.

Many older people could remain in their own homes or with family units if there were some help to assist them in their activities of daily living. Today this role is being met with greater and greater frequency by trained home health aides. These people are specially trained to give this assistance under supervision in the home.

General Hygiene

Hygiene, or practices conducive to health, is an important part of daily living. The scope of these practices does not essentially change with age. However, ways may need to be devised to make it easier for the elderly to care for themselves. Good hygiene plays a part in maintaining a positive self-image. It also supports general health. Behavioral patterns and attitudes are greatly influenced by hygiene. Conversely, hygienic practices sometimes give clues to inner feelings.

The elderly may have difficulty meeting their needs alone, figure 17-1. Review the nursing diagnostic categories in table 17-1 related to difficulties in meeting activities of daily living needs. You will frequently find them in nursing care plans. In some cases, the elderly may be unaware that their hygiene needs correcting. They may not realize that their clothes are soiled, their hair is unkempt, or their teeth need brushing. An older person's eyesight often becomes less sharp. Trembling hands are apt to spill food and misbutton sweaters. Bathing, eating, and caring for clothes, even dressing properly, may also take more effort and energy than the elderly have to give. The health care provider must not assume that because a person is not

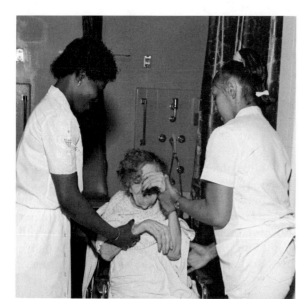

Figure 17-1 Residents may need help in carrying out their hygiene tasks.

always neat and clean that this is the way that he or she chooses to appear (review Unit 8 on physical changes).

The elderly are not children and cannot be

- Activity intolerance
- Alteration in comfort
- Alteration in elimination (bowel or urinary incontinence)
- Alteration in nutrition (overweight or underweight)
- Disturbance in self-concept
- Fatigue
- Ineffective breathing pattern
- Potential for injury
- Potential for joint *contractures* (shortenings)
- Potential impairment of skin integrity
- Self-care deficit (all or specific, such as bathing, toileting, feeding, dressing)
- Sleep pattern disturbance

Table 17-1 Nursing Diagnostic Categories Related to Alterations in Basic Activities of Daily Living

helped in the same way. A child takes dependency for granted; an adult cannot. Self-esteem is quickly lost when dependency is forced on an adult or unnecessary attention called to an obvious need for help. In being unnecessarily helpful, the health care provider may rob patients of what little dignity they have left. Assist patients only as needed in carrying out personal hygiene tasks. Be tactful in making them aware of any deficiencies and helping them improve.

Mental Hygiene

The elderly have psychosocial needs that must be met in order to ensure good mental health, figure 17-2. Stress is felt just as strongly by the older generation as it is by the younger. Yet older people have less stamina to deal with it. Interacting with others to maintain emotional stability is an activity of daily living engaged in by all age groups. The elderly are no exception. They just have fewer options.

Social activities that are mentally stimulating and satisfying contribute to positive mental health. But timing of activities is important. They cannot be enjoyed when the elderly are fatigued, when there is distracting noise, or when hearing aids or glasses are not in good condition. If older people are not able to control these details, the health care provider must assume responsibility. (Review Unit 3, Psychosocial Changes.)

The geriatric health care provider who is alert to the details of social activities can contribute to the good mental health of all residents. Routines give a sense of certainty to existence. The elderly are particularly upset by even minor changes in their routines. Moreover, people lose self-esteem when they feel they have no control over either the routine or the disruption. Try to maintain a routine, at least for major activities. When stress is not managed or pathology causes organic breakdown, mental illness develops. Satisfying social interactions help reduce stress. The problem of mental illness is discussed in Unit 21.

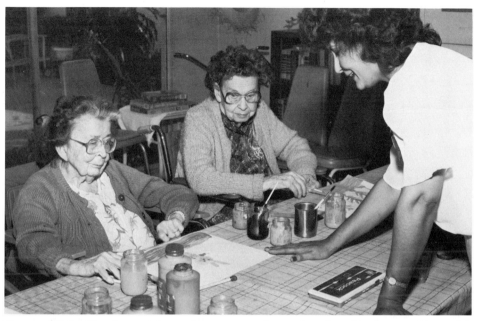

Figure 17-2   Psychosocial needs are met through enjoyable interactions with other people.

Selection of Apparel: Dressing

The old adage "clothes make the man" may not be true. But no one can deny that clothes confer a degree of identity. New recruits entering the military service lose some of their individuality when they give up their own clothes for a uniform. Hospitalized patients feel a sense of loss when trading in their own clothes for a hospital gown. Older people should wear their own clothes whenever possible to enhance their self-image, figure 17-3. Personal lockers, in which at least a few personal articles of clothing can be stored, should be readily available to each resident. When sharing another's home, the older person should have some personal area where his or her own clothing is kept.

Clothing should be chosen for its suitability to the kinds of activities the person participates in and, of course, the weather. Warm clothing should be lightweight. Layering of clothing traps body warmth and provides better insulation than a single heavy garment.

If you are in a position to help an older person select clothes, remember that the patient's personal preferences are the first consideration, as long as safety is not a factor. Long robes that could cause an older person to trip, or loose-fitting sleeves that could catch on fire, are inadvisable. The elder should be encouraged to select materials that are easily laundered, such as drip-dry fabrics. Soft, smooth fabrics such as flannel are best to provide warmth, rather than wool. Wool is apt to be irritating to dry, elderly skin. Color preference in clothing is very individualized. It is often influenced by culture. Some cultures wear white as a sign of mourning. Older women from some Mediterranean cultures wear black because they have earned the *right* because of their age. As a general rule, bright colors tend to lift the spirits and can be an added incentive to maintaining overall appearance.

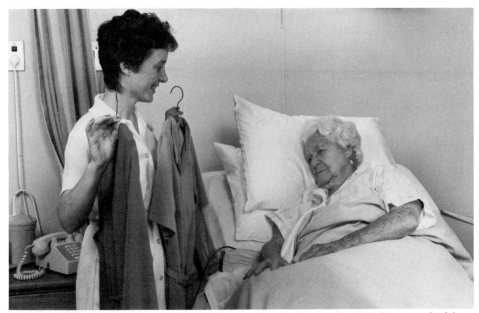

Figure 17-3   Older people should be encouraged to select their own clothing.

Keep in mind the older person's disabilities or energy levels. It can be fatiguing to struggle in and out of difficult clothing. Clothes should be easy to put on. Big buttons are more easily managed than small ones. Zippers and simple buckles are helpful ways to secure openings. Easy-stick (Velcro) fasteners that cling when pressed together form easy closures. This material can be purchased by the yard and in a variety of sizes and shapes. It can be sewn onto clothing, making openings easier to manage for the elderly. Fasteners on the front or side of a garment are more convenient than those in back.

It is very important that shoes and stockings fit, from an esthetic as well as a practical viewpoint. Shoes with tie laces or Velcro fasteners and low, broad heels are the safest. They offer the most support. Slippers that offer no support should be discouraged. Cotton socks, changed frequently, are best, because they help absorb perspiration. Support hose have value in that they stay up better than regular hose. But judgment must be exercised concerning whether the patient should wear them. Most of these stockings are made of nylon, which will not absorb

moisture as well as cotton. Moist feet are more susceptible to injury and infection. Care must also be taken that socks and stockings are not so tight that they interfere with circulation. Circulation to elderly feet is poor to begin with, and constrictions can cause serious complications. Round garters should not be worn for this reason. Rolling the stockings and twisting them to secure them is a poor practice. If stockings are loosely rolled they are apt to fall. If tightly rolled, they will interfere with circulation. A simple garter belt is a much safer method for securing stockings.

If pantyhose are preferred, the crotch should be cotton lined to reduce the possibility of vaginal infections. Support pantyhose are difficult for arthritic hands to manage. Such pantyhose require considerable strength to pull on correctly. Some elderly arthritic women who need support hose for circulatory problems (review Unit 24) use garter belts. Or they cut the crotch out of the pantyhose so that they can toilet themselves without struggling to get the pantyhose up and down.

Underwear should not be restrictive. It

should provide support when needed, because breasts, abdomens, and scrotums tend to sag with age. Many elderly women feel better when they are supported by bras and girdles or one-piece foundation garments. Some men prefer close-fitting underpants. Others prefer boxer (looser) shorts. They type of underwear, and whether a person even wears underwear, is also very individual. Often, small-breasted women will not wear a bra. Some women do not wear underpants, especially with pantyhose.

Underwear should be absorbent and should fit so that skin surfaces do not rub together. It should be made of materials that are easily laundered. Soiling and postvoiding dribbling are fairly common problems among the elderly. Nylon and synthetic fabrics can be used because they are easily washed and quickly dried. But cotton and cotton blends are preferred because they, too, are easily washed. Also, they are more absorptive and less likely to create skin sensitivity.

Whenever possible, the elderly should wear the clothes they are familiar with and in which they are most comfortable. Dressing encourages socialization. It may be the impetus to continence and greater involvement in self-care activities. Instructions for the elderly who are having difficulty dressing will be listed in the nursing care plan for the nursing diagnosis of Self-care Deficit: Dressing/Grooming.

Many times an elderly person can dress partially if the clothes have been laid out. Be sure to provide as much privacy as possible. Draw curtains, shut doors, and knock before entering. Let older people carry out this activity of daily living for themselves to the greatest extent possible.

Cleanliness: Bathing

Because of changes in aging skin, hair, and nails, less bathing is desirable. The skin becomes thinner and dryer, so a tub or shower bath once or twice a week is adequate. Partial baths for comfort can be given more frequently. People are usually more comfortable if they have face and mouth care, and if the hands, axillae, and *crotch* (perineal area) are washed. Lotion can be applied to the back and feet to further increase their comfort while protecting their skin. Nail care should be given as needed. If the nails are particularly thick, deformed, and horny, a podiatrist should be consulted. Hand washing and nail cleaning should be routine after toileting, before meals, and at other times as needed.

Care of teeth or dentures should be given regularly, figure 17-4. Dentures should be stored safely when out of the mouth. The mouth, like the skin and nails, should be inspected carefully. Anything unusual should be reported immediately to the nurse.

Basic cleanliness routines must consider individual preferences, physical limitations, and changes in condition. Be sure you check each patient's care plan daily for specific instructions that will be found to treat the nursing diagnosis

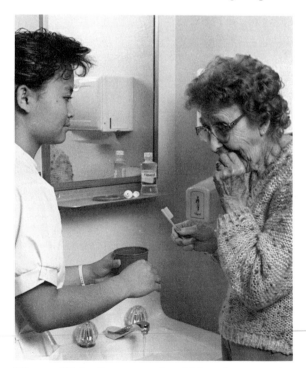

Figure 17-4 Dentures should be given regular care.

of Self-care Deficit: Bathing. One day a patient's condition might permit a tub bath. On another day, a bed bath might be more advisable. Specific care of skin, hair, nails, and dentures is detailed in Unit 26.

Nutrition: Feeding

Eating is another activity of daily living. Most older people are able to participate to some degree. Even if you must do the major part of preparation and feeding, encourage residents to do as much as possible for themselves.

In general, the elderly diet should be low in salt and certain kinds of fats and high in vitamins. It should be selected to meet the specific goals of providing adequate nutrition and stimulating elimination. Foods should be easy to chew and assimilate. Modifications in diet should take into consideration a somewhat slower metabolism, less physical activity, poorer intestinal muscular tone, and any specific limitations, figure 17-5.

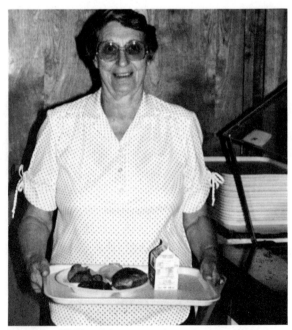

Figure 17-5 Diets need to be modified to accommodate the slower metabolism of the older person.

These might include poor dentures or chewing and swallowing problems.

Attention should also be given to food preferences, cultural habits, and individual eating patterns. The interventions for assisting elders having difficulty feeding themselves or suffering loss of appetite will be listed in the nursing care plan for the nursing diagnoses of Self-care Deficit: Feeding, Alteration in Nutrition: Less than Body Requirements, and *Anorexia* (loss of appetite). Unfortunately, in the institutional setting, individual preferences are not always considered. Older people often do better on several small meals rather than three large meals daily. Adequate fluids help maintain regularity and prevent dehydration. A more detailed discussion of nutritional needs is presented in Unit 16.

Rest and Activity

Activity and rest or sleep need to be balanced. They need to be considered when planning for a patient's activities of daily living. For example, a tub bath is refreshing and part of basic hygiene. It is also a way to encourage activity. Many joints can be exercised as patients assist in carrying out the bathing procedures. Shopping for foods to maintain nutrition, bringing them home, and preparing meals are action activities that increase circulation, ventilation, and joint mobility. These activities need to be interspersed with periods of rest and restoration.

The older person, in general, has less energy and stamina, is able to do less work, and requires more rest and relaxation. Therefore, activities need to be slower paced, figure 17-6. It takes older people more time to dress, to eat, and to eliminate. Geriatric health care providers must remember this and not be impatient. Perceived irritation or impatience on the part of a health care provider often results in older people giving up any attempt to maintain themselves.

Rest: Sleep

For the young, rest takes the form of nightly periods of refreshing sleep. For the elderly, sleep

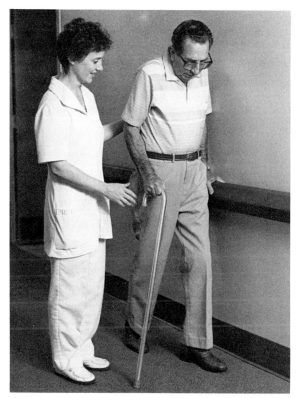

Figure 17-6 Activity must be appropriate for each resident.

patterns vary. The elderly frequently need more time to fall asleep, have more interruptions of their sleep, and sleep more lightly. Therefore, the older person needs less sleep and more rest periods.

Sleep occurs in cycles from deep to light, with and without dreaming. Sleep may be deep and refreshing even if not of long duration. People denied deep sleep become withdrawn, apathetic, depressed, and overly concerned with minor ailments. Often elderly people will nap deeply for short periods and awaken refreshed.

Everyone dreams during some sleep periods. Dreaming can be detected by rapid eye movements *(R.E.M.)*. Sleeping residents may cry or talk as they dream. Because dreaming is important for maintaining emotional integrity, do not awaken someone who seems to be dreaming. Dreamless sleep can lead to irritability, insecur-

ity, and disoriented behavior. Older people may sleep lightly at night and doze deeply during the day. Try not to disturb residents in either of these sleep states.

Symptoms of illness, such as shortness of breath or arthritic pains, stress, anxiety, and depression, can interfere with sleep. They can cause restlessness and sometimes confusion. Nursing measures such as warm fluids to drink, some friendly conversation, straightening the bedding, or giving a backrub should be tried before resorting to medication. Many medications only intensify restlessness. A firm mattress or a board under the mattress affords the best support. Bedding should be light and warm for comfort. An electric blanket, set on low, is comfortable. Although people may choose to use electric blankets in the home, electric blankets are not allowed in extended care facilities. Loss of sensation in the elderly may result in burns if the electric blanket malfunctions. More specific, individualized interventions for the diagnosis of Sleep Disturbance will be found in the nursing care plan.

The elderly should not be permitted to wander at night even if they are receiving adequate sleep during the day. Lowered lighting and shadows lead to confusion and accidents. There is no harm, though, in quiet activity such as reading in their room. Elderly sleep patterns may not be the same as they were in younger years. It is not unusual to find day and night activities almost reversed. Increasing daytime activity and stimulation may encourage more nighttime sleeping. But seniors should be given some leeway in developing their own sleep, rest, and activity patterns. Most extended care facilities maintain a limited staff at night. This may not be the best staffing pattern, considering the facts just discussed.

Activities: Mobility

Maintaining mobility is an important activity of daily living. Activities should be flexible, however, allowing for some degree of personal choice. Just getting out of bed and into a chair may be an opportunity to increase mobility in joints.

Chairs should provide good back support and allow the feet to rest flat on the floor. If the seat is too deep, it will press against the back of the knees and interfere with circulation. The chair should have arms for support. A tray affixed to the front can be used not only for support but also for eating and other activities. Such a chair, sometimes with wheels, is called a *geri chair*, figure 17-7. Seniors should not be left in any chair too long, because hip and knee contractures can develop. If the older person is in a chair for most of the day, he or she should be placed in a prone position for half an hour at least twice during that period. Prolonged sitting in bed or in a chair can predispose an elder to *pressure sores,* or *decubitus ulcers.* Decubitus ulcers are also known as *dermal ulcers.* It is important that the elderly person's position be altered in the chair every hour or so. If necessary, a supportive device such as a gelfoam pad or egg crate should be used (review Unit 26 on the integument). Geri chairs can be arranged for maximum interaction and sociability, which is a real advantage of their use. Extended care facilities are using geriatric chairs more and more. These recliners have wheels and trays and allow several different reclining positions.

Some seniors find that rocking in a rocking chair is a pleasant physical activity that also has beneficial musculoskeletal and circulatory effects to the lower extremities. Rocking chairs should also have supporting arms that can be pushed against when rising. The chairs can be stabilized by putting blocks under the rockers.

Walking, with assistance if necessary, can provide a means of exercising ambulatory muscles and of maintaining strength of the long bones. Simple crafts help maintain small hand muscle function.

Range of motion (R.O.M.) exercises, a part of basic nursing care, should be carried out by the nursing staff when patients are unable to perform these movements for themselves. Even seniors confined largely to bed or a chair should be encouraged to engage in exercise activities to

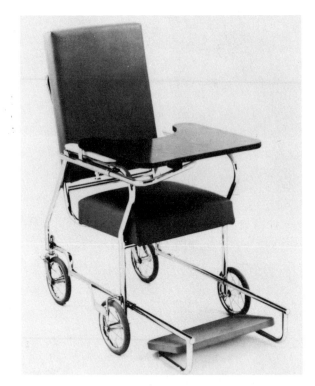

Figure 17-7   The geri chair offers good support as well as a tray for eating and activities.

the extent that they are able. These exercises are taught by the physical therapist or nurse. But the geriatric assistant plays a role in encouraging the patient to do the exercises several times each day and watching to be sure they are performed correctly. Exercises that can comfortably be done include deep breathing, posture maintenance, and flexion and extension of joints in the supine and prone position. Exercise, better posture and deep breathing can improve gas exchange (oxygen and carbon dioxide) and can be beneficial in improving ventilation.

Group exercises performed to music can be stimulating and fun, figure 17-8. Chair exercises can be performed with the senior sitting or standing beside the chair, using it for balance and support. Marching to music and dancing are two other activities that combine pleasure and exercise. Never forget that activities and rest must be balanced so that seniors do not become

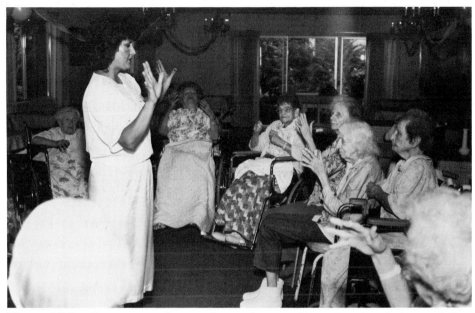

Figure 17-8 Group exercises performed to music can be stimulating and fun.

fatigued. Activity should not be painful. Keep individual limitations in mind.

Range of motion (R.O.M.) exercises that carry all joints through their designated movements are described in Unit 27. You may wish to review with your instructor the basic procedures related to assisting people in their activities of daily living.

Elimination

Elimination includes excretion of both solid and liquid wastes. Elderly people tend to be concerned about regular bowel *elimination*. Changes in the aging digestive tract may make elimination slower and less efficient but the frequency of bowel movements, or one's usual pattern, generally do not change with aging. Some older people believe there will be dire consequences if they fail to have a daily bowel movement. They fear constipation and often will use laxatives to ensure daily elimination. The consequences of constipation, however, should not be minimized. They include fecal impaction, diarrhea, laxative and

enema dependency, and urinary and fecal incontinence. Illness and changes in mobility and diet are often the contributing factors to alterations in bowel elimination. Specific interventions for bowel alterations will be found in the nursing care plan for the diagnosis, Alteration in Bowel Elimination: Diarrhea, Incontinence or Constipation. Exercise, a high-bulk diet, and adequate fluids can usually prevent elimination problems.

Elderly women tend to have more difficulty than men in managing changes in urinary function. There are several reasons for this. Women may not have enough upper body strength for transfers to and from the toilet, they may be unable to walk quickly enough to the toilet when they are experiencing an urge to urinate, or they may not move clothing quickly enough to prevent accidents. Elderly men often solve urinary problems by keeping a urinal nearby. Again, the importance of maintaining independence in A.D.L.s through body strength, mobility, and self-esteem cannot be overstressed.

Urinary complications are discussed in Unit 29 and solid elimination problems in Unit 28.

Summary

- Activities of daily living are all the actions taken to ensure personal comfort and a sense of well-being.
- Cleanliness, balanced rest and activity, proper diet and sufficient fluids to maintain regular elimination, and social interactions are important hygienic practices.
- Seniors who are living in the community maintain their own way of carrying out the activities of daily living, sometimes requiring some assistance. In the care setting, the health care provider must assume the tasks that elders can no longer do for themselves.
- Fatigue comes easily but can be avoided if judgment is used in planning the day's activities.
- It is sometimes difficult for the elderly to accept that their physical powers have diminished with age.
- Tact is needed to help them adjust to necessary changes in routine.
- Self-esteem and mental health are protected by careful choice of satisfying social interactions.

Review Outline

I. Behavioral Objectives

II. Vocabulary

III. Activities of Daily Living

    A. Basic activities of daily living (B.A.D.L.)
       1. Health—basic needs met
       2. Illness/Age—one or more needs unmet
       3. B.A.D.L.s include
         a. Hygiene
         b. Dressing
         c. Toileting
         d. Transfers
         e. Feeding

    B. Instrumental Activities of Daily Living (I.A.D.L.)
       1. Require interaction with others
       2. Include
         a. Shopping/cooking
         b. Laundry/housekeeping
         c. Money management
         d. Using transportation/telephone

IV. Assessment Scales

    A. Katz index measures level of dependency
    B. Barthel index measures needs assistance

V. Mental Hygiene

    A. Importance of routines
    B. Importance of social interactions
    C. Need to feel measure of control

VI.   Selection of Apparel

    A.   Own clothes preferred
    B.   Appropriate for activity
    C.   Safety considerations

VII.   General Hygiene

    A.   Less frequent bathing
    B.   Nail care
    C.   Teeth care

VIII.   Nutrition/Feeding

    A.   Diet
        1.   Easy to chew/digest
        2.   Low salt, low fat/high vitamins and minerals
        3.   Individual modifications
        4.   Several smaller meals daily
    B.   Assistance with Feeding

IX.   Rest and Activity

    A.   Sleep
        1.   Patterns vary
        2.   Short, deeper sleep
        3.   Frequent naps
    B.   Problem of nocturnal wakefulness

X.   Activities/Mobility

    A.   Must be flexible
    B.   Meet individual needs/abilities
    C.   Involve frequent change of position

XI.   Elimination

    A.   Includes liquid/solid wastes
    B.   Affected by aging changes
        1.   Incontinence
        2.   Diarrhea
        3.   Constipation
    C.   Cause for elderly concern

Review

I.   Vocabulary

Write the definitions of each of the following terms.

    1.   elimination
    2.   geri chair

     3. hygiene
     4. ventilation
     5. A.D.L.

II.   True or False

     1. Basic human needs are common to both young and old.
     2. A.D.L. stands for articles of daily living.
     3. A.D.L. are actions taken to ensure comfort and a sense of well-being.
     4. Hygienic measures include bathing, and full baths are necessary every day.
     5. Whenever possible, the elder should be given only limited choices in the selection of activities and clothing.
     6. Soft slippers do not offer firm support, so ambulation is safer in shoes.
     7. Large buttons on the side of a garment make it more difficult fo the elderly to dress themselves.
     8. Wearing one's own clothes helps one retain a sense of identity.
     9. Round garters should never be used to hold up stockings.
   10. Socks and underwear of cotton are best because they are most absorbent.

III.   Short Answers

     1. What is the value of a geri chair?
     2. Why should activities be spaced with rest periods for the elderly?
     3. What kinds of exercises should be encouraged for the bed patient?
     4. What is the difference between basic and instrumental activities of daily living? List the activities of each group.
     5. What consequences can result from not attending to a resident's complaints of constipation?

IV.   Clinical Situations

     1. A resident tells you she is worried because she hasn't had a bowel movement for three days. How do you respond?
     2. You pass by a resident's room and notice him mumbling in his sleep in the afternoon. How do you respond?
     3. An elderly resident asks you for help in writing out an order for crotchless pantyhose from an intimate apparel mail order house. How do you respond?
     4. An elderly man with severe tremors of the hands and head insists on feeding himself even though food spills all over him and the floor. What do you do?
     5. Several elderly people have been sitting in geri chairs playing a game for over two hours. What should your concern and action be?

Unit 18
Drug Therapy

Objectives

After studying this unit, you should be able to:
- Describe social and cultural influences that affect drug-taking behavior in the elderly.
- Describe the methods of medicating an elderly person.
- Identify unusual responses that need to be reported.
- Explain why medications may affect the elderly differently from other age groups.
- Discuss methods that can help the elderly take their medications at home.

Vocabulary

Learn the meaning and spelling of the following words or phrases.

analgesic
antibiotics
antihypertensives
cardiotonics
detoxify
diaphoresis
diuretics
glycemic
hyperglycemia

hypnotics
induration
ischemia
orthostatic
patient controlled
   analgesia (P.C.A.)
polypharmacy
reaction

sedatives
sleep apnea
somnifacient
steroids
tinnitus
tranquilizers
untoward
vasodilators

This is an age of wonder drugs and medications. Many of these can be easily purchased over the counter. New drugs of all kinds are continually being manufactured that promise relief from a wide variety of ailments. Having reached old age during these years of pharmaceutical improvements, some elderly have come to believe that the right pill or tablet can ease all their physical ills. Unfortunately, practitioners in the health care system have reinforced this belief. They tend to discuss problems with their elderly patients less often than they do with younger people, and they use drugs as a first-choice therapy. This has created a problem called *polypharmacy*. When residents see several health care providers for different problems, multiple medications may be prescribed that may have adverse reactions. Polypharmacy is a common problem in extended care facilities.

Aging increases health needs and decreases recuperative resources. The older generation is particularly susceptible to the glib, all-encompassing promises of advertisers. They frequently spend their meager funds on advertised "miracle drugs" and receive little value in return. It is estimated that the American public spends over $400 million each year on over-the-counter medicines, figure 18-1. A large part of that sum is spent by the elderly. Twenty-five percent of all prescriptions are written for the elderly, who represent slightly over 12 percent of the population. One danger of all this self-medication is that it delays proper diagnosis and treatment, may cause serious drug interactions, and may mask a serious problem until it is too late.

Sociocultural and economic factors influence attitudes toward taking drugs. Some elderly people do not like to take drugs of any kind and, indeed, refuse to do so. At the opposite extreme are those who believe that "if one is good, two are better." Their medicine cabinets are full of prescription and patent drugs. Some may be kept long after they are no longer effective. Those people at one extreme hoard pills and tablets. Those at the other refuse to take their prescribed medications, if possible. It is a fact, however, that as a person ages, failing body systems and multiple chronic illnesses need the support, stimulation, and correction that drugs can offer. It is a further fact that the elderly receive more prescriptions and spend more money on medicine and health services than any other age groups.

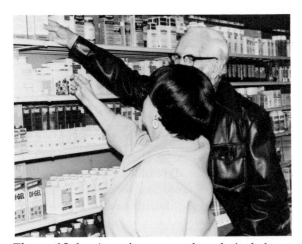

Figure 18-1 Americans spend a relatively large portion of their spendable income on over-the-counter medicines.

Drug Administration

By law, a person giving medications must be licensed to do so. This includes physicians, registered nurses, and licensed vocational or licensed practical nurses. Geriatric health care providers may not perform this function. For drugs to be administered safely, the nurse must know the drug to be given, its desired effects, its possible side effects, and possible interactions with foods and other drugs. The nurse must be able to explain these facts to patients and their families, figure 18-2.

Giving medications involves more than delivering drugs and seeing that they are consumed. The nurse must be constantly alert for changes in the patient's physical condition or mental responses that might indicate a side effect or interaction of the drug therapy. This means that the nurse must have a firm education in pharmacology. Nausea, vomiting, changes in pulse rate and rhythm, dizziness, and visual disturbances are common side effects. Mood swings, increased irritability, and insomnia may also be manifestations of drug reactions in the elderly. The most common adverse drug effects in the elderly are confusion, falls, incontinence, and immobility. Review table 18-1 for the diagnostic categories related to problems with medications.

Untoward (adverse) reactions may be demonstrated in unusual ways and may not develop as quickly as they did when the person was young. Drug reactions may sometimes continue despite withdrawal of the medication.

Although you may not actually dispense the medication, you also must be alert to changes in patient response or condition that might indicate a drug reaction. Any unusual responses must be immediately reported to the nurse.

Residents who are at greatest risk for untoward reactions to medications are those who have multiple illnesses, or have general allergies, or those who are frail or of small build. Those who have respiratory, renal, liver, or cardiovascular diseases are at extreme risk and need to be monitored carefully. Dehydration, conges-

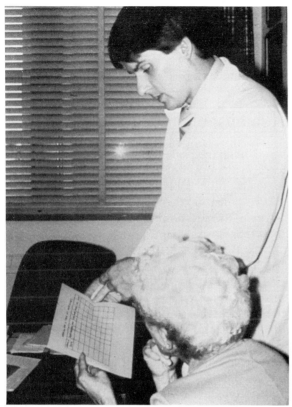

Figure 18-2 Facts regarding medications should be clearly explained to the patient and family members.

- Activity intolerance
- Alterations in health maintenance
- Alteration in thought processes: Confusion
- Alteration in urinary elimination: Incontinence
- Fluid volume deficit
- Impaired physical mobility
- Ineffective breathing pattern
- Knowledge deficit: Medications
- Potential for injury: Falls
- Sensory perceptual alteration: Vision, hearing, *gustatory (taste)*
- Sleep pattern disturbance

Table 18-1 Diagnostic Categories Related to Medication Problems

tive heart failure, and pneumonia also increase the risk.

People who live alone or who suffer from mental impairment may not manage their medications accurately. They are more likely to run into difficulties. Drug omission or overdoses are common. The most commonly misused medications are sleeping pills, anti-anxiety drugs, pain medications, laxatives, and antacids.

Drugs and their Actions

Drug	Action
Analgesic	Relieves pain
Antibiotic	Combats infection
Antihypertensive	Lowers blood pressure
Antiinflammatory compounds	Reduces inflammation
Diuretic	Promotes urine output
Hypoglycemic	Lowers blood sugar
Hypnotic	Induces sleep
Laxative	Promotes elimination
Sedative	Produces a quieting effect
Somnifacient	Produces sleep
Steroid	Decreases inflammation

Age-Related Changes

Age is a factor that affects the administration of drugs. Over the years an individual's reactions to drugs changes. Resistance to the expected effect and sensitivity to specific drugs both increase. Disease, malnutrition, and dehydration affect drug concentration in the body. The elderly also have more adipose (fat) and less muscle tissue, lower total body weight, and less body water than do younger people. All of these listed factors affect drug absorption, storage, and excretion. The aging body is no longer able to absorb or circulate medications as easily. The liver and kidneys are less efficient. Therefore, it is more difficult to metabolize, *detoxify* (remove harmful products), and excrete drugs. There is a greater tendency to retain sodium and water, thereby threatening electrolyte balance, particularly by the loss of potassium. Poor absorption by the intestinal tract can mean that drug intake may be erratic. Drugs are more apt to accumulate in the body fat, bringing on unpredictable complications. Reactions are apt to be more severe, because older people have a lower vital reserve. For these reasons, drug dosages are usually smaller for the elderly than they are for younger patients. To decrease the cumulative toxic effects, some extended care facilities practice "drug vacations" by omitting some drugs on weekends.

Drugs that are relatively nontoxic, do not cause easy addiction, and are specifically effective are best for the elderly person. Cost is another factor that must be considered. Meager finances must not be used up on expensive drugs if less expensive but equally effective ones are available. Elderly people may seem noncompliant in taking medications. The real problem may be that they cannot afford to buy the medications because of their expense or they cannot open the containers because of child-proof tops. Generic drugs can often be used instead of more expensive name brands. The use of generic drugs can often cause confusion. People may not believe or realize that two different generic drugs are the same. They may refuse to take the prescription because it is a different color or shape. They may also take both drugs, believing that they are different medications.

The nurse must be careful to report any omissions or refusals of medication and use good judgment when giving medications, especially with p.r.n. (as needed) orders. Be sure to document the results of the p.r.n. medication. Too vigorous drug therapy can be dangerous for an elderly person. For example, all analgesics, hypnotics, tranquilizers, and sedatives tend to inhibit respiratory function in the aged, some of whom may have *sleep apnea* (stoppage of brea-

thing during sleep), and many of whom already suffer from cardiopulmonary insufficiency. Observant nursing care by all staff members is essential if drug problems from overdosage and adverse interactions are to be avoided.

Administration of Drugs

Nurses responsible for giving medications are also responsible for knowing why the particular medication is being given and for assessing the response in the patient, both desired and adverse. Nurses should question medication dosages that do not seem appropriate for the size and body weight of the elderly person. Certain baseline information is also necessary in order to evaluate any suspected change in a client. This information includes usual pulse rate, blood pressure, mental status, sensory function, history of allergies, and so on. All medications should be checked against a drug compatibility chart to ensure safe drug-drug interactions. In some extended care facilities, patients who are capable administer their own medications, especially for pain (*patient controlled analgesia* or *P.C.A.*). It is very important to monitor the mental status in these patients to assure safety.

Following are some points that the nurse should keep in mind when administering drugs. The nurse must first identify the patient. Confusion or poor hearing may make patients respond to names other than their own. Any changes in medications should be explained to the patient before presentation. The older person is easily upset by unexpected changes in routine and may be reluctant to take a new medication. Because older people frequently suffer from more than one physical problem, they may be taking several drugs. Some of these may be prescribed. Others may have been purchased over the counter. The elderly sometimes visit more than one physician, obtaining prescriptions with each visit. Harmful interactions are apt to occur under these circumstances, figure 18-3. Therefore, it is extremely important to obtain a complete account of all medications being taken. This information

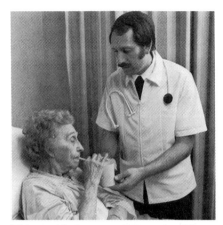

Figure 18-3 People who are frail and have multiple ailments are at greatest risk for drug interactions. (From Caldwell and Hegner, *Nursing Assistant, A Nursing Process Approach,* 5th edition, copyright 1989 by Delmar Publishers Inc.)

may come to other staff members. If so, it must be given to the medication nurse immediately.

Medications can be administered by a number of routes. The nurse must have permission before a route of drug administration is changed.

Parenteral Route

Parenteral medications may be administered intravenously, intradermally, subcutaneously, or intramuscularly. All require the use of needles to reach the correct site. Elderly skin is tough and difficult to penetrate. There is usually less adipose tissue than in a younger person, connective tissue is no longer resilient, and muscles may be atrophied. These factors are especially important when giving intramuscular injections. Because muscle loss is prominent in the thighs and buttocks, they are poor sites for injections. A much safer site is the hip (ventrogluteal) because it has three layers of muscles and no major nerves or blood vessels. It also has the advantage of almost always being accessible— sitting, standing, supine, prone, and sidelying.

Whether a patient is thin, normal size, or fat, the appropriate-length needle should be used. Frequently, the loss of elasticity will cause the injection site to bleed. Pressure and a small pressure dressing may control the bleeding. Closely inspect the area for local reactions. Localized reactions are seen more often in the elderly because of their poorer circulation. Be sure to report any reactions such as pain, *induration* (hardness), or inflammation that you may notice as routine care is given.

Oral Route

Medications administered by mouth pose some specific problems. The elderly patient, whose mucous membranes are drier, may have difficulty swallowing. A patient with cardiopulmonary problems may fear choking. Sometimes capsules remain in the oral cavity without the older person even being aware of them. Therefore, adequate fluids must be administered when giving oral medications to the elderly. Sometimes it will be necessary to check the patient's mouth to see that the medication has been swallowed. Be sure that the patient is positioned properly. Health care providers must make sure that the patient really takes medication.

If a drug is difficult to swallow or unpleasant to take, the nurse should ask the pharmacist whether the drug can be crushed and mixed with food. There may also be another form, such as a liquid, available. Remember never to crush enteric-coated tablets, time-release drugs, or capsules.

Crushing drugs and mixing them with foods often alters the effects of the drugs. In addition, it does not guarantee that the dosage is swallowed and absorbed. It is far safer to use other methods, such as positioning, offering plenty of fluid, reassuring the patient, and obtaining liquid forms of medications, if available. Medications should only be given with nourishment, if it is not contraindicated.

Capsules, of course, must not be broken open. The purpose of using a capsule covering is to mask the unpleasant taste of the drug. Oral hygiene can help prevent bitter or unpleasant aftertastes following medication.

The staff should watch stools for enteric-coated tablets, which may pass through the intestinal tract without breaking down. If tablets are noted in the stool, the specimen should be saved and the situation reported to the nurse.

Dermal Route

More medications are being given through the dermal (skin) route. Medication, such as nitropaste, a heart medication, is applied to a patch. The patch is placed against the patient's skin and the drug is absorbed into the patient's body. To be effective, it is important that the medicated patch remain in contact with the patient's skin. The geriatric health care provider should report loose patches or patches that have come off. Often a loose patch is secured with a piece of tape.

Rectal Route

Some drugs come commercially prepared in oil for rectal administration. Others may need to be dissolved in oil before administration. In either case, the routine is the same as for any rectal medication. Remember that circulation in the older person is not as efficient as it is in younger people. Therefore, drugs given as suppositories in the rectum or vagina may take longer to break down and become effective.

Geriatric Drugs

There are no drugs specifically indicated or contraindicated by age alone. However, certain types of drugs are given more frequently with advancing age.

As mentioned earlier in this unit, polypharmacy is particularly common in extended care facilities. The average resident receives six medications. The most commonly prescribed medications are tranquilizers and sedatives. All too frequently these drugs add to problems that, had they been investigated, could have been treated. Remember that elders do not show the same signs and symptoms of illness as younger people do. Most commonly, elderly people show signs such as confusion or incontinence.

Other commonly prescribed drugs for the elderly are sedatives, hypnotics, hypoglycemics, cardiovascular drugs, and diuretics. In addition, drugs given to the elderly include nutritional supplements, mood-altering drugs, laxatives, analgesics, antibiotics, and anti-inflammatory compounds.

Sedatives/Hypnotics

Sedatives are drugs used to treat anxiety states and help patients feel calmer. *Hypnotics* are used to treat insomnia (sleeplessness). These drugs cause general central nervous system depression. Patients tend to develop a tolerance to them with chronic use. There is also the potential for patients to develop psychological or physical dependence on them.

Drugs that reduce anxiety and induce sleep are frequently given in extended care facilities. Flurazepam (Dalmane) and chloral hydrate (Noctec) are the most-often-prescribed hypnotics. Others ordered include temazepam (Restoril) and triazolam (Halcion). Oxazepam (Serax) is ordered as a sedative.

Barbiturates are not recommended because the elderly have an increased sensitivity to them. These drugs tend to be stored in adipose tissue, which leads to a cumulative effect. Barbiturates are usually administered subcutaneously or orally. The cumulative effect is often bizarre and unexpected. The drugs tend to be habit forming. Therefore, they must be used carefully. Instead of the usual sedative effect, these drugs frequently cause patients to become confused. Agitation, persistent drowsiness, headaches, skin eruptions, an uneven gait, and itching are all side effects for which the staff should be alert. Interactions with other drugs such as narcotics, alcohol, or antihistamines can be dangerous. The potential for abuse of these drugs is great. Exercise care when administering them.

All nursing measures to ensure that the patient is relaxed should be employed before resorting to sedatives for sleep. A quiet, well-ventilated room free from drafts; a warm drink; a few minutes of conversation; a position change; and adequate lighting to eliminate shadows should be considered.

Hypoglycemics

Drugs that lower blood sugar levels are called hypoglycemic drugs. *Hyperglycemia* (excessive blood sugar) is a major problem for the elderly diabetic who most often suffers from the non-insulin-dependent form of the disease. Oral hypoglycemic drugs are usually prescribed to keep *glycemic* (blood sugar) levels controlled. When insulin is required, the dosages are kept very low. They are increased until effective levels are reached.

Commonly prescribed hypoglycemic oral agents are tolbutamide (Orinase), chlorpropadime (Diabenase), and glyburide (Micronase). Patients must be watched carefully for signs of hypoglycemia. The usual signs may be absent. Slurred speech and mental confusion may be noted first, figure 18-4.

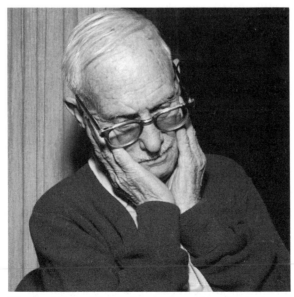

Figure 18-4 Slurred speech and confusion may be early indications of a hypoglycemic reaction.

All these oral hypoglycemic agents can interact with other medications. For example, alcohol, large doses of salicylates, and oral anticoagulants can increase hypoglycemic effects. Some diuretics (furosemide) and cortisone-like drugs can inhibit its actions.

Cardiovascular Drugs

Drugs that affect the circulatory system are often ordered. These include *cardiotonics* (heart stimulating), antihypotensive agents, and *vasodilators* to increase peripheral circulation. Because the conductive mechanism of the heart is less effective in the older patient, careful adjustment of the dosages is necessary. Sudden hypotension can precipitate a stroke.

Digitalis preparations such as digoxin are cardiotonic and are very commonly given, figure 18-5. Toxicity to this drug is a threat because the elderly require a lower dose and hypokalemia (common in the elderly) increases the possibility of toxicity. The drug is less effective when taken in conjunction with antibiotic therapy or in the presence of anemia. Signs of digitalis toxicity must not be missed. Signs of toxicity include nausea, loss of appetite, vomiting, mental confusion, changes in cardiac rate and rhythm, and visual disturbances.

Antihypertensives

Thiazide diuretics used alone or with other drugs are commonly ordered to control blood pressure. Specific hypertensive drugs that may be used alone or in combination include reserpine (Sandril), methyldopa hydrochloride (Aldomet), propranolol hydrochloride (Inderol), nadolol (Corgard), clonidine hydrochloride (Catapres), and nifedipine (Procardia).

Toxicity to reserpine results in serious depression. Therefore, patients must be monitored for withdrawal, agitation, and apathy. Hemolytic anemia and hepatitis may develop when methyldopa is prescribed. Insomnia, nightmares, nausea, vomiting, diarrhea, fatigue, dizziness, and psychotic behaviors may be observed when the patient takes beta-adrenergic blockers, prop-

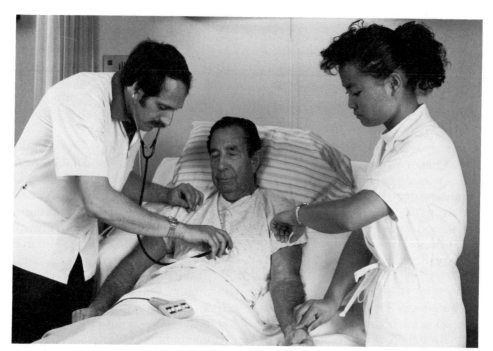

Figure 18-5 Apical pulse must be checked before administering digitalis preparations.

ranolol, and nadolol. Close observation and documentation of the patient's blood pressure and mental state must be maintained, figure 18-6. Antihypertensives and vasodilators often cause hypotension. This can result in dizziness, falls, and strokes. These patients especially need to move slowly from supine or sitting to standing positions so that their circulatory systems can adjust to the position change.

Vasodilators

Drugs such as nitroglycerin that relax smooth muscles and dilate blood vessels are frequently ordered for those suffering from myocardial *ischemia* (lack of blood flow). The anginal products come in various forms. Those who provide care must be familiar with the proper techniques of administration. Some products may be inhaled as vapors. Others are absorbed either through the skin or under the tongue. Side effects include dizziness, *orthostatic* (position

changing) hypotension, flushing, and throbbing headaches.

Diuretics

Diuretics are drugs that increase the output of urine. They do not all affect the body in the same way. The thiazide diuretics such as hydrochlorthiazide and bendroflumethiazide (Naturetin) inhibit sodium absorption while they increase the output of potassium and chlorides. Others such as the loop diuretics (furosemide and Lasix) block the reabsorption of sodium and chlorides in the kidneys. Potassium-sparing diuretics such as spironolactone (Aldactone) block aldosterone, a hormone that promotes sodium retention and potassium loss.

When diuretics are administered, the patient must be watched carefully for signs of dehydration and electrolyte imbalance. Dizziness, fatigue, muscle cramps or weakness, and nausea should be reported promptly. Daily patient

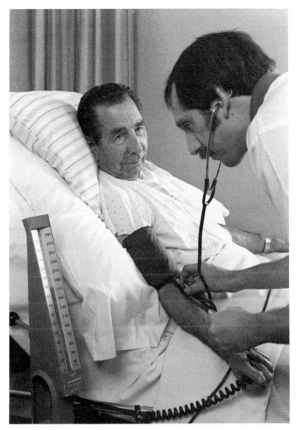

Figure 18-6 The patient's blood pressure must be observed and documented when the patient is receiving antihypertensive drugs.

weighing and accurate intake and output records help monitor the effectiveness of the drugs. Diuretics should be given early in the morning to interfere as little as possible with sleep. To counteract the loss of potassium, foods high in potassium should be included in the diet.

Incontinence may not be a signal of the onset of illness when diuretics are being given. The incontinence may only be the result of the bladder filling more quickly and creating stress before the patient is able to get to the toilet. Reassuring and helping the patient to wash and change clothes is the nonjudgmental way of handling the situation.

Nutritional Supplements

Vitamins and minerals are often needed by the elderly because they may be absorbed and utilized inadequately. Many older people may needlessly spend money on excessive amounts of these supplements and require advice about optimum levels. Vitamins A, D, and trytophan can cause serious problems if taken in large doses. More is not better when taking vitamins.

Mood-Altering Drugs (Hypnotics and Soporifics)

Some medicines are administered that affect the patient's mood, sensory responses, and degree of relaxation. Older persons experience depression and are assisted in coping with their situations. Antidepressants such as the tricyclic compounds are best, because they have fewer side effects. They cannot be used, however, if there is a history of a heart attack because they may precipitate another one. Amphetamines in some forms are widely used, but they can cause great mood swings. They should be given with caution and in minimal dosages. Tranquilizers, such as chlorpromazine (Thorazine) and thioridazine (Mellaril) reduce sensitivity to sensory annoyances while producing a degree of euphoria and relieving muscle tension. These drugs should not be given simply to reduce tension. Nursing measures such as taking or administering a backrub, a position change, or something to drink can often reduce tension without the aid of drugs, figure 18-7.

Patients receiving these drugs must be watched for hypotension and faintness. Watch for sudden mood swings or emotional responses that are inappropriate to the circumstances and report, figure 18-8. Also watch for blurred vision, urinary retention, constipation, *diaphoresis* (excessive perspiration), and dry mouth.

Many nursing and other experts recommend behavioral and environmental therapies instead of drug therapy to deal with behavioral problems in extended care facilities. These therapies are effective, do not make "chemical prisoners," and are much safer.

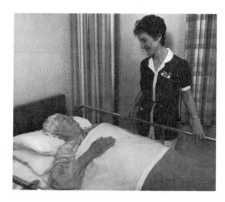

Figure 18-7 Tension can often be relieved without the use of drugs through simple nursing measures such as taking a few moments to talk. (From Caldwell and Hegner, *Nursing Assistant, A Nursing Process Approach,* 5th edition, copyright 1989 by Delmar Publishers Inc.)

The drugs are usually administered by mouth. These drugs have a cumulative effect. Reactions to them are often bizarre and unexpected. They tend to be habit forming and there-

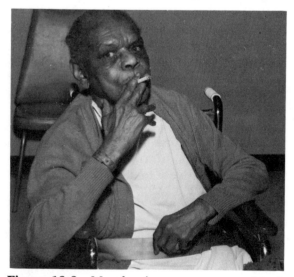

Figure 18-8 Mood swings can occur suddenly when patients are on mood-altering medications.

fore must be used carefully. Instead of the usual sedative effect, they frequently cause patients to become confused. Agitation, persistent drowsiness, slowed respirations, headaches, skin eruptions, an uneven gait, and itching are all side effects for which the staff should be alert. Interaction with other drugs such as narcotics, alcohol, or antihistamines can be dangerous. The potential for abuse of these drugs is great, so care must be exercised in their administration.

Alcohol

Alcohol is used for its relaxing and sedative effect. It is a mood-altering chemical. Its value lies in its cerebral depressant and vasodilator action. In small quantities, it acts as an appetite stimulant. There are mixed feelings in the profession about the use of alcohol in geriatric therapy. There is always the potential for alcohol dependence to develop. This danger cannot be minimized or disregarded. Many feel that the possibility of alcoholism is lower for the elderly than it is for the young. But an alcoholic at any age faces tremendous difficulties. Compounded by aging, those difficulties may be insurmountable. Here, as always in geriatrics, the emphasis should be on moderation. Alcohol as a therapy seems to have the best effect when used in conformity with the resident's usual habits.

Cocktail hours, a fairly recent innovation in some extended care facilities and residential facilities, have been effective in increasing the general morale and social responsiveness of the residents. All residents are served fruit and vegetable juices with alcohol on prescription. Some extended care facilities have experimented with afternoon meetings where beer, tea, and coffee are served. The residents have also accepted this type of gathering. The real value may lie in the congeniality that the event inspires rather than in the type of beverage served. Some health care providers may have some difficulty accepting alcohol as a legitimate therapy. This is especially true if they have been actively involved in the care and rehabilitation of alcoholics.

Laxatives

Laxatives and suppositories are used to promote bowel regularity. Bulk laxatives made from agar and psyllium seed, such as Metamucil, increase intestinal bulk and thus promote bowel movements. Such laxatives must be given with adequate fluid to prevent constipation.

Stimulant laxatives, such as castor oil and bisacodyl (Dulcolax), often cause abdominal cramping and urgency. With chronic use these laxatives may result in malabsorption of nutrients. Saline (salt) laxatives, such as milk of magnesia, can cause excessive fluid and electrolyte imbalance. Hyperosmotic laxatives, such as lactulose and glycerine, are probably safer in older people because of fewer reported side effects. Emollient laxatives, such as mineral oil, should be avoided in the elderly because they interfere with the absorption of vitamins A and D in the intestine and may result in anal leakage. Also, if vomitus with mineral oil is aspirated, pneumonitis may result. For these reasons, mineral oil is not usually recommended, but it is easily available and is used by many elderly persons.

Antibiotics

Antibiotics, now more commonly called antimicrobials, are one of the most important advances in treatment. They effectively treat infections, improve the quality of life for people, and make many other kinds of treatments possible, for example aggressive cancer chemotherapy, organ transplants such as lenses, bone and kidneys and other major surgery. Many elders would not have been able to benefit from these treatments without antimicrobials. If an infection is suspected based on the signs and symptoms and the history the elder provides, blood and culture tests may be performed and antimicrobials prescribed immediately. The reason drugs are not held until the laboratory results come back is because infections are best treated early before the organisms multiply so rapidly that a person is put at great risk. Generally, what is called a broad spectrum antimicrobial will be ordered. It is called broad spectrum because it is effective against many organisms, gram negative and gram positive. When the culture report is returned from the laboratory, the nurse and physician will look at the *culture* report to determine what organism is causing the infection and the *susceptibility* testing. Susceptibility means what antimicrobials are effective against the organism because it is *sensitive* to them and what antimicrobials are ineffective because the organism is *resistant* to them. There are some antimicrobials that are effective only against selected organisms that have developed resistance to the more commonly used drugs. These are used very cautiously because if resistance develops to them, there may be no other drug to use against the organism causing the infection. The *cephalosporins* are a group of broad spectrum antimicrobials.

Anti-inflammatory Drugs

Anti-inflammatory drugs are classified as nonsteroidal anti-inflammatory drugs (NSAIDS) and steroids. Salicylates are the most commonly used NSAID medication for arthritic conditions. (These are discussed in the section on analgesics.) Other nonaspirin drugs that produce fewer gastrointestinal complaints are also being used. These include ibuprofen (Motrin) and tolmetin (Rolectin). These drugs take longer to become effective and each has its own possible side effects. Patients taking motrin must be watched for drowsiness, dizziness, *tinnitus* (ringing in the ears), and blurred vision. Tolmetin side effects include hyperthermia, prolonged bleeding time, dizziness, visual disturbances, and sodium retention.

Rheumatoid arthritis is sometimes treated with gold salts. Responses develop over several months. Side effects include alterations in the blood cell production, bradycardia, inflammation of the liver and kidneys, and, in some cases, the severe reaction of anaphylactic shock.

Gout, a metabolic abnormality, is treated with colchicine. Colchicine therapy may cause nausea, vomiting, muscle weakness, confusion, and convulsions.

Steroids

Steroids are drugs used to decrease inflammation. They do so by improving the general protective function of the tissues and increasing protection against stress and degeneration. However, they decrease resistance to infection. Residents taking steroids must be carefully monitored, because these drugs tend to cause gastric ulceration with hemorrhage and perforations. Watch stools for color change (blackening), which would indicate bleeding in the gastrointestinal tract. Monitor the resident carefully for signs of infection.

Analgesics

Analgesics are drugs which reduce pain. The elderly experience pain for a variety of reasons other than disease. Constipation or an awkward position can cause much distress and pain. This pain can be alleviated without using medications. Therefore, efforts should be made to identify the cause of the discomfort.

The most common analgesic used by the elderly is aspirin (acetylsalicylic acid). Aspirin provides not only analgesia, but may also be used for its antipyretic and anti-inflammatory effects. Aspirin is frequently taken in combination with a buffer to reduce gastric distress. These products are readily available over the counter.

Residents ingesting aspirin must be watched for indications of gastrointestinal bleeding. They occasionally show signs of central nervous system disturbances, such as tinnitus.

A second type of commonly taken analgesic is acetaminophen. This analgesic is the main ingredient in a number of over-the-counter medications. These medications seem to produce fewer side effects compared to aspirin.

For stronger pain relief, codeine, either alone or in combination with aspirin, may be ordered. Residents frequently experience constipation and drowsiness when these products are taken.

Antacids

Because the elderly frequently suffer from gastrointestinal discomfort, they frequently take antacids. There are a variety of these preparations, each with different actions. Residents on sodium-restricted diets should not use sodium-based antacids. Those preparations with a calcium-carbonate base should be avoided by those with renal calculi or those who suffer from constipation. They should not be given with milk. Aluminum hydroxide and aluminum phosphate preparations can cause constipation.

The elderly often do not consider antacids as "medications." They fail to realize that drug interactions are possible.

Medications at Home

The elderly person who takes medicines and remains at home may pose a specific set of problems. Although the vast majority manage their situations well, a small percentage need help, figure 18-9. The rate of self-medication errors among elders is estimated to be between 25 and 50 percent. Most errors that occur in the home are the result of forgetfulness or misunderstanding of the directions. Errors may also be caused by the resident's denial of a diagnosis of illness or a change in his or her mental status. An inability to get to the store to get medications or a lack of understanding about the need for the medication are other reasons. Sensory impairment may be another factor causing errors.

Directions for taking medications should be simple and should be given both orally and in writing. Such directions should include the name and dosage of the drug, as well as the time and route of administration. The explanation should indicate any adverse reactions that may occur and should be reported.

Drugs such as digitalis, which must be taken daily at about the same time in order to maintain proper blood levels, figure 18-10, are sometimes forgotten. The elderly person may be interrupted or distracted at dosage time. The time to take the drug may be 9:00 A.M. If the telephone rings, the elderly person may not remember by the time the call has been completed whether or

WHEN and HOW to TAKE MY MEDICINES

NAME of DRUG	DIRECTIONS	SUN	MON	TUES	WED	THUR	FRI	SAT
Aldomet	3 times a day	8 12 6	8 12 6	8 12 6	8 12 6	8 12 6	8 12 6	8 12 6
Lasix	once a day	8	8	8	8	8	8	8
Chlortrimeton	twice a day	8 6	8 6	8 6	8 6	8 6	8 6	8 6

Figure 18-9 Patients sometimes need help remembering when to take their medications at home.

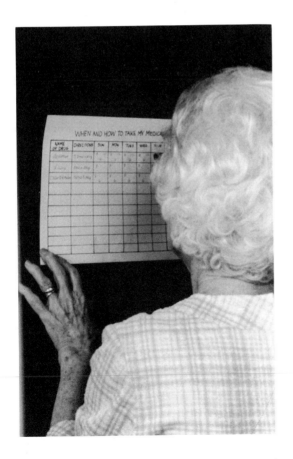

not the pill or medication was taken. Fearing overdosage, the client's tendency is to hold off. Thus doses of important medications are frequently missed. Errors also occur when bottles are mistaken for one another or labels are misread. Poor vision and poor legibility can combine, with disastrous results. Many elderly people become somewhat confused during the night hours, figure 18-11. This confusion leads to errors both in selecting and timing of medicines.

Ways must be devised to help such patients with medications. Suggestions may be made when the patient is prepared for discharge. First, the nurse must make a drug inventory. It should list all prescription drugs, over-the-counter drugs, and social drugs such as alcohol, caffeine, marijuana, and tobacco. The nurse needs to assess any possible interactions between them. For example, the client who is on a diuretic might be regularly taking sodium bicarbonate for its alkalizing effect. This may offset the full value of the diuretic.

The client's understanding of his or her condition and appreciation of the need for medications are significant factors in the maintenance of drug therapy. Talking with the client and with

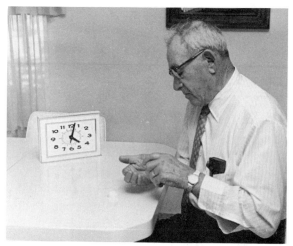

Figure 18-10 Some drugs must be taken at the same time every day to maintain proper blood levels.

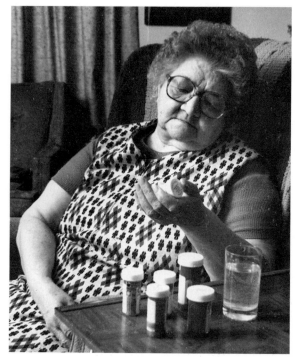

Figure 18-11 Confusion about proper drug consumption often occurs at night.

staff members who have observed the client can given the nurse valuable clues about how to help.

Labels should be checked for clarity. They must be printed in type large enough to be read easily. A cardboard tag can be attached to the neck of the bottle with wire so that extra-large print can be used. Coding the bottles with small strips of colored tape will also aid in identification. The client should be encouraged to keep medicines in a safe, easily accessible, well-lighted area. Some clients find it helpful to keep a large calendar on which the drugs and their times are marked for each day. As the medication is taken the client draws a line through the time. It takes time to set up such a chart, but many patients find it essential. If the patient is unwilling or unable to make such a record, a family member or home health aide may help.

For some patients, keeping only one day's supply of medicines on the nightstand helps them keep count. Others find it easier to take their medicines at a time that they associate with some important activity. For example, one elderly man remembered to take his daily digitalis when he made his first cup of coffee in the morning. A woman whose doctor had told her to take her pills regularly and to try to drink orange juice every day, simply combined the two activities. Another woman took her daily digitalis when an assurance caller telephoned each day. An alarm clock or timer can be used when a drug such as an antibiotic has to be taken at specific times. Whenever possible, medications that are compatible should be taken at the same time. These can be put out in a single container. When the container is empty, the older person knows that the medications have been taken. Many stores sell medication boxes with seven compartments labeled with the days of the week for medication storage and safe administration.

Clients are often ingenious when confronted with a problem. They should be encouraged to suggest solutions. If it is their own idea, they are more apt to follow it through. Some have found using egg crates to be an inexpensive and safe way to take their medications. The nurse should explain what the medications are supposed to do and any side effects that ought to be reported to the prescribing health care practitioner. The client is rarely as interested in the *how* of the drug reaction as in the net result and any special precautions that should be taken. The nurse should give directions and explanations to the client, another family member, and the home health aide at the same time. All should be given an opportunity to ask questions to be sure that they understand. Having them repeat the explanations is often helpful. Because questions may not arise until the client is at home alone, the directions should be written out for the client for referral. The nurse also needs to document on the client's record what was taught.

If you are providing home care, be sure to know what drugs are being taken (both prescribed and over-the-counter). Note any new medications that are added and be sure this information is conveyed to the supervising nurse. Try to become familiar with the common untoward reactions associated with the medications being taken by your clients. Note and report any unusual responses promptly.

Summary

- Elderly people tend to need the help that drugs can offer to their failing systems.
- Self-medication is common. Dangerous situations can arise when over-the-counter drugs are taken indiscriminately.
- Someone knowledgeable should check the client's total drug intake for compatibility and possible interaction.
- As a general rule, no drug is excluded for geriatric use. But drug dosages are lower and reactions are sometimes unexpected and extreme.
- Nurses are primarily responsible to see that drugs are properly administered in the agency and to help clients devise ways to take their medications safely at home.
- All members of the health care team must be on guard for any adverse reactions to medications.

Review Outline

I. Behavioral Objectives

II. Vocabulary

III. Elderly Drug Attitudes

    A. Medications are a panacea
    B. Tendency to self-medicate
       1. Overmedicate
       2. Neglect dosages
       3. Practice polypharmacy
    C. Influenced by culture
    D. Less compliant

IV. Age Factors Related to Drugs

    A. May be more sensitive
    B. Require more drugs

C.   More difficult to metabolize and detoxify
D.   Have bizarre and adverse reactions
    1.   Poorer nutrition
    2.   May be dehydrated
    3.   Less muscle tissue/more adipose tissue

V.   Drug Administration

A.   By licensed personnel only
B.   Variety of routes
    1.   Parenteral—subcutaneous, intramuscular, intravenous
    2.   Oral and sublingual
    3.   Dermal
    4.   Rectal or vaginal
    5.   Intrathecal
C.   Types often administered
    1.   Sedatives/hypnotics
    2.   Oral hypoglycemics
    3.   Cardiovascular drugs
        a.   Antihypertensives
        b.   Cardiotonics
        c.   Vasodilators
    4.   Nutritional supplements
    5.   Mood-altering drugs
    6.   Diuretics
    7.   Alcohol
    8.   Laxatives
    9.   Antibiotics
    10.   Anti-inflammatory drugs
    11.   Steroids
    12.   Analgesics
    13.   Antacids

VI.   Medications at Home

A.   Medication errors common
    1.   Poor vision
    2.   Confusion
    3.   Drug mixing
B.   Interventions
    1.   Large-print labels
    2.   Color coding
    3.   Administration in well-lighted areas
    4.   Calendar documentation
C.   Drug Inventory
    1.   Prescribed drugs
    2.   Over-the-counter drugs
    3.   Frequency of consumption

Review

I. Vocabulary

Complete the crossword puzzle using words from the vocabulary list at the beginning of the unit.

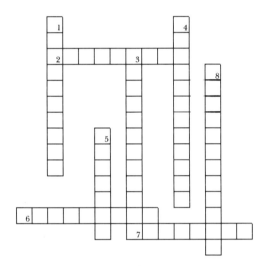

DOWN

1. Hardness
3. Drugs that reduce sensitivity to sensory annoyances
4. Drugs that increase peripheral circulation
5. Counteracts acidity
8. Strengthens heart actions

ACROSS

2. Drugs that increase urine output
6. Drugs that promote sleep
7. Responses

II. True or False

1. Drug reactions are more common among the elderly because their livers and kidneys are less metabolically active.
2. The elderly may overmedicate themselves when they find a small amount of drug to be effective.
3. The elderly spend less money on medicine and health services than other age groups.
4. Resistance to expected drug effects and sensitivity both decrease with age.
5. Before sedatives are employed, nursing measures should be tried.
6. Generic drugs may never be substituted for brand-name drugs.
7. Several types of drugs are specifically contraindicated by age alone.
8. Sudden mood swings may indicate intolerance to medications.
9. Medications may only be dispensed by someone licensed to do so.
10. When patients receive parenteral medications, the injection site should be carefully checked for reaction.

III. Short Answers

1. List ways to help patients relax without the use of drugs.
2. What are common changes in a resident's condition that need to be reported because they may be adverse drug reactions?
3. Describe the use of alcohol as a relaxant for older persons.

IV. Clinical Situations

1. In emptying a bedpan, you notice some red tablets in the stool. What do you do?
2. The medication nurse informs you that a resident's medication is to be given with the morning nourishment. What do you do?
3. Mr. Schwartz got out of bed quickly to go to the dining room for dinner. He had only taken two steps when he fainted and fell to the floor. What might have caused this, and how should he get out of bed or a chair to prevent this from happening again?
4. Mrs. Morales takes a bulk-forming laxative to help her move her bowels. She complains that she is still constipated. Is this really possible?
5. Ms. Hubbard has been on an antibiotic for a chest infection and has had diarrhea for the past three days. What should she take in sufficient amounts to overcome the diarrhea.

Unit 19
Care of the Terminally Ill

Objectives
After studying this unit, you should be able to:
- Discuss the various reactions of people to the thought of death.
- List the specific psychological steps that may lead to the acceptance of terminal illness and death.
- Describe the staff role with a patient during terminal illness and death.
- Explain the hospice philosophy.
- Describe the signs of approaching death.
- Carry out postmortem care.

Vocabulary
Learn the meaning and spelling of the following words or phrases.

acceptance
anger
bargaining
denial
depression

directive
durable power of attorney
euthanasia
hospice

living will
oncology
terminal

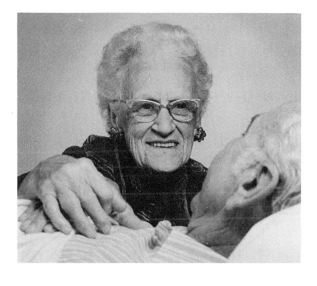

Death is part of the natural progression of life. It is a universal experience, one that may be postponed but never evaded. Every year about 6 percent of the older people in the United States can be expected to die. Death may arrive at any point in life, sometimes to the young but always to the old. As a geriatric health care provider, you will provide continuing care throughout the final living period. You will also care for the body immediately after death. Accepting the idea that death is a natural step in the life process may help you deal with your own feelings and those of your patients and their families.

It is a unique privilege to help patients prepare for death, to provide support during the final hours, and to help the family face the crisis. People differ widely in their ability and willingness to verbalize their feelings about death. Studies show that men tend to view death as an adversary. Women tend to see death in more peaceful terms. As a whole, society tends to avoid meaningful discussions of death. The Western culture negates the finality of death. Some people deny its very existence.

Death: A Progression of Life

Most older people gradually come to accept the reality of death, figure 19-1. Spouses and friends may be lost, bringing into sharper focus the realization that death comes to everyone. Some people continue to deny the fact and fill their lives with frantic activities so that they have no time to think about it.

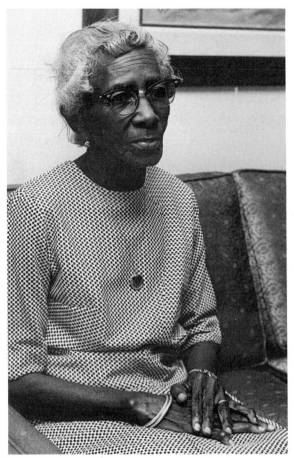

Figure 19-1 Even when well, the older person begins to contemplate the inevitability of death.

Retirement and release from the pressures of the working world often make more time available for introspection and reflection on the deeper meanings of life and death. Thoughts of death are not necessarily morbid and fearful. Some pleasure may be derived from thoughts of rejoining loved ones and making the necessary adjustments in one's own life. For some, death represents a final release from the loneliness and general physical infirmities of age. For other older people who are still relatively healthy, death lurks somewhere in the distant future. For the older person who is seriously or chronically ill, death is an ever-present reality.

Knowledge of Imminent Death

The knowledge of impending death comes to the patient directly from the doctor or indirectly from the staff. A diagnosis of terminal illness is difficult to conceal from the patient. Forced cheerfulness and evasiveness are just as revealing as other changes in staff behavior. Studies have shown that staff members make fewer actual contacts with dying patients. Yet, when questioned, staff members honestly believe their visits are more frequent or at least as frequently made. Uncertainty about how to handle questions is one reason for this fact, although few patients ever directly ask, "How soon am I going to die?" or "Am I going to die?" Even if they suspect what your answer might be, they are reluctant to confirm their fears.

Health care providers must recognize that most patients do eventually come to realize that death is part of their near future. They may or may not share their awareness with you. Each person reacts to this realization in a unique way. Their reaction is greatly influenced by personal belief about the hereafter, social situation, and perception of final circumstances, figure 19-2.

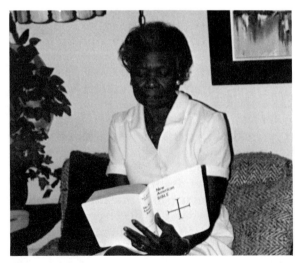

Figure 19-2 Many terminally ill persons find comfort in reading the Bible.

How many feelings they wish to share, and with whom, are personal decisions. They must not be forced to meet the comfort needs or expectations of the staff. All patients cannot be expected to react in the same way or feel the same degree of empathy with each staff member. The health care provider's reaction must be guided and directed by the patient.

Terminal Illness

A patient who is diagnosed as having a terminal (final) illness is assigned the social role of dying person. In this role, people are expected to be more dependent and exert less control over their lives. This may be an inaccurate expectation, because some terminal patients remain in control and active almost to the end.

Whether or not a patient is to be informed of a terminal diagnosis is a medical decision. Geriatric health care providers have an opportunity to closely observe and relate to the patient. Sometimes they can bring a point of view to the attention of the medical staff that will influence the decision. Whatever the decision, all staff members must accept it and adopt uniform behavior. Agreement should be reached about how to handle direct questions. This agreement is best made and communicated during a care planning conference. If specific information is not to be given to the patient, all must understand the extent of information that is permitted. If the patient is to be informed, all must know what was said and how the patient reacted. If unsure of what the patient has been told, staff members must listen carefully for clues to the patient's feelings. The staff must tactfully rephrase the patient's questions when necessary so that conversation is not cut off. Patients often know the answers to the questions they ask. But asking is a way of affirming their understanding and maintaining human contact.

Functioning in this way is difficult for the staff unless there is an opportunity to safely vent their feelings. A staff psychologist can be invaluable in helping staff members work through the stress that invariably develops under such trying daily interactions. If a psychologist is not available, nursing staff conferences focusing on staff needs can prove helpful. Emotional "burnout" can be high among staff on units where there are many terminally ill patients.

Patient and Family Response

Patients are apt to accept a terminal diagnosis more easily if they feel their life has been full and they have a secure belief in the hereafter. Strong convictions either in life after death or in life terminating with death make the patient less anxious. Lack of acceptance is demonstrated by anxiety, anger, and fear. There is fear of lingering pain, abandonment, humiliation, and loneliness. This is particularly true because many terminal diagnoses are of cancer. The patient may feel anxiety about the future and the security of loved ones or of work and dreams left unfinished or unfulfilled. The patient needs loved ones near and the security of a supportive and familiar staff, figure 19-3.

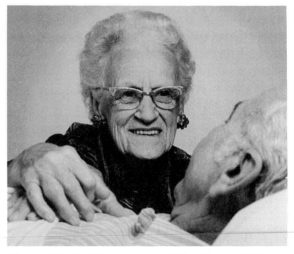

Figure 19-3   The support of family and friends is vital during the dying period. Liberal visiting hours are encouraged.

The Grieving Process

Elizabeth Kubler-Ross, a noted scientist, led research into the process of death and dying. This research has profoundly influenced current thinking on the subject. Prior to the work done by Kubler-Ross, little intensive research had been undertaken or published. From this research, we have learned much of the following information.

When they are told of the terminal diagnosis, patients and their families may proceed through several stages of grieving before finally accepting the inevitable. Kubler-Ross has identified five stages of grieving that people may undergo in preparation for death, figure 19-4. The five stages are denial, anger, bargaining, depression, and acceptance. Do not expect all people to experience each stage in sequential order. Patients often move forward to a new stage and then backward to a former stage. There is no set pattern of advancement. Both patient and family go through similar transitions.

Denial begins when a person is made aware that he or she is going to die and does not accept that this information is true. Statements such as, "This isn't happening to me" indicate that the patient is in the denial stage.

The stage of *anger* comes when the patient is no longer able to deny that death is inevitable. Blame for the illness may be directed toward those around the patient. It may include those who are giving care. Added stresses, however small, are likely to upset the patient who is in the anger stage. Statements such as, "It's all your fault. I should never have come to this hospital" and, "You are not making him comfortable enough" are typical of those in the anger stage.

During the *bargaining* stage of the grieving process, attempts are made to bargain for more time to live. Patients may ask to be allowed to go home to finish a task before they die. Or they may make private "deals" with God: "If you will let me live another two months, I promise I will try to be a better person." Basically, the patient in

Stages of Grief	Response
Denial	Reflect patient's statements, but try not to confirm or deny the fact that the patient is dying EX: "The lab test can't be right . . . I don't have cancer." "It must have been difficult for you to learn the results of your tests."
Anger	Understand the source of the patient's anger; provide understanding and support; listen; try to meet reasonable needs and demands quickly.
Bargaining	If it is possible to meet the patient's requests, do so; listen attentively.
Depression	Avoid cliches that dismiss the patient's depression ("It could be worse—you could be in more pain."); be caring and supportive; let the patient know that it is ok to be depressed.
Acceptance	Do not assume that, because the patient has accepted death, the patient is unafraid, or does not need emotional support; listen attentively and be supportive and caring.

Figure 19-4   The patient may exhibit various emotional responses to dying. The geriatric health care provider should be caring and supportive as the patient sorts out feelings.

this stage is saying, "I know I'm going to die and I'm ready to die, but not just yet."

Depression is the fourth stage, figure 19-5. During this stage, the patient comes to a full realization that death will occur soon. Patients are saddened by the thought that they will no longer be with family and friends and may not have accomplished some goals they had set for themselves. They may express regrets about not having gone somewhere or done something: "I always promised my wife that we would go to Europe and now we'll never go."

Acceptance is the stage during which the patient understands and accepts the fact that he or she is going to die. During this stage, the patient may strive to complete unfinished business. Having accepted the fact of eventual death, patients may also try to help those around them to deal with it.

If each of these stages is expressed with some degree of success, it is believed that all concerned are better able to accept the termination of life. Remember, not all people progress through these stages in sequence. In addition, movement from one stage to another does not mean that a previous stage will no longer be experienced. For example, a patient who displays anger one day may be full of optimism and denial the next. The family that is praising your care one day may be complaining on the next visit. The staff must be aware of the possible psychological positions and be able to identify the patient's and family's current reactions.

Many patients seek spiritual help during their terminal emotional struggle, figure 19-6. Arrangements must be made for clergy or lay visits whenever they are requested. Privacy must be provided. Patients may not be aware that members of the clergy are available for hospital counseling even when patients are not members of a specific church. These visits can be a source of great comfort to the patient and the family.

The Health Care Provider's Responses

The people most closely involved in the patient's resolution of the dilemma of death are the nursing staff. Their personal feelings and reac-

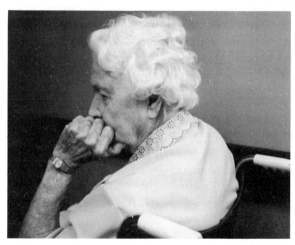

Figure 19-5 Depression is an important step that precedes final acceptance of a terminal diagnosis. (From Caldwell & Hegner, *Nursing Assistant, A Nursing Process Approach*, copyright 1989 by Delmar Publishers Inc.)

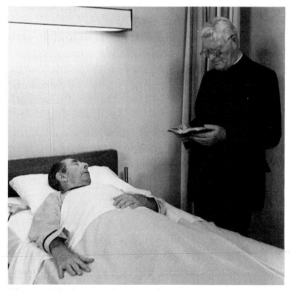

Figure 19-6 During the final dying stage, many people desire the support of clergy.

tions greatly influence the patient's success in working through personal feelings. Younger health care providers may find death and dying more easily denied than accepted. The medical and nursing staff are dedicated to preserving and protecting life. Death is the ultimate frustration of these goals. Yet all health care providers must come to terms with their personal feelings about death before the helping role can be truly fulfilled.

Unresolved feelings of guilt, frustration, and uncertainty can make the staff member avoid the types of contact that would help the patient most. The person with unresolved feelings avoids meaningful conversations and stifles the patient's attempts to discuss fears. Unconsciously, such a person avoids patient contacts or shortens the amount of time spent with the terminal patient. When in the patient's room, the health care provider with unresolved feelings becomes very involved with the mechanics of patient care. Conversation is stilted and artificial. One older woman, resigned to death, said, "That poor nurse, so young, so afraid to face life. How much easier if she could know that death is really just one more of life's experiences." How therapeutic and supportive had this health care provider really been?

A health care provider needs to find ways to compensate for feelings of helplessness and frustration in the confrontation with death. Social workers, other staff members, and the clergy are sources of comfort that should be readily accessible. The presence of terminal illness and death demands a professional reaction. The staff member must be available and must let patients know that they will not be abandoned, figure 19-7. Frequent visits to the bedside should be made even if the visits must be brief.

Signs of Approaching Death

As death approaches, body functions slow down and general control is lost. The body may appear limp and the jaw slack. Breathing be-

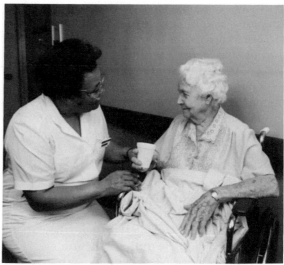

Figure 19-7 The geriatric nursing assistant can offer vital support by being a willing listener. (From Caldwell & Hegner, *Nursing Assistant, A Nursing Process Approach*, copyright 1989 by Delmar Publishers Inc.)

comes irregular and shallow. Involuntary voiding and defecation may also occur. Be prepared to change linen as necessary. As circulation slows, the blood pressure drops and the extremities become cold. Blankets should be added for warmth and comfort, figure 19-8. Profuse perspiration is common.

As death nears, the pulse becomes rapid and progressively weaker, the skin pales, and the eyes stare and do not respond to light. The patient may not be responsive. But this does not mean that he or she can no longer hear. Hearing is the last sense to be lost. In the presence of a dying patient, the health care provider should be careful in choosing words. He or she should speak in a well-modulated voice without whispering. Keeping the room cool adds to the patient's comfort because temperature tends to rise as death approaches. Keeping the room well lighted helps the patient maintain contact.

Mouth care is essential, figure 19-9. As respirations become more labored, oral breathing is more common and contributes to drying of the

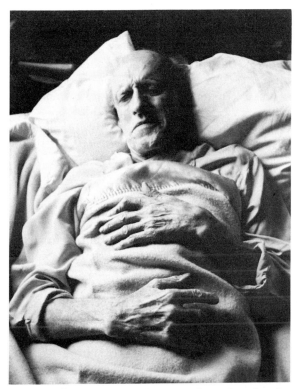

Figure 19-8   As death approaches, the circulation slows, blood pressure drops, and extremities become cold. Blankets should be added for warmth and comfort.

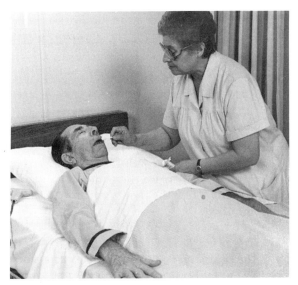

Figure 19-9   Mouth care and adequate hydration make the dying person more comfortable.

clare death. In some, the professional nurse may do so. Under no circumstance should anyone other than the nurse or doctor inform the family.

Nursing Responsibilities

In the period before death, the patient with a terminal diagnosis needs and receives the same care as the patient who is expected to recover. Attention is paid to both physical and emotional needs. The response of the staff must be guided by the attitude of the patient. This attitude may change from day to day. You must be open and receptive. Active listening becomes an important part of your function. Be sensitive to choice of words, body language, and voice inflections. Make sure you inform the nurse of incidents that reflect the patient's current moods and needs.

Health care providers should be quietly sympathetic without showing undue emotion. Duties should be carried out quietly and efficiently. Vital signs should be carefully monitored, recorded, and reported. If pain is present, be sure to report this to the medication nurse so relief can be given. This type of behavior instills

tongue and oral mucous membrane. If excess secretions such as mucus are present, suctioning may be needed. Position should be changed at least every two hours. Adequate administration of oral or parenteral fluids greatly helps make patients as comfortable as possible.

When breathing stops and the pulse is no longer felt, the nurse should be summoned and may summon the physician. Somatic death is based on the following criteria: lack of response to painful stimuli, absence of spontaneous heartbeat and respiration, permanent dilation of pupils and nonresponsiveness to light, and absence of brain waves as determined by two successive electroencephalograms within twenty-four hours. The time of death is a professional decision. In some states, only the physician can de-

confidence in both patient and family. Developing the proper attitude for this situation is not easy, but it will come with experience. Continue to allow the patient as many choices as possible.

All staff members must know if a "no code" order has been written. A "no code" order means that no extraordinary means of sustaining life, such as cardiopulmonary resuscitation or the use of a mechanical ventilator, are used.

When a patient's condition is critical, the doctor will officially place the patient's name on the critical list. Then the family and the chaplain will be notified.

If a Catholic patient appears in danger of dying, the priest must be called for the annointing of the sick. During this ritual, it is preferable that the family be present and leave the room only while the confession is heard. Practicing Catholics consider it a privilege to have the opportunity for confession while still mentally alert. Many patients recover completely, but this hope should not prevent the reception of this sacrament. The priest will decide after discussing it with the family.

Although most of the other religions do not have specific last rites, many families desire the support of clergy at this time. It is important to provide privacy for the patient and family. This does not mean leaving the patient and family entirely alone. Continue to perform your assigned care of the patient in a quiet, dignified manner.

For some time it has been recognized that the age-old practice of isolating the terminal patient is not the best way. In the past, it was thought that separating the patient from others provided the patient and family with needed privacy during the final days. It was also thought to protect other patients from depression. Families do need privacy during their bereavement, and the morale of other patients must be considered. But the dying patient has a great need for human contact and, when isolated, is far less likely to receive that contact. The patient should be near enough to the nurses' station to at least observe human activity. Only in the final hours

should additional privacy (but still not complete isolation) be provided, figure 19-10. No one should be alone just preceding and at the moment of death. Spiritual readings of the patients' faith, if requested, may be of some help during this crisis. Dying is lonely. Privacy, but not total solitude, should be the guiding rule.

Throughout a patient's illness, the patient's family has undergone a crisis of its own. If the illness has been prolonged, family members may have reached some kind of an adjustment. Still, the final hours bring a special crisis point. If the staff has been successfully supportive during the illness, the family will turn to them in this crisis period as well. Staying with the family to share their initial grief and allowing them to express their feelings is a therapeutic experience for both family and health care provider, figure 19-11.

Health care providers must be supportive during these trying times. This effort can take an emotional toll on the care provider. It is important to find a way of expressing the sorrow that you feel about the patient's death and to relieve the tension and stress that you may be feeling.

It is only natural that when you have known and cared for a person for some time, you make an emotional investment in their well-being.

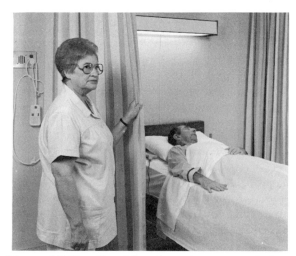

Figure 19-10   Provide privacy but not exclusion during the dying hours.

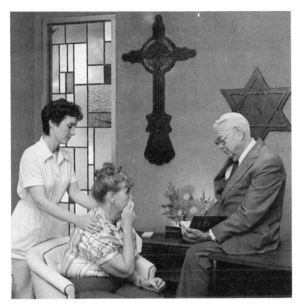

Figure 19-11 You can be of assistance to the grieving family.

Some health care providers experience feelings of grief, failure, guilt, and anger when the patient dies.

Repressing and denying these feelings is not healthy. It can lead to early burnout among staff members. Some facilities provide counseling for their staff. But even if this help is not available, you can help yourself. Discuss your feelings in a staff meeting. Simply verbalizing your emotional responses helps to relieve some of the tensions associated with them. Engaging in some kind of physical activity such as a brisk walk or aerobic exercise can prove very beneficial.

Remember that other patients may have become close friends with the deceased. Do not shut off discussions. Try, if possible, to direct them in positive terms, emphasizing the happy moments of the relationships.

Hospice Care

In recent years the movement for terminal care has developed rapidly. This movement is called hospice care and it provides care for those with a limited life expectancy. Beginning in England, the hospice philosophy spread to the United States and has become an important aspect of terminal patient care. The philosophy is based on a belief that death is a normal process that sould neither be hastened or delayed.

The first U.S. hospice was on the East Coast, but others have appeared all over the country. Growing numbers of people concerned about protecting the dignity and comfort of the terminally ill have developed units within hospitals and medical centers. Or they have founded specific care facilities. Hospice care can now be offered in individual family homes.

In 1974, Hospice Inc., of New Haven, Connecticut, was awarded the first contract from the National Cancer Institute to evaluate methods of providing pain control and psychological support for terminal cancer patients and their families. By 1978, a National Hospice Organization (N.H.O.) had been formed with a base in local and regional societies throughout the country. Setting standards and developing legislation are major tasks of the members.

Also in 1978, additional financing of demonstration projects was allocated by the U.S. Health Care Financing Administration, a branch the U.S. Department of Health and Human Services (formerly Health, Education and Welfare). These projects were designed to study various aspects of home and hospice care. Some of these projects continued into the mid-1980s. Reimbursement for care in similar programs is now made, at least in part, through Medicaid or Medicare and private insurance agencies.

With increasing pressure to base reimbursement through Medicare or Medicaid on disease-related groupings (D.R.G.s), there is an ever-greater need to deliver hospice care to the home, where vast amounts of this care are currently provided. When insurance is not available, many hospice programs waive fees. They depend on voluntary contributions to make up the deficit.

The goal of hospice care is to control pain so that the individual can remain an active participant in life until death. Psychological, spiritual, and social support, as well as legal and financial counseling, are available to both family and patient. Personal physical care for the patient is assured. A geriatric nursing assistant or home health aide provides most of the care under the direction of a professional hospice nurse.

Hospice care was first developed to meet the needs of terminal *oncology* patients (those with incurable malignant tumors). It has been naturally extended to include others with a life expectancy of six months or less. Support groups have been formed to visit terminal patients in conjunction with hospice teams. Many volunteers serve as "special friends." They make regular visits and work on a one-to-one basis with the patient and family.

Durable Power of Attorney

Sometimes people who feel that they may not be able to handle their own affairs or make decisions about themselves will sign a durable power of attorney. This act, in effect, makes someone else responsible for handling their affairs and making legal decisions on their behalf. At other times, the court will appoint a conservator if a person has already reached a point where he or she is no longer able to make decisions or conduct personal affairs.

The Directive and the Living Will

Technology has advanced to the point where machines can maintain vital life processes such as circulation and respiration despite the body's inability to recover. At great expense to families, this technology can hold off the death of terminally ill patients for extended periods. There is an increasing consensus that for the patient suffering from terminal cancer, these heroic measures are questionable. They only represent additional suffering on the part of the patient and additional hardship and financial loss for the family.

A *living will* is a request by an individual that life-sustaining procedures not be used in case of incurable injury or disease. It is signed before two witnesses and a copy is given to the physician and to the executor of the individual's estate. It is reviewed and initialled annually. A living will has no legal status, but it does indicate a person's desire and intent.

The Natural Death Act of California took effect in January 1977. It requires doctors to consider such a document valid when it conforms to specific requirements. The physician is bound to honor the document if it is signed at least fourteen days after the patient has been informed of a terminal illness and if a second physician has certified the terminal diagnosis. If the document was signed before the illness, when the individual was still in good health, the physician need only consider it. The legal document, known as the *Directive*, is effective for five years. It then becomes outdated. It must be witnessed by two adults who will not benefit from the estate. If the individual is in a skilled nursing facility, one of the two witnesses must be a patient advocate designated by the State Department of Aging. Neither the doctor nor the doctor's employees nor any hospital employees may sign as witnesses. The Directive can be revoked at any time in the final stages of terminal illness by either informing the doctor, destroying the document, or signing and dating a statement requesting that the Directive be revoked. Simply making a mark on the Directive also revokes it.

It is important to recognize that the Directive is a legal document under California law. The living will is not. The Directive is not equivalent to *euthanasia*, or mercy killing. It is merely a legal method of permitting a physician to respect the instructions of a patient and not interfere as death proceeds naturally.

Failure of a physician to carry out the Directive does not carry a penalty. However, it does constitute unprofessional conduct that could lead to license suspension. Cases are pending that are testing the validity of the Directive. Although legislation to allow euthanasia is introduced each year, none has ever been passed.

The living will and Directive are not uniform documents throughout the United States.

The procedures and requirements for each state may be different.

No Code

As mentioned previously, a "no code" order, when written, means that measures that simply maintain heart and lung activity are not to be started. Rather, the patient who has ceased cardiac and respiratory function is allowed to die with dignity.

It is often difficult to carry out a no code order when you have come to know and love the person. However, try to remember that life needs quality as well as quantity. The quality of life on support is very limited. Also recognize that the "no code" order agrees with the patient's wishes or the wishes of those legally acting on his or her behalf.

With today's technology, heart and lung function can be maintained as mechanical actions, despite the physical death of the person. At some point, we must accept death as a finality. It is important that all staff members know as soon as a no code order is written.

Postmortem Care

Postmortem care is the care given after death is pronounced. Immediately following death, make sure that the body is positioned with the limbs straight and that the bedding is clean and neat. Equipment should be moved out of the unit. Family members may wish to view the deceased. Attention to these details makes the experience easier.

Remain with the family if you feel that your presence is desired and could be supportive. After the family has viewed the body, it may be bathed. Dressings, tubings, and drainage equipment can be removed. Dentures should be returned to the mouth and belongings gathered and identified. The exact procedure varies with the facility, figure 19-12. Most often today the continued preparation of the body is under the direction of a mortuary. The body, once cleaned, is left until the mortician arrives.

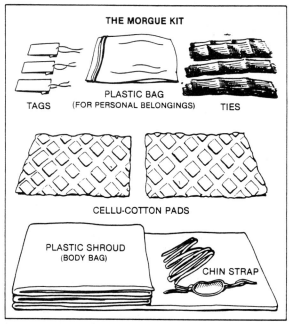

Figure 19-12   Some facilities use a postmortem kit when giving postmortem care.

Part of the staff responsibility during this period is to the other residents who are naturally concerned. The best approach is a direct and honest one. Use simple terms such as death instead of euphemisms such as "gone home." When a death occurs, staff behavior is watched closely by everyone. Death, like life, must be handled with dignity and caring.

PROCEDURE 9

Postmortem Care

1. Wash hands and assemble the following equipment:

shroud or clean sheet	identification cards (3)
basin with warm water	cotton bandages
washcloth	pads as needed
towels	

2. Remove all appliances and used articles.

3. Work quickly and quietly. Maintain an attitude of respect. If it is necessary to speak, do so only in relation to the procedure.
4. Place the body on the back, head and shoulders elevated. Close the eyes by grasping the eyelashes. Replace dentures. Jaw may need to be secured with light bandaging. Pad beneath the bandage.
5. Bathe as necessary. Remove any soiled dressings and replace with clean ones.
6. Pad between ankles and knees with cotton. Tie lightly.
7. Pad the anal area in cash of drainage.
8. Put the shroud on the patient.
9. Collect all belongings. Wrap and label. Valuables remain in hospital safe until signed for by a relative.
10. Fill out the identification cards and fasten:
    a. one on the body
    b. one on the patient's clothing and valuables (securely wrapped)
11. Close doors and empty corridor of patients and visitors. With assistance, place body on gurney. Cover with sheet and take to the morgue. The remaining identification card will be placed on the compartment in the morgue.

Summary

- Death is a universal, inevitable part of life.
- The aging person often becomes philosophical about the meaning of life and death and needs to verbalize personal feelings for clarification.
- Terminal illness brings death into sharper focus.
- When there is sufficient time, individuals and their families can often make a psychological adjustment to the situation.
- To help patients make this adjustment more easily, the health care provider's own personal feelings about death must be resolved.
- Both the patient and the family need emotional support throughout the illness and the final phases of life.
- Health care providers must find ways of reducing the stress they feel when death occurs.
- Hospice care is a way of providing comfort and support through the final living period.
- Physical care and emotional support must be maintained until death.
- Postmortem care must be carried out with dignity and respect.

Review Outline

I. Behavioral Objectives

II. Vocabulary

III. Death: A Progression of Life
   A. Growing awareness of death
      1. Loss of spouse or friends
      2. More time for introspection
      3. Varied reactions
         a. Acceptance as part of life
         b. Denial
   B. Most eventually come to terms with concept

IV. Knowledge of a Terminal Diagnosis

    A. Direct information
    B. Patient response
        1. More easily accepted if values firm
        2. Lack of acceptance
    C. Staff response
        1. Guided by patient attitude
        2. Must be consistent
    D. Need for support
        1. From family
        2. From staff

V. Grieving Process

    A. Elizabeth Kubler-Ross
    B. Stages
        1. Denial
        2. Anger
        3. Bargaining
        4. Depression
        5. Acceptance

VI. The Health Care Providers' Response

    A. Work most closely with patient
    B. Suffer feelings of their own
        1. Guilt
        2. Frustration
    C. Need outlets for their emotions
    D. Suffer high degree of burnout

VII. Signs of Approaching Death

    A. Slowing of body functions
    B. Involuntary responses
        1. Voiding
        2. Defecating
    C. Hearing last sense lost

VIII. Patient Care

    A. Maintain comfort/cleanliness
    B. Mouth care
    C. Meeting religious needs
    D. Need for personal contact
    E. Code/no code

IX. Somatic Death

    A. Based on specific criteria
    B. Professional decision
    C. Family informed by professional

    X. Hospice Care

        A.   Provides care for terminally ill
        B.   Durable power of attorney
        C.   The Directive or living will

   XI. Postmortem Care

        A.   Care of the body
        B.   Support of others
            1. Patients
            2. Family

Review

   I.   Vocabulary

Write each of the following words or phrases in a sentence that demonstrates your understanding of its meaning.

      a. Euthanasia _____
      b. Oncology _____
      c. Terminal _____
      d. Living will _____
      e. Directive _____

   II.   True or False

1. A diagnosis of terminal illness usually forces a person to think about death.
2. In our society, death is freely discussed.
3. Health care providers can help patients deal with feelings about death only if they are secure in their own feelings.
4. Older people seldom spend time reflecting on the meaning of life.
5. The thought of death frightens everyone.
6. People have the right to determine their own way of adjusting to the crisis of death.
7. Only certain health care providers should know what information has been given to a patient with a terminal diagnosis.
8. Patients with a terminal diagnosis should be isolated from other patients.
9. Dying patients no longer need human contact and emotional support.
10. Many patients need and seek spiritual help during their terminal illness.

  III.   Short Answers

1. Who was Elizabeth Kubler Ross?
2. List the stages of adjustment to the thought of death.
3. Describe the goals of the hospice movement.
4. Describe the Directive.
5. List the signs of approaching death.

IV.   Clinical Situations

1.   A person who appeared to accept his diagnosis of terminal illness suddenly becomes angry, saying you were too slow in answering his call light. What do you do?
2.   A patient expresses fears that since she is being transferred to a hospice, she will not receive good care and will die in pain. What do you tell her?

CASE STUDY

Mrs. Annie Hendricks, a ninety-two-year-old woman, was transferred from the extended care facility where she had been living for the past eight years to the community hospital. She had a diagnosis of terminal cancer complicated by acute pneumonia.

A little woman and frail, it was difficult to believe that she had raised six children and was grandmother to eleven, great-grandmother to seventeen, and great-great grandmother to two. Many of her family lived in the area and she received many visitors.

Her ovarian malignancy was diagnosed three years ago. Following surgery and a course of radiation, the malignancy was thought to be controlled. But it had now spread. When first diagnosed, Mrs. Hendricks had strongly made her wishes known with regard to her terminal care. She wanted no extraordinary measures used but wanted to die when her time came.

The pneumonia was vigorously treated with antibiotics, oxygen therapy, and expectorants. She began to respond favorably. Digitalis and diuretics were given daily in the extended care facility and were continued in the hospital. After two weeks of hospitalization, the lung fields were cleared and the patient was ready for discharge.

One of her great-grandchildren offered to have "Nana" come to her home rather than go back to the extended care facility. But she was afraid she wouldn't know how to handle the final days. Arrangements were made for the hospice unit to provide support. Mrs. Hendricks was discharged to her great-granddaughter's home.

The hospice nurse made visits to both client and family. Medications to alleviate pain were ordered. The family was told that a home health aide could be sent if necessary to assist in Mrs. Hendricks's personal care and that a nurse would be making regular contacts. The family requested a home health aide, who spent four hours each day in the home.

Death came peacefully just four days before Mrs. Hendricks's ninety-third birthday. Members of her family, her minister, and the hospice nurse were with her. Later, her great-granddaughter wrote a thank-you letter to the hospice nurse, which read in part: "You were there when we all needed so much help. Nana was kept comfortable and seemed alert and able to talk with us until almost the end. What a joy to have had her in our lives and how grateful we are to you for all your support. The hospice philosophy certainly made all our lives and her more comfortable. The suggestions you made about mouth care and frequent position change, about keeping the room cool but lighted, and about having one of us stay by the bedside and talk in normal tones all were so helpful to us. Our many thanks to you and your group."

1. Define the term *hospice* as both a place and a philosophy.
2. What disease prompted a terminal diagnosis in this case study?
3. What two drugs was Mrs. Hendricks receiving in the extended care facility for her condition of congestive heart failure?
4. Who came into the home to help with personal care?
5. List four measures the hospice nurse suggested that increased Mrs. Hendricks's comfort.

Section 5
The Geriatric Person and Health Alterations

Unit 20
Nervous System Alterations

Objectives

After studying this unit, you should be able to:

- Locate the parts of the nervous system.
- Describe senescent changes in the nervous system.
- Name the common pathologies of the nervous system.
- Discuss the difference between a small stroke and an acute cerebral vascular occlusion.
- Describe some of the functions of the health care provider in caring for patients with neurological conditions.

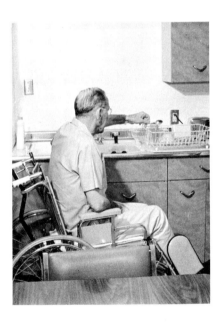

Vocabulary

Learn the meaning and spelling of the following words or phrases.

anesthesia
aneurysms
aphasia
autonomic nervous system (A.N.S.)
central nervous system (C.N.S.)
cerebrospinal fluid
cerebrovascular accident (C.V.A.)
cortex
fibers
hemiplegia
keratitis
meninges

nerves
neurons
neurotransmitters
paralysis
parasympathetic
peripheral nervous
   system (P.N.S.)

seizures
sympathetic
tic douloureux
transient ischemic attacks
   (T.I.A.s)
trigeminal neuralgia
viscera

The nervous system controls and coordinates all voluntary and involuntary body activities, even the production of hormones. The central nervous system is made up of the brain and spinal cord. The peripheral nervous system is composed of the cranial and spinal nerves.

Sensory receptors of the nervous system, such as the eye and ear, make us aware of our surroundings. Some parts of the nervous system maintain normal day-to-day functions. Other parts act during emergency situations and others control voluntary activities. Acute neurological conditions require highly specialized nursing care.

For easier study, the nervous system can be divided into two major parts: the central nervous system (C.N.S.) and the peripheral nervous system (P.N.S.). Remember, though, that it is actually one interwoven system, a complex of millions of neurons.

Structure and Function

Neurons

Cells of the nervous system are called *neurons*, figure 20-1. They are specialized to conduct electricity-like impulses. Neurons have extensions called axons and dendrites. Impulses enter the neuron through the dendrite and leave through the axon.

Although neurons do not actually touch each other, the axon of one neuron lies close to the dendrites of many other neurons. In this way, impulses may follow many different routes. The space between the axon of one cell and the dendrites of others is called a synapse. Special chemicals called *neurotransmitters* allow the impulse to cross the synapse. There are different kinds of neurotransmitters, but acetylcholine is the most abundant.

The Central Nervous System

The term *central nervous system (C.N.S.)* refers to the brain and spinal cord. These vital tissues are surrounded by bone and membrane *(meninges)*. They are cushioned by cerebrospinal fluid for protection. The brain and spinal cord are a continuous structure found within the skull and spinal canal. The spinal cord is about 17 inches long, ending just above the small of the back. Nerves extend from the brain and spinal cord.

The Brain

The Cerebrum   The largest portion of the brain is called the cerebrum. The outer portion *(cortex)* is formed in folds known as convolutions. It is separated into lobes that take their names from the skull bones that surround them, figure 20-2.

The outer portion, the cerebral cortex, is composed of cell bodies and appears gray. The

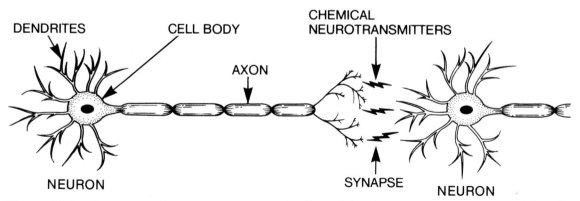

Figure 20-1   A neuron (From Hegner & Caldwell, *Assisting in Long-Term Care*, copyright 1988 by Delmar Publishers Inc.)

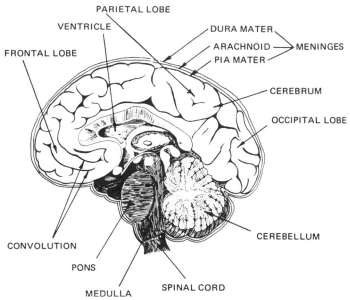

Figure 20-2   Cross-section of the brain (From Hegner & Caldwell, *Assisting in Long-Term Care*, copyright 1988 by Delmar Publishers Inc.)

inner portion is composed of axons and dendrites and appears white. All mental activities, such as thinking, voluntary movements, and interpretations of sensations and emotions, are carried out by cerebral cells, figure 20-3. Certain activities are centered in each lobe. In general, the right side of the cerebrum controls the left side of the body and vice versa.

Deep inside the cerebrum, special areas connect different parts of the brain. These areas must be functional if cerebral functions are to be carried out.

The Cerebellum   Beneath the occipital lobe of the cerebrum is the smaller cerebellum. It, too, has an outer layer of gray cell bodies. This portion of the brain coordinates muscular activities and balance. The cerebellum, brain stem, and basal ganglia (within the cerebrum) are interconnected.

The Brain Stem   The medulla, pons, midbrain, and diencephalon form the brain stem. They are composed mainly of neurons. Neurons serve as connecting pathways and as centers for controlling the involuntary movements of such vital organs as the heart, blood vessels, stomach, lungs, and intestines. Most of the cranial nerves enter and leave the brain stem.

The Spinal Cord

The spinal cord extends down from the medulla into the spinal canal. Spinal nerves entering and leaving the spinal cord carry impulses to and from the control centers. Certain reflex activities performed without conscious thought are controlled within the cord. Pulling your hand away from something hot is an example of this type of reflex activity.

The Meninges   Three membranes surround the brain and spinal cord. The outermost, the dura mater, is tough. The middle layer, the arachnoid mater, is loosely structured and filled with cerebrospinal fluid. The innermost layer, the pia mater, is delicate and clings closely to the surface of the brain and spinal cord.

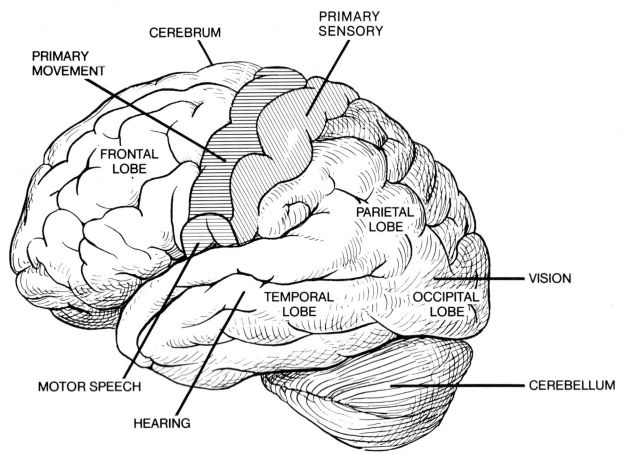

Figure 20-3 Functional areas of the brain (From Hegner & Caldwell, *Assisting in Long-Term Care*, copyright 1988 by Delmar Publishers Inc.)

Cerebrospinal Fluid Ventricles are cavities within the cerebrum that are lined with vascular tissue. This tissue is an extension of the pia mater and produces *cerebrospinal fluid*. The fluid flows from one ventricle to another. It finally reaches the central canal of the spinal cord and the area between the arachnoid mater and pia mater (subarachnoid space). The fluid is continually being produced in the ventricles and then returned to the general circulation. In normal amounts and freely circulating, the cerebrospinal fluid bathes the central nervous system and cushions it.

The Pheripheral Nervous System

The *peripheral nervous system (P.N.S.)* is formed of the twelve pairs of cranial nerves and the thirty-one pairs of spinal nerves. The cranial nerves have names and numbers and are attached to the under surface of the brain. The spinal nerves are attached to the spinal cord. The spinal nerves take their names and numbers from the point of their emergence between adjacent vertebrae.

Nerves

Nerves are bundles of axons and dendrites. Individual axons or dendrites are often referred to as *nerve fibers*.

Some axons and dendrites are long and others are short. The axons and dendrites of many neurons are found in bundles outside the brain and spinal cord. These bundles form the peripheral nerves which are held together by connective tissue. These bundles resemble telephone cables. They are called peripheral nerves. The axons and dendrites that make up the nerves are very long. Therefore, their cell bodies may be found at great distance from the ends of the nerves.

Sensory nerves, made up of dendrites, carry sensations to the brain and spinal cord. Feeling is lost *(anesthesia)* when these nerve impulses are interrupted. Motor nerves carry impulses from the brain and spinal cord to muscles. Loss of function *(paralysis)* occurs when these nerves are damaged. Peripheral nerves carry both sensory and motor impulses.

Autonomic Nervous System

The *autonomic nervous system (A.N.S.)* is concerned with involuntary body activities. The center of control for these activities is in the brain stem. The autonomic nervous system is made up of special nerves that carry messages to the body organs *(viscera)* and travel with cranial and spinal nerves.

The system is made up of two parts called the *sympathetic* and the *parasympathetic* divisions. Parasympathetic nerve fibers carry impulses to control heartbeat, digestion, elimination, respiration, and glandular activity. In times of stress or danger, the heart beats faster, blood pressure increases, the lungs work harder, and certain glands increase their production. These activities are brought about by stimulation of the sympathetic nerve fibers.

Senescent Changes

Throughout life a small number of neurons are lost, but not normally in sufficient numbers to inhibit adequate functioning. Although reaction time and cerebral processing are slower in the elderly, intelligence is not diminished.

There is some degeneration of end organs, reflexes are slower, sensory perception is somewhat diminished, and synthesis of information is slower, figure 20-4. It is difficult to determine exactly which changes are due to the aging pro-

- Degeneration of end organs
- Loss of neurons
- Reaction time increased
- Decreased tactile sensitivity
- Decreased sensory perception
- Memory changes

Figure 20-4 Senescent changes in the nervous system.

cess itself and which are the result of diminished or altered blood supply or inadequate production of neurotransmitters.

Some senescent changes and many organic alterations result in problems. Nursing diagnoses related to these alterations are listed in Table 20-1.

Organic Dysfunction

Increased Intracranial Pressure

Any pathology that increases intracranial pressure (pressure within the skull) will disrupt cerebral functioning. Tumors, occlusions of the

- Alteration in elimination: Bowel/urinary
- Alteration in health maintenance
- Alteration in home maintenance/management
- Altered thought processes: Confusion
- Fatigue
- Ineffective coping
- Impaired communication
- Impaired mobility
- Impaired swallowing
- Nutritional alteration: Less than body requirement
- Potential for injury
- Potential for violence: Self or others
- Self-care deficit (all or several)
- Sensory perceptual alteration: Visual, kinesthetic
- Sleep pattern disturbance

Table 20-1 Nursing Diagnoses Related to Neurological Alterations.

normal flow of cerebrospinal fluid, or intracranial accumulation of blood as in a stroke can so hamper cerebral action.

Intracranial pressure may also result in headache, vomiting, loss of consciousness and sensation, paralysis, and convulsions. Convulsions are uncontrolled muscular contractions, which are often violent. With increased intracranial pressure, the irises of the eyes may fail to respond to light. The pupil should normally become smaller when a flashlight is directed at each eye. The equality of the pupils and their ability to react to light are important signs of functions.

Almost any condition increasing intracranial pressure will produce these signs and symptoms. Toxins and high temperatures may also cause convulsions. How long the symptoms remain depends upon the extent and cause of damage to the brain cells. Loss of motor control is not always accompanied by sensory loss. Patients who have lost motor control should be moved with care. They may not only continue to feel, but be hypersensitive. It is important to keep a careful check on vital signs of any patient with a head injury. A special record (head chart) may be kept for recording all observations, figure 20-5.

Patients acutely ill with increased intracranial pressure require extremely skilled nursing care, figure 20-6. Level of consciousness and orientation, reaction to pain and stimuli, and vital signs must be monitored frequently. This is the nurse's responsibility. If, as you are assisting in the care, you should note any change in the patient's response or behavior, bring it to the nurse's attention immediately. Such changes might include incontinence, uncontrolled body movements, disorientation, deepening or lessening in the level of consciousness, dizziness, vomiting, or alterations in speech.

Once improved, the patient may be moved from a critical to an intermediate care unit, then to a long-term care facility for a prolonged period of convalescence. The nursing measures first established in the critical care unit must be maintained for an extended period.

Loss of sensation and decreased mobility make these patients especially prone to pressure sores, infection, and contractures. You must continue special skin care, range-of-motion exercises, and position changes. Early signs of infection should be reported immediately. Elimination must be monitored, because loss of muscle tone and inactivity may lead to constipation and impaction. Drainage tubes such as indwelling catheters must receive careful attention.

Patients recovering from these illnesses often experience anxiety and depression. Be alert to indications of mood decline and plan extra time to provide emotional support. Loss of sensory and motor functions often makes self-care difficult and frustrating. In response, your approach must be consistently calm and patient. The patient's expressions of irritability, fear, and depression as well as clumsy attempts at self-care must be accepted in a matter-of-fact manner. Remember that patients' ability to think is not necessarily impaired. Their frustration is even greater because they can no longer control their actions.

Incontinence causes the patient embarrassment and discomfort and makes skin care more difficult. Suppositories may be used to stimulate and control daily bowel movements. A catheter (sterile tube) may be inserted into the urinary bladder to drain the urine. Adult disposable diapers or garments may also be used, figure 20-7. Skin breaks down more easily because the lack of nervous stimulation decreases circulation to the part. Because pressure and pain cannot be felt, pressure sores and contractures can become serious problems. The skin must be kept clean and dry and inspected frequently. Regular turning and proper positioning are necessary to prevent contractures.

Success has been achieved in bladder and bowel retraining, but it requires consistent professional supervision. Specific care of the person who has experienced a cerebrovascular accident is described later in this unit.

Seizures

Seizures or convulsions are serious and require immediate attention. There are several types of seizures. They do not always follow the same pattern. They range from petit mal seizures, which are a momentary loss of contact, to

| NEUROSURGICAL WATCH RECORD | ☐ N.D. | ☐ D.D. | ☐ M.R. |

INSTRUCTIONS:
① Note date, time, and patient's BP and TPR.
② Check appropriate item in Sections 2 thru 5 (for orientation ask patient his name, address, and today's date—decerebrate means stiffening or flexing of limbs or extremities).
③ Grade ability to move: 4—normal, 3—slight weakness, 2—moderate weakness, 1—minimal, 0—no motion.
④ Pupils: draw actual size and shape.

DATE	4/22																
TIME	9A																
VITAL SIGNS:																	
BLOOD PRESSURE	130/84																
PULSE	88																
RESPIRATION	12																
TEMPERATURE	100³																
CONSCIOUS AND:																	
ORIENTED																	
DISORIENTED	✓																
RESTLESS	✓																
COMBATIVE	✓																
SPEECH:																	
CLEAR																	
RAMBLING																	
GARBLED																	
NONE	✓																
WILL AWAKEN TO:																	
NAME																	
SHAKING																	
LIGHT PAIN																	
STRONG PAIN	✓																
NON-VERBAL REACTION TO PAIN:																	
APPROPRIATE																	
INAPPROPRIATE																	
"DECEREBRATE"	✓																
NONE	✓																
ABILITY TO MOVE:																	
RIGHT ARM	0																
LEFT ARM	0																
RIGHT LEG	0																
LEFT LEG	0																
PUPILS:																	
SIZE ON RIGHT	●																
SIZE ON LEFT	⬤																
REACTS ON RIGHT	N																
REACTS ON LEFT	N																

Figure 20-5 Neurosurgical watch record (From Caldwell & Hegner, *Nursing Assistant, A Nursing Process Approach,* copyright 1989 by Delmar Publishers Inc.)

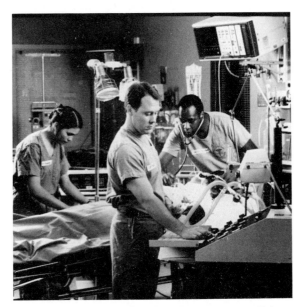

Figure 20-6   People suffering from conditions that cause increased intracranial pressure require the most skilled care. ("Be All You Can Be," courtesy U. S. Government, as represented by the Secretary of the Army.)

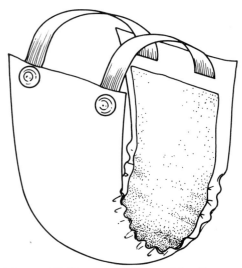

Figure 20-7   Adult disposable diapers or garments may be used with incontinent patients.

the more dramatic grand mal seizures, figure 20-8. A person with this type of seizure loses consciousness, falls, becomes rigid, is subject to uncontrolled movements and frothing at the mouth, and becomes cyanotic.

Jacksonian (focal) seizures usually result from a specific lesion. Initially moved are those parts of the body controlled by the affected brain area. However, these seizures may finally develop into the grand mal type.

Psychomotor seizures involve repeated motor movements such as grinding teeth or carrying out complex activities. There is no awareness or memory of any of the seizures.

The main nursing focus during a convulsion is to prevent injury and to maintain an airway. Clothing should be loosened, and any object the patient might hit should be moved away. No attempt should be made to move the patient, put something in the mouth, or restrain movements. A pillow should be placed under the head and the head turned to one side so that saliva may drain out. The patient should be carefully observed during and following the convulsion Breathing should be carefully monitored. Ring for assistance if possible, but do not leave the person who is convulsing alone. After the seizure, allow the person to rest in bed. Make sure siderails are secure. Report the length and type of seizure.

Tic Douloureux

After the age of forty-five, both men and women are more prone to the development of facial pain that follows the path of the trigeminal nerve (Cranial Nerve V), figure 20-9. This condition is called facial tic or *tic douloureux*. It is a fairly common nerve involvement among the elderly. Attacks become more frequent and severe with the advancing years. Its etiology is unknown. Some tics may be associated with malocclusion of the temperomandibular joint.

The trigeminal nerve carries sensations from the face, scalp, and teeth and conducts motor impulses to the chewing muscles. It has three branches: ophthalmic, maxillary, and man-

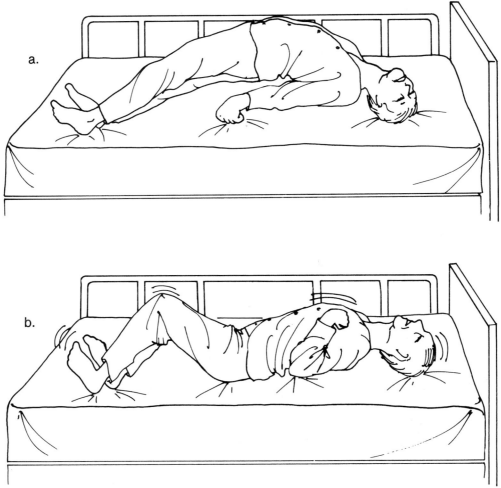

Figure 20-8   Grand mal seizures may be accompanied by (a) rigid posturing or (b) uncontrolled movements.

dibular. Tic douloureux is *trigeminal neuralgia* that usually affects the second and third (maxillary and mandibular) divisions. Paroxysmal or shooting pain is the chief symptom and may affect either side. But it is usually restricted unilaterally, at least at first. The pain may flash every few minutes for several hours or may stop for weeks or months. The pain is usually described as sharp and burning, similar to a red-hot corkscrew. Following an acute spasm, however, it may remain as a dull pain. It runs along one side of the face parallel to the jaw, causing severe

facial muscle spasms. Patients suffering trigeminal neuralgia look as if they are in severe pain, as indeed they are. Even when they are not in pain, they have a look of anxiety.

There are four common trigger points from which the pain can originate. They are the outer half of the lower lip, the side of the tongue, the nasolabial fold, and the outer side of the eyebrow. For each patient, some activity will precipitate the pain, although it is not always the same for each person. Facial movements, cold liquids, drafts, and even so light a pressure as the touch

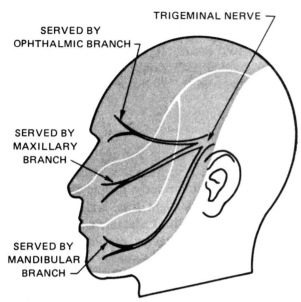

Figure 20-9 Areas of increased sensitivity and pain (trigeminal nerve)

of a finger or handkerchief against the sensitive area may trigger the pain. It is little wonder that these patients tend to be reluctant to have people touch or come near them.

Treatment and Nursing Care The treatment of tic douloureux includes both drugs and surgical intervention. Drugs used include analgesics. Carbamazepine is the drug of choice, but phenytoin and diphenythdantoin (dilantin) may also be effective. Surgical intervention has had varying degrees of success.

Preoperatively, the patient presents a picture of poor nutrition and generally poor hygiene, plus anxiety. For some time prior to surgery, the patient probably has not eaten and given little attention to the care of teeth from fear of triggering the pain. Frequently, this type of patient will complain of having slept poorly for some time. The patient will need encouragement to improve personal hygiene. It is unwise for the nursing staff to insist that the patient shave or wash the affected side. However, patients should be provided with warm water and applicators to clean their own mouth and teeth. Make sure that they are kept out of drafts. Try to learn from them what specifically precipitates the pain so that protection can be provided.

Food should be served attractively and at a warm temperature. Because chewing may be painful, foods should be pureed and fluids served with a straw. Since talking may trigger the pain, the patient may seem uncommunicative. The patient's needs must be anticipated to minimize the need for conversation.

Postoperatively, the head of the bed is slightly elevated. Watch for a yellowish drainage on the dressing, which indicates loss of cerebrospinal fluid, and for indications of cerebral hemorrhage. Adjusting to the change in sensations is difficult and takes time. A routine for oral hygiene after each meal needs to be supervised until it is well established.

Postoperative response depends on which branch of the nerve has been severed. If it is the upper branch (ophthalmic), the corneal reflex may be damaged or lost. To prevent corneal infection (*keratitis*) and possible ulceration, the eye is covered with a dressing or a shield. This will probably be in place when the patient returns from surgery. It will be left on until the patient recovers sufficiently so that the presence or absence of the reflex can be determined. No attempt should be made to elicit the reflex.

If a lower branch of the nerve has been severed, the mucous membrane and teeth will be less sensitive. The patient may complain of a feeling of coldness or numbness. He or she should be cautioned to avoid hot foods and to use extra care in shaving, because burns and cuts may go unnoticed. Careful dental examinations will be needed to determine the presence of dental cavities, since the pain of cavities will not be felt. If a herpetic rash develops, as it does in the majority of cases, it usually does so within twenty-four hours. It clears in about one week when treated with camphophenique or tincture of benzoin.

Coordinative Deficiencies

The inability to coordinate movements is commonly seen in the elderly person. It represents another form of senile nerve involvement.

The unsteady gait or trembling hand is seen so often that to many, they seem characteristic of the aged.

Senile tremors, or rhythmic movement at joints brought about by alternating contractions of antagonistic muscles, have different causes. Included are atherosclerosis, medications, and degeneration of the basal ganglia. The basal ganglia is the portion of the nervous system found deep within the brain. It is important in muscular coordination. Tremors, which are usually localized, may be slow (three to five movements per second) or fine and rapid (registering ten oscillations per second). The tremors are usually absent during sleep and increase when the patient is under emotional tension. The atmosphere should be kept as calm as possible, and attention must not be called to the tremors.

Parkinson's Syndrome   Parkinson's syndrome was first described by James Parkinson in 1817. The disease is also known as shaking palsy and paralysis agitans. The latter name is misleading, however, because there is no paralysis involved.

This condition affects more than one million people, most commonly those over fifty years of age of whom about 1 percent have the disease. It involves a decrease in the neurotransmitter dopamine and its metabolite which are produced in the basal ganglia, figure 20-10. Symptoms usually progress over a period of years, with progressive degeneration of the basal ganglia and their connecting pathways. Tremors, muscular rigidity, and slow execution of complicated voluntary movements (akinesia) are the three chief physical signs.

The tremors commonly affect the thumb and fingers, resulting in a pill-rolling type of movement. The tremors, which occur three to five times per second, may start in the fingers, gradually involving the hand, arm, and entire side. The head, jaw, and lower extremities may also be affected. The tremors begin on one side but usually spread and become bilateral. They are made worse by emotional tension and attempts to control them. They seem to dis-

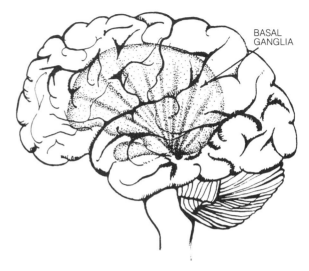

Figure 20-10   The basal ganglia are special cells deep in the cerebral hemispheres that produce essential neurotransmitters that control activity in the cells of the cortex and other brain areas.

appear when the patient is asleep or when gross movements are made. For example, leg tremors are less noticeable when the person walks. The muscle rigidity shows up in the slowness with which the patient moves and in the speech, which is slow and without expression. The gait is shuffling, with a tendency toward a forward running stance due to poor body balance, figure 20-11. The patient may also complain of a heaviness in the arms and legs which makes ambulation difficult.

The autonomic nervous system is involved as well, with a decreased blink reflex and decreased tongue movements. Facial expression is lost. Swallowing becomes difficult. Bowel and bladder efficiency is diminished. Salivary function may be disturbed, and drooling is common because of an inability to close the mouth adequately. The muscular rigidity results in eventual contracture, which draws the head downward and freezes the knees in a flexed position.

It is essential, therefore, to maintain proper alignment and to carry out range-of-motion activities. Rigid, unresponsive muscles and poor alignment make the person more susceptible to

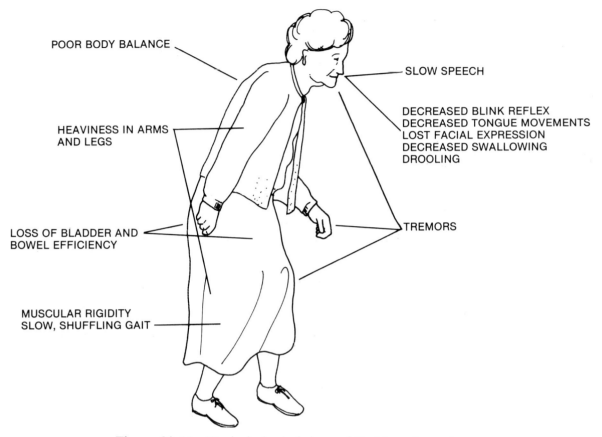

POOR BODY BALANCE

SLOW SPEECH

DECREASED BLINK REFLEX
DECREASED TONGUE MOVEMENTS
LOST FACIAL EXPRESSION
DECREASED SWALLOWING
DROOLING

HEAVINESS IN ARMS
AND LEGS

LOSS OF BLADDER AND
BOWEL EFFICIENCY

TREMORS

MUSCULAR RIGIDITY
SLOW, SHUFFLING GAIT

Figure 20-11   Typical physical signs of Parkinson's syndrome

falls and injuries. Special care must be taken to protect the patient when ambulating.

Treatment and Nursing Care   Treatment is directed to relief of symptoms. It includes drugs to control the symptoms and physiotherapy and exercise to retard the effects of muscle rigidity.

Emotional response to the condition is characterized by mood changes and, as the condition progresses, by despondency and melancholy. Personality changes are common. About 2 percent of patients require some form of psychotherapy.

In a limited number of cases, brain surgery is favored. The surgical approach attempts to destroy a small portion of the basal ganglia by electrocoagulation, or extreme cold. A fair amount of success in relieving the tremors has been achieved with this technique. Not all pa-

tients can be helped by surgery. It is most successful when used with younger patients.

Postoperatively, careful attention must be given to the vital signs, particularly the temperature, because the temperature control center may have been affected. Temporary hemiplegia, disorientation, and headaches are possible aftereffects. Steps must be taken to protect the patient from injury by using siderails, and from loss of muscle tone by regular passive and active exercises. Retraining may be needed to achieve control of elimination.

Drugs used today include L-dihydroxy-phenylalanine (L-dopa) and a synthetic compound, levodopa. Carbidopa may be used in combination with levodopa. Anticholinergic drugs, once the only drug available, are now given in combination with L-dopa.

Treatment with drugs such as levodopa and amantadine has shown encouraging results in diminishing the tremors, relaxing the muscle rigidity, and improving mental alertness. Side effects of the drug require daily observation and periodic blood examination. They include anorexia, nausea, and vomiting. Sinemet tablets are a combination of levodopa and carbidopa. The combination allows more levodopa to cross the blood brain barrier. Hence, it increases the potential effectiveness of the medication. Sinemet is being used more frequently than L-dopa alone.

Patients with Parkinson's disease require a great deal of emotional support and understanding. Special attention must be given to the patient's nutritional needs, because anorexia, swallowing difficulty, and drooling are common. Because of the diminished efficiency of the bowels, an adequate supply of roughage is essential to keep elimination regular. Special cups and spoons have been devised to help overcome the problem of spilling, but eating and maintaining the food in the mouth are troublesome. As with any chronic condition in which depression is a major factor, there is apt to be a lack of incentive to carry out prescribed exercises or to even take care of basic needs. Group exercises can be beneficial.

A prime nursing focus is to help the patient see the need for regular exercise and to promote self help activities as long as possible. The exercises include range-of-motion to maintain overall muscular ability, deep diaphragmatic breathing, singing and reading aloud to improve voice control, and exercises for specific muscle masses. For example, gait training can help control the shuffling walk that often develops. A calm, quiet environment is essential because symptoms are more intense when the person with Parkinson's is under stress.

Arteriosclerotic Brain Changes Men are three times more susceptible to brain changes due to arteriosclerosis than are women. Arteriosclerosis causes a narrowing of the blood vessels and subsequent cerebral hypoxia. The decrease in cerebral blood supply brings on confusion and incoherence. The arteriosclerotic patient tends to have lucid periods. That is, there are periods when there is less confusion and the patient is better oriented. Recent memory is limited, and errors in judgment are made. Lightheadedness, or so-called drop attacks in which the patient falls suddenly, is attributed to the hypoxia. Reflex reactions to danger are lessened. Therefore, the patient is usually admitted to custodial care for protection.

This type of patient has a shuffling walk with a tendency to maintain balance by leaning backwards. A male patient may also have a tendency to expose himself. The patient with arteriosclerotic brain change appears restless, spending the days walking or rocking to and fro. Because this patient's activities are disturbing to other patients, and because the patient tends to have little emotional control, aggressiveness and easy irritability can lead to frequent quarrels with others, figure 20-12.

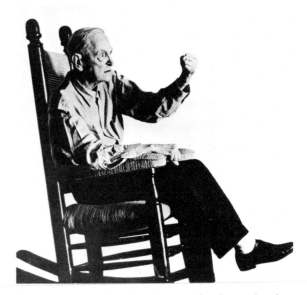

Figure 20-12 People with cerebral arteriosclerosis tend to have little emotional control. Aggressiveness and irritability lead to frequent quarrels with others.

Cerebrovascular Accident

Cerebrovascular accident, known also as stroke, shock, *C.V.A.*, and apoplexy, is usually classified as a neurological disease. It is covered here because of its etiology. The U.S. Public Health Service estimates that 1 percent of the population has suffered strokes. Of this group, 75 to 90 percent can learn to ambulate, and 15 to 20 percent can return to gainful employment. Cerebrovascular accidents stand in third place behind heart disease and cancer as a leading cause of death. Over two million people yearly are left handicapped because of the condition.

Etiology

A large percentage of C.V.A.s are due to either complete or partial thrombosis. The thrombosis frequently is a complication of atherosclerosis and hypertension. Other strokes are caused by rupturing of sclerotic vessels in the brain. Sometimes the walls of the vessels become weakened, forming blood-filled sacks called *aneurysms*. Aneurysms are more apt to rupture than healthy vessels. Many times the stroke will occur during sleep, when there is no hypertension. But it may also occur during periods of great activity when the blood pressure rises. A third mechanism leading to strokes is an embolism originating elsewhere, but coming to lodge in the cerebral vessels.

Small Strokes (T.I.A.)

Small strokes, or *transient ischemic attacks (T.I.A.s)* are usually due to multiple small thrombi. They occur frequently in the elderly. They may or may not cause loss of consciousness and cause little or no paralysis. These strokes are not usually death producing, although the condition is progressive. Repeated episodes result in deterioration of nervous tissue. They last from a few seconds to minutes, but never more than twenty-four hours.

The patient experiences any one or a combination of signs and symptoms. There may be nausea and vomiting, dizziness, a momentary loss of contact, confusion with behavioral changes such as forgetfulness or irritability, temporary interference with speech or vision, or transient weakness of a limb.

Because of the progressive nature of the condition, T.I.A.s may warn of an impending stroke. Strokes often occur within a month of the initial attack, so these patients need care and supervision. It may be possible for them to remain in the family unit, but the overall well-being of the family members may also necessitate custodial care. This is usually a difficult and stressful family decision.

Acute Cerebrovascular Occlusion

When circulation through a large cerebral vessel is completely interrupted, the situation becomes critical and requires immediate attention. There is a serious limitation to the cerebral circulation. The patient loses consciousness, respirations become labored, and paralysis of one side (*hemiplegia*) is definite. The blood pressure is elevated, and the patient may be incontinent. If the patient is conscious, speech and swallowing are difficult or impossible. Thought processes are deranged. Because the right side of the brain controls the left side of the body, the patient may exhibit right-sided hemiparesis if the ischemia is on the left, and left-sided paralysis if the ischemia is on the right.

Right-sided damage may result in deficits in thought, memory, comprehension, written computation, and correlation of event and time. Speech patterns may seem nearly normal, however. Behavior may be impulsive and judgment poor. The patient may ignore the left side of the body as if it didn't exist.

Left-sided damage, in addition to producing right-sided hemiparesis, affects the speech and communication centers. Aphasia complicates recovery greatly.

Inappropriate and quickly changing emotional responses are frequently seen. The patient may laugh or cry uncontrollably without reason. This is unsettling to both patient and health care provider.

Both long- and short-range goals need to be established. Short-range goals should focus on immediate physical care. Long-range goals should aim at increasing independence.

Immediate Treatment

First, an airway must be maintained. Occasionally, intubation is needed. Because the throat is partially paralyzed, gentle suction may be necessary to prevent aspiration of saliva. Careful skin care is essential if breakdown from the moisture around the mouth and face is to be avoided. Vital signs must be monitored accurately and frequently and level of consciousness must be assessed.

An indwelling catheter is inserted to manage incontinence, and oxygen is usually ordered. Nutrition must be maintained. A nasogastric tube may be inserted through which small quantities of liquid nutrients are given. Fluid levels are maintained with intravenous therapy. When the patient is able to take semisolid foods, care must

be taken to prevent choking. Check the patient's mouth after eating to be sure that no food has collected unswallowed in the affected cheek. During feeding, the patient should be placed in a sitting position with food directed to the unaffected side of the mouth.

The patient is placed on bed rest, and positioning is especially important. Patients must not be allowed to remain on the affected side more than twenty minutes four times a day. A trochanter roll will help maintain the affected leg in proper alignment, figure 20-13. The affected arm must be adequately supported, with pillows to prevent dislocation of the shoulder. Rolls can be used to support the hand in a functional position whether the patient is in the back, prone, or side-lying position. Adequate support is necessary for all limbs. Sandbags, pillows, and footboards can be used for this purpose, figure 20-14.

An affected eye that has a drooping or nonclosing eyelid must be protected to prevent dam-

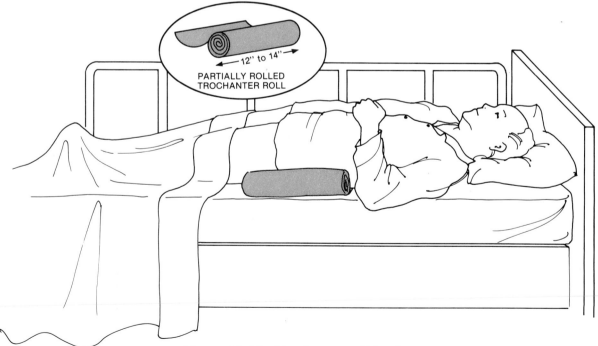

12" to 14"

PARTIALLY ROLLED
TROCHANTER ROLL

Figure 20-13 Trochanter roll in place

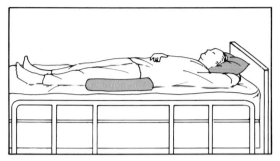

A. The patient's weak hand is tucked under the pillow with fingers open. Rolled sheet or bath blanket is used to maintain position of leg.

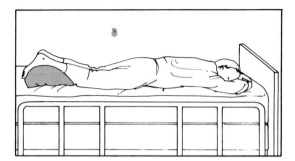

B. When it is not possible for the patient's toes to hang over the end of the mattress, a large pillow can be used to support the feet so that the toes do not touch the mattress.

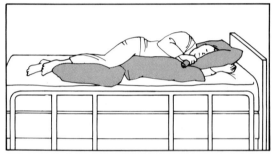

C. In this side-lying position, a pillow is used to support the weak arm. Another pillow is used to support the weak leg.

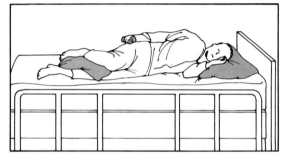

D. Here is one more side-lying position. The weak arm is placed on a pillow right behind the patient. Notice the rolled towel under the hand.

Figure 20-14 The stroke patient's affected body parts must be supported properly. (Side rails have been lowered for clarity of presentation.)

age to the cornea. Vision in that eye may also be affected. Saline irrigations and eyedrops are ordered for this purpose. A sterile dressing may be applied daily to keep the lid closed.

As soon as possible, range-of-motion exercises should be started to stimulate circulation and to prevent contractures. The affected muscles may go into involuntary contractions (spasms). If the muscles continue to maintain a single position, permanent shortening (contractures) will develop. As the coma lessens and the patient becomes more responsive, the real challenge of the patient's care begins.

Rehabilitation

The long-range goals are rehabilitative. The patient, therapy team, and family must all cooperate, and the therapy must be started at once. The nursing staff is of great assistance at this time, because reassurance can be a strong motivating force.

Bowel and bladder training is instituted immediately. Patients are gradually helped to feed themselves. Good oral hygiene is important, and when the swallow reflex is affected, special mouth care must be given carefully.

This is a frustrating time in the patient's life. Unable to communicate and unable to meet the most basic needs, the patient needs patience, understanding, and respect. The nursing staff must talk to the patient and explain each thing that will be done. This is true even when not sure just how much the patient is able to comprehend. Preventing contractures is perhaps the staff's greatest immediate responsibility. Simple range-of-motion exercises four to five times a day early in the care lay the groundwork for more specific

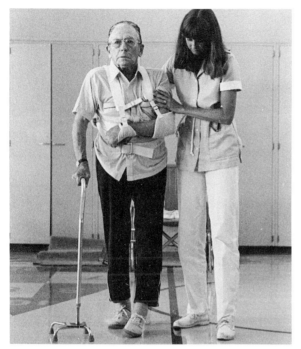

Figure 20-15   Muscle strengthening exercises are supervised by the physiotherapist. (Courtesy of Long Beach Memorial Medical Center)

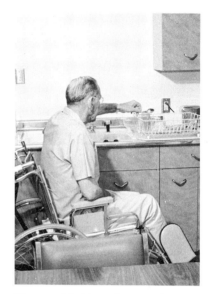

Figure 20-16   The stroke patient must be retrained in activities of daily living.

exercises by a therapist at a later date, figure 20-15.

Setting exercises that tighten the gluteal and quadriceps muscles are started early. The muscles will be important when the patient is ambulatory. Therapy resources should be made known to the patient and family, and use should be made of the multiple services they offer. Most patients need specialists in the fields of family services, physical rehabilitation, and speech therapy. Families can be advised of help available from the American Speech and Hearing Association and the American Heart Association.

Stroke patients need retraining in the activities of daily living, figure 20-16. Evaluation by a trained therapist can direct the patient in a thorough program. Exercises are prescribed to protect range of motion and to strengthen special muscle groups. It must be remembered that the stroke patient has an altered body image. Learning to balance and walk again is difficult and frustrating. Practicing standing and then walking

in front of a mirror helps the patient become reoriented to a bilateral body.

The trend today is for early ambulation. In addition to preventing the complications of hypostatic pneumonia, thrombophlebitis, and decubiti, early ambulation results in a more rapid clearing of the sensorium. Training in basic transfer activities begins as early as possible. These basic activities include transferring safely from bed to chair, wheelchair to toilet, and chair to tub, figure 20-17. Commercial equipment is available to assist in these activities. But home equipment can often be adapted satisfactorily with far less expense. Siderails and handrails placed strategically around tub and hallways aid mobility. A raised toilet seat makes transfer from a wheelchair or standing position much easier. Lapboards or wheelchairs with adjustable trays, figure 20-18, make it possible for the stroke victim to carry on independent activities. Steps may be replaced by a gently sloping ramp to make wheelchair operation a possibility. It is also possible to adjust the level of household equipment such as stoves, tables, and storage areas so that the person in a wheelchair can use them. The therapist often goes into the home to determine

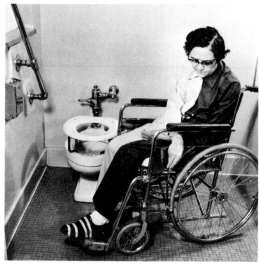

A

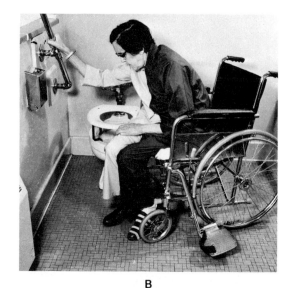

B

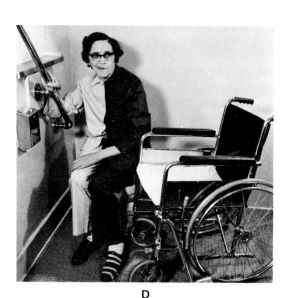

C   D

Figure 20-17   Being able to transfer from wheelchair to toilet is an important step in rehabilitation of the stroke patient.

ways that equipment can be arranged to better meet the individual's needs.

Aphasia

Aphasia means language impairment. Some patients have no useful language after a stroke, and for them the prognosis is poor. They have no useful means of communicating through reading, writing, or speaking. These patients are unable even to gesture meaningfully. Other patients have retained some useful language ability and with patience and help can improve. Their problems may be expressive or receptive. Expressive aphasia means inability to express

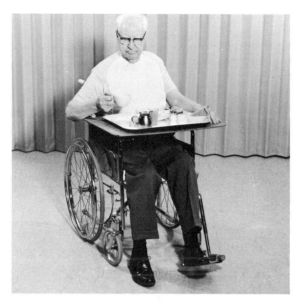

Figure 20-18 Wheelchairs with adjustable trays make it possible for stroke patients to carry on some activities of daily living.

thoughts coherently. Receptive aphasia means inability to understand the spoken word or printed information. These patients make errors in reading and writing, misuse words, and confuse related expressions, figure 20-19. Words that sound alike and number and time concepts also confuse them. Their visual fields may be imperfect, figure 20-20, so that items in that section of their visual fields are disregarded when reading. They still have some basic skills that can be developed, however. "Automatic speech" or words (profane) that have no real meaning or relationship are common to both types of aphasia.

A positive nursing approach to the aphasic patient can contribute greatly to the patient's recovery. Patience is essential. Expect failures and aim for small successes. Short, precise sentences must be used, speaking slowly to give the patient time to comprehend. Raising one's voice is of no value. The problem is one of comprehension, figure 20-21. Gestures or simple pictures can help convey meaning. Pictures or cards with printed words that the patient can point to can be

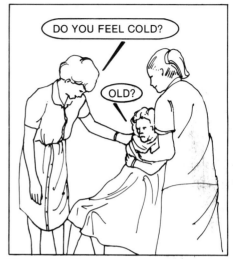

Figure 20-19 The aphasic patient understands only part of the question and therefore may answer incorrectly.

a valuable aid to communication. Too often, nurses fail to talk to aphasic patients because of the lack of significant response, but the aphasic patient needs examples to emulate. The nurse must talk to the patient.

When communicating, try to minimize noise and external distractions. Supply other sensory and orientation stimuli, such as a radio, television, clocks, and calendars. Provide positive feedback

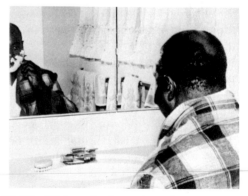

Figure 20-20 This aphasic patient does not see objects to his left. Therefore, he may not shave the left side of his face.

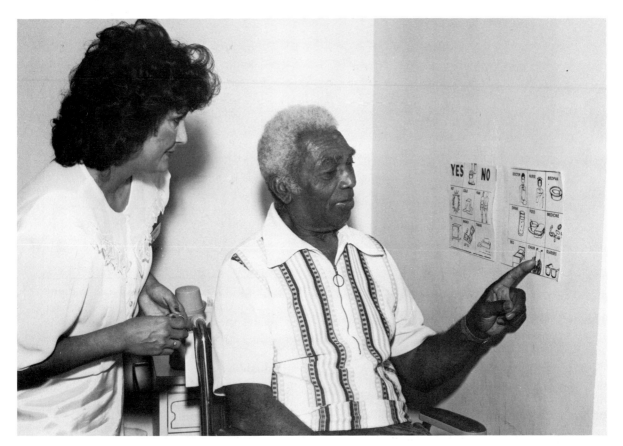

Figure 20-21   This stroke victim has language impairment. He uses picture cards to help convey his thoughts and needs.

for all progress. Actual speech therapy requires the services of a competent speech therapist. The therapist will begin the training by evaluating how much of the patient's intellect remains. The patient must start at the beginning to reacquire oral and written communication skills. This is a tremendous task that requires much training and skill on the part of the teacher.

The primary retraining cannot be done by the family, but families can help lend emotional support. The psychological needs of the aphasic patient are great. Fears, frustrations, and anxieties can undermine attempts to communicate. Group sessions, where patients and their families meet similar patients and families, have proved helpful. The sessions present an opportunity for participants to recognize similarities in their problems and to evolve ways of handling them more satisfactorily.

Summary

- Organic changes in the complex nervous system may be due to the aging process or to disease.
- Organic neurological conditions commonly seen in the older person include arteriosclerotic brain changes, Parkinson's syndrome, and trigeminal neuralgia.

- Any condition that increases the intracranial pressure interferes with normal neurological function and predisposes to the development of seizures.
- Both professional and supportive nursing interventions need to be taken to assure the safety and well-being of those suffering neurologic deficits.
- A combination of dedicated nursing care and special therapy has helped stroke victims recover a large measure of their abilities.

Review Outline

    I. Behavioral Objectives

   II. Vocabulary

  III. The Nervous System

       A.   Controls and coordinates
       B.   Divided for easier studying
          1. Central nervous system (C.N.S.)
             a. Brain
             b. Spinal cord
          2. Peripheral nervous system (P.N.S.)
             a. Cranial nerves
             b. Spinal nerves
       C.   Neuron—Functional unit
          1. Dendrites
          2. Axons
          3. Cell bodies
       D.   Transmission
          1. Synapses
          2. Neurotransmitters
       E.   Cerebral spinal fluid
       F.   The meninges
       G.   Autonomic nervous system (A.N.S.)

   IV. Senescent Changes

       A.   Reaction time slower
       B.   Cerebral processing slower
       C.   Intelligence not diminished

    V. Organic Dysfunction

       A.   Increased intracranial pressure
       B.   Seizures
       C.   Tic douloureux
       D.   Coordination deficiencies
       E.   Parkinson's syndrome
       F.   Senile dementia
       G.   Arteriosclerotic brain changes
       H.   Strokes (C.V.A.)

Review

I. Matching

1. Nerve cell
2. Seizures
3. Bundles of nerve fibers
4. Source of dopamine
5. Composed of brain and spinal cord
6. Loss of sensation
7. Loss of motor control
8. Cushions the central nervous system
9. Trigeminal neuralgia
10. Fifth cranial nerve

a. Trigeminal
b. Neuron
c. Nerves
d. Autonomic nervous system
e. Anesthesia
f. Convulsions
g. Cerebrospinal fluid
h. Tic douloureux
i. Paralysis
j. Basal ganglia
k. Central nervous system

II. A.   Identify the functional areas indicated in figure 20-22.

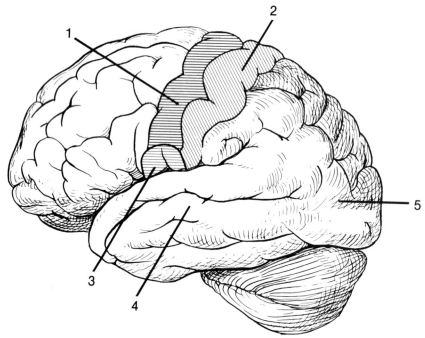

Figure 20-22   (From Hegner & Caldwell, *Assisting in Long-Term Care*, copyright 1988 by Delmar Publishers Inc.)

1. Control of movement
2. Pain and other sensations
3. Speech
4. Hearing
5. Vision

B.   Identify the structural areas indicated in figure 20-23.

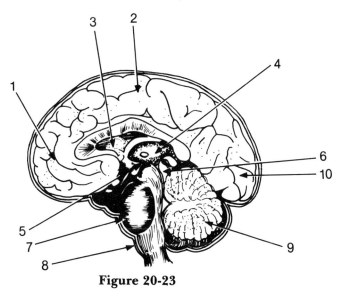

Figure 20-23

1. Frontal lobe
2. Parietal lobe
3. Ventricles
4. Thalamus
5. Hypothalamus
6. Midbrain
7. Pons
8. Medulla
9. Cerebellum
10. Occipital lobe

III. List six normal senescent changes related to the nervous system.

IV. Nursing Care

Select the one best answer to complete each of the following. These statements relate to the patient with arteriosclerotic brain changes.

1. The patient with arteriosclerotic brain changes suffers from
   a.   cerebral edema.
   b.   decreased cerebral blood flow.
   c.   dilation of cerebral blood vessels.
   d.   cerebral hypoxia.
2. This patient needs protection because
   a.   the gait is rapid, with closely spaced steps.
   b.   reflex reactions to danger are diminished.
   c.   of lucid periods.
   d.   judgment is generally improved.
3. This patient needs careful supervision because he or she
   a.   appears restless and disturbs others
   b.   has an easygoing personality.

    c.   may experience "drop attacks" and fall.

    d.   both a and c.

4.   Which of the following observations regarding the patient with increased intracranial pressure should be reported at once?

    a.   Stable vital signs

    b.   Equal pupillary reflexes

    c.   Decreased level of consciousness

    d.   Unchanged verbal response to stimuli

5.   Which of these observations needs to be reported?

    a.   Constipation

    b.   Uncontrolled body movements

    c.   Stable level of consciousness

    d.   Consistent speech

6.   Which of the following is the responsibility of the geriatric health care provider when the patient is incontinent?

    a.   Keep the patient clean and dry.

    b.   Insert a sterile catheter.

    c.   Tease the patient about lack of control.

    d.   Handle drainage tubes carefully.

7.   Which of the following are true for a patient with tic douloureux?

    a.   Pains follows the optic nerve pathway.

    b.   The condition is more common before age forty-five.

    c.   Maintaining proper nutrition and hygiene is often a problem.

    d.   It is caused by a virus.

8.   This patient seems reluctant to have you assist with his care. You should

    a.   insist that he let you brush his teeth for him.

    b.   offer warm water and applicators for mouth care.

    c.   try to engage him in conversation to take his mind off his troubles.

    d.   sit him by an open window to stimulate his interest in his surroundings.

9.   You enter a patient's room and find him on the floor in a seizure. Your first action is to

    a.   turn his head to one side.

    b.   leave and summon help.

    c.   restrain the arm or leg movements.

    d.   force something between the teeth.

10.   The patient has momentary lapses of contact. You recognize this as a seizure known as

    a.   Jacksonian.

    b.   grand mal.

    c.   psychomotor.

    d.   petite mal.

V. Clinical Situations

What should you do in the following situations?

1.   Your patient who has had a C.V.A. seems irritated and frustrated with attempting to feed himself.

2.   Your patient has Parkinson's syndrome, and muscular rigidity is developing.

3.   Positioning the patient with paralysis is important. In the diagrams that follow, select the picture that demonstrates the best positioning and explain why it is the best.

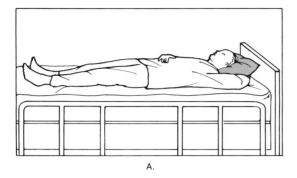

A.

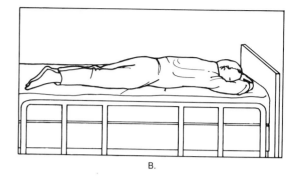

B.

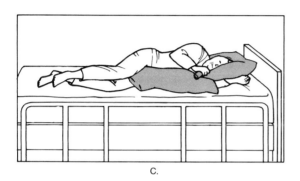

C.

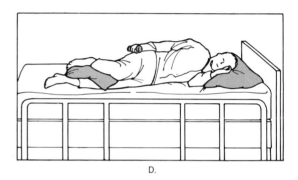

D.

CASE STUDY

Ms. L. R., age seventy-eight, is a resident of an extended care facility. She can frequently be seen sitting by the big window in the dark room watching the activities of those passing by. The right side of her body seems to be more affected by her disease process than her left, and she exhibits tremors. Sometimes the tremors are demonstrated by a rolling motion between her thumb and forefinger. At other times, they seem to be more generalized. When she is asleep, the tremors tend to be absent. She often falls asleep in her chair by the window. Sometimes she is responsive, and at other times when you approach, she seems disturbed and depressed.

When spoken to, Ms. L. R. seems to have a blank facial expression and tends to drool.

Her speech is slow and lacks the affectation that might be expected. She is still able to walk, but her gait is slow and shuffling and she complains of a feeling of heaviness in her arms and legs. Ms. L. R. is being treated with levadopa. Your assignment includes assisting her to ambulate, socialize, and eat.

Her diagnosis is Parkinson's syndrome.

1. What area of her brain is affected by the disease process?
2. How many people are affected by this condition?
3. What is the name of the neurotransmitter that is deficient?
4. Why must Ms. L. R. be protected against falls?

5. Why is making sure that Ms. L. R. has adequate nutrition a challenge?
6. How might you encourage socialization and at the same time promote activity?
7. What kind of an environment should you maintain?
8. What possible side effects should you watch for from the drugs that Ms. L. R. is taking for her condition?
9. What affect might the side effects have on Ms. L. R.'s appetite?
10. What are the two primary nursing care focuses for this patient?

Unit 21
Mental and Behavioral Alterations

Objectives

After studying this unit, you should be able to:

- Describe common mental disorders among older people.
- Recognize the need for treating confusion early.
- Explain the important differences between depression, delirium, and dementia.
- Describe ways to help elders with mental and behavioral problems feel more secure and safe.

Vocabulary

Learn the meaning and spelling of the following words or phrases.

alert
chemical restraint
confusion
delirium
delusion
dementia
depression
disorientation

hallucination
hypochondriasis
illusion
lethargic
multi-infarct
paranoia

paraphrenia
psychosis
reality orientation
schizophrenia
S.D.A.T.
validation therapy

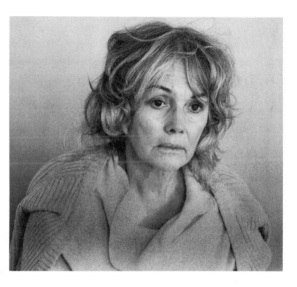

The majority of elderly people—70 to 80 percent—are mentally *alert* and competent, active in the community, and living independently or making their homes with their families. Others with keen minds are in homes or other facilities that provide them with necessary physical support. Only 5 percent of the elderly population need custodial care, and only 1 percent are found in mental hospitals.

Behavior Patterns

The behavior patterns indicating changes in mental health vary greatly. Some are subtle, taking place gradually. Others occur abruptly and are rather severe.

People of all ages adjust emotionally to stress situations in ways that have proven successful in the past. Aging does not alter this expectation. If anger and tantrums have worked in younger days, there is no reason for a person to believe that they will not continue to do so. In the same manner, if withdrawal or rejection has been effective in achieving goals, the individual will choose this method of handling the situation. Too many people fail to take these facts into account when they view the behavior of the elderly. They see an old man talking to himself and don't consider that this same man talked to himself when he was younger. They see an irritable, demanding old woman as emotionally unstable when in fact she was irritable and demanding all her life. They believe that the old woman crying in the corner is having a mental breakdown. They don't make the effort to learn whether her circumstances justify the brief period of tears. An old person is often judged by preconceived stereotyped notions of how one should behave or react, figure 21-1. It is important to understand also that an elderly person may have less resiliency and flexibility. The ability to adjust to stress and change may be greatly diminished.

In addition, people of all ages base their actions on what they think others expect them to do. They tend to fill the roles others establish for them. For example, if older patients see the nursing staff as authority figures, the staff tends to behave authoritatively. Similarly, one must expect a patient who is treated in a condescending manner, as if a child, to behave childishly.

Some patients exhibit definite changes in personality and behavior, figure 21-2. Organic brain damage resulting from cerebral arteriosclerosis is common. Emotional or functional changes become more pronounced when the elderly find that they can no longer manage situations and relationships in the same old ways. Both their authority and independence have been eroded by age. They have less emotional reserve, and incidents passed over in former days suddenly precipitate a crisis.

It takes less strain to produce disturbed behavior in an elderly person than in a younger one. This is especially true if early life adjustments were immature, deficient, or disordered.

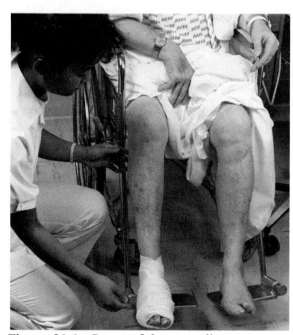

Figure 21-1 Be careful not to discount a patient's complaints of pain and simply attribute their complaints to the patient's feelings of depression.

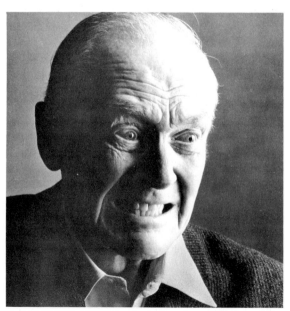

Figure 21-2 Change in behavior may signal the onset of a problem.

Factors Contributing to Mental Health Problems

The proportion of people with mental illness increases directly with age. *Senile psychosis* (mental illness associated with the aged) is more common among women than men.

Many factors can contribute to a mental health problem. Essentially, a problem indicates that the elderly person is unable to adjust to a specific stress. The pressure of chronic, incapacitating conditions such as arthritis can be distressing and lead to intense depression. Sometimes the pressures of chronic illness are borne until they are compounded by an acute condition such as a fractured leg. Avenues of emotional support are cut off when means of communication are limited. This can occur when hearing or sight fail or speech is lost through laryngectomy.

In general, emotional stress is great for the elderly person. At this time in life, personal losses are apt to increase as spouses and old friends become infirm or die. Loneliness may be intense, and the sense of personal value may decrease. Intrafamily relationships may crumble and the elderly person feels hurt and rejected. Once the pattern of rejection is firmly entrenched within the family unit, it is usually irreversible.

The older person has less stamina and reserve to handle these stresses and so responds with outbursts, anger, and resentment. Social pressures exert an influence as well. There may be less money available, and physical limitations inhibit the frequency and extent of social contacts. Loss of social contact is a significant factor in a high percentage of mental health problems.

Signs of Impending Mental-Emotional Problems

There are often advance indications of a psychotic episode. In some cases, deterioration takes place gradually over a number of years. If these changes are noted and appropriate steps taken immediately, it is sometimes possible to minimize the problem.

There may be changes in social behavior. A usually responsive patient may become apathetic or withdrawn. A quiet one may begin to chatter. Loss of interest in food or personal appearance may be an early clue. Antisocial behavior may intensify. For example, a person who is somewhat resistive may become frankly negative and increasingly irritable and suspicious.

Regressive behavior may be a forerunner of a problem, for example, soiling, hoarding, or cradling a doll or pillow. Confusion may increase, attention span may decrease, and signs of mental and physical fatigue and muscular weakness may become evident. Insomnia may prevent rest at night and make the patient wake early, and the patient may be found wandering about. Depression, expressed in tears and agitation, sometimes precedes the actual breakdown.

Mental and Behavioral Disorders

Although most older people experience few mental and behavioral changes, about 15 percent, or three million, have psychiatric problems (breakdowns). Approximately 5 percent, or one million, have dementia. The sad news is that these people are often undiagnosed and untreated. Those who may be diagnosed are often undertreated. Younger health care providers seem to think that psychiatric problems are the usual response to physical changes and ailments. Thus, many older people may be robbed of their productivity. For example, a seventy-four-year-old man told his physician he was "feeling down" because the pain in his shoulder kept him from doing things. His physician told him that depression was normal with arthritic pain. Fortunately, during discussions with the geriatric clinical nurse specialist, it became apparent that he was worried about finishing a roof-shingling job. He was then diagnosed as having a traumatic bursitis (inflamed shoulder joint) from hammering shingles on a roof for three days without rest. Obviously, it is important to keep normal behavior patterns in mind and be able to recognize changes in these patterns that might indicate mental or behavioral problems.

It is often difficult, even for professionals, to distinguish among individual idiosyncracies, temporary emotional crises, psychotic states, and dementia. For example, an elderly woman may be observed hoarding various things—bits of food from a tray, carefully wrapped in toilet tissue and tucked under her pillow; and items picked up from other rooms and stacked methodically in her closet. It would be almost impossible, without a full evaluation, to decide whether this woman was fulfilling her own basic need to save and be tidy, experiencing temporary confusion, or exhibiting true psychotic behavior. Nursing diagnostic categories frequently associated with mental and behavioral alterations are listed in table 21-1.

A major problem in treating mental and behavioral disorders is that they often occur in conjunction with physical illnesses and confuse the clinical picture. This makes it very difficult for the physician, nurse practitioner, or physician's assistant to diagnose and treat the problem or problems. Certain disorders, though, occur commonly in old age. *Depression*, (a state of marked sadness) for instance, is the most common mental health problem in older people. However, there may be other psychological problems as well. These may include schizophrenia, paraphrenia, hypochondriasis, and paranoia. These problems

tend not to be characterized by as much confusion as is present with depression, delirium, and dementia.

Depression, Delirum, and Dementia

Confusion   Periods of *confused* (disorganized) behavior are often transient and temporary. Many factors may be responsible for bringing about a confused state. A person transported to unfamiliar surroundings, for example, when hospitalized away from the familiar landmarks of home, can quickly become confused, disoriented, and even delirious. Such a move overtaxes the person's capacity to adjust. This behavior is particularly common at night. The patient may wake up in the darkness and, instead of seeing familiar furniture and pictures of loved ones, see a dark room and rails at the bedside. It is no wonder that the patient becomes frightened and confused.

Physical factors may also bring about periods of temporary confusion. A full bladder, constipation, hunger, and dehydration can operate in this way. Correcting an electrolyte imbalance or bringing down an elevated temperature can clear the confusion. The older person is also likely to have adverse reactions to drugs. Confusion is one of the common signs associated with overmedication or toxicity, particularly with barbiturates and alcohol.

Although the brain constitutes only 2 percent of the total body weight, it consumes 20 percent of the oxygen. Therefore, cerebral hypoxia, whatever the cause, produces confused, disoriented behavior. Temporary confusion can also result from undetected infections and diabetes mellitus. An eighty-four-year-old woman was admitted to a general hospital with a primary diagnosis of cardiac failure. She was confused and disoriented. Throughout the initial phases of therapy, she remained confused. Then a bladder infection was discovered and treated. Hypoxia, unfamiliar surroundings, and dehydration, all possible contributing factors to the confusion, had been given prescribed therapy. The condition did not abate, however, until the bladder

- Alterations in health maintenance
- Alteration in thought processes
- Impaired mobility
- Ineffective coping
- Potential for violence
- Self-care deficits
- Sensory perceptual alterations
- Sleep pattern disturbance
- Urinary incontinence

Figure 21-1   Nursing diagnostic categories associated with mental and behavioral alterations

infection was discovered and brought under control.

Because four out of five persons over sixty-five have one or more chronic illnesses, you will encounter many elderly confused individuals in long-term care facilities. The confusion of these patients is secondary to a primary health diagnosis. In some cases, unearthing the cause of the confusion and helping these patients to become oriented is an even greater challenge than basic nursing care. In some cases, attempts to help may only compound the dilemma. Isolating and restraining patients, failing to make an honest attempt to communicate with them, and keeping rooms in semidarkness are far more detrimental than helpful.

Types of Confused Behavior   Degress of confusion may vary from mild to severe, figure 21-3. Delirium is a mental condition in which the patient's speech is incoherent, and illusions, delusions, and hallucinations are experienced. An *illusion* is a false sensory interpretation. The person sees or hears or feels or tastes one thing and believes it is something else. A shadow on the wall may become a frightening form, figure 21-4. A *delusion* is also a false interpretation, but it cannot be corrected with reason. The person hangs on strongly to a false thought even when the error is explained. A *hallucination* is an idea or perception that is not based on reality but on things present only in the person's own mind.

It is important to recognize the differences in confused behavior and to use the correct term when charting the incident. Inaccurate charting may confuse the diagnosis. For example, illusions must not be mistakenly described as hallucinations. The confused patient must be observed closely. The patient's nursing needs must be assessed on an individual basis. Mild confusion is exhibited by incoherent speech and

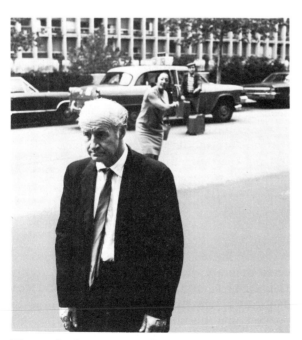

Figure 21-3   Degree of confusion varies from mild to severe.

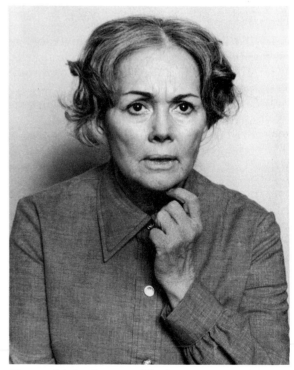

Figure 21-4   Sensory illusions cause patients to become agitated. (Courtesy Sandoz Pharmaceuticals Inc.)

immediate memory loss. Often the patient becomes apathetic and withdrawn, and appetite decreases. Patients who are normally responsive become irritable and negative and may resist staff attempts to position or feed them.

From mild confusion, patients may deteriorate into a more severe form. Time is distorted, familiar people are no longer recognizable, and patients do not know where they are or why they are there. Hallucinations may make the patient cry out, attempt to get out of bed, and sometimes attempt to assault the staff. Continent patients become incontinent and, if put on Foley drainage, struggle to pull out the catheter. All of this hyperactivity quickly leads to exhaustion.

Nursing Care The geriatric health care provider must intervene when confused behavior is first noticed. With prompt attention, much can be done to relieve the confusion and prevent further deterioration. Health care providers must meet three important objectives:

1. To limit the patient's disorientation by providing for basic physical needs and avoiding those factors known to precipitate an episode
2. To provide protection for the patient during periods of abnormal behavior
3. To help the patient become better oriented to reality

Limit Disorientation and Confusion. Disorientation is frequently accompanied by a high degree of agitation. When disorientation is first observed, steps must be taken to reduce the agitation. Warm, soothing baths and massages will help the patient relax. The room should be well lighted so that dim shadows or outlines are not misinterpreted. Reality must be stressed at every opportunity. The patient should be called by name and the approach should be gentle, cautious, and positive.

Orient the person to time and place by referring to familiar belongings, figure 21-5. Do not stress these patients by asking them to make decisions. Carry out activities in a routine way. Generally, one should not enhance the disori-

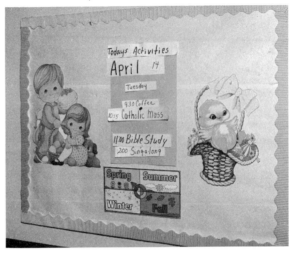

Figure 21-5 Signs and posters help patients stay oriented to reality. (From Hegner & Caldwell, *Assisting in Long-Term Care*, copyright 1988 by Delmar Publishers Inc.)

entation by "going along" with incorrect ideas and interpretations. Physical needs must be monitored, remembering that dehydration or a full bladder can cause or enhance confusion.

If possible, daytime activity should be increased so that the patient is more apt to sleep during the night. Sedatives can be given as needed, but they should not be relied upon solely. Other measures are equally important. The environment should be calm and quiet. Activity and noise around the patient's unit should be minimized, because excess stimulation makes the confused or delirious person hyperactive. It is best to place these patients where they can observe activity while not being disturbed by it.

Provide Protection. Patients need to be protected when they are disoriented or confused, figure 21-6. They should be placed in an area where they can be closely observed. They should be isolated only if absolutely essential for the wellbeing or protection of others. When isolation is necessary, frequent contact must be made with the patient. Simple observation is not enough.

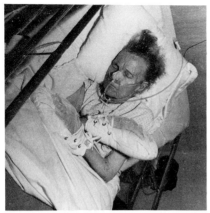

Figure 21-6   Hand restraints have been applied so the patient will not injure herself by pulling out her nasogastric tube.

Sometimes just having a family member sit quietly beside the bed will have a quieting effect. Sometimes a *chemical restraint*, a medication, will be ordered. The purpose of the medication is to calm and reduce agitation. This, combined with the presence of a friend or family member, may be very helpful to the confused, frightened client. It may make the use of physical restraint unnecessary.

Physical restraint should be used only after all other methods have been tried. Use of restraints contributes to an increase in agitation. Struggling against these restraints leads to exhaustion. Even the confused and disoriented patient interprets their use as punitive, and communication is decreased accordingly.

By tending to immobilize patients, restraints increase the risk of pneumonia, stasis of circulation, and skin breakdown. There are times, however, when restraints are the only way to keep a patient from dislodging intravenous injection needles and pulling out tubes. Soft restraints are best. They should be removed as soon as possible. The nurse should explain why it is necessary to use them and reassure the patient even if it is thought that the patient cannot understand.

Restraints must be removed every two hours for at least ten minutes. The affected areas should be inspected carefully for signs of irritation and circulatory impairment. Watch positioning and alignment carefully, and give careful attention to the skin. The basic physiological needs of hydration and elimination must also be anticipated. Patients who are restrained cannot provide for themselves.

It is often possible to remove restraints when someone is with the patient. If a member of the family can stay with the patient, use of restraints can sometimes be avoided altogether. Remember, restraints may not be used without a specific order.

Reorient to Reality. The entire staff must work to reorient the patient. A calm, unhurried approach will help. Glasses, dentures, and hearing aids should be returned to the patient as soon as possible. These aids are designed to keep a person in touch with reality, yet often their return is neglected.

Sensory stimulation can be provided. As the sensorium begins to clear, it is helpful to talk with the patient. Give the patient an opportunity to verbalize on familiar subjects. Call the patient by name and insist that you be called by yours and not confused with family members. Use short, concrete sentences, and tell the patient the time and day while giving care. Repeat this information patiently. A calendar, digital clock, and large, simple, printed signs giving day and date are helpful in the reorientation process. Even a well-oriented person loses touch with time when left alone with no sensory stimulation and no clock or calendar. All staff members must be consistent in their approach. Lack of caring nursing intervention can result in more permanent mental, emotional, and physical losses.

Depression   Depressive reactions among elders can be mild or major. They may also be the result of illness or medication. Older people have had to adjust to many changes and losses, some of which occur in rapid succession. With milder depression, elders may be sad, fatigued, or feel discouraged. They may have some difficulty managing activities that they usually do easily. In more severe depression, elders may have difficulty communicating, be unable to pay attention, appear very *lethargic* (without energy), have hallucinations, and be confused. Suicide threats by elders are rarely idle threats. Suicide rates are very high among elders, especially men, and most attempts are successful. Fortunately, depression can be treated with therapy and medications, often with very good results.

Depression may be difficult to diagnose because the client may be disoriented or confused or not answer questions. Sometimes a health care provider may diagnose senile dementia in error, and the client is not treated for depression. Therefore, a psychiatrist should be called in so a correct diagnosis can be made. Also, many of the common signs of depression—such as insomnia, loss of appetite, and changes in elimination found in younger, depressed persons—are what elders experience as normal aging changes. They are not very helpful in diagnosing depression. Therefore, many practitioners now use a mental status examination and one of several special depression instruments for elders to try to make an accurate diagnosis.

Depression is reversible. Without diagnosing it accurately, lack of interest in daily activities, appearance, socializing with others, and managing health problems can lead to serious or fatal consequences. Depression is treated with antidepressants, sometimes electroshock therapy (ECT), and some type of talk therapy. Often, a mental health clinical nurse specialist, psychologist, or psychiatrist will support and counsel the client through this painful period. Staff can assist in the client's recovery by finding opportunities to encourage family and friends to visit, encouraging an elder to reminisce or share memories (life review), and communicating their caring. These activities help build feelings of self-worth. All staff must be aware of the depressed client's needs and observe behavior. Anger and hostility, often the basis of depression, may be expressed in the form of self-violence or suicide.

Suicide Prevention When suicide is threatened,

the nursing staff has the responsibility to protect the patient against self-destruction. Careful, unobtrusive observations and removal of environmental hazards such as sharp knives, razor blades, matches, and cords are essential.

Helping the patient to direct feelings of hostility and aggression outward is somewhat more difficult. Allowing patients to verbalize complaints without the staff's own emotional involvement is one possibility. Activities that allow the patient to pound, hit, and mold can release pent-up feelings. Using clay in occupational therapy may be helpful. If the physical condition of the patient permits, playing table tennis or shuffleboard may also be helpful. Watch and listen carefully. Any abrupt changes in mood, good or bad, should be reported immediately.

Delirium Delirium is also known as an acute confusional state. Cerebral function is impaired, and the elderly client's alertness waxes and wanes. This condition is very different from depression and dementia. It is extremely important to be very accurate in describing any client whom you think is confused. An accurate diagnosis depends on it. At least one-third to one-half of all older clients will experience delirium at some point if they are hospitalized. Remember, confusion may be the only sign of a serious illness, and 33 percent of confused people die within one month if they are not treated correctly.

Delirium is different from depression and dementia in that it occurs fairly suddenly, figure 21-7. It lasts for hours, days, or weeks, and is worse at night. Delirium manifests itself with confusion, agitation, and restlessness; loss of recent memory; hallucinations; and fear. It may be caused by infection, trauma, cardiac problems, or drugs. When the cause is treated quickly, the effect on delirium is dramatic.

Dementia Approximately 30 percent of the public mental health beds are occupied by people over sixty-five who suffer from some form of dementia.

Dementia means a loss of mental faculties such as judgment and memory and a personality change. It also includes specific losses in occupa-

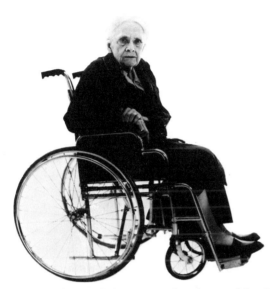

Figure 21-7 Delirium may develop suddenly.

tional and social functioning. Senile dementia, known also as Alzheimer's disease *(S.D.A.T.)*, is an incurable disease, so far, in which a person becomes progressively more dependent. Fortunately, only about 7 percent, or one to two million, of people over sixty-five years of age are afflicted by it. Other dementias include *multi-infarct* (series of strokes and TIAs) and mixed. All are irreversible and progressive. The demented patient forgets recent happenings but may remember in detail episodes in the distant past. Patients suffering from dementia usually tend to repeat themselves. You may explain that it is too early for a patient's daughter to visit, only to be asked the same question again within five minutes. The patient is simply unable to retain the information.

Adjustment to new situations is particularly difficult. This is often noted when an elderly person is newly admitted to a mental health facility. A person who may have been forgetful and confused at home may be totally disoriented af-

ter arriving at the unit. The patient will slowly regain the previous level of behavior. Regressive behavior, such as hoarding and emotional outbursts, is common and occurs with little or no provocation. It is not uncommon to see elderly patients pouting or whimpering. Tears are easily evoked.

Dementia is different from depression or delirium in that it comes on insidiously over months and years. In addition, it does not usually affect a person's alertness or orientation in the early years. Later, memory is very affected, emotions vary from apathy to wide mood swings, and the sleep-wake cycle is disrupted by insomnia and confusion. The last year of about a ten-year course of the disease is characterized by apathy, general body wasting, inability to communicate, contractures, and emaciation. The decision to place a forgetful patient in a long-term care facility is a difficult one for all concerned. The patient feels rejected, and the family members are often overwhelmed with guilt feelings.

Dementia is usually progressive and was at one time attributed solely to arteriosclerotic brain changes. Now it is believed to result from too little of an enzyme called acetylcholine. This may be caused by an abnormal gene, a virus, or a chemical.

Alzheimer's Disease Alzheimer's disease strikes 100,000 Americans each year. Up to three million Americans are already affected. This degenerative brain disorder is by far the greatest cause of senile dementia. The average onset is between forty-five and sixty years of age.

Alzheimer's is recognized as a form of dementia that begins slowly, with an inability to name familiar objects. Within three to ten years, patients with Alzheimer's disease become unable to reason, care for themselves, or control their basic functions. Most of these patients are elderly. It is the fourth leading cause of death among those over age sixty-five, following heart disease, cancer, and cardiovascular accidents.

Early indications of Alzheimer's disease may be confused with general aging as memory patterns grow less distinct, figure 21-8. Gradually,

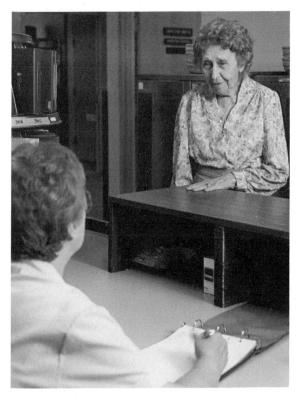

Figure 21-8 The patient with Alzheimer's disease may ask the same questions repeatedly. (From Hegner & Caldwell, *Assisting in Long-Term Care*, copyright 1988 by Delmar Publishers Inc.)

however, there is such loss that social and work relations are strained. Language problems develop, such as being unable to name familiar objects or express specific thoughts. Personality changes are also observed. Depression is a major factor in the early stages.

Early stages of Alzheimer's disease can be mistaken for depression because symptoms such as withdrawal, apathy, and mood changes may be present. Depression can also be mistaken for Alzheimer's disease, and an elderly client may not get the proper and needed treatment for the depression. Both can co-exist, but medication for depression can make Alzheimer's disease worse. Treatment when both exist is difficult.

The symptoms are progressive, and judgment and reasoning abilities are gradually lost.

In the later stages, speech and motor control are lost and contractures of face, arms, and legs can develop. The progress of the disease follows a fairly steady decline. If losses are rapid in the beginning, they continue at the same rate.

Since 1976, federal government spending on research into Alzheimer's has increased from less than $4 million to more than $37 million. In 1984, the National Institute on Aging designated five medical schools as Alzheimer Research Centers.

Research in the 1960s identified physical changes within the brain tissues of the Alzheimer's victim. A few of these changes can be seen in the aging brain, but not all together and not as extensively. Three specific changes were noted with the Alzheimer patient. The first is the presence of neurofibril tangles, with neuron loss, particularly in the areas of memory and cognition. The second change is the presence of aggregates of starchlike (amyloid) protein adjacent and within cerebral blood vessels, which normally are not present. The third abnormality is neuritic plaques of cellular debris irregularly scattered in the tissues. In addition, there is a decrease in the amount of neurotransmitter (acetylcholine) in the lower brain segments.

Several areas of Alzheimer's research are currently being investigated. Each has merits and defects. They include the possibility of a genetic predisposition, an examination of the abnormal proteins, the possibility of an infectious agent called a prion, the potentially toxic effect of the salts of aluminium, and the faulty utilization of glucose as an energy source for the brain. The most widely accepted hypothesis has developed since 1976. Research identified a great reduction in the amount of an enzyme (CAT or choline acetyltransferase) necessary for the formation of the neurotransmitter acetylcholine in the brain.

The area of the brain where this enzyme is deficient is the hippocampus, deep in the cerebral cortex. Since 1978, the chemical licithin—which the body breaks down to form choline, which can then be converted to acetylcholine—has been experimentally used with Alzheimer's patients. Initial results show some improvement in cognitive ability. Some theorists are looking into the possibility that there may be more than one form of Alzheimer's. There may also be more than one factor that causes the disease to develop.

Nursing Care   Whatever the cause of senile dementia, the essential care is the same. The use of medications is very controversial. Certain tranquilizers in very low doses may be necessary to control extreme agitation and restlessness. Drugs should never be used for the convenience of staff or to make clients more comfortable in place of using particular interventions that have been found to help patients with dementia.

The interventions recommended include a structured environment, social support, *reality therapy* (techniques to keep the person oriented regarding self, one's surrounding, time, and the use of objects in the environment), *validation therapy* (techniques to promote feelings of self-worth), touch, and family support. Maintaining the proper environment is important, and much can be done to help the patient. Consistency and patience are the key words. Set, well-known routines and simple words should be used. The health care provider's attitude should be positive, letting patients know that it is assumed they are able and willing to do as requested. The health care provider's voice should be well modulated and words formed carefully. Loud or sudden noises should be avoided. This type of patient has a tendency to overreact to sudden loud noises because the central nervous system is more vulnerable to stress. Sometimes patients know they are confused and rambling. The health care provider can help patients orient themselves by gently bringing them back to the present when they begin to ramble.

A calm, consistent environment can only be maintained if all personnel cooperate. When a patient dies, or there is increased pressure because of staff conflicts or patient care load, the tension is measurably greater. This is felt by the patients, who become more agitated. Even happy occasions such as holidays can have a disruptive effect if the activities are involved or prolonged. This does not mean that occasions cannot be observed, but their observance should be kept moderate.

Because these patients are confused and forget easily, they cannot be relied upon to give valid information about eating, drinking, and eliminating. It is essential, therefore, that the nurse carefully check these activities, as well as supervise all other activities of daily living. Shoes may be put on the wrong feet or left untied, and articles of clothing may be completely neglected.

Simple crafts and music can give pleasure. All patients should have the opportunity to participate within the limits of their abilities.

Psychological Disorders

Psychosocial and physiological aging changes may manifest themselves in a variety of psychosocial problems late in life. Some of these problems have been discussed in earlier units. Therefore, focus here will be on the problems of schizophrenia, hypochondriasis, and paranoia.

When an elderly person has a diagnosis of *schizophrenia*, it means that the disease usually occurred before the person was forty-five years old. After that, the disease is called *paraphrenia*. People with this diagnosis suffer from illusions and hallucinations. They are fearful and agitated; think, speak, and behave inappropriately; and may have some confusion. These elders need intensive supervision and support to help them feel safe and decrease their suspiciousness.

The psychologically disordered person has feelings of impending doom and suffers from anxieties, phobias, and compulsions. Self is the focus of concern. Each physical ailment is greatly magnified, as in the person with *hypochondriasis*. These complaining patients continue to function marginally on a social level even though they often prove to be a trial to themselves and their friends. They do not really want their imagined physical problems to be cured so much as they want understanding.

Experts believe that hypochondriasis is an expression of depression or stress, and that it serves as a means of warding off more serious mental illness. Although these elders may not have a physical illness or disease, they do have a serious problem. These clients need to be reassured that they are taken seriously and that the geriatric health care provider is trying to understand and help. These clients, however, should not be encouraged in believing that they are ill.

The psychologically disordered person is overwhelmed by guilt, withdraws from social contact, and feels all is lost or hopeless. The further from social contact the patient withdraws, the less hopeful the prognosis. When the behavior is accompanied by delusions and intractable insomnia, treatment is very difficult.

A third breakdown reaction is *paranoia*. These patients feel that everyone is "picking" on them or "out to get them." The fears are based on deep feelings of guilt and unworthiness. Contact with reality is lost.

Paranoia is part of other mental problems and exists as a problem by itself. Remember that elders who have a hearing loss and those with paraphrenia may feel suspicious and suspect plots against them. Common signs are having delusions that may be frightening or comforting, receiving messages through a radio or television, and accusing others of plots. Because paranoid people are minimally confused and convinced that their beliefs are accurate interpretations of reality, the problem is difficult to treat. Their behavior tends to drive away family and friends, even though they need the social contacts. Explaining to loved ones that the behavior is a disease often helps them to continue visiting and caring.

Therapy

With any of these problems, there is rapid deterioration among the elderly without therapy. However, the response to therapy is about the same as it is for any group. About one-third nearly recover, one-third improve vastly, and the rest either remain the same or grow worse.

Therapy employs a combination of drugs, electric shock, and psychotherapy. Ataractics are used for their tranquilizing effect, and antidepressants are given to elevate the mood. Both have the effect of making the patient calmer and more responsive. Electroconvulsive therapy has much the same effect as medication. Psychotherapy is conducted both on an individual and a group basis. The objectives of psychotherapy must be short term. An effort is made to improve the patient's self-concept and to reestablish feelings of worth. Groups are kept small, and sessions are brief and spaced. Role-playing has been used somewhat successfully. Where social interaction is possible, it is encouraged. Throughout treatment, the patient must be protected from self-destruction, and provisions must be made to reduce environmental hazards.

The role of the geriatric health care provider is continuous as day-to-day care is provided. The health care provider can help the patient achieve a more realistic, positive self-concept by listening without being judgmental. The better aspects of the patient's personality and health can be stressed, and ways in which the patient's life is still of value can be suggested.

The patient's family can suggest familiar routines that may be instituted, because these can have a quieting effect and can be used to forge a bridge to reality. The geriatric health care provider can reinforce the bridge by telling patients about themselves, their environment, and their therapy. Aggressive and hostile behavior does not disappear overnight even with therapy. There are times, however, when the patient can be helped to express this type of behavior in more acceptable ways.

Summary

- Mental alertness does not necessarily decrease with age. Organic changes and emotional stresses, however, can bring about mental and behavioral changes.
- It is not always easy to determine the nature of and basis for many of these changes.
- Neurological pathologies can affect the central nervous system and the peripheral nervous system.

- Much can be done to limit or prevent confused behavior by carefully controlling the environment and factors that are apt to precede an episode.
- Mental illnesses occur more frequently with advancing age, and not without some justification.
- Physical illness, social deprivation, and personal loss combine to create situations that strain emotional stability.
- Under such stress, depressive, paranoid, and psychologically disordered reactions are common.
- Suicidal reactions among those over age sixty-five are more common than they are among other age groups. They must be guarded against.
- Elderly people with emotional breakdowns have approximately the same response to therapy as do their younger counterparts.
- Senile dementia, with a gradual deterioration of the mind and self-care abilities, is most often due to Alzheimer's disease.
- Alzheimer's is under intensive investigation in hopes of alleviating the suffering of its victims and their families.

Review Outline

I. Behavioral Objectives

II. Vocabulary

III. Behavioral Patterns

    A. Indicate changes in mental health
        1. Subtle
        2. Abrupt and severe
    B. Develop over a lifetime
    C. Expectations tend to be self-fulfilling
    D. Elderly have less stamina for stress
    E. Need to differentiate responses
        1. Normal
        2. Abnormal

IV. Factors Contributing to Breakdown

    A. Fewer reserves
    B. Chronic incapacitation
    C. Acute crisis
        1. Illness
        2. Loss

V. Signs of Impending Breakdown

    A. Changes in social behavior
    B. Regressive behavior
    C. Insomnia
    D. Confusion

VI. Temporary States of Confusion

    A. Due to temporary stress

    B.   Due to physical problem
       1. Full bladder
       2. Dehydration
       3. Poor oxygenation
       4. Infections

VII. Degress of Confusion

    A.   Mild
    B.   Suffering from illusions
    C.   Suffering from delusions
    D.   Experiencing hallucinations

VIII. Nursing Intervention

    A.   Limit disorientation
    B.   Provide protection
    C.   Reorient to reality
    D.   Prevent suicide

IX. Delirium

X. Dementia

    A.   Alzheimer's disease
    B.   Arteriosclerotic brain syndrome

XI. Psychological Disorders

    A.   Manifestations
       1. Schizophrenia
       2. Paraphrenia
       3. Hypochondriasis
       4. Paranoia
    B.   Therapy

Review

I. Vocabulary

Write the definition of each of the following.

1. Lethargic_____
2. Paranoia_____
3. Hallucination_____
4. Paraphrenia_____
5. Confusion_____
6. Hypochondriasis_____
7. Dementia_____
8. Depression_____
9. Illusion_____
10. Schizophrenia_____

II. True or False

1. The majority of elderly people are not mentally alert and competent.
2. People usually react to stress when they are old in the same ways they did when young.
3. Our expectations influence the behavior of others.
4. It is usually easy to tell the difference between individual idiosyncracies and abnormal behavior.
5. The elderly person has less energy and flexibility than the younger person to adjust to stress.
6. Organic brain damage is often due to arteriosclerosis.
7. The most common cause of senile dementia is Alzheimer's disease.
8. Confused behavior is seldom symptomatic of cerebral arteriosclerosis.
9. Physical factors can bring on confused behavior.
10. An illusion is false sensory perception.
11. Sensory stimulation is not necessary to keep a person oriented.
12. The rate of response to therapy among the elderly is lower than it is for other age groups.
13. The therapy employed to help psychotic elderly people includes drugs, electric shock, and psychotherapy.

III. Short Answers

1. List three objectives to keep in mind while caring for the disoriented patient.
2. Explain why restraints should be used only as a last resort.
3. Describe the current areas of research into Alzheimer's disease.
4. List the differences between delirium, depression, and dementia.

IV. Clinical Situations

1. A resident who has Parkinson's syndrome is sitting withdrawn and depressed in her room. What do you do?
2. The family of a patient with Alzheimer's disease wishes to have a big celebration for the patient's seventieth birthday. What do you do?
3. Over the past three weeks, Mrs. Alvarez has been very agitated, restless, awake at night, and, at times, seems to be in a dreamlike state. What should be done?

CASE STUDY

Mrs. J. R., eight-one years of age, is admitted to the hospital with a primary diagnosis of fractured left hip. She is a pleasant person with some previous history of congestive heart failure and atherosclerosis. She makes a satisfactory adjustment until two days after surgery, when she is moved to a new room. During the evening of the second post-operative day, she becomes confused. Although offered the bedpan, she has not voided since early morning. She has had no visitors, her roommate was discharged, and busy nurses have hurried with their procedures. There is no radio or television in the room, and as night approaches, no light is left on. An indwelling catheter is inserted and 560 ml of urine is obtained. Mrs. J. R. pulls at the catheter, and restraints are applied. As the hours pass, she cries out loudly and, because she disturbs other patients, is moved to a room alone at the end of the corridor. By morning, she has taken no fluids, has an elevated temperature, and is delirious. Records reveal that she has had no bowel movement for three days. She is totally exhausted, and oxygen is ordered to relieve her dyspnea and cyanosis.

1. Identify eight factors that might have contributed to the emotional breakdown of this patient.
2. List two things that might have been done to avoid this situation.

Unit 22
Sensory Alterations

Objectives
After studying this unit, you should be able to:
- Review the normal anatomy and physiology of the senses.
- List the senescent changes occurring in the senses.
- Demonstrate nursing care for a blind person.
- Recognize and use appropriate vocabulary.
- List measures that health care providers can use with hearing impaired people to assist with communication.

Vocabulary
Learn the meaning and spelling of the following words or phrases.

accommodation
blindness
choroid
cochlea
cones
conjunctiva
cornea
cryosurgery
densities
diathermy
diplopia
ectropion
entropion
eustachian tube
fistulizing
hyperopia

iridencleises
iris
macula
mydriatics
myopia
O.D.
O.S.
ossicles
pinna
presbycusis

presbyopia
pupil
refracted
retina
rods
sclera
semicircular canals
tonography
trabeculectomy
tympanic membrane

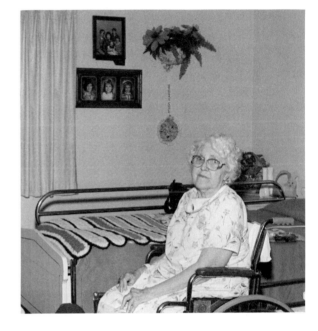

Functional nerve pathways and centers and responsive receptors are vital for healthful living at all ages. The five senses are necessary for self-care, for warning of possible dangers, and for experiencing the pleasures of life.

Successful social interactions are largely dependent upon the ability to see and hear accurately, figure 22-1. Because mental growth continues throughout life, the importance of maintaining the health of the eyes is easily under-

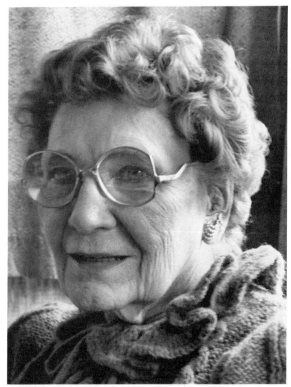

Figure 22-1 Diminished senses require artificial aids such as glasses and hearing aids to assure safety.

stood: 85 percent of all learning takes place through them.

Sensory Receptors

The ends of the dendrites carrying sensations to the central nervous system are found throughout the body. Some end in joints and bring information about body positions to the brain (proprioceptors). Others end in the skin and carry sensations of pain, heat, pressure, and cold (exterioreceptors).

The sense of smell originates with stimulation of dendrites in the lining of the nose. The sense of taste is due to stimulation of dendrites in the tongue. Sensory dendrites also receive stimulation through two special end organs, the eye

and the ear. All of these structures are called sensory receptors because they carry information about the outside world to the brain.

The Eye

The eye is a hollow ball filled with a semiliquid, figure 22-2. The wall of the eye is made up of three layers. A tough, white, fibrous outer coat (the *sclera*) has a vascular layer called the *choroid*. Its job is to nourish the eye. The innermost lining, the *retina*, is made up of dendrites highly sensitive to light. There are two kinds of these special receptor cells. The rods and the cones are named because of their shapes. The *cones* are most centrally concentrated near the macula. They carry information transmitted by bright light and color. The *rods* are concentrated more laterally in the retina. They are stimulated by dim light and are especially important for peripheral (side) vision.

The retina is normally held firmly against the choroid layer by the vitreous body. This is a jellylike fluid that fills the posterior cavity of the eye. The area of most acute vision is the *macula*, which is close to the optic nerve. The neurons in each eye join together and leave the eye as the optic nerve. The two nerves cross beneath the brain and carry their impulses to the occipital lobe of the cerebrum, where vision is interpreted.

Light enters the eye through the cornea. The amount of light entering the eye is controlled by the colored portion of the eye, the *iris*. It is found behind the cornea. Fluid between the cornea and iris, called aqueous humor, helps to bend the light rays and bring them to focus on the retina. This fluid is constantly being produced and absorbed through the small canal of Schlemm at the base of the cornea and iris.

The opening in the iris is the *pupil*. The pupil appears black because there is no light behind it. Directly behind the iris is the lens. Light rays travel in a straight line until they reach the eye. As they pass through the different *densities* (thicknesses) of the eye structures and fluids, they are bent *(refracted)* so that they come to focus on the areas of most acute vision. The lens,

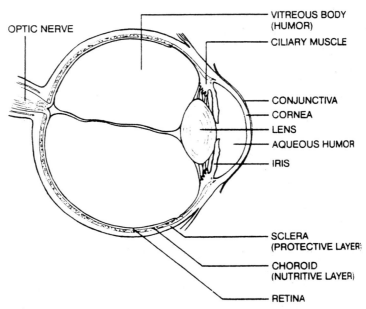

Figure 22-2A Internal structure of the eye (From Hegner & Caldwell, *Assisting in Long-Term Care,* copyright 1988 by Delmar Publishers Inc.)

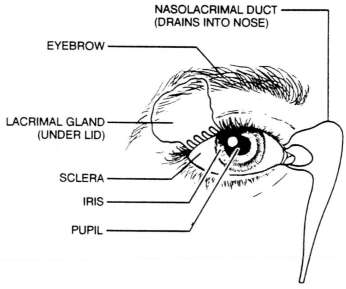

Figure 22-2B External structures of the eye (From Hegner & Caldwell, *Assisting in Long-Term Care,* copyright 1988 by Delmar Publishers Inc.)

by changing its shape and density, bends the light rays most effectively. This action by the lens is called *accommodation*. Refraction is needed to get the rays to focus correctly.

Small muscles pull on either side of the lens to change its shape. The changing shape of the lens makes it possible to adjust the range of vision from far to near and vice versa.

The eye is held within the bony socket by muscles that can change its position. A mucous membrane, the *conjunctiva*, lines the eyelids and covers the eye. Conjunctivitis is an inflammation of this membrane. The eyelids, eyelashes, and tears protect the eye. Tears are manufactured by the lacrimal gland that is found beneath the lateral side of the upper lid. Tears wash across the eye, keeping it moist, and drain into the nose.

The Ear

As the eye is sensitive to light, the ear is sensitive to sound. The ear has three parts: the outer ear, the middle ear, and the inner ear. The outer ear consists of the visible parts: the *pinna* (external ear) and the external auditory canal that direct sound waves to the middle ear, figure 22-3. At the end of the canal is the eardrum *(tympanic membrane)*. Sound waves entering the ear cause the eardrum to vibrate. Three tiny bones called *ossicles* form a chain across the middle ear from the tympanic membrane to a membrane-covered opening in the inner ear. These bones carry the sound waves across the middle ear and, by pushing against the opening of the inner ear, start fluid moving in the inner ear. A small tube, the *eustachian tube*, leads from the nasopharynx into the middle ear. Air carried through this tube helps to keep pressure equal on both sides of the eardrum.

The inner ear is a complex structure having two main parts. One looks somewhat like a coiled snail shell and is called the *cochlea*. Within the cochlea are the tiny dendrites of the auditory

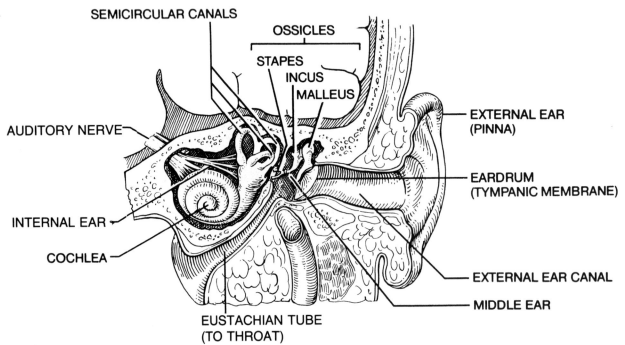

Figure 22-3   Internal view of the ear (From Hegner & Caldwell, *Assisting in Long-Term Care,* copyright 1988 by Delmar Publishers Inc.)

(hearing) nerve. Fluid covers the dendrites. When the fluid is set in motion by the vibrating bones of the middle ear, it stimulates the dendrites with sound sensations. The auditory nerves, one from each ear, carry the sensations to the temporal lobe of the cerebrum, where sound is interpreted. Also found in the inner ear are three *semicircular canals* that also contain liquid and nerve endings. Stimulation of these nerve endings sends impulses to the brain about the position of the head. These impulses are critical to the sense of balance.

Senescent Changes

Aging brings about changes in both the structure and the functional abilities of the human nervous system. There are changes in the cytoplasm and nuclei of the neurons. In some instances, there are changes in the relationship of the neurons to the surrounding cells. Death of some nerve cells may occur.

In general, sensory receptors are less reactive in the elderly, and stronger stimulation is needed to elicit a response, figure 22-4. For example, the threshold of pain is raised, and more illumination is needed to stimulate the sensory receptors of the retina of the eye.

As the person ages, the number of taste bud receptors diminishes. It becomes more difficult to distinguish between salty and sweet tastes. Smell receptors also become less acute. Because the ability to smell is closely related to the sense of taste, this also hampers the appreciation of food. Smoking and abnormalities of the mouth may make adequate nutrition a problem.

The older person may use excessive sugar and salt to improve the flavor of food. Ways of improving food flavor without these spices should be sought. However, you should not assume that all elderly limit their dietary spices. The loss of smell receptors can place the elderly at risk for fire injuries because they may not be able to smell smoke. Smoke detectors can be a valuable safety factor for them.

With aging, the lens of the eye becomes less able to change its shape and bend the light rays passing through it. The problem is called *presbyopia,* described as a loss of accommodation, This usually results in *hyperopia* (far sightedness). A person who has been nearsighted *(myopia)* for many years may find that vision improves. A condition frequently seen in elders is *entropion* or *ectropion.* Entropion is a turning in of the eyelid and eyelashes, frequently causing irritation. Ectropion is a turning out of the eyelid to expose the conjunctiva to infection and drying. Foot and eye coordination decrease, leading to increased chance of accidents. In general, the elderly will experience less acute vision at night and when lighting is dim. The twilight hours can be an especially hazardous time.

Nursing diagnostic categories related to sensory problems are listed in table 22-1.

- Degeneration of end organs
- Decreased sense of taste
- Decreased sense of touch
- Decreased sense of temperature
- Decreased sense of smell
- Decreased hearing ability
- Decreased sight

Figure 22-4 Senescent changes in sensory organs

- Alteration in health maintenance
- Alteration in nutrition
- Anxiety
- Diversional activity deficit
- Health management deficit
- Potential for injury
- Sensory perceptual alteration: Visual, hearing, gustatory, etc.
- Social isolation

Table 22-1 Nursing diagnostic categories related to sensory problems

Geriatric Eye Conditions

Proper care of the eyes is a lifelong task. Early care can safeguard precious sight. Changes in vision tend to take place slowly. Thus, periodic examinations by an ophthalmologist are important.

As a person ages, vision assumes greater importance because of increased leisure time and a decrease in physical stamina. These factors make less strenuous activities desirable. The eyes are used more and more for such leisure-time activities as reading or hobby work. Emotional problems associated with diminishing visual acuity are great. The fear of blindness, dependency, and social isolation hangs like a dreaded sword. So great is the fear that many people are reluctant to recognize danger signs and may react with hostility when finally forced to admit to them.

General Signs and Symptoms

The services of an ophthalmologist should be sought whenever changes in eye structure or vision are noted. Redness, irritation, burning, and excessive watering of the eyes should not be neglected. Dry eyes or ineffectual tearing should be investigated. Other signs to watch for include sensitivity to light, frequent headaches, and visual disturbances.

The variety of visual disturbances is wide. Some may complain of seeing spots, halos of light, or blurred images. Others may notice a loss of side vision or an inability to adjust to darkened rooms. Any of these signs or symptoms warrants treatment by a competent eye specialist. Drugs such as digitalis may also cause visual symptoms. The major focus for nursing care when sight is impaired is to maximize the vision that remains and to help the person to remain as independent as possible.

Senile Cataracts

Senile cataracts are the single most important cause of blindness in old age, figure 22-5. They account for 22 percent of all lost vision.

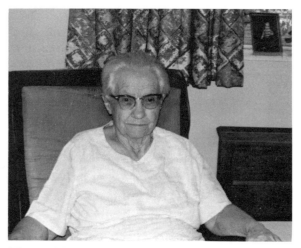

Figure 22-5   This woman has lost some of her vision because of cataracts, but surgery will soon restore much of her sight. (From Hegner & Caldwell, *Assisting in Long-Term Care*, copyright 1988 by Delmar Publishers Inc.)

Visual loss is due to a gradually increasing opacity of the lens. The lens is originally a clear, crystalline body enclosed in a capsule that changes its shape to bend the light rays to focus on the retina. If the lens is opaque (not transparent), light cannot pass through it and so vision is lost. Sometimes double vision *(diplopia)* may occur and the ability to assess color values may diminish. The cause of cataracts is unknown. However, they are frequently associated in later years with endocrine disorders such as diabetes.

Throughout life, gradual changes in the lens eventually lead to senile cataracts. The lens gradually increases in size. As fibers grow around the outer part of the lens (cortex), the inner (nuclear) fibers become compressed and hardened. In early phases, this causes shortsightedness, but eventually distance vision is also limited. Degeneration begins in the cortex and moves inward until the entire lens is involved. Central vision is lost first, but peripheral vision is eventually affected.

Senile cataracts are usually found in people over seventy years of age. Cataracts generally can be managed by surgery. A new method utilizing ultrasonic vibrations to remove the cataract holds some promise. The vibrations are applied to the lens with a hollow needle. This fragments and emulsifies the lens, which is then aspirated. The lens may be removed at any stage of opaque development. The choice of time depends largely upon the needs of the individual patient.

Treatment and Nursing Care. Cataract extractions (surgical removal of the lens) restore useful vision in 90 percent of the cases. Most surgery is now done on an outpatient basis.

Sometimes a man-made lens transplant is possible. The replacement lens is slipped into a lens capsule after the original lens is removed. The new lens will then function as the original lens. In other cases, corrective lenses will be needed to carry out accommodation. These may be either contact lenses or glasses.

Cataracts may be removed under local or general anesthesia. If both eyes are involved, which is often the case, one eye is done at a time. Both eyes can be done during a single hospitalization, however. The affected eye or possibly both eyes are bandaged when the patient is returned from surgery. Gauze bandaging over the unaffected eye lessens excessive eye movements during the first twenty-four hours. Many times only the affected eye is covered.

Nursing care begins with admission. Because the patient will probably return from surgery with both eyes bandaged, preparation for this temporary blind period begins at once. The nurse carefully acquaints the patient with the room and the available services. Proper orientation can make a great deal of difference in the early postoperative period. It can lessen anxiety and feelings of isolation. When deprived of their sense of sight, the elderly are easily confused and disoriented.

Preoperatively, the nurse may have orders to apply antibiotic drops as a precautionary measure. The nurse will also have orders to administer eyedrops to dilate the pupil preoperatively. The abbreviations *O.D.* (right eye) and *O.S.* (left

eye) are in common usage, and orders may be written in this way. The drugs ordered are called *mydriatics.* Cyclopegic drugs, such as homatropine, are also used. These drugs dilate the pupil, but in addition they cause paralysis of accommodation. Both of these drugs may be administered postoperatively as well.

It is essential that the nurse administer eyedrops accurately. The patient must be in a sitting position, and the nurse's hands must be washed thoroughly. The nurse should gently separate the lids of the proper eye and, as the patient looks upward, draw the lower lid outward and place the medication on it. The eyedropper must not touch the eye.

The patient should then close the eye to disperse the medication. If the nurse rests the hand holding the eyedropper on the patient's forehead, there is less danger of accidentally hurting the eye with the tip of the dropper, figure 22-6.

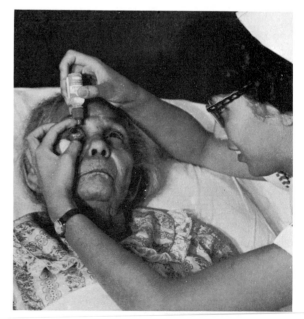

Figure 22-6 The nurse rests her hand against the patient's forehead as the drop is placed inside the lower lid. (Reprinted from *Care of the Adult Patient* by Smith and Gips)

Postoperatively, patients are usually transferred from the operating-room table immediately to their own bed or a reclining chair in one move. The head of the bed is usually elevated 30 degrees to reduce strain. Side rails must be up for general safety. This is especially important because the patient may become disoriented following surgery.

Cataract surgery patients may be discharged on the day of surgery. However, each physician writes specific orders for postoperative care. These orders must be followed exactly for about one month. The dressing is usually changed postoperatively the day after surgery in the surgeon's office.

The patient is usually cautioned to keep the eye shield on to protect the eye at all times. He or she is also advised to avoid activity that increases intraocular pressure, which would put a strain on the suture line. Patients are also advised not to rub the eye, not to allow it to become wet, and to lie on the nonoperative side.

In general, the patient requires much psychological support, especially if both eyes are bandaged. The health care provider must be available to meet the patient's physical needs for water, food, and elimination, as well as to give the comfort of frequent personal contact.

Antiemetics may be ordered to control nausea. Vomiting, like coughing or sneezing, puts undue stress on the incision.

Orders for care of the patient may vary. Some require that the pupil of the patient's eye be kept dilated with atropine for the first twenty-four hours. Most permit ambulation on the first postoperative day.

You must watch the patient for signs that the iris is not being maintained in its proper position. Watch for bulging of the wound or changes in the shape of the pupil. Report immediately any complaints of sharp pain in the eye.

The nurse must keep in mind, in all cases, that any elderly person deprived of sensory stimulation can quickly lose contact with reality. The importance of repeated personal contacts and of other stimuli, such as a radio, cannot be overstressed.

Initial ambulation requires assistance, especially if both eyes are bandaged. The eyes are used to help maintain balance. When the patient is deprived of sensory stimulation, ambulation is difficult. Even if only one eye is affected, adjustment is required.

General activity is limited for some time. A quiet type of occupational therapy is of value. Eyeglasses are prescribed. Temporary glasses are used during the adjustment period of six weeks to three months. The permanent lenses are usually bifocals so that the patient can once more see at different distances. Contact lenses are intraocular lens replacement are two other means of correcting visual problems. But these are more commonly used with younger people. In old age, recovery from cataract surgery depends in large part on the morale of the patient. A positive attitude by the caregiver will lend emotional support.

Glaucoma

Glaucoma is a disease primarily of old people. It affects approximately 2 to 4 percent of the adult population, although many are unaware that changes are taking place in their eyes. The condition usually develops slowly between the ages of forty and sixty-five. It is to some extent hereditary. It may affect only one eye, but usually both eyes are involved.

There are two liquids or semiliquids in the eye, the vitreous humor and the aqueous humor. The aqueous humor in the normal eye is continually being produced by the ciliary body. It flows into the posterior chamber between the iris and lens and then into the anterior chamber (in front of the iris). It is reabsorbed by way of the canal of Schlemm. The pressure is kept constant in this manner.

In glaucoma, the fluid is continually produced, but the drainage system no longer functions adequately. The result is an accumulation of fluid that increases the intraocular pressure. The pressure is exerted throughout the eye and specifically against the optic disk, causing it to "cup" against the retina. The retina then becomes ischemic and atrophies. Peripheral vision is lost first and then central vision, giving rise to the sensation of tunnel vision. Early diagnosis and treatment can control the condition and prevent further damage.

Glaucoma may be classified as secondary or primary. The secondary type follows disease or injury to the eye. Most cases are of the primary type (glaucoma simplex), which develops insidiously with no relationship to previous pathology. Early indications include headache, nausea, blurred vision, dull eye pain, and the appearance of halos around lighted objects. Glaucoma simplex may be acute, causing severe damage and accompanied by nausea and intense pain in the eye and head. The pupils become dilated and do not respond to light. Sometimes the primary form is described in relation to changes in the anterior angle (that point of juncture formed by the ciliary body, iris, and cornea).

The disease may then be classified as chronic open angle glaucoma and narrow angle (angle closure) glaucoma. The chronic open angle form affects about 90 percent of glaucoma patients. The angle is open, but drainage is inadequate. This is caused by changes in the porous meshwork of tissues that form the angle and through which the aqueous humor filters back into general circulation. There seems to be a genetic predisposition to this condition. In narrow angle glaucoma, drainage is blocked because of the iris, which occludes the canal of Schlemm.

Diagnostic Tests.   Intraocular pressure, which is greatly raised in glaucoma, can be measured by digital palpitation and by an instrument called a tonometer. *Tonography* is the technique of measuring intraocular pressure. The preferred technique employs the tonometer and a recording device to measure the outflow of the aqueous fluid. An ophthalmoscope is used to observe the optic disk for signs of cupping due to increased pressure.

Visual acuity tests measure the extent of peripheral and central vision. The peripheral vision test plots the moment that a moving object moves into the patient's visual field. The central vision test makes use of the familiar eye chart at a distance of twenty feet. Charting these findings helps to determine the extent of nerve damage.

Treatment and Nursing Care   Treatment of glaucoma depends in part on the extent of damage to the drainage system and whether drainage can be reestablished. If this is impossible, treatment focuses on decreasing the amount of aqueous fluid that is produced. In general, treatment includes drugs to decrease the production of aqueous fluid and to increase its drainage, narcotics to relieve pain, bedrest, and sometimes surgery.

Four types of drugs are used, figure 22-7. *Miotic* drugs, which constrict the pupil, are given to contract the pupil, allowing an increase in the outward flow of the aqueous fluid. Carbonic anhydrase inhibitors are used to decrease production of the aqueous fluid by the carbonic anhydrase enzyme. Osmotic agents increase the water-drawing power (osmolarity) of plasma and, in turn, bring about a decrease in the intraocular pressure. Adrenergic agents are also used to reduce intraocular pressure in cases where dilation of the pupil will not create a problem in combination with another drug, especially a miotic.

Surgery may be the treatment chosen. *Diathermy* (extreme heat) or *cryosurgery* (extreme cold) can be used to shrink the ciliary body, providing more room for drainage. A *fistulizing* procedure (also called *trabeculectomy*) may also be done to allow drainage into the suprachoroidal space or externally through the conjunctival tissues. An *iridencleises* may be performed. In this surgery, part of the iris is cut and inverted to a form a wick into the subconjunctival space to promote drainage. Argon laser surgery (trabeculectomy) is being employed in selected cases.

During acute attacks of glaucoma, the patient should be kept quiet. Sedatives and analgesics are given to ensure rest. The remainder of the time, the patient must use the prescribed eye medicine four to six times daily. As with any chronic condition that can be controlled by relatively simple means, there is a tendency for

DRUGS USED TO TREAT GLAUCOMA

Drug	Form
Miotics—Cholinergic drugs	
Acetylcholine chloride-miochol®	Solution (drops)
Pilocarpine nitrate	Solution (drops)
Carbachol—Daryl®	Solution (drops)
Miotics—Cholinesterase inhibitors	
Physostigmine salicylate—Eserine	Solution (drops)
Demecarium—Humorsol®	Solution (drops)
Echothiophate—Phospholine®	Solution (drops)
Isoflurophate—DFP Floropryl®	Solution (drops)
Neostigmine bromide—Prostigmine®	Solution (drops)
Adrenergic agents	
Epinephrine—Adrenalin®	Solution (drops)
Epinephrine—Eppy®	Solution (drops)
Epinephrine—Epitrate®	Solution (drops)
Carbonic anhydrase inhibitors	
Acetazolamide—Diamox®	Tablets
Methazolamide—Neptazane®	Tablets
Ethoxzolamide—Cardrase®	Tablets
Dichlorphenamide—Daranide®	Tablets
Osmotic agents	
Glycerine	In solution w/orange juice
Urea—Urevert®	Solution (intravenously)
Mannitol—Osmitrol	Solution (intravenously)

Figure 22-7   Drugs for glaucoma

patients to become lax in carrying out the basic regime. The elderly person may simply not remember to insert the drops. The fact that the drops cause momentary discomfort and must be instilled regularly means that many patients require encouragement to carry out the treatment. A family member should be thoroughly familiar with the medication routine and be prepared to assume responsibility if the patient does not.

Bending and lifting should be avoided. These activities tend to raise the intraocular pressure. Tight clothing and emotional tension such as quarreling may also have this effect. Patients with glaucoma are advised to avoid stimulants such as caffeine, to space their fluid intake, and to have regular checkups.

During ophthalmologic checkups, several of the tests already described—tonometry, tonography, visual field, and central vision acuity—may be performed. One of the biggest nursing responsibilities is to help interpret the disease, its treatment, and its control to the community, and especially to the individual glaucoma patient.

Macular Degeneration

Macular degeneration is associated with hardening and obstruction of the retinal arteries. Small hemorrhages can develop within the eye. The hemorrhages may be related to hypertension, diabetes, or multiple sclerosis. Central vision is lost, but total blindness doesn't usually develop because peripheral vision is maintained. Vision aids may be helpful. This form of pathology affects 30 percent of those over age sixty-five. Treatment for this condition is as yet unsatisfactory.

Diabetic Retinopathy

This condition is often seen in Type II (NIDDM) diabetes patients. Occurrence is related to longevity of the diabetes. The condition is further aggravated by hypertension. Retinal hemorrhage and white or yellow exudates hamper macular function. There is a growth of new blood vessels even into the vitreous body, with subsequent hemorrhage and sometimes retinal detachment. The patient experiences blurred vision; both eyes are involved. Laser surgery may be used to destroy the new vessels and slow the process of blindness that usually occurs.

Retinal Detachment

Retinal detachment can be a complication of diabetes mellitus or a result of trauma. Flashes of light and blurred vision often precede the detachment. As part of the retina loses contact, a veil or cloud seems to cross the visual field. Vision can be lost completely. Laser surgery has proved successful. Diathermy or cryotherapy can also be used.

Hemianopia

Hemianopia is an inability to see the entire visual field. Affected persons are unable to see half of what they are looking at, figure 22-8. A cerebral vascular accident is the most common cause of this problem.

These patients must be helped to be aware of the entire visual field. For example, a man may only see and therefore eat only one half of the food in front of him. He may be injured by running into an object because he cannot see where it extends beyond his visual field.

Teach the patient to slowly turn his head to the affected side to bring the object into view. Place materials such as clothing to be put on in the visual field.

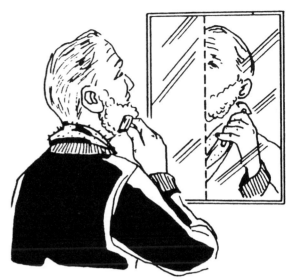

Figure 22-8   Hemianopia causes a person to see only part of the visual field.

This situation may be temporary or permanent, depending on the cause. But as long as it exists, it can be extremely frustrating for the patient.

Blindness

Cataracts, glaucoma, and other retinopathy can lead to *blindness* (loss of vision) of varying degrees, from partial to total. Blindness is defined legally as 20/200 vision in the better eye when wearing corrective lenses. Not all those who are blind are totally unable to see. Those who are legally blind may have some sight. In caring for blind patients, the staff should be guided by what the blind person needs and wants. Individual differences must be recognized. Each patient must be permitted as much independent activity as possible. In general, the blind need to have their other senses stimulated. A radio is almost a necessity.

The approach to caring for a blind person depends in part of the degree of blindness. An elderly person who has been blind all or most of his or her life will be relatively self-sufficient and independent. However, a newly blind person must make a difficult adjustment to a new and terrifying situation. Adjustment to blindness is both physical and psychological. The patient may go through the same series of psychological adjustments made by the dying person.

A directory of agencies for the blind is published by the American Foundation for the Blind. It describes the many services available. Another source of information is the Vocational Rehabilitation Administration, Department of Health and Human Services, Washington, D.C.

Health care providers must always make a blind patient aware of their presence by speaking before touching the patient. Safety can be ensured by keeping the environment unchanged and advising the patient of any required change. The blind use familiar objects to help orient themselves. If those objects are moved, these patients may become confused or have an accident, figure 22-9.

Orient the blind patient to any new room, and try to maintain the furnishings in a standardized way. Have some method, such as raised letters, to identify special doors such as those to bathrooms or hallways. Keep personal articles in the same place and return them to the same location after use.

The staff should escort blind patients until they gain familiarity with the surroundings. This is best done by walking slightly ahead of the person with his or her hand on your arm. Make sure that no obstacles such as cleaning equipment, wheelchairs, or unused chairs are left in the way. Doors should be left fully opened or fully shut. Unit 16 describe special considerations when providing food for the blind.

Refer to figure 22-10 to review the actions to be performed at the beginning and end of each patient care procedure.

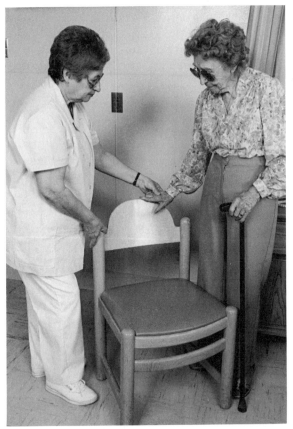

Figure 22-9   Never rearrange furniture without informing the blind person. (From Hegner & Caldwell, *Assisting in Long-Term Care,* copyright 1988 by Delmar Publishers Inc.)

- Politely ask visitors to leave. Tell them where they can wait.
- Identify the resident.
- Provide privacy by drawing curtains around bed and closing door.
- Explain what you will be doing, and answer questions.
- Raise bed to comfortable working height.

Beginning Procedure Actions

- Wash your hands.
- Assemble all equipment needed.
- Knock on door and pause before entering resident's room.

Procedure Completion Actions

- Position resident comfortably.
- Leave signal cord, telephone, and fresh water where resident can reach them.
- Return bed to lowest horizontal position.

- Raise side rails, if required.
- Perform general safety check of resident and environment.
- Clean used equipment and return to proper storage, according to facility policy.
- Open privacy curtains.
- Wash your hands.
- Tell visitors that they may reenter the room.
- Report completion of procedure.
- Document procedure following facility policy.

Figure 22-10   Beginning procedure actions and procedure completion actions.

Procedure 10

Caring for Glasses

1. Wash your hands.
2. Assemble the equipment you will need:

   patient's eyeglasses
   cleaning solution
   clear water
   soft cleaning tissues

3. Identify the patient.
4. Explain what you plan to do. Allow the person to do the procedure or assist as able.
5. Handle glasses only by frames.
6. Clean with cleaning solution or clear water.
7. Dry with soft cleaning tissues.
8. Return eyeglasses to case and place on bedside stand or return to resident.

Procedure 11

Caring for a Patient with an Artificial Eye

1. Wash your hands.
2. Assemble the equipment you will need:

   eyecup lined with gauze

   cotton balls
   washcloth
   lukewarm water
   cleansing solution if ordered

3. Identify the patient.
4. Explain what you plan to do. Allow the person to assist as able.
5. Assist person into bed.
6. Close curtains for privacy.
7. Have person close the eyes and turn head to side of the prosthesis.
8. Wash external eye with warm water.
9. Use one cotton ball at a time. Stroke once only from medial eye to outer eye.
10. Remove eye by depressing lower eyelid with your thumb while lifting upper lid with your finger.
11. Collect eye in your hand and place in eyecup.
12. Place eyecup and prosthesis in center of overbed stand or bedside stand.
13. Clean eye socket in the same manner, using warm water and cotton balls. Dry area around eye gently.
14. Carry eyecup to bathroom and half fill sink with lukewarm water.
15. Place folded washcloth in bottom of sink as added precaution against breakage.
16. Remove all secretions from the prosthesis. *Do not use* abrasives or general solvents.
17. Empty water from eyecup.
18. Place a fresh gauze square on the bottom and place the wet eye on the gauze.
19. Add water if eye is to be stored in the drawer of the bedside stand.
20. Wash your hands.
21. Return to the bedside to reinsert the eye.
22. Raise the upper lid with one finger and insert the eye into the socket with notched edge toward the nose.
23. Depress lower lid and slip over prosthesis.
24. Clean, replace, or dispose of equipment according to facility policy.
25. Wash your hands.

26. Report completion of procedure and record the following:
    - The date and time of procedure
    - Procedure: prosthetic eye cleaned and reinserted/stored
    - Type of solution used
    - Patient's reaction

Hearing Loss

More than three million people in the United States suffer some degree of hearing loss. Thirty percent of those over age sixty-five suffer from this handicap. Thirteen percent of them would benefit from professional help, but many deny that help is needed. Loss of hearing is twice as common in men as it is in women, and it may develop gradually over a period of time. The incidence of hearing loss is expected to increase dramatically as those who listen to rock music at very loud levels age. The inability to hear can cause great emotional stress because of missed communications. Elderly people who are hard of hearing may have suffered ear infections or ear diseases in childhood or middle life and have carried this handicap into their later yers. Hearing problems can result from limitations in ossicle movement (conduction loss) or may be due to damage to the eighth cranial nerve (nerve loss). Probably the most common cause of hearing problems is otosclerosis. In otosclerosis, the tissues of the labyrinth and middle ear become hardened, and hearing is gradually diminished. Extreme tones are lost first, with the greatest loss in the high-pitched range. Patients with otosclerosis may also be disturbed by distressing inner ear sounds.

Hearing aids, which amplify sounds, can help these people, figure 22-11. Hearing aids must be properly fitted to the individual. The patient should be instructed carefully in their use and care. Not all patients can be helped by hearing aids. the aids should not be purchased indiscriminately.

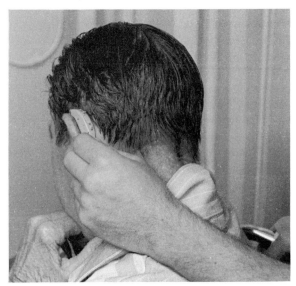

Figure 22-11   Hearing loss can be improved by the use of a hearing aid. (From Hegner and Caldwell, *Assisting in Long-Term Care,* copyright 1988 by Delmar Publishers Inc.)

Careful handling of a hearing aid is important to protect it from damage, figure 22-12. Be sure it is stored safely in the bedside stand when not in use, with the battery out. Before applying the device, always check the ear mold for cleanliness and the ear itself for any abnormalities. Check for battery failure and immediately report the need for new batteries. Make sure that the hearing aid is identified according to facility policy. Therefore, if it is misplaced, it can be promptly returned to its owner.

Presbycusis

Presbycusis, also known as senile deafness because of the frequency of its occurrence in the elderly, is the only ear condition that is more common to this age group than to any other. Also known as eighth-nerve-damage deafness, it is caused by damage to the eighth cranial or auditory nerve, which is responsible for conducting sound waves. Senescent changes in the nerve, probably due to degeneration, make perception

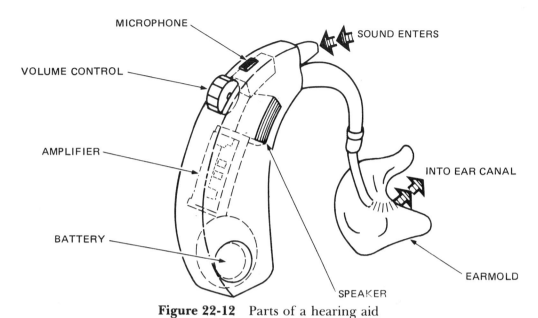

MICROPHONE

SOUND ENTERS

VOLUME CONTROL

AMPLIFIER

INTO EAR CANAL

BATTERY

EARMOLD

SPEAKER

Figure 22-12 Parts of a hearing aid

and conduction more difficult. Because hearing aids essentially increase the sound that still must be carried by the auditory nerve, they are of little value when the auditory nerve itself no longer functions.

In presbycusis, there is a progressive, bilateral hearing loss. The condition affects the ability to hear high-pitched sounds and the sound of consonants such as *f, s, th, ch,* and *sh*. With increased loss, it becomes increasingly difficult to distinguish the sounds, and background noise further impedes the hearing process.

You may wish to review procedures related to the eye and ear with your instructor.

Emotional Adjustment

Emotional reaction to hearing loss is apt to be severe. The sense of social isolation is extreme. When the problem has developed over the years, the adjustment in old age is usually better. Older people experiencing initial hearing loss tend to deny it and blame others for not speaking clearly. They often become withdrawn, exhibiting fear and suspicion of those around them. This is understandable, because they can-

not comprehend what is being said to them or take part in conversations around them. The person with a hearing loss may also be labeled "confused" or "senile" because they answer questions incorrectly or not at all.

Communication

Communication with a deaf person takes skill and practice, but it is well worth the effort. Be alert to recognize the signs of hearing loss. The person may have difficulty following directions, may frequently ask you to repeat, or may turn the head so the ear is closer to you while watching your mouth as you speak.

Pay particular attention to those in your care who seem somewhat withdrawn or less willing to participate. Their reluctance may be due to an inability to hear. Because the deaf person must use the sense of sight for help, the health care provider must stand directly in front of the patient to be clearly viewed, figure 22-13. Many patients learn lip reading. Conventional sign language is an almost universal means of communication. However, each of these requires practice, and some elderly people lack sufficient

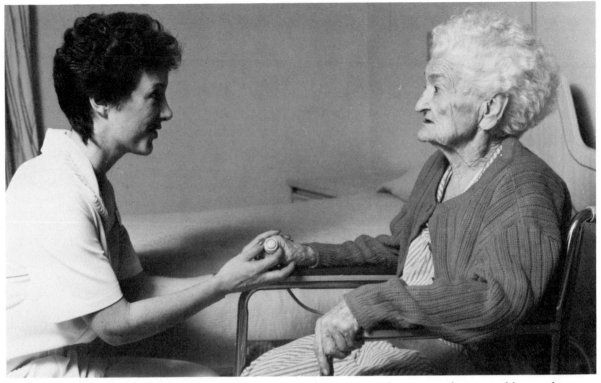

Figure 22-13A   Sit directly in front of the hearing impaired person when speaking to her.

motivation to learn. Also, much of the hospital nomenclature is not included in basic sign language. Body language such as pointing to the object being discussed can be very helpful. Facial expressions can also convey many messages. Deaf patients need to be encouraged to answer verbally, because they tend to respond only with a nod or shake of the head.

---

1. Speak slowly and distinctly.
2. Form words carefully; keep sentences short.
3. Rephrase words as needed.
4. Face the listener.
5. Make sure any light source is behind the listener.
6. Use facial expressions or gestures to help express your meaning.
7. Encourage lip reading.
8. Diminish outside noise or distractions.

Figure 22-13B   Summary of techniques to use when communicating with those who are hearing impaired.

PROCEDURE 12

Caring for a Patient with a Hearing Aid

1. Wash your hands.
2. Identify the patient.
3. Check the hearing aid to be sure the batteries are functioning.
4. Check the patient's ear for wax buildup or any abnormalities.
5. Handle the aid carefully. Do not drop it or allow it to get wet.
6. When not in use, store it carefully in the off position.

7. Hand the aid to the patient so that you support the appliance as the resident inserts the earmold into the ear canal.
8. Adjust the volume.
9. Wash your hands.
10. Report completion of assignment.

Summary

-   Sensory losses are experienced as aging progresses.
-   Taste, smell, and touch all require more intense stimulation.
-   Adequate hearing and sight are essential if a person is to function independently.
-   Many elderly people suffer from either hearing or sight loss, and frequently from both. Cataracts and glaucoma are the most common causes of blindness.
-   Otosclerosis and eighth-nerve damage are responsible for most hearing loss.
-   The major nursing care focus for people with sensory deficits is to maximize the remaining function.
-   Health care providers can do much to help the hearing and sight impaired live more independent lives in a safe environment.

Review Outline

I.   Behavioral Objectives

II. Vocabulary

III. Sensory Receptors
   A. Skin
       1. Heat
       2. Cold
       3. Pressure
       4. Pain
   B. Joint—body position
   C. Nose—smell
   D. Tongue—taste
   E. Eye—vision
   F. Ear—hearing

IV. The Eye
   A. Basic anatomy and physiology
   B. Senescent changes
   C. Geriatric conditions
       1. Ectropion
       2. Entropion
       3. Cataracts
       4. Glaucoma
       5. Macular degeneration
       6. Diabetic retinopathy
       7. Retinal detachment
       8. Hemianopia
       9. Blindness

    V.   The Ear

        A.   Basic anatomy and physiology
        B.   Senescent changes
        C.   Geriatric conditions
            1.   Hearing loss
            2.   Presbycusis

Review

    I. Vocabulary

    Matching

1. Thickness	a. Glaucoma
2. Treatment using extreme cold	b. Trabeculectomy
3. Farsightedness	c. Density
4. Double vision	d. Cataract
5. Lens becoming opaque	e. Hyperopia
6. Technique of measuring intraocular pressure	f. Refraction
7. Bending of light rays	g. Miotics
8. Increased intraocular pressure	h. Cryosurgery
9. Fistulization procedure	i. Tonography
10. Drugs that constrict the pupil	j. Diplopia

  II. Basic Anatomy and Physiology

    Label the diagrams.

      A.   The Eye

    1. Vitreous body
    2. Ciliary muscle
    3. Conjunctiva
    4. Cornea
    5. Lens
    6. Aqueous humor
    7. Iris
    8. Sclera
    9. Choroid
    10. Retina

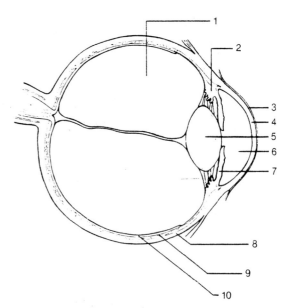

Figure 22-14 (From Hegner & Caldwell, *Assisting in Long-Term Care,* copyright 1988 by Delmar Publishers Inc.)

B.   The Ear

1.   Eustachian tube
2.   Middle ear
3.   External ear canal
4.   Tympanic membrane
5.   Pinna
6.   Ossicles
7.   Semicircular canals
8.   Auditory nerve
9.   Internal ear
10.   Cochlea

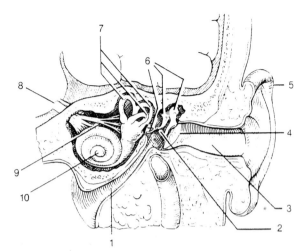

Figure 22-15   (From Hegner & Caldwell, *Assisting in Long-Term Care*, copyright 1988 by Delmar Publishers Inc.)

III.   Short Answers

1.   Describe how light rays reflecting the image of an object being seen are brought to focus on the fovea centralis.
2.   Explain how sound waves reach the cerebrum for interpretation.
3.   Describe the problem of glaucoma.
4.   Describe the problem of cataracts.
5.   Explain why the person who is hard of hearing may seem withdrawn.

IV.   Nursing Care

Select the one best answer to each of the following.

1.   Your patient has reddened, watery eyes. Your best action is to

a.   ignore the condition because this is a sign of aging.
b.   report the condition to your supervisor.
c.   suggest that the person read in better light.
d.   clean the person's eyeglasses so there will be less eye strain.

2.   Your patient informs you that as he looks at the light, he sees a halo around the bulb. You report this because you suspect he may have

a.   a cataract.
b.   glaucoma.
c.   otosclerosis.
d.   presbycusis.

3.   Following surgery for a cataract, you should

a.   encourage the person to exercise freely.
b.   keep the head of the bed flat.
c.   encourage the patient to cough.
d.   none of these.

4. Your elderly patient has a diagnosis of glaucoma. You will need to be sure

   a. to perform tonometry regularly.
   b. the patient is kept in dim lighting.
   c. that prescribed eyedrops are administered.
   d. you perform visual acuity tests routinely.

5. When caring for a person with an artificial eye, you should

   a. wash the external eye with warm water, stroking in a medial to lateral direction.
   b. clean the socket with cold water after removing the eye.
   c. remove the eye by depressing the upper lid.
   d. hold the eye while cleaning the socket.

CASE STUDY

Mrs. Yvonne Bean is eight-eight and has just been admitted to your unit. She is a widow who lost her sight at age fifty-seven as the result of diabetic retinopathy. Before that time, she had raised a family of five boys and one girl while working as a legal secretary.

Her children have all moved out of the area and her arthritis makes caring for herself very difficult. What kind of care must you provide for her?

Unit 23
Endocrine System

Objectives
After studying this unit, you should be able to:
- Describe the function of the endocrine glands.
- Name and locate the glands in the endocrine system.
- List the factors that influence the incidence of diabetes mellitus.
- Name the two types of diabetes mellitus.
- List the common complications of diabetes mellitus in the elderly.

Vocabulary
Learn the meaning and spelling of the following words or phrases.

acidosis
decaliter
D.K.A.
H.H.N.C.
hyperglycemia
hypertrophy
hypoglycemia
I.D.D.M.
Ketoacidosis

ketosis
lipodystrophy
N.I.D.D.M.
obesity

polydipsia
polyphagia
polyuria
thyroxine

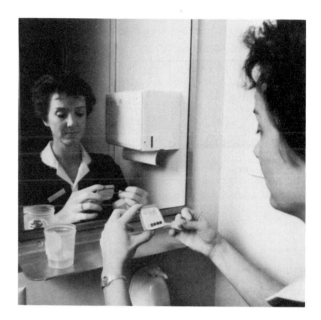

Endocrine glands are special tissues found throughout the body. These glands produce chemicals called hormones that enter the bloodstream directly and so are quickly carried to all parts of the body, figure 23-1. Endocrine glands do not have ducts. This makes them different from exocrine glands, such as those that produce digestive enzymes or perspiration.

Hormones regulate and control body activities and metabolism. There are seven distinct endocrine glands, some of which work in pairs. Some endocrine glands secrete several hor-

mones. In addition to the glands discussed in this unit, there are glandular cells scattered throughout the body that secrete minute amounts of regulatory hormones.

Structure and Function

Pituitary Gland
This gland has two portions (lobes). Each secretes more than one hormone. It is surrounded by bone and located under the brain. The hormones secreted by this gland control

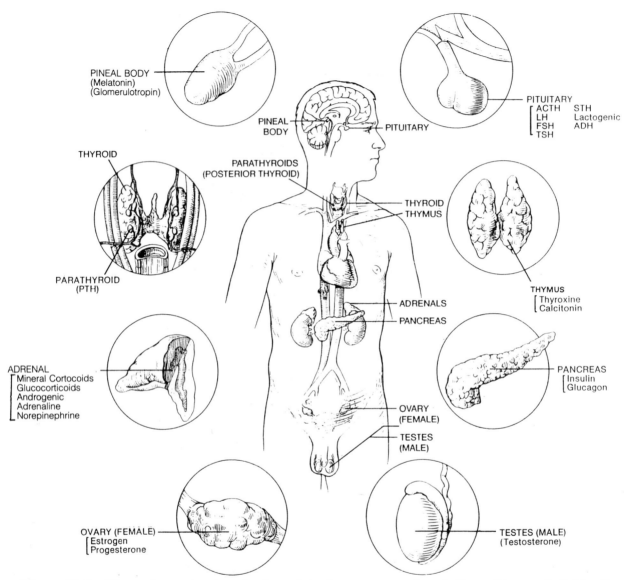

Figure 23-1   The major endocrine glands and the hormones produced (From Hegner & Caldwell, *Assisting in Long-Term Care,* copyright 1988 by Delmar Publishers Inc.)

growth, urine production, and the contractions of involuntary muscles. They also influence the activity of all the other glands. Because it controls the activities of the other glands, the pituitary is called the "master gland." The pituitary gland is controlled by a portion of the brain called the hypothalamus. With aging, the weight of the gland is believed to decrease somewhat, although the concentrations of all hormones, except the

follicle stimulating hormone (E.S.H.), seem to be the same.

Pineal Body

This is a small gland also located in the skull beneath the brain. Little is known about it. It is thought to be related to sexual maturation because it tends to atrophy at puberty.

Adrenal Glands

There are two adrenal glands, located on top of the two kidneys. Each gland has two distinct portions that secrete separate hormones, e.g. adrenaline and cortisone. In general, the adrenal hormones control the release of energy to meet emergencies, and water and salt usage by the body. They also secrete small amounts of male and female hormones. These glands do not seem to change appreciably with aging.

Gonads

These are the male and female sex glands. The female gonads are the two ovaries located within the pelvis on either side of the uterus. When stimulated by the pituitary gland, they produce two hormones, estrogen and progesterone. After menopause, they atrophy and no longer produce estrogen. Only the adrenals continue to produce small amounts of estrogen. Progesterone continues to be produced in small amounts.

The male gonads, the two testes, are located outside of the body in a pouch called the scrotum. They produce the hormone testosterone.

The male and female gonads are responsible for secondary sex characteristics. They also produce gametes (ovum and sperm), which unite to form a fetus. Review Unit 30 for a discussion of reproductive changes.

Thyroid Gland

This gland has two lobes and is found in the neck, anterior to the larynx. *Thyroxine* is the main hormone secreted by this gland. It helps to regulate the metabolism of all body cells. It is also related to the ability of the cells to pick up and use oxygen. In order for the thyroid gland to produce thyroxine, sufficient iodine must be present. Although there do not seem to be any age-related changes, this gland's function is affected by other changes in the body.

Parathyroids

These are several tiny glands embedded in the thyroid gland in the neck. The hormone they manufacture controls the body's use of two minerals, calcium and phosphorus. Research reports present conflicting information about age-related changes in these glands. Increased parathyroid hormone levels are seen in osteoporosis.

Pancreas

The pancreas, in the abdomen, is both an exocrine and an endocrine gland. The islets of Langerhans are small groups of cells within the pancreas. They produce the hormones insulin and glucagon. These hormones are important in regulating the level of glucose in the blood stream. Glucagon causes blood sugar to rise. Insulin must be present in order for the cells to use glucose, thereby lowering the blood sugar level. Insulin is also needed to convert excess glucose to glycogen for storage. With these glands, too, evidence is conflicting as to whether they change with age.

Some changes in pancreatic function suggest that insulin production or utilization decreases as the body ages. A higher level of glucose seems to be needed to trigger insulin release. Glucose intolerance may also be related to a higher level of blood fat (hyperlipemia) and to less exercise. As a result of these changes, glucose accumulates in the bloodstream at higher-than-normal levels *(hyperglycemia)* and may be excreted in the urine (glycosuria), depending on the renal threshold for glucose.

Diabetes Mellitus

The United States has the highest rate of diabetic morbidity and mortality in the world. Each year 250,000 new cases of diabetes mellitus are added to the more than four million known cases. Many new cases are discovered during routine physical examinations. In addition, it is estimated that millions more are unaware that they are diabetic.

There are two types of diabetes mellitus, Type I or insulin-dependent diabetes mellitus *(I.D.D.M.)* and Type II or non-insulin-dependent diabetes mellitus *(N.I.D.D.M.)*. Only about 15 percent of all adult diabetics have insulin-dependent diabetes. This means that they need insulin injections to prevent ketoacidosis and death. *Ketoacidosis* is a very serious complication of diabetes in which ketones accumulate in the blood stream and the pH of the blood drops. This condition is also called diabetes acidosis. Most adults have non-insulin-dependent diabetes and do not require insulin because the pancreas still produces some insulin. These adults are characteristically overweight, inactive, eat too many sweets made from refined sugar, and may smoke—all factors that contribute to N.I.D.D.M.

Although forms of the condition can appear at any age, it is more common in the middle and later years. About 80 percent of all diabetics are over forty years of age. As many as 5 percent of those over sixty-five require treatment.

Factors that seem to play a role in the incidence of diabetes are heredity, *obesity* (excess weight), sex, and age. Diabetes is transmitted as a recessive characteristic. In addition, the disease seems to appear at an earlier age with each succeeding generation. In the age range from fifty-five to sixty-four, there are twice as many diabetic women as men. There is a more even distribution of cases between the sexes after the age of sixty-five.

Insulin-Dependent Diabetes Mellitus

In this type of diabetes, the normal metabolism of fats, carbohydrates, and proteins is unbalanced. Normally when carbohydrates are absorbed into the bloodstream, the blood sugar level rises. The pancreas responds to an increase in glucose by secreting more insulin. Insulin is the hormone that is primarily responsible for lowering the blood sugar level by allowing glucose to cross the cell membrane. Insulin increases glucose oxidation by the tissues, stimulates glucose conversion to glycogen by the liver, decreases glucose production from amino acids and promotes glucose conversion into fat for storage.

In diabetes, there is insufficient insulin for these metabolic functions. Glucose cannot be properly used for energy. Fats and proteins are incompletely broken down. This leads to ketosis, an accumulation of ketone bodies in the forms of acetone and diacetic acid. This can lead to a decrease in blood pH *(acidosis)*. The excess glucose is eliminated along with water and salts through the kidneys, causing both dehydration and electrolyte imbalance. The characteristic symptoms of excessive thirst, hunger, and urination are directly related to the loss of fluids and electrolytes.

Type I (juvenile onset) or I.D.D.M. (insulin-dependent diabetes mellitus) first appears in youth and in those under forty years of age. The disease tends to be severe and unpredictable, and it usually requires insulin. Typical signs and symptoms are *polyuria* (excess urine output), *polydipsia* (excess thirst), *polyphagia* (excess hunger), and glycosuria.

Non-Insulin-Dependent Diabetes Mellitus

Type II non-insulin-dependent diabetes, also known as ketosis-resistant diabetes, usually begins in later years. It is more difficult to diagnose because classic signs and symptoms are not generally present. Common signs and symptoms are shown in figure 23-2. Often only one or two symptoms are apparent in the elderly person. The person may complain of constant fatigue or have a skin lesion that takes an unusually long time to heal. Vision changes, attributed to general aging, may be far advanced before their relationship to a diabetic condition is recognized.

Complications

Retinopathy (small blood vessel pathology of the eyes) is common in longstanding diabetes. Frequent eye examinations are necessary as are

---

- Easy fatigue
- Skin infections
- Slow healing
- Itching
- Pruritus vulvae (itching of the vulva)
- Burning on urination
- Pain in fingers and toes
- Vision changes

Figure 23-2 Common signs and symptoms of non-insulin-dependent diabetes

precautions for diminished vision. Little can be done to halt blindness once its progression is under way.

Nephropathy, another type of small blood-vessel damage, occurs in the kidneys and leads to renal failure. Both of these problems can be made worse by large blood-vessel changes, atherosclerosis, and arteriosclerosis. Because the large blood-vessel changes can cause hypertension, increased blood pressure will also affect delicate blood vessels in the kidneys and eyes. The primary cause of death in diabetics is a myocardial infarction.

Neuropathy, or changes in the sensory nerves, usually involve the legs and feet. Diabetics may experience numbness, burning, and tingling that seems to be worse at night. Diminished sensation in diabetics requires vigilance by geriatric health care providers to prevent accidents and to treat injuries promptly to prevent infection. Neuropathies can also affect many other body systems with various results. These may include changes in taste, slower stomach emptying after eating that causes a feeling of bloating, diarrhea, problems urinating, and changes in sexual sensations leading to impotence in men.

Poor circulation and high glucose levels favor the growth of bacteria. Infections are frequent and difficult to treat because the wounds heal slowly and poorly. Bladder and foot infections occur frequently. Remember that infection can precipitate coma. Therefore, observation and exacting attention must be given to the principles of safety, as well as to skin and foot care. A small blister or cut on the foot that becomes gangrenous and is then followed by amputation is a common ordeal for the elderly diabetic, figure 23-3.

Amputations

Single-toe, foot, or leg amputations, the result of diabetes and vascular problems, are not uncommon. Routine care of the stump, with careful checking for hemorrhage, infection, and blood glucose levels, is indicated in the early phases. Preventing flexion contractures by

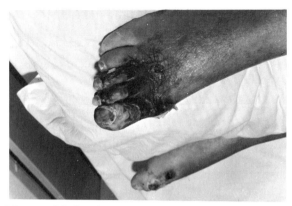

Figure 23-3 Gangrene of the toes and foot often means eventual amputation.

hyperextending the stump and having the patient lie in a prone position several times daily is vitally important. The prosthesis, if one is used, is fitted by the physician and limb fitter. Shrinking of the stump necessitates adjustments, sometimes for as long as ten years. The patient is encouraged to start wearing the prosthesis at once, and careful explanations of its care should be given. Follow-up care at home is planned by the public health nurse.

Rehabilitation

Successful rehabilitation of an amputee depends in large part on emotional adjustment. The importance of a good patient-staff relationship should not be underestimated as a motivating factor. The patient's general condition and overall prognosis combine with this traumatic experience to create feelings of anger, grief, and frustration. The nursing staff needs patience and understanding in helping the patient develop the shoulder and arm muscles necessary to achieve crutch-walking. A supportive approach does much to help the patient through a difficult period of adjustment.

Diabetic Coma

Ketosis-resistant diabetes is three times more common in people over sixty than in the forty-to-sixty age group. The incidence of the disease increases with advancing years. The disease in the elderly is much more stable than it is in the young, however. There are fewer incidents of diabetic ketoacidosis *(D.K.A.)*. However, the elderly are at risk for hyperglyccmic, hyperosmolar, nonketotic coma *(H.H.N.C.)*. This occurs when blood glucose levels are very high and there are no ketones in the blood. It may occur with illness and is often seen in debilitated elders who are mentally and physically impaired. Adequate fluid intake is essential to prevent dehydration, circulatory collapse, and death. Insulin is not always necessary for this type of coma. It is essential for D.K.A., however. Review the characteristics of D.K.A. and H.H.N.C., figure 23-4. Geriatric health care providers will see H.H.N.C. more often than DK.A. Nevertheless, the consequences of insulin shock or diabetic coma to the elderly person can be severe, resulting in heart attacks and strokes. Because this form of diabetes is more predictable, less than half the patients require insulin. The majority are treated successfully with diet and hypoglycemic agents. If the elder is obese, weight reduction alone may be sufficient to bring the condition under control.

Care of the diabetic is largely directed toward managing the long-term problems related to diabetes. Three areas of the diabetic's life need to be balanced. They are diet, exercise, and use of oral antidiabetic agents, and sometimes, insulin. Review the nursing diagnostic categories related to diabetes mellitus in table 23-1.

- Alterations in bowel elimination: Constipation or diarrhea
- Alterations in nutrition: More than or less than
- Altered physical mobility
- Altered sensory/perception
- Altered sexual function
- Altered thought processes
- Anxiety
- Coping deficit
- Disturbance in self-concept
- Impaired tissue perfusion
- Knowledge deficit
- Noncompliance

Table 23-1   Nursing Diagnostic Categories Related to Diabetes Mellitus

Treatment of Diabetes Mellitus

Diet

Diet is an important part of diabetic treatment. Physicians are not in full agreement about how rigidly the elderly most follow a diet. For the obese, weight reduction is necessary. The goal is to maintain ideal body weight (I.B.W.). Occasionally diabetics are underweight, and then the goal is to reach close to optimal body weight. Any diet should include basic nutritional elements. Carbohydrates are about 55 to 60 percent of calorie intake and are individualized to the elder's blood glucose and lipid levels. Refined sugars should be decreased and unrefined carbohydrates increased. Proteins comprise approximately 20 percent and fats less than 30 percent of the diet. Less than 10 percent of fats should be saturated because of the problem of large blood-vessel disease. The most important goal for residents with N.I.D.D.M. is control of weight with balanced, regularly scheduled meals.

The use of lists based on the exchange system has simplified the task of measuring food by weight. Measurements can now be made using a standard 8-ounce measuring cup, teaspoon, and tablespoon. The exchange system was formu-

H.H.N.C.	D.K.A.
• Coma	• Coma
• Decreased urination	• Dehydration
• Dehydration	• Flushed face
• Elevated temperature	• Fruity breath odor
• Low blood pressure	• Kussmaul breathing
• Mobility changes	• Lethargy
• Possible seizures	• Nausea and vomiting
• Sensory changes	
• Weak pulse	

Figure 23-4   Characteristics of H.H.N.C. and D.K.A.

lated by a committee with representatives from the American Diabetic Association and the diabetic branch of the U.S. Public Health Service.

The nurse must be sure that the elder and those preparing the meals understand how the exchange lists are used. An older person may be bewildered by such a list but reluctant to admit it. An opportunity to discuss the exchange list and plan a day's menu around the elder's usual dietary habits is helpful.

Appetite diminishes with age, and making food attractive is important. Foods should be selected from usual family menus rather than prepared separately. Diebetic foods are available, but most elderly people do not want them. Elders need to have the diet slowly and thoroughly explained and have an opportunity to ask questions. A list of instructions should be given to be taken home and some provision made for a follow-up visit. Many times questions and problems do not come up until the patient is at home.

Changing eating habits is difficult for young and old alike. Geriatric health care providers need to consider a person's food preferences, activity levels, medications, and life-style when planning meals. Residents will need encouragement to eat according to the plan and to exercise to maintain or improve their health.

Exercise

Exercise is extremely important for maintaining ideal body weight (I.B.W.) and for treating hyperglycemia. Exercise helps glucose cross into muscle cells. It also helps increase the number of sites that insulin can attach itself on the cells to metabolize the glucose. Therefore, exercise seems to help decrease the insulin resistance that so many elders have. Before any exercise plan is developed, the physician, nurse practitioner, or physician's assistant must complete a cardiovascular assessment. Exercise physiologists or physical therapists can help plan an exercise program based on the physical condition and preferences of the elder. Even those who are on bedrest can exercise in bed. By letting elders know that their own insulin can work better in their bodies if they exercise, motivation is often increased.

Antidiabetic Drugs

Diabetes is treated with one of two main drug groups. One is administered subcutaneously, whereas the other is given orally. N.I.D.D.M. is treated with oral hypoglycemics when diet and exercise are not successful in controlling diabetes. Rarely is insulin used with elders who have N.I.D.D.M. When it must be used, it is to relieve symptoms such as fatigue, depression, blurred vision, and dizziness caused by failing beta cells (insulin-producing cells in the pancreas).

Insulin Insulin is essential for people with I.D.D.M., because they cannot produce their own insulin, and for the very few with N.I.D.D.M. whose symptoms cannot be relieved. Most manufactured insulin is prepared from pork or beef pancreas. Pork more closely resembles human insulin. Because it is still a foreign substance introduced into the human body, antibodies can be formed. This makes the use of insulin by the body less effective. A newer insulin, humulin and some other brand names, more closely resembles human insulin and is often prescribed to reduce insulin resistance. These insulins have slightly different effects in the individual. Therefore, they should not be interchanged without a physician's order.

Currently, there are seven types of insulin, which vary in their speed of action, duration, and potency. The different types of insulin are injected subcutaneously and measured in units, figure 23-5.

The chances for error in administering insulin are high for the elderly person. Poor eyesight, trembling hands, and forgetfulness may make measurements inaccurate, sterilization faulty, and handling of the equipment difficult, figure 23-6. The elderly person may break syringes and expel insulin prematurely from the syringe because of poor coordination.

Although insulins vary in concentration

Type	Onset	Peak	Duration
Rapid Acting			
Regular	< 1 HR	2-4	4-6
Crystalline	< 1 HR	2-4	5-8
Semilente	< 1 HR	4-7	12-16
Intermediate			
NPH	1-2	8-12	18-24
Globin Zinc	2-4	6-10	12-18
Lente	1-4	8-12	18-24
Slow Acting			
Protamine Zinc	4-8	16-18	36+
Ultralente	4-8	16-18	36+

Glyburide (Micronase)	1.5-20 mg
Glipizide (Glucotrol)	2.5-40 mg

Figure 23-5   Commercially available insulins

(strength), the strength most often used is U-100, or 100 units per milliliter. For the few people requiring very small doses of insulin, U-40 may be ordered. The shift toward using U-100 insulin has helped reduce medication errors such as incorrect concentrations (U-40, U-80, U-100) being drawn up in the wrong syringe. Some elders, however, may still be using glass syringes or different unit syringes, and error is still possible. As a safety precaution, the patient should take the older syringe to the store so that a direct comparison of old and new can be made. The same precaution should be taken when purchasing new insulin. The old bottle should be taken along when a new bottle is purchased.

A Cornwall syringe, with a plunger that can be locked at a prescribed level, can be helpful when hands are unsteady. But its cost may be

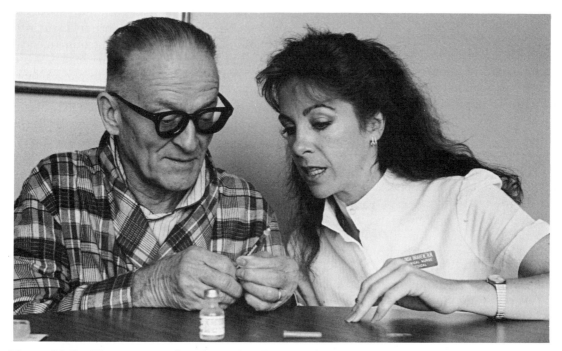

Figure 23-6   The nurse teaches the patient how to measure insulin accurately. (Courtesy Long Beach Memorial Medical Center)

prohibitive. The Tru-set syringe has a metal marker that can be set at a desired level, thereby preventing an overdose. Its barrel is larger than the regular insulin syringe and so is easily handled. A small magnifying glass helps those with poor vision. One (the C-Better Magnifier) is available that can be attached to the syringe. Disposable syringes are safe and convenient. Again, however, they may prove too great an expense for an elderly person who must take insulin regularly.

There is additional danger when two types of insulin are required. To equalize the pressure in the vials of insulin, the sterile needles must first be placed in the top of each bottle. The syringe is then attached to each needle in turn without injecting air. The exact amount of insulin is then withdrawn from each bottle. Trembling hands and poor vision makes this a difficult and complicated procedure. Some elders with poor eyesight or coordination purchase several syringes and have a family member, neighbor, or community health nurse prefill their syringes to avoid mistakes. These, unlike bottles of insulin, need to be refrigerated to decrease possible bacterial growth.

Repeated injections of insulin can cause changes in the subcutaneous tissue of some patients. These changes are referred to as *lipodystrophy* and *hypertrophy*. Lipodystrophy, loss of subcutaneous fat in injection sites, is thought to be caused by giving injections in the same site repeatedly, impure insulin, and faulty injection technique. Hypertrophy is scar tissue formation in the injection site. These sites tend to be used more often because nerve endings are sparse or nonexistent, and the injection is painless. Absorption of insulin from hypertrophied sites can be slow and irregular. Both can be avoided by rotation of injections using multiple sites on the arms, legs, buttocks, and abdomen. The nurse must carefully rotate the injection site, figure 23-7, when giving insulin and must urge the patient to do so also. The older patient is apt to forget the site of the last injection and needs help

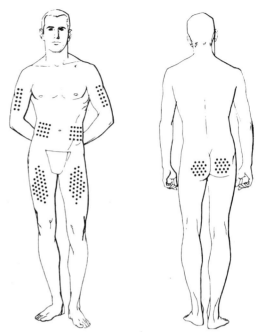

Figure 23-7 Sites of insulin injection must be changed daily.

in following a routine of site rotations, figure 23-8

Insulin pumps are battery-operated, portable machines that deliver insulin through tubing and a needle in subcutaneous tissue. They are used primarily with people who have I.D.D.M. and need very close control of their blood glucose. The pumps are very expensive, and not all insurance companies reimburse for their cost. Their use also requires that the diabetic be well educated for safe and effective use and for avoiding complications.

Oral Antidiabetic Agents Oral hypoglycemics are drugs that, when taken into the body by mouth, lower the blood glucose level. They are particularly useful in treating non-insulin-dependent diabetes. They are not substitutes for insulin.

One drug group, the sulfonylureas, figure 23-9, is remotely related to the sulfa drugs but is not a true sulfa. It will not produce sulfa reac-

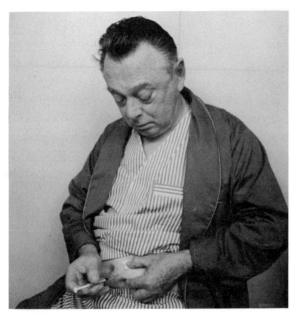

Figure 23-8 When patients take their own insulin, you must check the administration site carefully. (From Caldwell & Hegner, *Nursing Assistant, A Nursing Process Approach*, copyright 1989 by Delmar Publishers Inc.)

tions. Tolbutamide (Orinase) was the first of the sulfonylureas. Since then, others that differ in potency and duration have been developed. Newer oral hypoglycemics are more powerful and require smaller doses. Review the drugs in figure 23-9 and compare dosages among them.

This group of drugs stimulates the pancreas to increase its own insulin production. In some way, it also influences the release of glucose from the liver. There must be functional beta cells (those producing insulin) in the pancreas for the sulfonylureas to be effective. Of the patients, most of them elderly, who do have some functional tissue, 80 percent are helped by these drugs.

Less than 5 percent of those taking these agents have adverse effects, but some do occur. Adverse reactions to the sulfonylureas include papular or maculopapular skin eruptions, visual disturbances, gastrointestinal complaints, and depression of thyroid and liver functions. These drugs are normally excreted by the kidneys. Therefore, when kidney function is limited, hypoglycemia may occur. When alcohol is consumed, there may be flushing and headache. Patients are usually advised to limit intake of alcoholic beverages. Interactions with other drugs being taken may increase or decrease the hypoglycemic effect.

The same guidelines for controlling diabetes must be followed when taking oral hypoglycemics. Elders need to follow their diet plans, exercise, maintain meticulous skin care, and monitor their glucose levels.

Hypoglycemia

Hypoglycemia occurs when the blood glucose level is 60 mg or less per decaliter (10 liters) of blood. It occurs far less commonly when oral antidiabetic agents are given. When hypoglycemia results from an overdose of insulin, it is referred to as insulin reaction or insulin shock. Hypoglycemia also occurs when there is more insulin in the body than there is food intake or

SULFONYLUREAS

Drug Name	Usual Daily Dose	Duration (Hours)
Tolbutamide (Orinase)	0.25-3 gm (divided doses)	6-12
Acetohexamide (Dymelor)	0.25-1.5 gm (divided doses)	12-24
Tolazamide (Tolinase)	0.1-0.5 gm (single dose or divided doses)	12-24
Chlorpropamide (Diabinese)	0.1-0.5 gm (single dose)	Up to 60

Figure 23-9   Some oral hyopglycemic agents

exercise. This may occur with elders who do not follow their meal plans or eat their snacks because of a diminished appetite. Unusual activity, stress, vomiting, diarrhea, or the interaction of an oral agent with an antibacterial sulfonamide can also create a hypoglycemic state.

In contrast to ketosis, which develops slowly, hypoglycemic reactions are apt to occur rapidly. Signs and symptoms of hypoglycemia (insulin shock) include hunger, sweating, dizziness, drowsiness, blurred vision, and erratic behavior. Staggering, mental confusion, and disorientation are commonly observed, as well as pale, moist skin.

The signs and symptoms of hypoglycemia and ketosis are similar in their early stages. Because the patient will progress more rapidly into insulin shock, the patient should be treated for hypoglycemia if there is doubt about which reaction is taking place. Although hypoglycemic reactions are unusual in patients with N.I.D.D.M., consequences can be severe. Cerebrovascular accidents, increased anginal symptoms, and myocardial infarctions have resulted.

Familiarize yourself with the signs of hypoglycemia, figure 23-10, and report immediately to the nurse if patients show evidence of them. Blood glucose level should be determined immediately. The elder or any geriatric health care provider should obtain a blood glucose reading with a glucose monitoring device, not a urine glucose level because it is not as accurate. Orange juice or other easily assimilated sources of carbohydrates are usually kept easily accessible for emergency use. Every staff member should be aware of their storage location.

The hypoglycemic patient is treated with sugar in some form. A food containing sugar is given orally if the patient is conscious. Many patients carry with them at all times some easily assimilated form of carbohydrates such as hard candy or crackers. Glucagon, a crystalline polypeptide extracted from the pancreas, was developed in 1960 and is now commonly used for the treatment of hypoglycemia. It may be stored at home and injected either intramuscu-

Hypoglycemia (Insulin Shock)	
History	Excessive insulin; unusual exercise; too little food
Onset	Sudden; minutes
Skin	Pale, moist, cool, sweating, tingling sensation; numb lips and tongue
Behavior	Excited, irritable, confused, nervous, dizzy, weak, tremor, may act intoxicated, convulse, coma
Respiration	Normal to rapid; shallow
Pulse	Rapid; full bounding
Blood Pressure	Normal
Nausea/Vomiting	Absent
Hunger	Present
Thirst	Absent
Urinary Acetone	Absent
Treatment	Give sugar, orange juice, candy, cola immediately if patient conscious; call doctor or emergency hospital
Response to Treatment	Rapid

Figure 23-10   Signs and symptoms of hypoglycemia

larly or subcutaneously. Someone in the family should be taught to dissolve glucagon in the fluid that is supplied with it, and to inject it. The dosage (0.5 mg to 1.0 mg) can be repeated in 15 minutes, and there are no harmful side effects.

Glucose Monitoring

Monitoring glucose levels in the body is essential for good control of diabetes. Most people are capable of monitoring their own glucose levels using blood glucose monitoring devices, figure 23-11, or testing their urine for sugar and acetone. Blood glucose monitoring devices may not be accepted by or be suitable for some diabetics because of their expense, good vision needed

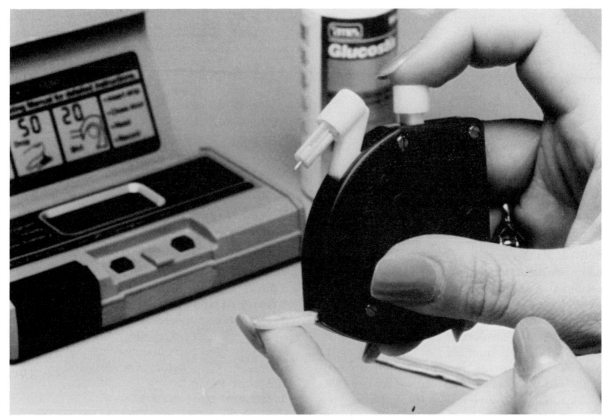

Figure 23-11   Self-monitoring kit for blood glucose levels (Courtesy Miles Inc., Diagnostics Division)

to read scales, neuropathies, and discomfort from pricking. Some believe that there is no reason to change methods, because they have successfully managed their diabetes without blood glucose monitoring.

Many more people are now monitoring their glucose levels in blood rather than urine. Urine testing is not very accurate. The renal threshold for "spilling" sugar may be quite high, so that a urine test might be negative, while glucose in the bloodstream may indicate hyperglycemia. Decisions for monitoring insulin injections are more safely made with blood glucose monitoring. Urine testing for glucose is still done but, more important, urine testing for ketones should be done. All I.D.D.M. and ill diabetics should have their urine tested for ketones daily.

PROCEDURE 13

Blood Glucose Monitoring

1. Wash hands and assemble the following equipment:

   blood glucose monitoring device
   alcohol wipes
   glucose oxidase strips

2. Prick the side of the distal part of the finger.
3. Obtain a drop of blood.
4. Prepare the specimen of blood according to the manufacturer's directions.
5. Carefully time and read the scale.
6. Report and record results.

Testing procedures for blood glucose, and urine for sugar and acetone, vary according to the equipment used. It is very important to follow the instructions very carefully to avoid an incorrect reading. Also, sugar in the urine should be reported in percentages, not plus (+) signs. Different testing products plus marks (+) do not correspond with percentages. Percentages are the most accurate way to report glycosuria. Most urine testing for sugar is done as a five-drop procedure, although on occasion a two-drop method may be used.

PROCEDURE 14

Testing Urine for Sugar with Reagent Tablets

1. Wash hands and assemble the following equipment on a tray:

   freshly voided urine in specimen container
   test tube
   medicine dropper
   Clinitest tablet
   Clinitest color chart
   water
   Acetest tablet or powder or Ketostix strips
   plain white paper
2. Read manufacturer's directions carefully.
3. Place five drops of urine in a clean, dry test tube with medicine dropper. Hold medicine dropper upright so that urine does not touch the sides of the test tube. Rinse medicine dropper in cold water.
4. Add ten drops of fresh water to test tube with dropper. If you miscount drops, empty tube and begin test again.
5. Remove fresh Clinitest tablet from wrapper. Do not touch it with the fingers. Drop it into test tube. If bottle of tablets is used, drop tablet into test tube from cover of bottle. Cover bottle immediately.
6. Watch reaction carefully. After the reaction has stopped, wait fifteen seconds and

shake the test tube gently. Compare resulting color with Clinitest color chart. Do not handle tube during reaction. Time the waiting period with second hand of watch.
7. Clean and replace equipment according to hospital policy. Drain test tube in test tube rack.
8. Report and record results.

PROCEDURE 15

Testing Urine for Acetone with Acetest

1. Place one acetone tablet on white paper. Do not touch tablet with fingers.
2. Place one drop of urine on acetone tablet with medicine dropper. Use only enough urine to moisten tablet.
3. Wait thirty seconds. Compare resulting color with color chart.
4. Discard tablet, paper, and urine.
5. Clean and replace equipment according to hospital policy.
6. Report and record results.

PROCEDURE 16

Testing Urine with Ketodiastix Strip Test

1. Wash your hands.
2. Assemble the equipment you will need:

   Ketodiastix reagent strips
   sample of freshly voided urine
3. Identify the resident and ensure that the sample is from that resident.
4. Dip one end of the Ketostix strip into the urine.
5. Remove strip and hold horizontally. Note the exact time.
6. After fifteen seconds, compare the strip with the color chart on bottle label for ketone.

7. Continue to thirty seconds and read the chart for glucose.
8. Dispose of urine specimen if it is not to be saved.
9. Clean and store equipment according to facility policy.
10. Report completion of test. Record results according to facility policy.

Summary

- There are two forms of diabetes mellitus: non-insulin-dependent diabetes and insulin-dependent diabetes.
- Non-insulin dependent diabetes (N.I.D.-D.M.) is a more stable form of the disease.
- N.I.D.D.M. is fairly common in people over forty years of age and becomes more frequent with advancing age.

- Obesity, heredity, and sex are factors in the development of N.I.D.D.M.
- Frequent complications include retinopathy, arteriosclerosis, neuritis, and gangrene.
- Amputations are common in N.I.D.D.M., because minor injuries heal poorly and gangrene is apt to develop, especially in the feet.
- N.I.D.D.M. is controlled primarily through a well-planned diet and exercise.
- Oral hypoglycemic agents are used when control of N.I.D.D.M. has not been achieved. Insulin is used very rarely, but primarily for relieving symptoms.
- The focus of nursing care is on supervision and administration of diet and medication, with special attention to skin and foot care.
- Blood and urine testing gives information about the level of sugar balance being achieved.

Review Outline

   I. Behavioral Objectives

  II. Vocabulary

 III. Endocrine System

     A. Formed of glands
       1. Scattered throughout body
       2. Produces secretions (hormones)
       3. Secretions go directly into bloodstream
     B. Individual Glands
       1. Pituitary
       2. Pineal
       3. Adrenal
       4. Gonads
         a. Ovaries
         b. Testes
       5. Thyroid
       6. Pancreas

 IV. Diabetes Mellitus

     A. Incidence
     B. Types
       1. I.D.D.M.
       2. N.I.D.D.M.

C.   Signs and symptoms
   1.   Classical
   2.   Nonclassical
D.   Complications
   1.   Retinopathy
   2.   Nephropathy
   3.   Neuropathy
   4.   Amputations
   5.   Hyperglycemic reactions
   6.   Hypoglycemic reactions
E.   Diet
F.   Exercise

V. Antidiabetic Drugs

A.   Insulin
B.   Hypoglycemics

VI. Glucose Monitoring

Review

I. Vocabulary

Fill in the proper terms to match the definitions given.

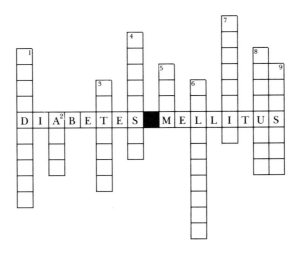

1.   Excessive thirst
2.   Letters used to identify the hormone that controls the adrenal cortex
3.   States of excess ketones in the blood
4.   A decrease in blood pH
5.   Letters used to describe the diabetic condition requiring insulin
6.   Excessive hunger
7.   Glucose in blood
8.   Excessive urination
9.   Condition of being overweight

II. Short Answers

1. What four major factors influence the incidence of diabetes?
2. How does I.D.D.M. compare with N.I.D.D.M.?
3. What is another name for old-age diabetes?
4. How do oral antidiabetic agents affect the blood sugar level?
5. What four precautions should be taken when administering insulin?
6. List two different problems that can occur when the patient suffers from N.I.D.D.M. Describe their causes, signs and symptoms, treatment, and the speed with which they develop.
7. Why does the elderly diabetic who is receiving A.C.T.H. or cortisone require special attention?
8. Why does nursing care of the elderly diabetic patient stress foot and skin hygiene?

III. Clinical Situations

1. You notice that one of the residents who is a diabetic seems confused and disoriented. What do you do?
2. You pick up trays after dinner and note that one of the diabetic residents has not eaten half of the meal. What do you do?
3. Mrs. Chavez has returned from an outing with the recreational therapist, and you notice that she is limping. She tells you that the little sore on her foot is nothing. She is a well-controlled diabetic. What do you do?

CASE STUDY

John Martinez, age seventy-eight, is a somewhat obese, gray-haired man. He was a resident in a boarding house where older people each maintained their own living space. Each unit had a small sink, stove, and combination living room-bedroom. A bathroom at the end of the hall was shared by four people. Mr. Martinez had always been active. He often bowled several times a week after operating a jackhammer all day in his younger years.

Lately, he had been feeling tired and had lost a little weight, even though he was no longer working. He spent most of his time sitting and talking to friends, drinking coffee and eating doughnuts at the neighborhood senior center. A bruise on his left little toe was slow to heal, so he cut the leather of his old worn shoe to relieve the pressure.

As part of the senior services, a podiatrist occasionally visited the center. Although not too concerned, Mr. Martinez thought he might have the podiatrist take a look at his foot.

The podiatrist treated the injured area. He asked Mr. Martinez if he was drinking more water than usual or voiding more often. When Mr. Martinez admitted to both of these facts, the podiatrist suggested that Mr. Martinez talk with the nurse at the center, since he suspected that Mr. Martinez might be a diabetic.

During the nursing conference, Mr. Martinez had his urine tested for sugar and acetone and his blood glucose level tested. Both tests were positive. The nurse suggested that he see his physician. His physician ordered a fasting blood sugar test and a glucose tolerance test. These tests were to determine the current level of blood sugar and how well insulin production would respond in its management. Both tests were positive for diabetes mellitus. The physician diagnosed Mr. Martinez's condition as non-insulin-dependent diabetes, which meant that the condition could probably be controlled by diet and exercise.

Mr. Martinez was greatly relieved to learn that he probably would not need insulin injections. The therapeutic regime prescribed included a diet balanced in fats, proteins, and carbohydrates, and moderate exercise.

He was taught the importance of proper foot care and how to test his own urine for sugar and acetone. The signs of diabetic coma were carefully outlined, and he was cautioned to report any indication he noticed and to seek treatment for infections. Learning to manage his food intake was troublesome. A visiting nurse made visits to his home until he felt secure.

Despite treatment, the discoloration of his little toe continued and eventually amputa-tion was necessary. He was prescribed an oral hypoglycemic. A new pair of well-fitting shoes offered protection to his vulnerable feet. He was cautioned to report any signs of irritation promptly. Mr. Martinez still spends most of his time visiting with friends. But he has stopped eating doughnuts and uses an artificial sweetener in his coffee.

1. What three early indications of diabetes mellitus did Mr. Martinez ignore?
2. Why did the podiatrist suspect diabetes mellitus?
3. What two urine tests were done in the senior center that helped establish the diagnosis of diabetes mellitus?
4. What therapy in addition to diet was prescribed for Mr. Martinez?
5. What probably made it necessary for him to take an oral hypoglycemic?

Unit 24
Cardiovascular System Alterations

Objectives

After studying this unit, you should be able to:

- Locate and describe the function of the organs of the circulatory system.
- Describe how normal aging affects the cardiovascular system.
- List the signs and symptoms of peripheral vascular disease.
- Name ways to safely stimulate circulation to the extremities.
- List the life-style adjustments a person with cardiac disorders must make.
- Describe the difference between left-sided and right-sided heart failure.

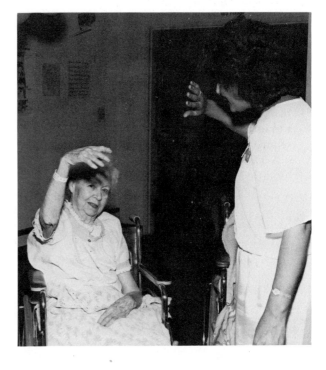

Vocabulary

Learn the meaning and spelling of the following words or phrases.

anemia
arteriosclerosis
arteries
ascites
atherosclerosis
atrium
blood pressure
capillaries
cardiac cycle
central venous pressure
   (C.V.P.)
claudication
cyanosis
decompensation
diastolic

edema
erythrocytes
hemoptysis
hyperkalemia
hypokalemia
hyponatremia
ischemia
leukocytes
lumen
Mockberg's
   degeneration

orthopnea
peripheral vascular disease (P.V.D.)
phlebotomy
plasma
pulmonary arterial wedge pressure
   (P.A.W.P.)
septum
systolic
thrombocytes
veins
ventricle

The circulatory system may be thought of as a transportation system. It takes nourishment and oxygen to the cells and carries away waste products. Without this process, the tissues become less functional and then die. The system is kept in motion by the force of the heartbeat.

Structure and Function

The circulatory system is made up of the heart (central pumping station), blood vessels, lymphatic vessels, lymph nodes, spleen, and the blood itself. It is a continuous network.

The Heart

The heart is a muscular organ. It is hollow inside and divided into four chambers (cavities): the right *atrium*, the left atrium, the right *ventricle*, and the left ventricle. It is separated into right and left sides by a wall *(septum)*. One-way valves separate the chambers and guard the exit point of the pulmonary artery and aorta. The pulmonary artery carries blood high in carbon dioxide to the lungs for oxygenation, figure 24-1. The aorta carries freshly oxygenated blood away from the heart and through its many branches to

the cells. Nerve impulses make the heart contract regularly according to body needs.

The Cardiac Cycle

The heart pumps blood through the body by a series of movements known as the *cardiac cycle*. The upper chambers of the heart (atria) relax and fill with blood as the lower chambers (ventricles) contract. This forces blood out of the heart through the aorta and pulmonary arteries. The lower chambers then relax, allowing blood to flow into them from the upper chambers. Then the cycle is repeated. The blood, pushed by the heart contractions, causes pressure in the vessels called *blood pressure*. Two different amounts of pressure are measured. The *systolic* blood pressure reading indicates the period when the pressure within the heart is the greatest, during con-

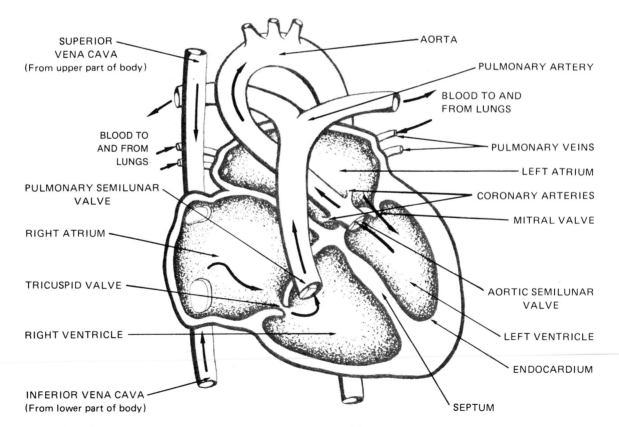

Figure 24-1 The arrows indicate the circulation of blood through the heart.

tractions. The *diastolic* reading indicates the lowest point of pressure, between contractions. The coronary arteries, branches of the aorta, carry nourishment and oxygen to the heart muscle itself.

Major Vessels

Many large *arteries* and *veins* take their names from the bones they are near. Others are named for the part of the body that they serve.

For example, the femoral artery and vein run close to the femur (thigh bone), figure 24-2. The cerebral arteries go to the brain. The coronary arteries go to the heart.

Arteries have muscular, elastic walls. Their linings are normally smooth. They branch, first to form smaller vessels (arterioles) whose walls are not as thick. Then they form *capillaries*, whose walls are only one cell thick. Fluid (serum) carrying nutrients and oxygen bathes the cells. Waste

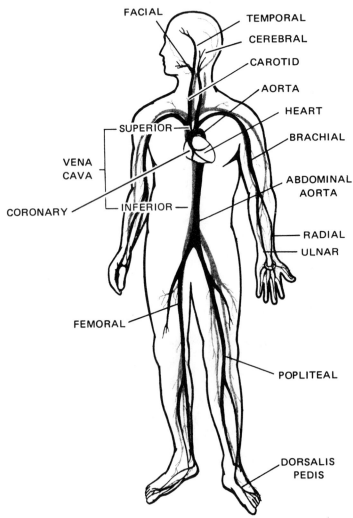

Figure 24-2   General plan of circulation (arteries are black, veins are gray).

materials and products of cellular activity pass from the cells into this "tissue fluid" and then back into the bloodstream.

The capillaries merge to form tiny veins (venules). Much of the tissue fluid flows directly back into the general circulation. Some tissue fluid is drained off into open-ended tubes (lymphatic vessels). These tubes carry it to the lymph nodes and larger lymphatic vessels before it is carried through the general circulation. There are two reasons for this bypass. First, some of the strain is removed from the veins, which are not nearly as muscular as the arteries. Second, impurities may be removed as the lymph passes through the lymph nodes. Sometimes this fluid carries abnormal (cancer) cells into the lymph nodes and throughout the body, where they reproduce. Serum, tissue fluid, and lymph are similar. They are all derived from blood and ultimately return to the general circulation.

Veins, which carry the blood to the heart, are formed from the venules. Small cuplike valves within the veins help to keep the blood moving forward. They sometimes become weakened and distended, resulting in varicose veins.

The Spleen

The spleen is a small organ in the upper left quadrant of the abdomen. It produces some of the white blood cells and destroys worn-out red blood cells. The spleen always has large quantities of blood passing through it. Therefore, it acts as a blood bank.

The Blood

If the blood vessels are the highways carrying nutrients and wastes, the blood may be thought of as the trucks and cars traveling along the highways. A person has 4 to 6 liters (quarts) of blood, depending on size, sex, age, and general health. Both the quality and quantity of blood are indicative of the status of a person's health.

Blood consists of a liquid portion and cells. The liquid portion is called *plasma*. Plasma is the carrier of water, nutrients, and waste products. It carries fibrinogen, which helps the blood to clot. It also carries gamma globulin, which helps protect against certain infections, and albumin, a protein. Serum is plasma from which the fibrinogen, gamma globulin, albumin, and other materials have been removed.

There are three kinds of blood cells, figure 24-3. They are:

- Red blood cells *(erythrocytes)*, which are produced in bone and carry oxygen to the cells and carbon dioxide away from them.
- White blood cells *(leukocytes)*, some of which are produced in the bone and some in the lymph nodes and spleen. These cells protect the body by surrounding and destroying germs and other foreign materials.
- Platelets *(thrombocytes)*, which are produced in the bone and are important in blood clotting.

Senescent Changes

Changes taking place in the cardiovascular system include changes in the size and walls of the blood vessels. With a resultant decrease in blood flow to vital organs, the heart muscle is less effective in pumping the blood. The changes in the vascular beds increase the blood pressure. Refer to figure 24-4.

Anemia   *Anemia* is the result of a decrease in the quantity or quality of red blood cells. It has several causes, such as poor diet, low production of new red blood cells, and blood loss as in hemorrhage. The anemic person has little energy and is usually pale. Dizziness, digestive problems, and dyspnea may be present when anemia is severe. Treatment is aimed at improving the quantity and quality of the blood and eliminating the basic cause of the disease. Whole blood transfusions are sometimes necessary. Nursing care includes providing rest, adequate diet, and special mouth care. Vital signs are checked frequently. Any signs of bleeding should be reported promptly.

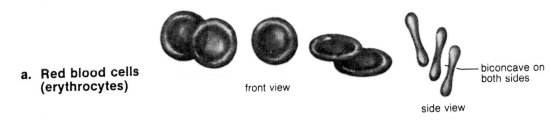

a. Red blood cells (erythrocytes)

front view

side view

biconcave on both sides

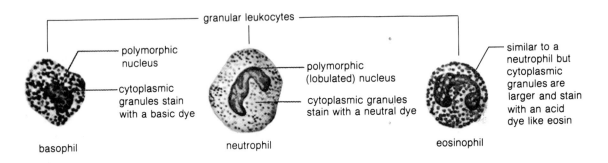

granular leukocytes

polymorphic nucleus

cytoplasmic granules stain with a basic dye

basophil

polymorphic (lobulated) nucleus

cytoplasmic granules stain with a neutral dye

neutrophil

similar to a neutrophil but cytoplasmic granules are larger and stain with an acid dye like eosin

eosinophil

b. White blood cells (leukocytes)

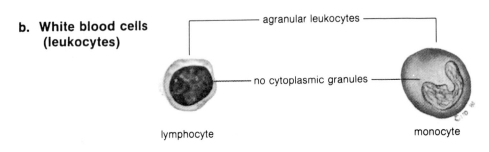

agranular leukocytes

no cytoplasmic granules

lymphocyte

monocyte

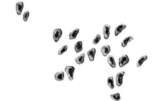

c. Platelets (non-cellular cytoplasmic fragments)

Figure 24-3   The blood cells (From Fong, Gerris, and Skelly, *Body Structures and Functions*, copyright 1989 by Delmar Publishers Inc.)

Heart Disease

Heart disease is the major health problem in our nation today. Every year, 900,000 lives are lost to this killer. In fact, there are three times as many deaths from heart disease as from cancer, and ten times as many as from accidents. In the last decade, the incidence of arteriosclerotic heart disease has risen to 20 percent. It is so common among the elderly that it is referred to

- Fibrotic changes in vascular walls
- Narrowing of vascular lumen
- Increase in blood pressure
- Atrophy and fibrotic changes in myocardium
- Cardiac output decreased
- Less efficient chemical conversions

Figure 24-4 Senescent changes in the cardiovascular system.

as senile heart disease. As many as 18 percent of those over sixty-five have some limitation due to heart disease.

Factors that contribute to heart disease can be divided into two categories: those that a person can change and those that cannot be changed. Those that can be changed involve diet, exercise, weight, smoking, stress, and alcohol intake. The major factor that cannot be changed is genetic, that is, a family history that makes a person susceptible to heart disease.

Disease affecting the blood vessels exerts a profound influence on the ability of the heart to perform. The heart can compensate for increased peripheral resistance, sometimes for years. Eventually, however, a state of decompensation or failure occurs. Cardiac stress also increases when there is pathology in other major systems such as the lungs, kidney, or liver.

Nursing diagnostic categories related to circulatory problems are listed in table 24-1.

Personal Adjustments

A person faced with a cardiac diagnosis must make a deep personal adjustment. Usual activities must be curtailed or at least adapted. Most patients fear permanent disability and are concerned about the future. This is particularly true for the elderly person who is already trying to cope with failing health and financial problems. Fears and anxiety are enhanced by enforced idleness. Patients often become ill-tempered as thoughts turn inward.

Family relationships undergo reevaluation. Family members' responses to such a major illness vary. They range from concern over ability

- Activity intolerance
- Alteration in cardiac output
- Alteration in comfort: Pain
- Alteration in health maintenance
- Alteration in tissue perfusion
- Alteration in sexual patterns
- Anxiety
- Disturbance in role performance
- Fear
- Fluid volume deficit
- Fluid volume excess
- Health maintenance deficit
- Ineffective breathing patterns
- Knowledge deficit
- Potential for injury
- Potential noncompliance

Table 24-1 Nursing Diagnostic Categories Related To Circulatory Problems

to provide adequate care to smothering overprotectiveness. Resentment of the additional burden may show up in signs of hostility. It may also be buried in a sense of guilt.

For the elderly person living alone, a cardiac diagnosis may mean the end of independent living. The current trend is to hospitalize the cardiac patient during phases of acute heart failure and to provide for routine convalescent care at home.

The patient and patient's family require the coordinated efforts of social services and both private and public nursing agencies. This will provide adequate care and suitable living accommodations.

Heart Attack

The term "heart attack" refers to a period in which the heart suddenly cannot function properly. There are different kinds of heart attacks. They differ in their severity and probable outcome (prognosis). Remember that the heart is muscle tissue and may become tired just as any muscle may tire. The cells of the heart require nourishment and oxygen just as all other cells do.

Heart Block

Heart block occurs when there is an interference with the electrical control of the heartbeat. Although this situation may develop from an unknown cause, a frequent cause is scarring from a previous heart attack (coronary occlusion).

To overcome this loss of control, an artificial electronic device called a pacemaker is implanted surgically. The site of implantation varies, but it is often under the chest muscle. Small wires reach from the device to the heart muscle. They send electrical impulses directly into the myocardium to control the heartbeat.

There are two kinds of pacemakers: the fixed rate and the demand. The fixed-rate pacemaker sends out impulses at set intervals. The demand pacemaker sends out impulses only when the heart contractions fall below a preestablished rate.

In caring for persons with a pacemaker, remember not to allow them within 10 feet of a microwave oven. This may disturb the pattern of electrical impulses. Heart rates should always be checked apically. Any change in heartbeat below the preset rate, pain or discoloration over the implant site, or hicupping may indicate problems. These signs should be reported immediately. Most people with pacemakers function well as long as the operation of the pacemaker is monitored.

Refer to figure 24-5. Refresh your memory of the beginning procedure actions and the procedure completion actions.

PROCEDURE 17

Measuring the Apical Pulse

1. Wash your hands.
2. Assemble the equipment you will need:
   stethoscope
   alcohol swabs
3. Identify resident.
4. Explain what you are going to do.
5. Use an alcohol swab to clean stethoscope earpieces.
6. Place earpieces in ears.
7. Place stethoscope diaphragm or bell over the apex of heart.
8. Listen carefully for the heartbeat.
9. Count the beats for one minute.
10. Check radial pulse for one minute. Another health care provider may take radial pulse at the same time that apical pulse is being checked.
11. Compare the results.
12. Chart apical pulse over the radial pulse.

    Example: $\dfrac{\text{A108}}{\text{R82}}$

    Be sure to indicate character as well as rate differential. Pulse deficit may also be charted in this way: 26 (108 − 82 = 26)
13. Clean earpieces as in step 5.
14. Return stethoscope to proper storage.
15. Wash your hands.
16. Report completion of procedure. Record apical/radial differential.

Myocardial Ischemia (M.I.)

The main cause of death among the elderly is disease of the blood vessels that nourish the heart. Myocardial *ischemia* (deficient blood supply to the heart) occurs when there is interference with the circulation to the heart muscle (myocardium). Arteriosclerotic or atherosclerotic changes in the coronary vessels account for 77 percent of the deaths caused by heart disease. These changes may occur slowly over a period of years. Slow development sometimes allows for a collateral circulation to develop. At some point, however, the lumens (channels) narrow to such an extent that insufficient blood reaches the heart. The heart muscle differs from ischemia. The myocardial ischemia may increase gradually as the vessel lumens close with atherosclerosis. It may also develop suddenly but temporarily, as in angina. It may be complete and more permanent as in coronary occlusion because of a clot. When there is generalized narrowing of the blood vessels and the heart has labored with a decreased blood supply for some time, almost continual vasodilation is necessary.

Angina Pectoris. The pain of angina occurs with exertion or stress, figure 24-6. It is dull with

Beginning Procedure Actions

- Wash your hands.
- Assemble all equipment needed.
- Knock on door and pause before entering resident's room.
- Politely ask visitors to leave. Tell them where they can wait.
- Identify the resident.
- Provide privacy by drawing curtains around bed and closing door.
- Explain what you will be doing, and answer questions.
- Raise bed to comfortable working height.

Procedure Completion Actions

- Position resident comfortably.
- Leave signal cord, telephone, and fresh water where resident can reach them.
- Return bed to lowest horizontal position.
- Raise side rails, if required.
- Perform general safety check of resident and environment.
- Clean used equipment and return to proper storage, according to facility policy.
- Open privacy curtains.
- Wash your hands.
- Tell visitors that they may reenter the room.
- Report completion of procedure.
- Document procedure following facility policy.

Figure 24-5   Beginning procedure actions and procedure completion actions.

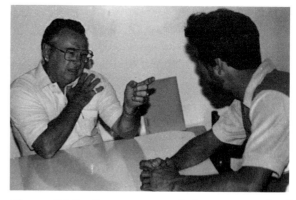

Figure 24-6   Stress can precipitate an attack of angina.

increasing intensity, located in the substernal area and radiating down the left arm and to the jaw. The individual may grow pale or flushed. Profuse perspiration is common. Symptoms vary from patient to patient. But they are always the same in the same patient. Older persons may experience weakness or fainting, especially in cold weather or when under stress. Diagnosis is based on the patient's history and an electrocardiogram, preferably performed during an attack. Stress causes an immediate need for increased coronary blood supply. The patient must be taught not to ignore this warning pain.

The intense pain that accompanies the insufficiency can be relieved with nitroglycerine tablets or Isordil. Most angina patients carry these tablets with them at all times. Nitroglycerine may also be administered in a lanolin-petrolatum base through the skin or in nitroglycerine "patches." This form of administration is becoming more and more common. Many older persons do not experience pain, but rather a feeling of discomfort that they are unable to describe. Some do not experience anything, yet they are undergoing ischemic changes. This is called "painless angina." Its consequences are just as serious. Sometimes the patient will take a nitroglycerin tablet prior to anticipated exertion. The effect lasts about one-half hour. The tablets are taken sublingually in 0.4-mg (1/150-gr) doses. They are not habit forming and can be used without diminishing effect. Relief is experienced within two to three minutes. There may be headache, but there are relatively few other side effects from this medication, and it is not expensive. The usual dosage of Isordil (isosorbide denetrate) is one or two 5-mg tablets every two to three hours. Common side effects include headache, transient dizziness, and weakness. Signs of cerebral ischemia associated with postural hypotension may also occur.

Three other drugs may be ordered if changes in life-style and nitroglycerin are not adequate. They are beta-adrenergic blockers such as propanolol hydrochloride (Inderal), calcium ion antagonists or calcium channel blockers, and angiotensin converting enzyme (A.C.E.) drugs. The beta-adrenergic blockers lower the heart's need for oxygen. They inhibit the heart's response to sympathetic nervous stimuli so the heart rate and blood pressure are also lowered.

The calcium ion antagonists (nifedipine and verapamil) dilate the coronary arteries and reduce the workload of the heart by reducing the systemic arterial pressure. The ACE drugs inhibit the conversion of angiotensin that causes blood vessels to contract.

Calcium channel blockers and A.C.E. inhibitors have far fewer side effects than the other hypertensives, and patients are more compliant with drug therapy. Calcium channel blockers and A.C.E. inhibitor drugs however, are much more expensive.

Patients taking these drugs may also suffer from depression and a decreased sex drive. These are side effects of the medication.

The patient with angina needs help in learning to live with its limitations and to avoid those factors known to precipitate an attack. These factors differ with each patient. Several generally common factors are emotional stress, heavy meals, sudden cold, and heavy exertion, figure 24-7. Keeping an adequate supply of vasodilators on hand is important. An elderly person who is forgetful may need reminding. Rest is also important. The patient should be encouraged to keep activity within reasonable limits and to rest following an attack. Smoking, a vasoconstrictor in itself, is forbidden.

When symptoms cannot be controlled through drug therapy, precutaneous transluminal angioplasty may be performed. A balloon is inserted into the narrowing artery and, with controlled pressure, is inflated. The purpose is to flatten the obstruction against the vascular wall, thus allowing more blood to flow. Not all people are candidates for this procedure. Eventually, a more permanent surgical bypass may be needed.

Acute Coronary Occlusion   Acute coronary occlusion is the most common medical emergency. The occlusion may develop gradually as the lu-

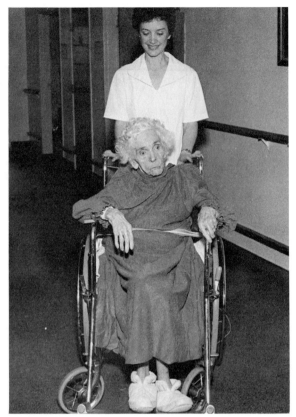

Figure 24-7   The patient must be protected against too much activity that would stress the existing congestive heart failure.

men narrows and finally closes or it may develop more dramatically as the lumen is blocked by an embolus. The size of the blocked vessel and its location determine the extent of the symptoms and the resulting damage. If the narrowing is gradual and a collateral circulation has had time to develop, the occlusion may cause little damage and present minor symptoms, or no symptoms at all. These "silent coronaries" often occur in patients with diabetes mellitus. Unrecognized, they may be discovered during a routine cardiogram. The acute coronary, affecting a large vessel, is more often due to thrombosis following years of atherosclerotic changes. The resultant myocardial infarction may cause death.

The signs and symptoms of myocardial infarction include chest pain that is crushing or vise-like, radiating down arms and up into the neck. It is sometimes described as similar to indigestion. The skin is clammy and pale or ashen. There is profuse sweating (diaphoresis), nausea, and vomiting. Feelings of weakness, anxiety, and panic are expressed. The pulse is barely perceptible. Shock and collapse follow. In the elderly, myocardial infarctions are more apt to be "silent."

Treatment and Nursing Care Treatment and nursing care are designed to combat shock, prevent collapse of the circulatory system, and relieve pain. Preparation for eventual discharge must be started early. Residents in extended care facilities will probably be transferred immediately to the intensive care unit of an acute hospital.

Immediate care in the coronary care unit includes the administration of morphine sulfate or meperidine hydrochloride, oxygen at 3 L/min, and complete bed rest in the semi-Fowler's position. Intake and output, vital signs, enzyme levels, and electrocardiograms are monitored carefully.

If no complications develop, activity is gradually increased. Transfer to an intermediate care unit is usually made by the end of the first week. In uncomplicated cases, discharge to home occurs after the third week. Patients and their families are counseled regarding both the potentials and limitations associated with the health status.

Anticoagulants are occasionally administered for three to four weeks to keep the prothrombin level at 30 seconds or 10 percent of normal. Subcutaneous heparin is frequently used for M.I. patients. The nursing staff must watch carefully for any signs of bleeding. Note bleeding gums as mouth care is given. Watch for petechiae (small pinpoint skin hemorrhages) or changes in the color of the urine. Even though bed rest is essential, passive exercises must be scrupulously carried out to prevent the complications inherent in enforced immobility. Cardiac rupture, ventricular fibrillation, and acute pulmonary *edema* (abnormal collection of fluids in the tissues) are all possible complications. Be alert for

changes in cardiac rate or rhythm and for the symptoms of shock or congestive failure. Be sure to report any of these findings to the nurse.

Congestive Heart Failure (C.H.F.)

The normally aged heart has lost elasticity and the muscle fibers have atrophied. Prolonged peripheral resistance due to sclerotic vascular changes increases cardiac stress. Stress is also felt in the pulmonary network.

Cor Pulmonale This is a condition arising from prolonged pressure within the pulmonary artery due to chronic chest conditions such as emphysema. Cor pulmonale increases the cardiac stress, with eventual hypertrophy and failure of the right ventricle. These factors all contribute to eventual cardiac insufficiency and failure. The prognosis is poor.

Congestive failure (decompensation) is sometimes discussed in relation to the ventricle that fails first.

- *Left-sided failure:* The signs and symptoms of left-sided failure are mainly in the respiratory tract. They include cough, dyspnea or *orthopneia* (inability to breathe except in an upright position), *cyanosis,* (bluish skin due to oxygen deficit), and *hemoptysis* (spotting blood). Fluid is retained in the lungs. The elderly person is constantly fatigued and, with increased hypoxia, may become confused. Low levels of oxygen may help reduce the confusion.
- *Right-sided failure:* The signs of right-sided failure occur throughout the body. They are largely based on the accumulation of fluid. Fluid may accumulate in the abdomen *(ascites),* chest, subcutaneous tissues, and around the heart itself, figure 24-8. The veins of the neck are distended. Patients complain of gastrointestinal disturbances and a feeling of heaviness in the abdomen. The symptoms increase when acute failure is pending. Edema and dyspnea are evident. Fatigue increases. Sleeping becomes difficult, probably due to unrecog-

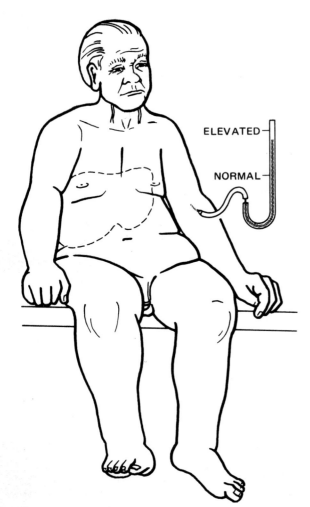

ELEVATED

NORMAL

Figure 24-8 In right-sided failure, accumulated fluid enlarges the liver, abdomen, and lower extremities.

nized orthopnea. Positioning the patient in a more upright position may be more effective than sedatives in promoting rest and sleep.

Acute Failure   Acute failure is an urgent situation. If unrelieved, acute failure will lead to shock, cardiac rest, and death. A small dose of morphine is given slowly to relieve anxiety. Vasodilator drugs such as isosorbide denitrate (venous dilator) or nitroprusside (arterial dilator) may be administered to reduce the cardiac work load.

Rotating tourniquets may be ordered to relieve the acute pulmonary edema, figure 24-9. Tourniquets are applied, or blood pressure cuffs are inflated, just above the venous pressure points. The tourniquets or cuffs are applied to three limbs at a time and rotated at regular intervals (usually ten to fifteen minutes). *Phlebotomy* (blood letting) may be necessary if use of the rotating tourniquets is unsuccessful.

Oxygen at 8 L/min is provided via nasal cannulas or intubation. Respiratory secretions can be removed via an intubation. Intermittent positive pressure ventilation can utilize the same mechanism. Digitalis improves cardiac function and promotes diuresis. Rapid diuresis is also needed to reduce the fluid load.

Patients in acute failure should be in an intensive care unit, where close observation and intervention is possible.

Chronic Failure   Patients can live for years in some degree of chronic failure. In general, they need rest but not immobility. They need a quiet, unexciting environment. A limitation should be placed on visitors, although having a member of the family sit with the patient can have a quieting influence. It may be more beneficial to give nursing care with the patient positioned in a chair.

Pressure Measurement   One of the best ways to assess cardiac function is to measure changes in the pressure within the cardiac cavities. Measuring *central venous pressure (C.V.P.)* provides some information. A more definitive measurement can be gained through one of the Swans-Ganz flow-directed, balloon-tipped catheters. These are small catheters with an inflatable balloon. The balloon is introduced into a vein and advanced into the right heart and up into the pulmonary artery to become wedged within a pulmonary arteriole. In this position, the pressure within the left heart can be measured and compared to the norm. A direct relationship exists between the *pulmonary arterial wedge pressure (P.A.W.P.)* and the pressure found in the left

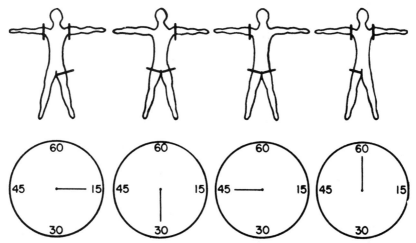

Figure 24-9 Tourniquets are rotated every fifteen minutes to limit the need for the heart to pump blood to the entire body at one time.

ventricle at the end of diastole. An increased P.A.W.P. indicates a decrease in myocardial sufficiency.

Nursing Care Armchair nursing is becoming an increasingly accepted means of caring for the cardiac patient. Maintaining the patient in a supported upright or semiupright position seems to decrease strain on the heart. More blood flows to the extremities, thus decreasing the engorgement of the pulmonary vessels. This position can, of course, be achieved with the patient in bed. But the chair offers the psychological advantages of being out of bed. If chair nursing is selected, remember that the patient's feet must reach the floor and the head and back must be well supported. The best chair is low, deep, and padded. A broad, low footstool may be used to support the feet.

Whether in chair or bed, the patient's position must be changed frequently. Pillows carefully placed can support the head, shoulders, and arms and maintain the patient at a 60° to 90° elevation. Changes in position should not be made suddenly, however. That may bring about a corresponding change in venous pressure, with an increase in pulmonary congestion and dyspnea.

Padded footboards help keep the weight of the bedding off the feet. The patient should be encouraged to press the feet against the footboard to promote venous return. Sitting exercises can be used to maintain muscle tone as well as to promote venous return. Elastic stockings or bandages help channel blood to the deeper vessels. The stockings must be checked often and reapplied every six to eight hours. The nurse must carefully observe the extremities for circulatory impairment. Pitting edema is common. Remember that in this position, weight on the buttocks and shearing force put the patient at extreme risk for decubiti.

Personal Hygiene. Cardiac patients tend to be mouth breathers and oxygen therapy tends to be drying. Therefore, special mouth care is essential.

Complete bathing is fatiguing. Partial baths, which still can stimulate circulation and provide comfort, are a desirable substitute. Special attention must be given to the skin, because the presence of edema gives it a tendency to break down.

Bowel hygiene is important. Straining at the stool is to be avoided. A bedside commode is convenient and less tiring for the patient than a bedpan. Bulk laxative and mineral oil are often prescribed. Ascites may cause a decrease in peristalsis, resulting in constipation. There is some disagreement regarding the use of small enemas and suppositories as bowel aids. Stimulation of the rectal sphincter may stimulate the vagus nerve, which in turn may slow the heart rate.

Diet. Several small, low-bulk meals are suggested for the cardiac patient, because consuming them is less fatiguing. There is also disagreement about the degree to which sodium and fluid should be restricted. Some physicians strictly limit sodium, whereas others limit only the addition of salt. If sodium levels drop too low *(hyponatremia)*, water is usually restricted. For many patients, the limitation of salt is one of the greatest hardships associated with this condition. Salt substitutes can be used if *hyperkalemia* (excess potassium) is not a problem. However, not all patients are able to adjust to their use. During the acute phases, low-sodium milk and distilled water can be used to further reduce sodium intake. To help prevent potassium depletion and an electrolyte imbalance, potassium-rich foods are included in the basic diet. These include bananas, orange juice, peaches, apricots, carrots, seedless raisins, prunes, and fresh raw tomatoes. Pamphlets on sodium-restricted diets are available from the American Heart Association and American Dietetic Association to help patients and their families with menu planning.

Intake and output must be carefully recorded. Daily weighings are sometimes considered an even better indication of fluid retention. Portable scales brought to the bedside may be used, figure 24-10. In some hospitals, a large scale can be positioned to weigh the patient in bed.

Whether patients are in bed or in a chair, they will have little stamina and will tire easily. Plan and organize your work so that the patient has a balance between activity and rest. For example, allow a rest period between breakfast and bath.

Drugs

Drugs are an important part of cardiac therapy. When heart stimulants and diuretics are ordered, it is especially important to keep a care-

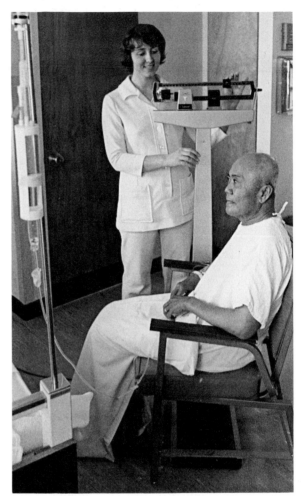

Figure 24-10   The chair scale can be used to determine the weight of the patient without causing undue stress. (Courtesy Long Beach Memorial Medical Center)

ful record of intake and output or to make daily weighings to indicate how much fluid is being retained. It is also important to watch for signs of potassium depletion *(hypokalemia)*. Weakness, unusual fatigue, anorexia, excessive thirst, nausea, and cardiac arrhythmias should be reported at once. Serum potassium levels are determined periodically. Potassium salts in liquid or tablet form are sometimes given with diuretics as a preventative. Gastric irritation, bowel ulceration, and strictures are possible side effects of potassium salt therapy.

Diuretics

Diuretics are among the most commonly used drugs today, figure 24-11. They should be given in the morning so that there will be as little interference with sleep as possible. The object of diuretic therapy is to remove excess extracellular fluid without endangering the metabolism.

The greatest danger of diuretic therapy is too rapid diuresis. Diuretics may also result in hyperglycemia or decreased glucose tolerance. They may cause water and electrolyte imbalance and serious states of hypokalemia or hyponatremia. Several types of diuretics are in current use and have different modes of action and effect. The nursing staff must understand the action of the drugs being administered.

Thiazides and Related Drugs

Bendroflumethiazide (Corzide, Naturetin, Rauzide)
Benzthiazide (Exna) (NaClex)
Chlorothiazide (Aldochlor, Diupres, Diuril)
Chlorothiazide sodium (diuril sodium)
Chlorthalidone (Chlorthalidone, Clonidine, Combipres, Hygroton, Regroton, Thalitone)
Hydrochlorothiazide (Aldactazide, Aldoril, Amiloride, Esidrix, Hydrochlor, HydroDIURIL, Lopressor, Oretic)
Hydroflumethiazide (Diucardin, Saluron)
Metalazone (Diulo, Zaroxolyn)
Methyclothiazide (Aquatensen, Diutensen, Enduron)
Polythiazide (Minizide, Renese)
Quinethazone (Hydromox)
Trichlormethiazide (Trichlormethiazide)

Nonthiazide Diuretics

Amiloride (Midamor)
Bumetanide (Bumex)
Ethacrynic acid (Edecrin)
Furosemide (Aquamed, Lasix)
Indapamide (Lozol)
Spironolactone (Aldactazide, Aldactone)
Triamterene (Dyazide, Dyrenium, Maxzide)

Figure 24-11 Diuretics

Mercurial diuretics interfere with kidney reabsorption of sodium and chloride. They act in one to three hours and have a duration of twelve to twenty-four hours. With continued use, they may lose their effectiveness. They cannot be used in the presence of kidney disease. Many of the mercurials have been replaced by other types of diuretics.

The nonthiazides, ethacrynic acid (Edecrin) and furosemide (Lasix), act by decreasing the reabsorption of sodium and chlorides in the proximal tubules of the kidney. Because potassium is also excreted, there is danger of hypokalemia developing. The loss of potassium in a patient receiving digitalis can bring on arrhythmias. Irregularities of heartbeat should be reported immediately. These drugs act in approximately two hours, with a duration of six to twelve hours.

Antialdosterone compounds (Aldactone) block the action of the sodium-retaining adrenal steroid alsosterone. Triamterene (Dyrenium) conserves potassium while it promotes the elimination of sodium and chlorides. Xanthine compounds (caffeine, theophylline) increase the rate of excretion of both sodium chloride and water.

Each of these drugs influences in some way the chemistry that controls the loss or retention of fluids and electrolytes. The nursing staff must be alert in observing patients receiving diuretics. Changes in heart rate of rhythm, edema, weakness, or apathy should be called to the attention of the professional nurse.

Cardiac Stimulants

Some form of digitalis is given to the patient with chronic heart insufficiency. It increases cardiac output and slows the heart rate while increasing the strength of its contractions. It decreases venous pressure and has a diuretic effect.

The elderly person has increased sensitivity to drugs of all kinds. Digitalis is no exception, especially since this drug is given over such long periods. In addition, the hepatic congestion often found in cardiac patients makes detoxification of drugs more difficult. Therefore, toxicity is more likely to occur. Side effects in the elderly are unexpected and often bizarre. The nursing staff may see cardiac arrhythmias such as premature ventricular contractions, bradycardia, and, in some cases, heart block. Other effects to be watched for are nausea, anorexia, visual disturbances such as blurred or greenish-yellow haze, and mental confusion. Be sure to note and report any sign of arrhythmia. Watch for signs of hypokalemia. The apical-radial pulse must be taken for one full minute prior to administration of the drug. If the pulse is under 60 or over 100, the drug should be withheld and the physician contacted.

Vascular Disease

Circulatory impairments due to pathology of the blood vessels are more common among people over fifty years of age. These peripheral vascular diseases have become a leading cause of death as well as of chronic long-term conditions. The symptoms are slow to become evident. Much vascular damage can take place before symptoms call attention to the disease process. Pain is usually associated with *peripheral vascular disease (P.V.D.)*. Change takes place within the blood vessels themselves, as well as within the areas that are served.

The brain and the extremities are most profoundly and most often affected by diseased blood vessels. Peripheral vascular disease is also frequently associated with cardiorenal disease and diabetes. Changes in the vascular system seem to be accelerated by a diabetic condition. Over a long period, the constant pain of P.V.D. exerts a demoralizing influence on the elderly, increasing the emotional stress they face. Because this additional painful problem comes at a time when they are taxed to their limits with other problems, it is not surprising that these patients can be irritable and demanding.

Arterial Obstruction
Damage to the arterial vessels results in ischemia of the tissues served. It leads to hypoxia,

ulcerations, and severe pain. Vascular damage is due most often to arteriosclerosis obliterans, atherosclerosis, embolism, diabetes mellitus, and cardiorenal disease. Diabetes accelerates the degeneration process. Pulses in the affected areas may be absent or weak, and they should be checked frequently.

Patients with arterial peripheral vascular conditions exhibit changes in their skin and nails. The skin hardens, becoming dry and scaly or shiny. The pigmentation deepens, and the skin is cold to the touch. The color becomes pale or cyanotic, and there may be swelling. The nails become hardened, thick and brittle. Ridges or fissures develop. There is a loss of hair, noticeable on the great toe. Diminished sensory perception in the area leads to injuries that may be overlooked until there is extensive tissue damage.

The pain associated with P.V.D. may develop suddenly or gradually. It is often described as constant and gnawing. When ulcerations are developing, the pain is steady and throbbing. With arteriosclerosis obliterans, there are severe nocturnal cramps. Increased pain in the legs with exercise *(claudication)* requires that exercise be alternated with rest periods. The pulse in the legs and feet may be absent.

When cerebral tissue changes take place in response to vascular disease, the condition is referred to as chronic brain syndrome or cerebral vascular arteriosclerosis.

Venous Obstruction
Damage to the venous vessels is usually due to thrombosis or phlebitis, and elderly people are predisposed to a greater incidence of varicosities. The areas drained by the disease or obstructed veins become congested, swollen, hot to the touch, and tender. Deep vessel involvement is serious. It can lead to a pulmonary embolus and eventual ulcerations. Keep the patient quiet during the acute inflammatory phase, increasing exercise as the condition abates.

Nursing Care

When there is diminished arterial flow, the nursing focus is to prevent further damage to ischemic tissues, promote increased blood flow, and relieve pain. When there is obstruction to venous flow, the nursing care centers around maintaining bed rest with a gradual increase in activity, preventing emboli, and assisting the patient to avoid those practices that promote varicosities.

Attention to the general hygiene of the peripheral vascular patient is important in order to help maintain circulation and prevent infections. Full baths two or three times a week are usually sufficient. Patients must be taught to use a bath thermometer to avoid burns. It may be necessary to have another family member take responsibility for checking the temperature of the bath water. Loss of sensitivity makes it possible for the elderly not to realize that the water is too hot.

Care of the Feet Care of the feet and nails is extremely important. Shoes and socks should fit well and offer firm support. Stretch socks should not be used because they may interfere with circulation. Cotton socks should be changed daily, more often if feet perspire greatly. The feet must be bathed daily and a softening lotion of lanolin applied if the skin is dry. The area between the toes should be dried carefully. A light dusting of powder may be used. Too much powder may cake, act as an irritant, and cause breaks in the skin, however.

The feet should be soaked in lukewarm water before the nails are cut. The nails should be cut straight across, but not too closely to the toe. a good-quality nail clipper offers the best protection. If the nail tends to curl under, a wisp of cotton may be placed under the corner to retrain the growth. The cotton should be changed frequently.

Toes and feet can be lost from injuries or infections that fail to heal because of poor circulation that leads to gangrene. Therefore, feet should be checked frequently for any abnormalities. Corns, calluses, and fungus infections should be treated by a podiatrist. Elasticized hose may be applied to support existing varicosities.

PROCEDURE 18

Applying Elasticized Stockings

1. Wash your hands.
2. Take elasticized stockings of proper length and size to patient's bedside.
3. Identify patient.
4. Explain what you are going to do.
5. With patient lying down, expose one leg at a time.
6. Grasp stocking with both hands at the top and roll toward toe end.
7. Adjust stocking over toes. Place opening at base of toes (unless toes are to be covered). Remember that the raised seams should be on the outside.
8. Apply stocking to leg by rolling upward toward hips.
9. Check to be sure stocking is applied evenly and smoothly. There must be no wrinkles, figure 24-12.
10. Repeat procedure on opposite leg.
11. Report completion of procedure.
12. Record:

   - Date and time
   - Procedure: Application or reapplication of elasticized hose
   - How patient tolerated procedure
   - Any unusual observations

Diet Dietary control may be needed to keep weight within normal limits. If weight loss is necessary, it should be gradual and under medical supervision. The regular diet should be high in protein, vitamin B, and vitamin C. Protein should be increased to prevent tissue breakdown; vitamin B, to maintain healthy blood vessels; and vitamin C, to help healing and prevent bleeding.

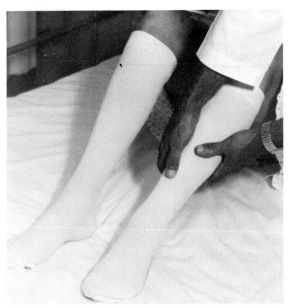

Figure 24-12   Both hands are used to smooth the hose into place and to remove any wrinkles. (From Simmers, *Diversified Health Occupations*, copyright 1988 by Delmar Publishers Inc.)

Water intake should be increased to approximately 3,000 ml daily. This level increases the elimination of wastes and decreases the viscosity of the blood. Smoking or tobacco in any form is forbidden because tobacco causes vasoconstriction vasospasm.

Temperature Control   When there is an interference with circulation, as there is in peripheral vascular disease, patients complain of coldness in their extremities. The temptation to use external heat in the form of hot water bottles or heating pads is strong. But it must be resisted, for two reasons. First, heat increases cellular metabolism. The constricted blood vessels cannot dilate in response to the increased needs. Therefore, the oxygen and nutritional debt is felt even more drastically. Second, decreased sensitivity increases the hazard of burns.

Providing indirect warmth is much safer. Room temperature should be kept at 70°F. Warm, nonconstricting clothing and warm drinks help. Warm baths at body temperature and, for bed patients, heat cradles thermostatically controlled at 86° to 95°F can be used. A warm, not hot, water bottle or heating pad to the abdomen can help by reflexly dilating the leg vessels.

Stimulation and Maintenance of Circulation

Some form of exercise is essential for the elderly. Frequent position changes are the minimum requirement. The exercise program depends upon the general condition of the individual and the specific degree of pathology.

Elevation or lowering of the feet may not always be desirable. For example, in venous deficiency, lowering the feet increases the pooling of blood. In arterial deficiency, elevation may cause severe ischemia. The order regarding general and special exercises must be understood fully. Special postural exercises may be ordered. The length and frequency of the exercises will vary. They may include elevation of the extremities 45° to 60°, lowering the extremities to the side of the bed, and placing legs flat on the bed. These positions are prescribed for specific periods of time.

The oscillating bed, figure 24-13, and tilt table are valuable aids in stimulating circulation. Walking is encouraged because it helps to develop collateral circulation. Patients must be taught to avoid anything that will constrict their circulation. Tight clothing, round garters, sitting for long periods, sitting with legs crossed, and even tight shoelaces are to be avoided at all times.

Surgical Treatment

A lumbar sympathectomy (cutting of the lumbar ganglionic nerve fibers) may be prescribed to improve circulation. It is especially useful in improving ulcerations and localized gangrene. The procedure produces permanent dilation of the peripheral vessels in the lower extremities. The nursing care following this procedure is similar to that for any abdominal surgery. A rectal tube is effective in relieving abdominal distension. Elastic stockings are used to relieve the feelings of warmth and fullness in the legs.

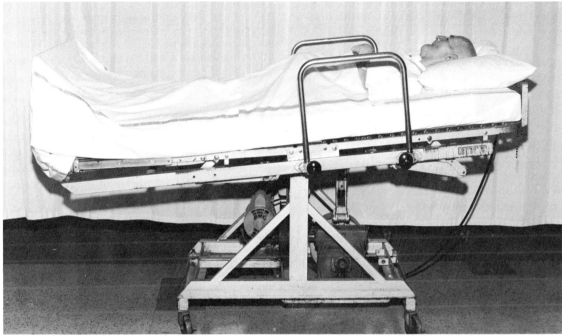

Figure 24-13   Oscillating beds are a valuable aid in stimulating circulation.

Drug Therapy

The pain associated with any ischemia is severe, and analgesics are ordered for relief. Direct vasodilators, which cause the smooth muscles in the walls of the blood vessels to relax, and adrenergic blocking agents, which inhibit sympathetic nerve impulses, are given to increase the circulation.

Sympathetic nerve impulses cause vasoconstriction. Sometimes drugs that interfere with these impulses (adrenergic-blocking agents) are given to produce the opposite effect. Whenever there is interference with the normal blood flow, the possibility of clot development is always greater. For this reason, anticoagulants are ordered in some cases to increase the clotting time.

Complications

Decreased circulation predisposes the individual to ulcerations known as "stasis ulcers," figure 24-14. the ulcers form from even minor trauma. A scratch or a bump can easily deterio-

rate into an ulceration because of poor circulation. Ulcerations of this kind are difficult to cure. Their treatment may last many months, causing a physical and economic strain. Frequently they become secondarily infected, making their cure even more difficult.

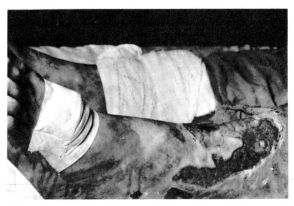

Figure 24-14   Ulcers on legs of patients with peripheral vascular disease (Reprinted from *Care of the Adult Patient*, by Smith and Gips)

The medical management of these ulcers includes frequent cleansing of the area with lukewarm water. The area is then dried gently. An antibiotic ointment is applied if infection is present. If there is necrotic (dead) tissue in the ulceration, an enzyme type of ointment is used. This breaks down the necrotic tissue, which then sloughs off. Continuous saline compresses may be ordered to help reduce the inflammation.

A technique employing gold leaf has shown promising results in treating ulcerations of this type. The thin sheet of gold is placed directly on the ulceration, where it stimulates the formulation of new granulation tissue and healing.

Usually these more conservative medical treatments are attempted first. For some patients, however, the surgical approach provides a better result and skin grafting is performed.

The geriatric health care provider must be constantly on the alert for any indications that new ulcerations are developing. Legs that tire easily, feelings of heaviness in the extremities, and night cramps may be early warning signals. All necessary precautions must be taken to avoid injuries of any kind to the extremities.

Specific Pathologies

Arteriosclerosis is a general term meaning hardening of the arteries that leads to ischemia of the tissues served. There are several different forms.

Atherosclerosis   *Atherosclerosis* is characterized by deposits of fatty materials (atheromas) that narrow the vessels. The vessels of the heart, brain, and legs are most often affected.

Although the mechanism of atherosclerosis is not completely understood, a number of factors seem to contribute to its development and progression. These include diets high in fats and refined sugar, heredity, stress, excess weight, lack of exercise, and cigarette smoking.

Mockberg's Degeneration   *Mockberg's degeneration* (a special form of arteriosclerosis) affects middle-sized vessels such as the radial tibial. Calcium deposits develop in the middle muscular layer of the vessels. This makes the vessels unable to deliver needed blood when the tissues are stressed.

Arteriosclerosis Obliterans   Total occlusion of an artery, caused either by vascular inelasticity due to Mockberg's degeneration or by development of the plagues of atherosclerosis, is known as arteriosclerosis obliterans. This condition is more common among men than among women. Pain, especially severe cramps at night, is the most prominent symptom. Temperature changes are evident, and trophic changes such as ulcerations may develop. If the pain is extreme, amputation may be the only means of relief, figure 24-15.

Hypertension   Atherosclerosis changes the capacity of the vascular beds, causing an increase in blood pressure. This increase is known as hypertension. Hypertension is a serious complication of P.V.D. and of other diseases such as renal and liver disease. The persistent pressure elevation damages the vascular linings, especially in the heart, eyes, kidneys, and brain. This predisposes the person to strokes, renal failure, coronary occlusion, and congestive heart failure.

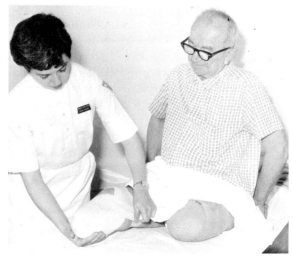

Figure 24-15   Arteriosclerosis obliterans sometimes leads to amputation.

A blood pressure reading over 140 mm Hg systolic and 90 mm Hg diastolic usually indicates hypertension. The normal limit for the elderly is 160/95. When the blood pressure rises above 160/100 mm Hg, the mortality rate from heart attack or stroke increases 200 percent. About 20 percent of hypertension is related to pathologic changes in the body. But most hypertension is related to unknown causes and is called "essential hypertension." Unless hypertension is brought under control with weight reduction, dietary control, and antihypertensive drugs, the prognosis is poor. Approximately 50 percent of hypertensives succumb to congestive heart failure. Twenty percent die of myocardial infarction or stroke and another 10 percent die of kidney failure.

The most obvious indication of hypertension will be revealed when you take the blood pressure, but look for other signs as well. These include disoriented behavior, flushed face, dizziness, headache, and nosebleeds. The individual may complain of blurring of vision, or you may note changes in speech patterns. If you notice any of these signs or symptoms, check the blood pressure and report all findings to your supervisor.

The treatment of hypertension includes correction or treatment of any underlying pathology, dietary control of salts and cholesterol, weight reduction, elimination of tobacco, and an exercise program. When conservative approaches are ineffectual, drug therapy including vasodilators, diuretics, and adrenergic inhibitors may be started. It is extremely important that blood pressure readings be accurately made according to the ANA guidelines of 1988.

Summary

- Cardiovascular disease is commonly seen in the elderly.
- Many patients suffer from some form of myocardial ischemia due to atherosclerosis or complete coronary occlusion.
- Changes in the tissue of the heart combine with a lifetime of systemic disease to produce stress and cause the heart to fail.
- Many elderly persons have some degree of cardiac insufficiency.
- Circulatory impairments are also common among the elderly.
- Various forms of atherosclerosis cause changes in the blood vessels and in circulatory patterns.
- Changes in the peripheral vessels can result in painful ischemias and ulcerations. Changes in the cerebral vessels can cause strokes.
- Atherosclerosis can also lead to hypertension and its complications.
- Nursing care of the cardiovascular patient includes ensuring good general hygiene, increasing the blood flow to ischemic areas, and reducing the strain on already damaged tissues.

Review Outline

B. Major blood vessels
  1. Arteries
  2. Veins
    a. Structural differences
    b. Naming
C. Spleen
D. Blood
  1. Components
  2. Function

IV. Senescent Changes

V. Heart/Blood Diseases

A. Anemia
B. Heart attack
  1. Heart block
  2. Myocardial ischemia
    a. Angina pectoris
    b. Acute coronary occlusion
  3. Congestive heart failure
    a. Acute failure
    b. Chronic failure

VI. Drug therapy

A. Diuretics
B. Cardiac stimulants

VII. Vascular Disease

A. Arterial obstruction
  1. Atherosclerosis
  2. Mockberg's degeneration
  3. Arteriosclerosis obliterans
B. Venous obstruction
C. General nursing care
  1. Foot care
  2. Diet
  3. Temperature maintenance
  4. Stimulation of circulation
  5. Drug therapy
D. Complications
E. Hypertension

Review

I. Vocabulary

Match the terms on the left with the definitions on the right.

1.	Arteriosclerosis	a.	Removal of venous blood
2.	Veins	b.	White blood cells
3.	Atrium	c.	Fluid accumulated in the tissues
4.	Hemoptysis	d.	Hardening of the arteries
5.	Decompensation	e.	Cardiac failure
6.	Ascites	f.	Vessels carrying blood toward the heart
7.	Edema	g.	Fluid accumulating in the peritoneal cavity
8.	Ischemia	h.	Spitting up of blood
9.	Phlebotomy	i.	Diminished blood supply
10.	Leukocytes	j.	Upper heart chamber

II. True or False

1. Smoking is forbidden to all peripheral vascular patients because it slows the heartbeat.
2. Direct heat to the extremities of peripheral vascular patients is dangerous because it may cause burns and because it increases the need for blood.
3. Three ways to stimulate circulation to the extremities are to use a tilt table, use an oscillating bed, and walking.
4. A major factor that cannot be changed in the potential for heart disease is genetic.
5. Anemia is the result of an increase in the number or quality of the red blood cells.
6. Angina patients need help learning to accept the limitations of the disease and avoiding those factors that precipitate an attack.
7. Myocardial infarction that is not accompanied by symptoms is known as a "silent coronary."
8. The primary treatment of a patient with myocardial infarction is designed to relieve the pain, combat shock, and prevent collapse of the nervous system.
9. A heart patient being given some types of diuretics may develop a degree of potassium depletion known as hyperkalemia.
10. Drugs prescribed to treat congestive heart failure are diuretics to help eliminate fluids, and stimulants to increase cardiac contractibility.
11. As the heart ages, the cardiac output increases.
12. Cardiac disabilities can be stressful for both the patient and family.
13. Essential hypertension is a well-understood pathology.
14. Ascites would be most associated with left-sided failure.
15. When there is peripheral vascular disease, there will be changes in skin and nails.

III. Short Answer

1. Identify the parts of the body shown in figure 24-16.
   a. Left atrium
   b. Left ventricle
   c. Interventricular septum
   d. Pulmonary artery
   e. Aorta

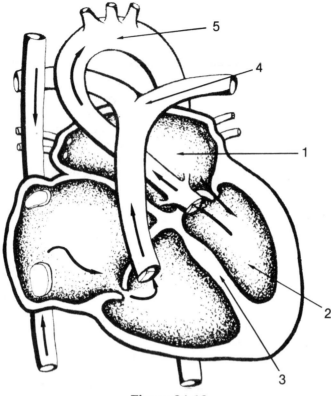

Figure 24-16

2. Why is foot hygiene particularly important for patients with peripheral vascular disease?
3. How does a warm water bottle or heating pad held to the abdomen aid circulation in the extremities?
4. Why do ulcerations in peripheral vascular patients require long-term treatment?
5. Why may elasticized hose be used in varicosities?
6. Clinical Situations
   a. Your patient with a diagnosis of peripheral vascular disease complains of cold feet and asks for a hot water bottle. What do you do?
   b. Your patient further complains that the weight of the bedding hurts his feet. What do you do?

CASE STUDY

   She looked much older than her seventy-four years. She could easily have been classed among the truly frail elderly. Her face was drawn and slightly cyanotic against the raised pillows. Despite the 8 L/min of oxygen reaching her through cannula, she seemed to have difficulty breathing. Her hands and arms were thin. Under the bedding that covered her, the mound of a swollen, fluid-filled abdomen and thin legs were clearly outlined. It was an effort for her to speak, but the nurse seemed to understand as she gently fed the patient ice chips and gave her parched mouth care.

The central venous line that measured her venous blood pressure was checked. Rales, due to fluid in her lungs, were clearly audible on auscultation. Her arterial blood pressure was 156/110. Her apical pulse was 92 and radial pulse 76, indicating a severe pulse deficit.

A urinary catheter, coiled flatly under the linen, dropped straight down into a drainage bag. A padded footboard raised the bedding to prevent undue pressure. Antiembolism stockings smoothly covered her legs. A bedside commode stood in the corner, but at this time the effort of its use could have proved fatal.

Until two days ago, Mrs. Partridge has lived at home with two older sisters. She had been married early in her twenties, raised a family of three, and become a widow at fifty-four. Her husband, a fireman, had succumbed to a massive heart attack six months before retiring. Alone, her family grown and moved to distant parts of the country, Regina Partridge had decided to move back into the family home with her older sisters.

For the past fourteen years, the three sisters had been relatively comfortable. During that time, however, it was discovered that Mrs. Partridge had emphysema. This eventually led to cor pulmonale and right-sided failure. As a young child, allergies had plagued her, a situation gravely compounded by heavy smoking since her teens.

Her diagnosis of congestive heart failure (C.H.F.) was well established by her first hospitalization three years ago. Since then there had been five such admissions, usually associated with the stress of a respiratory infection.

Following each admission, she had rallied enough to be discharged home to limited activity, a sodium-restricted diet, digitalis, and diuretics. This time, however, discharge would be to a long-term care facility, because her sisters, now seventy-eight and eighty-one, were no longer capable of providing the necessary help and care.

As the days passed and cardiac function improved, diet and exercise were increased. The liquid sodium diet was replaced by soft salt-free foods, and sitting exercises were supplemented with getting out of bed and gradual ambulation. Bulk laxatives were given as a bowel aid to reduce straining. Removal of the catheter and use of the commode were instituted.

Mrs. Partridge was watched carefully for signs of hypokalemia and toxicity of digitalis. Intake and output measurements were made, and she was also weighed daily to determine fluid retention.

It was a day of mixed emotions as Mrs. Partridge said goodbye to the staff and, with her sisters by her side, was transported by ambulance to her next residence. A cardiac diagnosis requires a major adjustment for both the patient and those who care for her.

1. What three signs were evident in Mrs. Partridge that were the result of her congestive heart failure?
2. What is fluid in the lungs called?
3. What was Mrs. Partridge's pulse deficit?
4. What disease condition contributed to early heart stress?
5. What two factors probably contributed to the lung problem?
6. What three therapies were prescribed for the congestive heart condition?

Unit 25
Respiratory System Alterations

Objectives

After studying this unit, you should be able to:

- Describe the structures and function of the respiratory system.
- List five safety measures in the use of oxygen therapy.
- Explain the changes that take place as the respiratory system ages.
- Name the conditions that are most likely to develop into chronic obstructive pulmonary disease (C.O.P.D.).
- Assist patients with C.O.P.D.

Vocabulary

Learn the meaning and spelling of the following words or phrases.

antipyretic
arrested
asthma
chronic bronchitis
chronic obstructive pulmonary
  disease (C.O.P.D.)
cold
compressed air
emphysema
expiration

hypoxia
inspiration
malignancies
narcosis
paroxysmal
phlegm
pneumonia
postural drainage

pulmonary emphysema
senile emphysema
spirometer
sputum
stoma
tubercle
ventilator

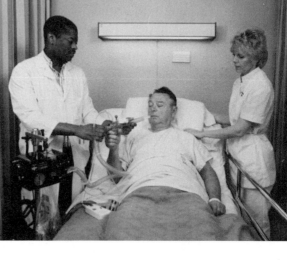

The respiratory system is sometimes referred to as the lifeline of the body. Without the oxygen it carries, life cannot be maintained. Diseases of the respiratory tract that interfere with the vital exchange of oxygen and carbon dioxide bring acute distress. All nursing care is directed toward making breathing easier.

Structure and Function

The respiratory system extends from the nose to the tiny air sacs (alveoli) that make up the bulk of the lungs. Organs of respiration include the nose, pharynx (throat), larynx (voice box), trachea (windpipe), bronchi, and lungs, figure

25-1. The sinuses, diaphragm, and intercostal muscles between the ribs are called auxiliary structures. The nasal cavity is the normal route of air flow for breathing. When there is an obstruction to nasal breathing, the mouth is used. Mouth breathing is drying to the oral cavity and makes special mouth care essential. Mouth breathing also bypasses some important defense mechanisms. This predisposes the person to the greater likelihood of infections.

The air is warmed, moistened, and filtered as it passes through the nasal cavities. The nasal cavities are separated by the nasal septum. The air passes through the pharynx, a common passageway for both air and food, into the larynx, trachea, bronchi, and alveoli. It is at the level of the alveoli that gaseous exchange takes place. Carbon dioxide is brought to the lungs by the pulmonary artery. It passes through the tiny capillaries that surround the alveoli, through the walls of the alveoli, and is exhaled. Oxygen is absorbed by the blood and carried back to the heart by the pulmonary vein. It is then pumped through the general circulation.

There is such an intimate connection between the cardiovascular system and the respira-

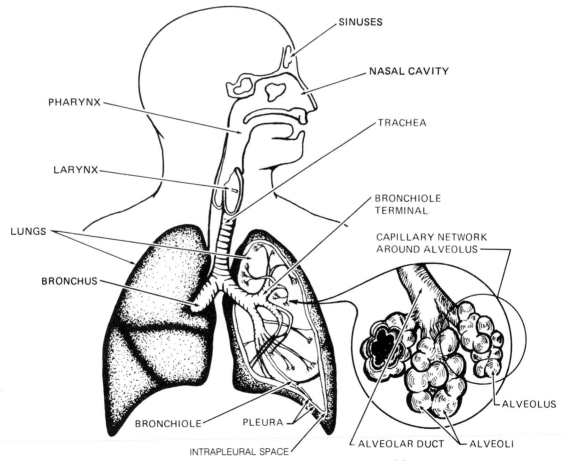

Figure 25-1   The respiratory system and normal lung anatomy

tory system that the two are sometimes referred to as the cardiopulmonary system. Disease and stress in one part (heart or lungs) will inevitably cause disease in the other. This is called cor pulmonale.

The two lungs are found in the thoracic cavity. They resemble cones and are made up of millions of small air sacs, the alveoli. The pointed surface of the lung is called the apex. The broad surface is called the base. Double-thick pleural membranes cover the lungs, separated from the lungs by a small amount of fluid. The base of the lungs is attached to the diaphragm. When the diaphragm and intercostal muscles contract, the thoracic cavity enlarges, pulling the lungs downward and out, and air rushes in *(inspiration)*. When these muscles relax, the thorax becomes smaller, reducing the space available for the lungs, and forcing air out *(expiration)*. Inspiration plus expiration equals respiration.

The contraction of the diaphragm is under the automatic control of the phrenic nerve. This nerve responds to the amount of carbon dioxide in the blood, which thus determines the breathing rate. Exercise such as running makes the body cells work faster and put out more waste products, such as carbon dioxide. Therefore, running increases the breathing rate. The body requires a constant supply of oxygen. Any decrease in gaseous exchange stresses the body and threatens life itself.

Voice Production

Expiration rids the body of excess carbon dioxide. As it passes through the larynx, it may be used to produce sound. Two folds of tissue (vocal cords) extend across the inside of the larynx. Changes in the length of these folds and of the opening (glottis) between them, as air passes outward, produce the sounds used to speak. These sounds are further changed by being bounced against the walls of the sinuses and shaped by the tongue and lips. During a *cold*, when the sinuses become filled with mucus, changes in the voice are easy to detect.

Senescent Changes

Conditions involving the respiratory tract are becoming increasingly common among elderly people, figure 25-2. Such conditions are caused by normal aging of the organs combined with the results of a lifetime of trauma. Improved techniques make more accurate diagnoses possible.

Lung tissue becomes less elastic with age. There is a decrease in the recoil ability of both chest and lungs as the chest wall tends to become more rigid. Lung volume decreases and the alveoli enlarge. The overall rate of gaseous exchange diminishes. Sclerotic changes are evident in the pulmonary blood vessels. The regulation of ventilation is impaired. The cough mechanism becomes less effective, allowing secretions to accumulate in the bronchial tree.

The term *senile emphysema* is sometimes used to refer to a pulmonary condition in which pulmonary elasticity is decreased, but functional impairment is minimal. Obstructive pulmonary disease may develop simultaneously with the aging process and be mistaken for it. Because certain changes are to be expected in the elderly, signs and symptoms of obstructive pulmonary disease may be ignored or simply overlooked. Obstructive pulmonary disease is often associated with arteriosclerotic and hypertensive heart disease.

Nursing diagnostic categories related to respiratory problems are listed in Table 25-1.

- Decreased lung volume
- Reduced elasticity of lung tissue
- Diminished breathing capacity
- Enlarged alveoli
- Fibrotic changes in diaphragm and chest shape
- Diminished rate of gaseous exchange
- Changes in larynx
- Drier mucous membranes

Figure 25-2   Senescent changes in the respiratory system

- Alterations in health maintenance
- Activity intolerance
- Anxiety
- Fluid volume deficit
- Fluid volume excess
- Impaired gas exchange
- Impaired mobility
- Ineffective airway clearance
- Ineffective breathing pattern
- Noncompliance
- Potential for suffocation
- Self-care deficit
- Sleep pattern disturbance

Table 25-1 Nursing diagnostic categories related to respiratory problems

Malignancies

Malignancies (cancerous tumors) can occur anywhere along the respiratory tract. The lungs and larynx are most commonly involved, however. The etiology of malignancies is not completely understood, although some carcinogenic factors have been identified. These include the chronic irritation of smoking. The initial lesion is a cluster of abnormal cells that continue to grow and spread at the expense of the body by competing for available nutrients.

Chest X rays can detect the presence of cancers of the lung. Because early cancer of the lung may be largely asymptomatic (without symptoms), the contribution made by diagnostic X rays is significant. Cancers of the lung may be treated with surgery, radiation, or chemotherapy, or a combination of all three.

Cancer of the Larynx
Cancers located in the larynx may necessitate removal of that organ.

Laryngectomy There are approximately 30,000 laryngectomy patients in the United States with 2,000 more joining their ranks yearly. After a laryngectomy, breathing is done through a tracheostomy, figure 25-3. Special methods of communication must be learned. Although elderly patients can appreciate the lifesaving value of this procedure, they can hardly be expected to accept this drastic change in their lives easily. Cancer of the larynx occurs most commonly in white males over sixty years of age. More than 75 percent of these men are smokers. For some men, the loss of their voice may be psychologically equated with castration. Their very masculinity is threatened.

Establishing Communication Preoperatively, plans for communicating, suctioning, and feeding are discussed with both family and patient. Following surgery, communicating is difficult. The patient must be allowed sufficient time for the feelings of frustration to decrease. Most patients use writing as their basic form of communication until they can learn esophageal speech. This is tedious and tiring, and patients become discouraged easily. The nursing staff must refer to the loss of communication skill as temporary and convey confidence that a suitable form of communication will develop. Approximately 80 percent of laryngectomy patients learn

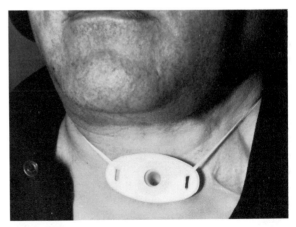

Figure 25-3 The trachea stoma is an opening in the trachea. (From Hegner & Caldwell, *Assisting in Long-Term Care*, copyright 1988 by Delmar Publishers Inc.)

esophageal speech after the operative area has healed.

Esophageal speech is achieved by learning to swallow air and then regurgitate it. This is not easy, and motivation is extremely important. The patient must have privacy to practice in the beginning and then sufficient opportunity to communicate with others as confidence is gained. Patients who have difficulty learning esophageal speech may learn to use an electronic type of artificial larynx, figure 25-4. At times, patients will use a combination of the two methods.

Even though speech is now a possibility, patients need time and encouragement in order to adjust. Speech centers can offer the specialized kind of assistance needed. The Lost Chord Club is a group of laryngectomy patients formed to offer mutual assistance.

Postoperative Adjustment   Postoperatively, the patient may appear apathetic and depressed or resentful and demanding. The patient's basic hostility is aimed toward the surgeon, the perpetrator of this mutilation. But as social custom demands that the patient-physician relationship be one of respect, this avenue for release of feel-

ings is closed. The patient's hostility is more easily directed to members of the family and staff. Families find this behavior particularly upsetting and difficult to understand.

The Stoma   The tracheostomy opening is called a *stoma*. Care of the stoma is a primary focus of basic nursing care. It must be kept clear, clean, and protected from trauma and aspiration. Water-soluble lubricants or petroleum jelly can be used on the skin around the stoma to protect it. Lint is particularly dangerous. Only lint-free clothes should be used around the face and neck. Shaving can pose a serious problem. Be sure that shaving cream does not inadvertently find its way into the stoma. An electric razor is probably safest. The stoma must be kept moist; increased room humidity will be an aid. Making sure that the patient has adequate fluids is very important in keeping body secretions thinned. A wire cage with gauze can be used to maintain the moisture and protect the entrance. Various types of stoma guards are shown in figure 25-5.

After a laryngectomy, there is a tendency for crusts to form in the mouth. Halitosis is common. Special mouth care and frequent toothbrushing and rinsing of the mouth will help. Because the nose can no longer be blown, it must be kept

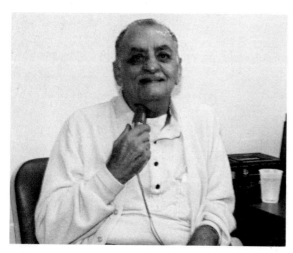

Figure 25-4   Electronic devices help laryngectomy patients to communicate. (From Huber & Spatz, *Homemaker/Home Health Aide*, copyright 1989 by Delmar Publishers Inc.)

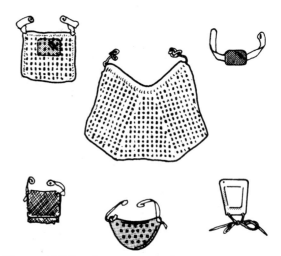

Figure 25-5   Stoma guards prevent foreign materials from entering the trachea.

clean manually and by suctioning. The catheter used in the nose must be kept separate from the catheters used to suction the trachea.

Suctioning of the trachea is a nursing procedure. It should be done gently but firmly. Sterile gloves and equipment are needed. A sterile catheter attached to a *Y* or vented connector offers the best suction control. The tip should be moistened with normal saline or a water-soluble jelly before insertion. Position the patient upright to make passage of the tube easier. No suction is applied during the passage of the tube. Once in place, the tube is gently rotated and suction is applied for about fifteen seconds at a time. No suction is applied as the tube is withdrawn. The nursing staff must be properly instructed before attempting tracheal suction, as the procedure is not always included in basic programs.

Feeding   Initial feedings are through a nasogastric tube, which is inserted before the patient leaves the operating room. It usually remains in place approximately one week. Feedings must be at room temperature to prevent nausea and abdominal cramps. The approved technique for gavage must be followed. Once the tube is removed, care must be taken to prevent food from dropping into the tracheostomy. The patient may complain that the senses of taste and smell are lost. The patient may be encouraged by learning that this is only temporary and that they will gradually be regained.

Infections of the Tract

Respiratory infections are common in the elderly. Infectious organisms are always present in the nose and throat. However, the normal defenses of the healthy body help to limit the damage that these pathogens can cause. The elderly are less active and have weaker defenses. Therefore, they become ill as the germs move further down into the respiratory tract.

Influenza and pneumonia are common and can be life threatening. Some infectious diseases can develop into chronic conditions.

Acute respiratory infections such as *pneumonia* (acute inflammation of the lungs) need to be treated early with antibiotics, oxygen, and supportive care so that complications do not develop. The signs and symptoms of pneumonia are not always as dramatic as they are with younger people. They may be missed. Cough, fatigue, tachypnea (rapid, shallow breathing), confusion, and restlessness may indicate inadequate oxygen stemming from a hidden respiratory infection. Treatment of respiratory infections includes antipyretics (drugs to lower temperature) and antibiotics and oxygen therapy as needed.

Tuberculosis

Pulmonary tuberculosis in the elderly is becoming increasingly common and almost endemic in extended care facilities. It usually is not a new infection, but a reactivation of a primary tuberculosis infection that occurred years before and was contained. Diagnosis may be difficult. Symptoms are often not recognized and may mimic the normal changes of the aging process.

Tuberculosis, one of the oldest known infectious diseases, still ranks high as a cause of death. It is caused by a microorganism that is easily transmitted to others by sneezing and coughing.

The organism usually attacks the lungs, but other parts of the body may also be invaded. If the number of invading organisms is not too great, they may be surrounded by white blood cells and are either destroyed or walled off. A walled-off area is called a *tubercle*. The condition is then said to be *arrested* (confined) alive within the tubercle. Sometimes bodily resistance is lowered because of fatigue or strain, or another infection. In this case, the organisms may again become active. This is particularly true of the elderly or poorly nourished people and those affected with HIV infections (AIDS).

Diagnosis may be made based on the symptomatology, a positive Mantoux test, chest X ray, and sputum culture. Symptoms to look for are loss of appetite, weakness and loss of weight, afternoon temperature, and night sweats. In elders, the only symptom may be fatigue and infection elsewhere in the body. When the process becomes advanced, there may be hemoptysis (spitting up of blood) and, if the pleura become involved, pleuretic pain.

Treatment of pulmonary tuberculosis with drug therapy (Isoniazid, Rifampin, and PZI) can make the patient's disease noncommunicable within two weeks. The drugs, however, must be taken regularly over a period of months. Presently, the recommended time is six to nine months with these three drugs.

Extra precautions must be taken when caring for the patient who has tuberculosis. This disease is transmitted primarily through respiratory secretions. In addition to the usual infection control technique, masks may be needed to prevent transmission. Also, you should turn your head so that the patient doesn't breathe directly in your face as you give care. Be sure to properly dispose of any respiratory secretions such as soiled tissues.

Other Respiratory Conditions

Asthma

Asthma is a disorder of respiration characterized by labored breathing, shortness of breath (S.O.B.) and dyspnea and wheezing. There is constriction of the muscles of the bronchioles, with swelling of the mucous membranes. The production of large amounts of mucus fills narrowed passageways, leading to extreme respiratory distress.

People who suffer from asthma may experience an attack when they come in contact with the allergen or when they are under emotional stress. Some common allergens include pollen, medications, dust, feathers, and foods such as chicken, eggs, or chocolate. If a patient has known allergies, they should be posted in the health record and at the bedside. Treatment includes bronchodilating drugs, beta 2—adrenergic agonists, adrenalin, and antihistamines.

Chronic Bronchitis

Chronic bronchitis is a condition that stems from inflammation in the bronchi because of infection or irritants. The bronchial tissues become swollen and red, narrowing bronchial passageways. There is a persistent cough, which may or may not produce sputum. There may be signs of respiratory distress.

Treatment includes avoiding irritants and using antibiotics to control infection, mucolytic drugs to loosen phlegm, and techniques to improve urination and drainage.

Emphysema

Emphysema is a common chronic obstructive pulmonary disease in which the terminal bronchioles become plugged with mucus. The American Lung Association estimates that 75 million Americans suffer from chronic respiratory distress. That number includes 2.3 million with emphysema, 8 million with asthma, and 10 million with chronic bronchitis. Emphysema deaths have increased fourfold in the past decade. It is second only to heart disease as a cause of disability among men over forty. The incidence of emphysema among women is advancing as the numbers of women with long standing histories of smoking increase.

Contributing Causes of Emphysema *Pulmonary emphysema* is characterized by enlargement of the air spaces distal to the terminal bronchioles, with destruction of the alveolar walls. The etiology of emphysema is unknown at present. However, several factors are known to influence its development or to aggravate an already existing condition.

Chronic respiratory conditions such as asthma, pneumonia, and chronic bronchitis are a major factor in long-term changes. Another factor considered important is air pollutants. Pollutants exacerbate the condition by causing bronchial spasm, edema, and increased airway resistance. Figure 25-6 shows the typical position of a person with emphysema. Cigarette smoke, coal

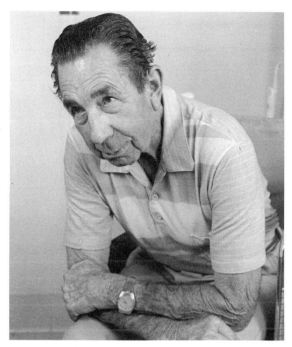

Figure 25-6   Characteristic position of a patient with emphysema

dust, wood and coal smoke, auto exhaust, and industrial smoke and fumes are the specific pollutants that have been indicated. Abrupt changes in temperature, such as sudden exposure to cold air, or dampness and chilling of large areas of the body are also detrimental.

Emphysema is 50 percent more common among whites than among blacks. In late 1988, a new drug (alpha-proteinase inhibitor) was released for long-term replacement therapy for patients with progressive emphysema associated with congenitally low levels of alpha-antitrypsin. Scientists are investigating the possibility of a genetic link in the etiology of this disease. Cases of emphysema are increasing because of the increasing number of elderly people, the increased consumption of cigarettes, and improved survival rates from other conditions such as tuberculosis because of better therapy.

Treatment of emphysema includes antibiotics, bronchodilators, and mucolytic drugs. In ad-

dition, treatment includes postural drainage, special breathing exercises, avoidance of stress, and adequate fluids and nutrition. Coughing is the major mechanism to clear the respiratory tract. Encouraging the patient to cough is a major responsibility of the health care provider.

Chronic Obstructive Pulmonary Disease (C.O.P.D.)

Chronic obstructive pulmonary disease is frequently referred to as *C.O.P.D.* The pathology involves blocking of the bronchial airway. Chronic pulmonary inflammation results in the narrowing and irreversible destruction of the bronchioles and alveoli and the pulmonary blood vessels. There is an increasing loss of lung elasticity.

Signs and Symptoms of C.O.P.D.

The earliest signs of obstructive pulmonary disease are fatigue and a progressive increase in dyspnea upon exertion. Mouth breathing, coughing with or without *phlegm*, (mucus) and bronchial spasm are common. There is a feeling of constriction or "tightness" in the chest and frequent acute respiratory infections.

Inadequacy of ventilation lowers oxygen availability. Exertion may lead to dizziness and restlessness. Cyanosis may be observed at the base of the fingernails and in the conjunctiva.

Laboratory Diagnosis   Laboratory diagnosis is based on the findings of pulmonary function tests. The most valuable measurement is the degree of expiratory airway obstruction. A recording *spirometer* (respirometer) is used to measure lung volumes and the relationship of time needed to move a specific volume of air into and out of the lungs. Usual diagnostic findings include increased residual volume, decreased expiratory reserve, and reduced vital capacity. In addition, arterial blood studies that reveal a decrease in oxygen pressure and saturation and an increase in carbon dioxide pressure clearly demonstrate the ventilation problem. Chest X rays show enlarged lungs with large interstitial air spaces, widened intercostal spaces, and a low, flat diaphragm. The pathological changes that take place in C.O.P.D. vary, but ventilation is affected early and prominently.

Treatment of C.O.P.D.

Treatment of chronic obstructive pulmonary disease is basically supportive. It focuses on the need to preserve and improve existing lung function and to help patients adapt to their limitations.

In larger facilities, many of the procedures related to improving ventilation are administered by the respiratory care therapist. In others, the nurse carries out these techniques or assists the patients in doing so.

Drug Therapy Bronchospasm is relieved by administering bronchodilating drugs such as Bronkosol with equal parts of saline, Adrenalin Chloride solution, aminophylline, Bronkephrine, and detergent-like drugs such as acetylcysteine. If the bronchospasm is prolonged or *paroxysmal*, adrenal corticosteroids may be ordered.

Bronchodilators can be administered topically with a hand nebulizer. A nebulizer is equipment that can turn the medication into a fine vapor. When inhaled, the vapor can more easily reach deeper areas of the lungs. Sometimes the nebulizer is driven by hand by squeezing the attached bulb. At other times, the apparatus is attached to an oxygen source or to *compressed air* equipment, figure 25-7. The air or oxygen pressure increases the ability of the equipment to ventilate the lungs. The patient usually operates the nebulizer, but it may be necessary for a member of the family to assist with this procedure. The nebulizer must not be overfilled with the aerosol nor allowed to run dry. The patient is taught to exhale fully and then inhale deeply. The vaporized stream of the drug is directed well back toward the sides of the throat. The hand bulb is compressed rapidly several times. Temporary relief is often immediate. If the nebulizer

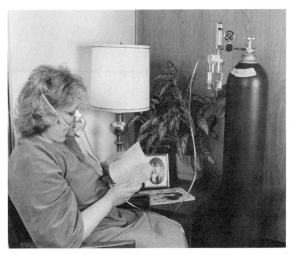

Figure 25-7 Nebulizer attached to oxygen tank. (Courtesy of Puritan-Bennett)

is overused, it tends to lose its effectiveness and can cause sudden death. A pressurized hand cartridge with a premeasured dose of drug is now available.

When secretions tend to be retained, an intermittent positive-pressure breather (I.P.P.B.) or a *ventilator* is most effective. Through this machine, oxygen and vaporized drug are forced into the lungs at intervals under pressure. The machine can be set to cycle at the patient's own respiratory rate or at a preset rate. Available equipment varies. The nurse must completely understand how to operate a particular machine before assuming responsibility for patient care. In general, the patient is asked to breathe through the mouth. Nasal passages are covered. The patient exhales fully and then inhales gently to activate the machine. The patient should be encouraged to relax as much as possible during the treatments. They are frequently ordered for fifteen-minute periods three times a day.

The medication may also be given intravenously or subcutaneously. When necessary, it can also be given as a rectal suppository. When excess secretions are present in the bronchi, a saturated solution of potassium iodide (S.S.K.I.) is prescribed. Increased humidity may add to the patient's comfort. Myloytics, sodium bicarbonate, or sodium chloride may help loosen secretions.

Palliative Measures Coughing, which may or may not be productive, can be fatiguing to the patient and may cause vomiting. If the cough is nonproductive, instruct the patient to take short, rapid breaths to decrease the cough reflex. A soothing cough syrup may be given if ordered.

If the cough is wet and productive, the patient should be encouraged to take deep breaths, hold them, and cough fully. Coughing should not be forced, however. Both the character and amount of sputum brought up should be noted. *Sputum* refers to matter that is brought up by mouth, usually after coughing. This matter comes from the lungs. Sputum specimens are frequently taken from people who have chest conditions. Some tests on specimens may be done by the health care provider in the utility room.

PROCEDURE 19:

Collecting a Sputum Specimen

1. Wash hands and assemble the following equipment:
   disposable gloves
   container and cover for specimen
   glass of water
   tissues
   emesis basin
   label including patient's full name, room number, hospital number, date and time of collection, doctor's name, examination to be done, and other information as it is requested
2. Identify the patient and explain what you plan to do. Screen the unit.
3. Put on disposable gloves.
4. Have the patient rinse the mouth. Use emesis basin for waste.
5. Ask patient to cough deeply and expectorate (spit) into the container. Ask patient

to cover mouth with tissue to prevent spread of infection. Collect one to two tablespoons of sputum unless otherwise ordered.
6. Remove gloves and dispose of them according to facility policy.
7. Wash hands. Do not contaminate the outside of the container.
8. Cover container tightly and attach completed label.
9. Clean and replace equipment according to facility policy.
10. Take or send specimen to appropriate area immediately.
    Note: If a twenty-four-hour specimen is being collected, leave the container at the person's bedside.
11. Record procedure on patient's chart. Be sure to include a description of the specimen, such as odor and color.

Positioning Positions permitting expansion of the lungs and a straightened airway are helpful to patients with respiratory distress. Expiration is difficult. Therefore, patients with emphysema characteristically lean forward with shoulders raised as they try to force the carbon dioxide out of their lungs, figure 25-6.

In high Fowler's position, the patient is in a sitting position with the backrest elevated. Three pillows may be positioned behind the head and shoulders. The knee rest may be adjusted. The feet should be kept in proper alignment with pillows or footboards.

The orthopneic position may be used as an alternate to the high Fowler's position. The position of the bed remains the same. The bedside table is brought across the bed and a pillow or two placed on top. The patient leans forward across the table with arms on or beside the pillows, figure 25-8. Another pillow is placed low behind the patient's back for support.

Breathing Exercises An attempt is made through breathing exercises to improve pulmonary ventilation in order to overcome *hypoxia*, or lack of oxygen supply. Emphasis is on increasing

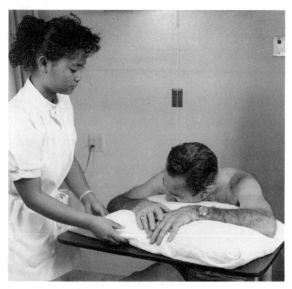

Figure 25-8   Orthopneic position

the expiratory phase. This is referred to as "pursed lip breathing." These exercises are taught by the physiotherapist and supervised by the nurse. The exercises are designed to strengthen abdominal muscles. This helps the diaphragm elevate during expiration, improves aeration, increases exercise tolerance, and encourages productive coughing to expel the accumulated sputum.

The patient is first taught the basic breathing pattern. The patient learns to breathe in deeply through the nose to the count of "one," allowing the abdomen to rise. Air is forced out of the lungs through pursed lips, in a blowing manner, to the count of "two" and "three" as the abdomen is drawn inward. Exercises are done in supine, sitting, and walking positions.

Activities that increase vital capacity include walking a treadmill and riding a stationary bicycle. Speed and length of time are adjusted to the individual patient and are gradually increased. Oxygen may be given if necessary during these activities.

Specific exercises include blowing a candle out at varying distances, blowing against water resistance in a bottle, and blowing a feather or tennis ball across the table. In each of these exercises, the patient blows with pursed lips to develop skill in the expiratory movement. This movement is essential to diaphragmatic breathing. Practicing the basic breathing pattern with a weight on the abdomen is also helpful.

Figures 25-9 through 25-12 show different exercises to help improve pulmonary ventilation.

Incentive Spirometer   Incentive spirometers are frequently used to improve ventilation. Incentive devices help patients visualize the effects of their respiratory efforts. Breaths are taken slowly and deeply through the mouth. A respiratory volume goal is preestablished. The patient is encouraged to inhale until the goal is reached and to sustain it three to five seconds before exhaling.

Improving Drainage   Percussion and vibration are techniques employed to loosen thick secretions. These techniques are used in conjunction with thinning aerosols, ventilators, and positional drainage.

Percussion means to tap the chest with cupped hands to loosen secretions in each lung area. Vibrators are electronically operated and hand held. They are placed against the chest wall and shake loose the secretions within the lungs.

Types of Drainage   Rotary and *postural drainage* are employed to rid the respiratory tract of trapped sputum by encouraging drainage by gravity as the patient's position is changed. Drainage is not always effective. The sputum may be tenacious and there may be abnormalities of the bronchial tree. Also, it is difficult for the elderly to assume postural drainage positions for long periods. Each position change should be made slowly.

Rotary or postural drainage should be preceded by inhalation of a bronchodilator or mucolytic (mucus thinning) drug. The drug should be taken at least fifteen minutes prior to the treatment. *Postural drainage* is best undertaken at least forty-five to fifty minutes after meals to avoid possible nausea. It is recommended that the patient cough continuously with small, un-

1. Sitting erect on the side of the bed, the patient inhales deeply, allowing the abdomen to expand against a small pillow or book.

1A. The book is pressed in firmly as the patient exhales. This helps elevate the diaphragm, improves aeration, and encourages cough to dislodge accumulated sputum.

2. Each leg is raised alternately as the patient exhales. This strengthens and improves tone of abdominal muscles.

3. The head and shoulders are raised from the bed as the patient exhales. This is a more strenuous exercise of the abdominal muscles.

4. With inhalation the patient puffs out the abdomen as far as possible. As he exhales he pulls in the abdomen, bringing the book as close as possible to the spinal column. This teaches synchronization of the abdominal and diaphragmatic muscles with breathing.

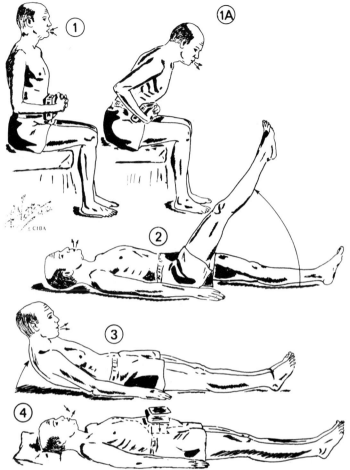

Figure 25-9 Breathing exercises improve ventilation. (Copyright 1988 CIBA-GEIGY Corporation. Reproduced with permission from the *Clinical Symposia*, illustrated by Frank H. Netter, MD. All rights reserved.)

strained coughs. The chest should be tapped with cupped fingers throughout the procedure to help loosen the secretions, figure 25-13.

Use of a tilt table for postural drainage offers the older person the greatest degree of security and requires the least effort. Several different positions can be assumed. Positions are chosen specifically for each patient, figure 25-14.

If a tilt table is not available, the knee break of the bed may be raised and the patient positioned over it for the final drainage position. The foot of the bed may also be elevated twenty-one inches. The ideal final drainage position is over the edge of the bed with head and arms on the floor. But this is usually too strenuous for the elderly person. The length of time that the individual exercise positions are held varies. However, an attempt is made to gradually increase the length of time in each position. The patient should be encouraged to breathe deeply and cough during this final phase to help raise the sputum that has been loosened. Tissue and an

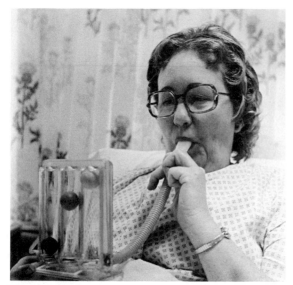

Figure 25-10 Respiratory exercises improve the patient's ventilation. (Courtesy Long Beach Memorial Medical Center)

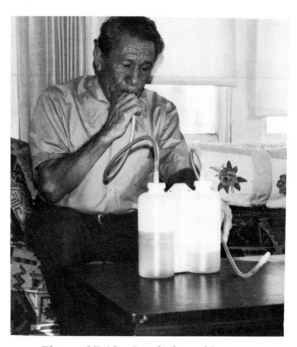

Figure 25-12 Bottle breathing

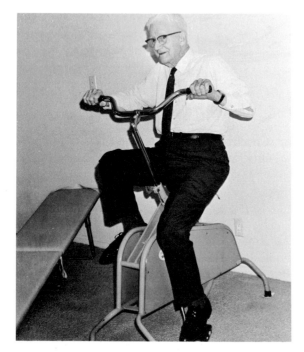

Figure 25-11 Riding a stationary bicycle helps to strengthen muscles and aids the respiratory effort.

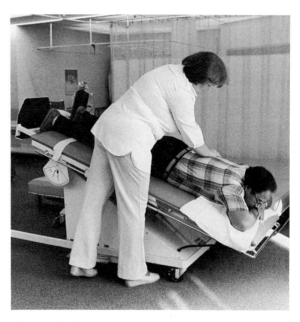

Figure 25-13 Postural drainage and percussion loosen and drain respiratory secretions. (Courtesy Long Beach Memorial Medical Center)

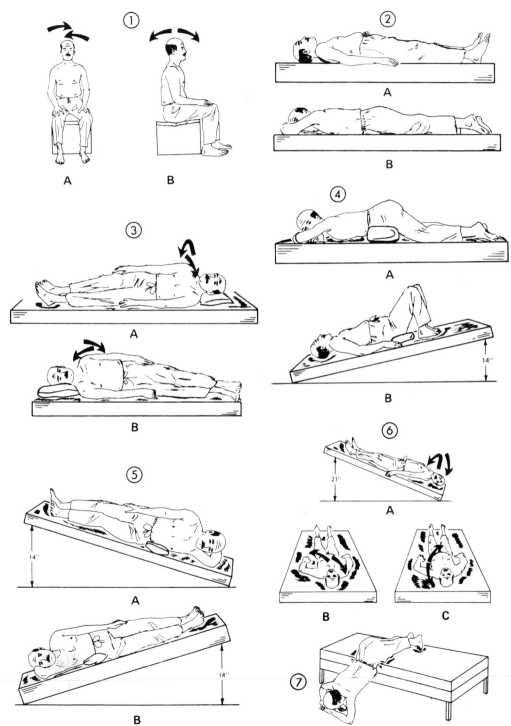

Figure 25-14   Postural drainage exercises help to clear respiratory passageways.

emesis basin should be at hand. Note and report the color and amount of sputum.

Whichever final drainage position is chosen, the patient must be watched closely for signs of fatigue. Oxygen therapy can be helpful when there is real respiratory distress or simple hypoxia such as occurs during exercise. The lowest flow rate to relieve the oxygen debt or dyspnea should be used. A high oxygen flow rate can lead to acute respiratory insufficiency in some patients with chronic pulmonary disease, as hypoxic drive is lost.

Supportive Care   In addition to the specific nursing measures described, attention must be given to fluid intake and diet. Ten glasses of fluid are recommended daily. The extra fluids can be offered in fruit juices, sherbets, gelatin, and soups. Adequate fluid intake is especially important during a period of respiratory infection to reduce the sputum viscosity. An intake and output sheet should be kept. Large meals, which distend the stomach, increase respiratory embarrassment. Frequent, small meals are preferred and will be taken more easily. They should be high in protein. Gas-producing foods should be avoided to prevent abdominal distension. Milk, which tends to make secretions more viscous, should be eliminated. Shortness of breath makes eating a serious problem. The act of eating may be fatiguing, so the patient should be encouraged to eat slowly.

Weight should be maintained at or just below ideal. It is important that clothing not be allowed to restrict respirations in any way. Medications, especially narcotics, sedatives, and tranquilizers, must be given with extreme caution. The majority of patients are not improved by moving to a dry, warm climate. Good results can be achieved, however, by maintaining the immediate environment at a constant temperature, slightly lower than usual, with good ventilation.

Immediate disposal of secretions and use of a chlorophyll deodorizing stick will control the unpleasant odors sometimes associated with C.O.P.D. Oral hygiene is important, because mouth breathing is common. Lemon and glycerine inside the mouth, and petroleum jelly or a commercially prepared lipstick applied to the lips, can provide comfort. Chewing gum and hard candy help to keep the mouth moist. Mouthwashes used every four hours and before meals improve the taste in the mouth and may make food more palatable. The care and rehabilitation of patients with C.O.P.D. requires a team of professionals that includes the physician, nurse, physiotherapist, psychologist, and social worker.

Preventative Measures   Patients with C.O.P.D. must be protected from acute respiratory infections. They must be taught to avoid groups when infections are prevalent. Acute bronchitis is usually viral and pneumonia is bacterial in nature. Both place stress on an already overtaxed respiratory system. Broad-spectrum antibiotics are prescribed promptly for a minimum of one week. Annual immunization against the flu virus is recommended as a precautionary measure. Pneumonia vaccine (pneumovax) is available to protect against pneumococcal pneumonia. It may be administered every three years.

In general, defensive measures should include protection from chills and avoidance of known bronchial irritants and of crowds during epidemics. These patients should be encouraged to stay indoors when temperatures outside are 35° to 40°F or lower. The patient must stop smoking, which may prove to be one of the most difficult adjustments that must be made. It may even be necessary for the C.O.P.D. patient to seek other employment if bronchial irritants are associated with work. Proper diet, adequate rest, and an annual physical that includes a forced expiratory spirogram and chest X ray help check early and mild forms of C.O.P.D.

Carbon Dioxide Narcosis

In advanced C.O.P.D., there is increasing evidence of respiratory distress. It climaxes in the signs and symptoms of ventilatory failure, carbon dioxide *narcosis* (stupor) and eventual coma. As carbon dioxide blood levels rise, the patient becomes lethargic, may appear dazed or belligerent, or may exhibit psychotic behavior.

The head of the bed should be elevated 30° to 40°. A pillow should be positioned so that the head is tilted slightly backward to maintain an airway. The bed can be lowered every two to three hours for fifteen minutes to help change positions. Total position change should be made every three hours to prevent decubiti and pulmonary congestion. The orthopneic position may be used, or the patient may be positioned with pillows in an upright position in bed or a chair.

Intubation or tracheostomy may be needed when respiratory distress increases and sputum is retained because the cough is ineffective. An I.P.P.B. machine, figure 25-15, is used to assist and control ventilation. Sunctioning of the endotracheal or tracheostomy tube must be done carefully. A disposable sterile catheter must be used each time. If the nose and pharynx need suctioning, a separate catheter must be used. The tracheostomy site must be dressed and the inner cannula kept clean. The tracheostomy cuff is released every four hours for fifteen minutes to reduce pressure on the trachea. The cuff is reinflated with 5 to 10 milliliters of air.

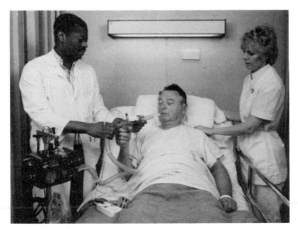

Figure 23-15 Intermittent positive pressure breathing using a ventilator aerates the lungs.

Continued respiratory failure must be handled with vigorous artificial ventilation. Vital signs and emotional and physical response to therapy must be observed carefully.

Emotional Adjustment

Both the C.O.P.D. patient and the family need emotional support. They need help in accepting a progressive, chronic, debilitative condition and in formulating realistic goals. The emotional response to such an illness can be extreme. It is common for patients to be self-centered, irritable, and impatient. Fear of death or of being abandoned makes them anxious and unhappy.

The nursing approach needs to be realistic, calm, and supportive. Encourage the patient to keep activities within the limits of dyspnea and fatigue. As always, the patient needs to cooperate in the medical-social planning. Progress and attitude will be affected by the patient's employment status, ability to make the necessary work adjustments, and family finances. Being able to contribute to the well-being of the family will do much to enhance feelings of self-worth. The patient's past responses to illness and the stability of interpersonal relationships with other family members will, in a large part, determine the success or failure of adjusting to the present situation.

Oxygen Therapy

Oxygen is often ordered by the physician at very low levels (2 to 4 liters per minute). Older patients usually receive oxygen by nasal cannula, catheter, mask, or I.P.P.B. Nasal cannulas are small tubes placed at the entrance to the nose, figure 25-16. Nasal catheters are small plastic or rubber tubes inserted into the nose.

When patients receive oxygen therapy by these methods, keep the patient's face free of any nasal discharge. Make sure that there are no kinks in the tubing. Be sure that straps holding cannulas in place are not constricting or irritating and check behind the ears for signs of irritation.

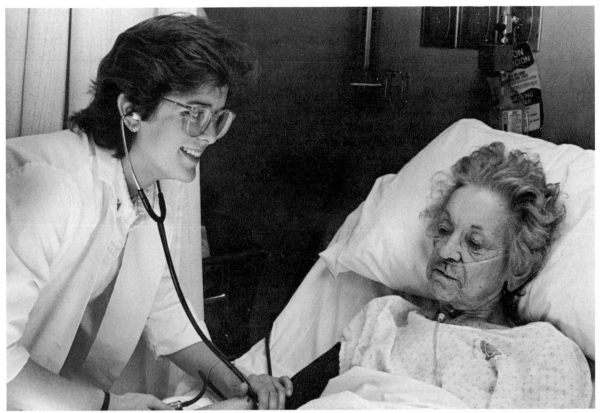

Figure 25-16   Oxygen can be delivered to the patient through a nasal cannula. (Courtesy Long Beach Memorial Medical Center)

A cuplike mask may provide oxygen when held in place over the nose and mouth by hand or by straps around the head. If mask oxygen is given, be sure the straps are secure but not too tight. Remove the mask periodically. Wash the area under it, dry carefully, and lightly powder the area.

Oxygen given by I.P.P.B. is administered by professional personnel. This technique helps to expand the lungs.

Preventing Fire

Although oxygen doesn't explode, burning is more rapid and intense when oxygen is present. Therefore, anything that might result in fire must be eliminated when oxygen is in use. The following safety measures must be taken:

- Health care provider and patient should wear cotton clothing.
- Cigarettes and matches should be removed from the room.
- No smoking is allowed in an area of oxygen use. Signs should be posted.
- No open flames, such as smoking or candles, are permitted.
- Provide a hand call bell instead of an electric one. Do not use woolen blankets.
- Before using electrically operated equipment at the bedside, such as an electric razor, discontinue the flow of oxygen.

If a fire occurs, safety of the patient is paramount. Sound the alarm by using the signal that connects the patient to the switchboard. Manual alarms may also be activated. Give the location and the nature of the fire. Then move patients out of the area as quickly as possible. Bed patients are moved in their beds. Ambulatory patients are escorted and directed to safe areas.

Be prepared to follow instructions when a nurse or other person in authority assumes control. In the meantime, carry out the safety policies of your facility. Once the patients are safe, check to be sure oxygen is shut off and electrical equipment is disconnected. Shut doors and fire doors if they are part of the safety equipment. Be sure to keep all exits accessible. If you have been trained in the use of a fire extinguisher, if may be used on small fires. In all situations, get patients to safety, follow hospital policy, and keep calm.

Maintaining an Oxygen Source

In some facilities, oxygen is piped from wall units directly into the patient's room, figure 25-17. In others, the oxygen source is a tank brought to the patient's room when therapy is ordered, figure 25-18. If a tank is used, be sure that:

- There is sufficient oxygen. Check gauge each time you go to the bedside.
- An additional oxygen tank is readily available.
- Empty tanks are marked and returned to the proper area promptly.
- The tank is secure and cannot fall. Straps may hold it to the bed, or it may stand in a tank holder.
- Oxygen is always moisturized before reaching the patient. It can be very drying to mucous membranes.

To help keep the patient ambulatory and to promote more independence, an oxygen tank can be mounted on a wheelchair, figure 25-19.

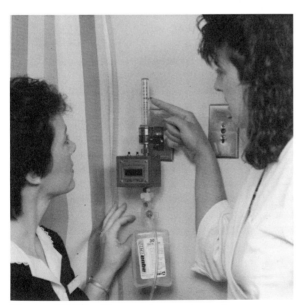

Figure 25-17 Oxygen users must have a constant source of oxygen. One source is to have oxygen piped directly into the room. (From Caldwell & Hegner, *Nursing Assistant, A Nursing Process Approach*, copyright 1989 by Delmar Publishers Inc.)

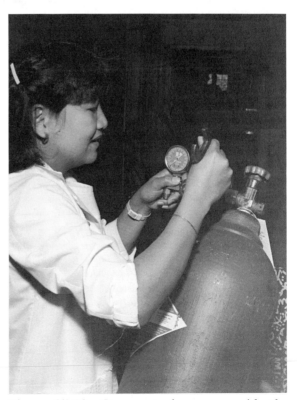

Figure 25-18 Oxygen tanks may provide the oxygen source.

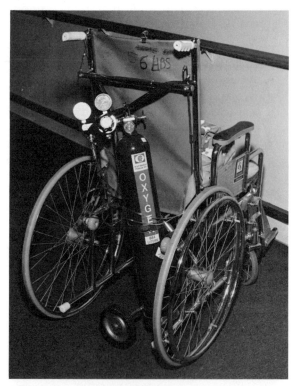

Figure 25-19   An oxygen tank can be attached to the back of a wheelchair to allow the patient with a respiratory problem more mobility.

Summary

- The organs of respiration function to take in oxygen, exchange it with carbon dioxide, and expel carbon dioxide.
- Diseases that affect the respiratory tract make breathing difficult.
- The most common chronic obstructive pulmonary disease is emphysema, although chronic bronchitis and asthma are also common.
- The elderly have a high incidence of these conditions. Early-life lung conditions, as well as the aging process, have made them more susceptible.
- The care and treatment of the patient with C.O.P.D. includes basic hygiene and nutrition, breathing exercises to improve ventilation, drugs to decrease and liquefy secretions, and postural drainage procedures.
- When carbon dioxide narcosis develops, more extreme measures of tracheostomy and artificial ventilation are necessary.
- The patient's emotional response and willingless to participate in medical and socioeconomic planning determine to a large extent the success or failure of rehabilitation.

Review Outline

I. Behavioral Objectives

II. Vocabulary

III. Respiratory System

    A.   Structure
    B.   Function
    C.   Voice production
    D.   Senescent changes

IV. Diseases

    A.   Malignancies of the larynx
        1.   Laryngectomy
        2.   Establishing communciation
        3.   Adjustments
        4.   Stoma care

    B.   Infections of the tract
        1. Tuberculosis
        2. Emphysema
        3. Bronchitis
    C.   Asthma

V. Promoting Improved Ventilation

    A.   Drug therapy
    B.   Ventilators
    C.   Positioning
    D.   Breathing exercises
    E.   Incentive spirometers
    F.   Vibrators
    G.   Drainage techniques
    H.   Supportive care

Review

I. Vocabulary

Match the word or phrase on the right with the phrase on the left.

1. Inflammation of the lungs   a. Emphysema
2. An example of C.O.P.D.   b. Hypoxia
3. Thick respiratory secretions   c. Pneumonia
4. Inadequate oxygen   d. SOB
5. Shortness of breath   e. Tubercle
                                      f. Phlegm

II. Select the one answer that best completes each sentence.

    1. Patients with respiratory disease should
        a. cover the nose and mouth when coughing.
        b. turn face toward others when sneezing.
        c. wash hands only after toileting.
        d. dispose of soiled tissues by dropping them in the nearest trash can.
    2. To assist the patient with ventilatory difficulty, you had best
        a. keep the bed flat.
        b. elevate the bed to a high Fowler's position.
        c. keep the patient on the left side.
        d. keep the patient on the right side.
    3. Your patient is receiving oxygen. You should
        a. monitor intake and output.
        b. know the ordered rate.
        c. check the flow rate once each shift.
        d. check the flow rate every three hours.
    4. When administering oxygen by mask, in addition to routine care and precautions, you should
        a. make sure that the straps are not too tight.
        b. remove the mask periodically to wash and dry under it.
        c. powder lightly.
        d. all of these.

5. When a patient is receiving oxygen through a cannula, you should
   a. make sure that the straps are very tight.
   b. check behind the ears for signs of irritation.
   c. make sure cannula tips are in the mouth.
   d. none of these.
6. When caring for the patient with a laryngectomy stoma,
   a. special mouth care is needed.
   b. remember that lint is not a problem.
   c. use the same catheter to suction both the trachea and the nose.
   d. serve food very hot or very cold.

III. True or False

1. The respiratory system extends from the nose to the alveoli.
2. The lungs become more elastic as they age.
3. In asthma, there is increased production of mucus that blocks the respiratory tract.
4. Chronic bronchitis frequently leads to C.O.P.D.
5. In the high Fowler's position, the patient leans forward across the overbed table.
6. The flow rate is ordered by the physician.
7. Oxygen need not be moisturized before reaching the patient.
8. Elderly patients with tuberculosis always demonstrate typical signs and symptoms such as cough and weight loss.
9. People with chronic respiratory obstruction care become overly dependent on the use of nebulizers.
10. Always post a sign when oxygen is in use.

IV. Clinical Situations

1. You notice a patient who suffers from C.O.P.D. behaving strangely and seeming confused. What do you do?
2. You notice a patient in the dorsal recumbent position having some difficulty breathing. What do you do?
3. A patient is using a hand nebulizer for the first time. What instructions do you give?
4. A patient asks how the I.P.P.B. machine will help. What do you say?
5. A patient has been taught the basic breathing pattern. What is it?
6. A patient has been told to vibrate his chest with finger tapping to loosen secretions during rotary drainage. What do you tell him to do?

CASE STUDY

Mr. R. C., eighty-six years old, was a regular visitor to a neighborhood geriatric day center. He lived with his divorced daughter and her two children. Since the daughter worked and the children were in school, he became rather lonely. When a mass screening by a mobile unit suggested the need for further chest evaluation, Mr. C. was referred to the local general hospital with a diagnosis of "possible emphysema."

A team of professionals discussed the case after the examination and diagnostic tests were completed. The team developed a program of rehabilitation designed to improve the patient's ventilatory status. It was decided that the program could be conducted on an outpatient basis.

Arrangements were made for Mr. C. to come to the rehabilitation department twice a week for therapy. Three times a week he would continue to visit the day center, which was his major source of socialization.

After one week of therapy, Mr. C. confided to the center nurse that he had skipped his last session because he felt it was too much effort. He had to take the bus back and forth because his appointment was at a time when his daughter was at work. Besides, he felt he was not making any progress. His daughter couldn't see any difference either. "Anyway," he continued, "what's the use? An old man like me isn't worth all that bother."

The center nurse listened carefully and then made some suggestions. She let Mr. C. know that he was a valued member of the center. She suggested that when he had better respiratory control, he would be able to participate more fully in center activities. She suggested he might concentrate first on learning the proper method of inhaling and exhaling to the count of three. She showed real pleasure when he demonstrated that he was already beginning to learn. She told him she would contact the rehabilitation department to see whether his appointment could be made in the morning when his daughter would be available to drive him. She expressed the hope that he would continue therapy because there was much he still could contribute. But she was careful not to insist.

Identify at least three factors in geriatric rehabilitation that the nurse recognized in talking to Mr. C. List the ways the nurse responded to each. For example, one factor is that elderly people resist change. The nurse responded by making positive suggestions but carefully not insisting.

Unit 26
Integumentary System
Alterations

Objectives

After studying this unit, you should be able to:

- List the functions of the skin.
- Provide decubitus ulcer care.
- Provide denture care.
- Describe skin care necessary for the elderly person.
- Review the characteristics of the aging integumentary system.
- Provide nail care.

Vocabulary

Learn the meaning and spelling of the following words or phrases.

bath itch
constrict
cyanotic
debridement
decubitus ulcers (dermal ulcers)
dilate
epidermis
pallor

rubra
shearing force
tactile

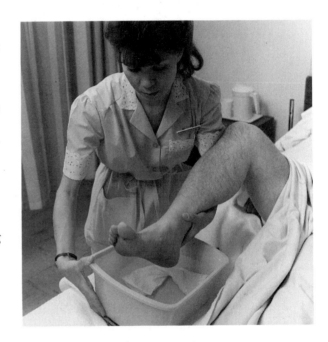

The skin tells much about the general health of the body. A fever may be indicated by hot, dry skin. Unusual redness (*rubra*) or flushing of the skin often follows a very warm bath. *Pallor* (less color than normal) is a sign associated with many conditions. The oxygen content of the blood can be noted quickly by the color of the skin. When the oxygen content is very low, the blood is darker and the skin appears bluish (*cyanotic*).

Structure and Function

The skin is one of the most important organs in the body. The integumentary system includes the skin and accessory structures: hair, nails, nerves, and sweat and oil glands, figure 26-1. The oil glands lubricate the hair. The sweat glands eliminate waste and control heat. The *epidermis*, the thick top layer of skin cells, is con-

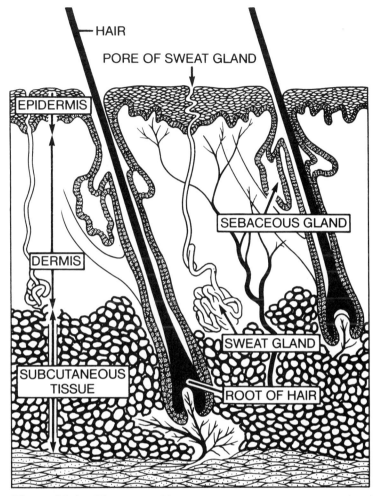

Figure 26-1 The normal integumentary system (From Hegner & Caldwell, *Assisting in Long-Term Care*, copyright 1988 by Delmar Publishers Inc.)

stantly being washed or worn away and renewed. The dermis lies directly under the epidermis and contains many blood vessels and nerve endings. It is sometimes called the true skin. Subcutaneous tissue, which is largely fat, lies directly under the dermis. Functions of the skin include:

- Protection: The healthy skin is a mechanical barrier to injury and disease. The constant shedding of the outer layer removes bacteria.

- Heat regulation: Many small blood vessels are present in the deeper part of the skin. When they *dilate* (become enlarged) with blood, heat is brought to the surface, where it escapes from the body. When heat needs to be conserved, these vessels *constrict* (become narrowed), thereby preserving heat within the body.
- Storage: Energy in the form of fat as well as some vitamins are stored in this vital area.
- Elimination: Some waste products as well as

excess water and salts are cast off (excreted) as perspiration through the activities of the sweat glands.

- Sensory perception: Many nerve endings are found in the skin. They quickly respond to external changes in heat, cold, pain, and pressure. This provides our sense of touch (*tactile* sense).

Senescent Changes

As a person ages, there are changes in the integumentary system, figure 26-2, just as there are changes in all the other parts of the body. These changes include:

1. The activity of the sweat glands decreases.
2. Loss of elasticity and fatty tissue causes wrinkling. The eyelids tend to drop and the skin is drier, as oil glands slow down their secretions.
3. Areas of pigmentation seem more pronounced. The skin takes on a more sallow or yellowish, less pink coloration. Skin tabs and moles are more common.
4. The hair loses its color, becoming first gray and then white. Less oil causes the hair to become dull and lifeless. The amount of hair, especially in men, diminishes.
5. Nails on both fingers and toes thicken, becoming more brittle. They often split.
6. Skin insulation is poorer.

In addition to normal changes due to aging, a number of pathological conditions can also affect the integumentary system. A few of the more common conditions are described in figure 26-2.

Nursing diagnostic categories relating to problems of the integumentary system are listed in table 26-1.

Skin Care

Cleanliness of the skin is essential. However, a daily bath for the older person is neither necessary nor advisable. In fact, most elderly are reluc-

- Altered nutrition
- Altered tissue perfusion
- Comfort alterations
- Impaired skin tissue integrity
- Potential for infection
- Self-care deficit
- Sleep pattern disturbances

Table 26-1   Nursing Diagnostic Categories Related to Integumentary Problems

tant to bathe daily. Aging skin has less oil. Dryness from frequent baths causes itching, sometimes referred to as *"bath itch,"* in which the skin develops pinpoint red spots. The skin of an elderly patient is easily damaged and takes a long time to heal because of inefficient general circulation.

Lotions should be applied to dry areas to protect them. Bath oils lubricate the skin but are dangerous because they make the bathtub slippery. It is better to apply lotions directly to dry areas.

Skin areas that touch must be kept free from perspiration and should not be allowed to rub together. Whenever moisture, perspiration, urine, or feces are present, skin breakdown is possible. After gently washing and drying local areas, a light dusting of powder or cornstarch is sufficient. Too much tends to cake and cause irritation.

Although a daily bath is unnecessary, frequent sponging of specific areas is necessary. The face, groin, underarms, and other body creases need regular cleaning and care. Elderly people tend to be sensitive to deodorants, so care should be used when applying them. Soaps may be drying. Superfatted soaps are less drying and less irritating to the skin of the elderly.

More skin tabs, moles, and warts become noticeable as the skin ages. Care must be taken not to disturb them. Any change in color, size, or texture should be reported immediately. Cancer of the skin, often seen in the elderly, has an excellent cure rate (93 percent) when treated early. Skin cancer tends to grow slowly and the cells tend not to spread. These lesions are usually

Condition	Description and Contributing Factors	Therapy and/or Nursing Care
Senile Keratosis	Found on exposed areas such as ears, hands, and lips. Flat or raised, gray to black in color. May be premalignant.	Biopsy and remove with freezing agents or cauterization. Routine postoperative care.
Basal Cell Epithelioma	Cancer of the skin, usually found on face, trunk, occasionally on the extremities. Lesion resembles a small nodule of varying size. It tends to break down (ulcerate) and then crust over. Slow growing and rarely spreads (metastasizes).	Removal by electro-dessication and curettage, X-radiation, and excision. Routine postoperative care.
Leukoplakia	White to silvery lesions found inside the mouth, on gums, tongue, and lips. Chronic irritation from smoking, poor dentition, and local infection contribute.	Soothing mouthwash such as Dobell's Solution. May need to be surgically removed and biopsied.
Onychomycosis	Fungal infection of the nails. Nails become thickened and deformed. Particularly common in diabetics.	Careful removal of the infected toenail. Application of ointments to break down the underlying overgrown tissue.
Pruritis (Itching)	Pruritis accompanies many types of skin conditions including allergies to food or chemicals or systemic problems such as renal or liver disease, diabetes, and infections. In addition, the dryness of the older skin makes it more sensitive to many contacts tolerated in youth. Scaling, redness, or rashes may be local or generalized.	Pruritis often responds poorly to therapy. Antipruritic powders, lotions, and colloidal baths may help. Tranquilizers, steroids, antihistamines and vitamins may be tried. Diversion therapy is a helpful nursing measure.
Stasis Dermatitis	Edema of the lower extremities leading to poor circulation and ischemia of the legs and feet. Skin becomes dry, pigmented, and cracked Itching and scratching lead to ulcerations (stasis ulcers).	Elevate legs. Check to be sure nothing interferes with circulation. Adequate fluids and nutrition are important.

Figure 26-2 Description and contributing factors for various conditions of the integumentary system

painless. Many derive from precancerous dermatosis. All skin lesions are suspect. The health care provider must be alert to follow through when changes are noted. The skin should be dried by patting gently rather than by rubbing. All contact with the skin must be gentle. Even pulling a sheet from under a patient too rapidly can cause trauma.

Bed baths clean the skin but are a rather passive activity for the patient. Therefore, a tub or shower bath is desirable two or three times a week to stimulate the patient. General safety factors and the patient's physical limitations should be considered before giving a tub or shower bath. Placement of handrails and availability of tub and shower seats or hydraulic lifts should be checked. Be sure you know how to use the hydraulic lift before trying to use one with the patient. Whirlpool baths can improve circulation and can be stimulating, figure 26-3. Warm baths

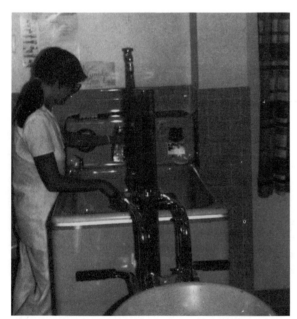

Figure 26-3 The whirlpool bath provides a stimulating means of cleaning the skin. (From Hegner & Caldwell, *Assisting in Long-Term Care*, copyright 1988 by Delmar Publishers Inc.)

may decrease cerebral circulation, which can lead to confusion. They may best be given just before the patient retires.

Refer to figure 26-4 for a review of beginning procedure actions and procedure completion actions.

Beginning Procedure Actions

- Wash your hands.
- Assemble all equipment needed.
- Knock on door and pause before entering resident's room.
- Politely ask visitors to leave. Tell them where they can wait.
- Identify the resident.
- Provide privacy by drawing curtains around bed and closing door.
- Explain what you will be doing and answer questions.
- Raise bed to comfortable working height.

Procedure Completion Actions

- Position resident comfortably.
- Leave signal cord, telephone, and fresh water where resident can reach them.
- Return bed to lowest horizontal position.
- Raise side rails, if required.
- Perform general safety check of resident and environment.
- Clean used equipment and return to proper storage, according to facility policy.
- Open privacy curtains.
- Wash your hands.
- Tell visitors that they may reenter the room.
- Report completion of procedure.
- Document procedure following facility policy.

Figure 26-4 Beginning procedure actions and procedure completion actions.

PROCEDURE 20

Assisting with the Tub Bath or Shower

1. Wash hands and assemble the following equipment:

soap	bath powder
washcloth	chair or stool
2–3 bath towels	gown, robe, and
bath blanket	slippers
bath thermometer	bathmat

2. Identify resident and explain what you plan to do.

3. Take the supplies to the bathroom and prepare them for the bath. Make sure the tub is clean.

4. Fill tub half full with water 95-105°F or adjust shower flow. If a bath thermometer is not available, test the water with an elbow. The water should feel comfortably warm.

5. Assist resident with robe and slippers.

6. Place a towel in the bottom of the tub to prevent slipping.

7. Help resident undress.

8. Assist the resident into the tub or shower.

9. Wash the back. Observe the skin for signs of redness or breaks. The resident may be left alone to wash the genitalia. If the patient shows signs of weakness, remove the plug and let the water drain out or turn off the shower. Allow the patient to rest until feeling better before assisting out of the tub or shower. Keep the resident covered with a bath towel to prevent chilling.

10. Hold the bath blanket around the person who is stepping out of the tub. A male resident may choose to remove wet towel under bath blanket.

11. Help the resident to dry, powder, dress, and return to the unit.

12. Return supplies to the unit.

13. Clean the bathtub. Wash hands.

14. Report completion of task to nurse.

15. Record on chart the date, time, tub bath/shower procedure, and resident's reaction.

PROCEDURE 21

Giving a Bed Bath

1. Wash hands and assemble the following equipment:

bed linen	gown or night
bath blanket	clothes
laundry bag or	alcohol or lotion,
hamper	powder
bath basin: on	equipment for oral
filling, the water	hygiene
should be 105°F	nail brush and
bath thermometer	emery board
soap and soap dish	brush and comb
washcloth	bedpan or urinal
face towel	and cover
bath towel	

2. Identify the resident and explain what you plan to do and how you can be assisted.

3. Make sure windows and door are closed to prevent drafts.

4. Screen the unit.

5. Put towels and linen on chair in order of use. Place laundry hamper conveniently.

6. Offer bedpan or urinal. Empty and clean before proceeding with bath. Wash hands.

7. Lower the back of the bed and the near side rails if permitted.

8. Loosen top bedclothes. Remove and fold blanket and spread. Place bath blanket over top sheet and remove sheet by sliding it out from under the bath blanket.

9. Leave one pillow under the head. Place other pillow on chair.

10. Remove night wear and place in laundry hamper.

11. Fill bath basin two-thirds full with 105°F water.

12. Help the resident move to the side of the bed nearest you.

13. Fold face towel over upper edge of bath blanket to keep it dry.

14. Form a mitten by folding washcloth around hand. Wet washcloth. Wash eyes, using separate corners of cloth. Do not use soap near eyes.

15. Rinse washcloth and apply soap if desired. Squeeze out excess water.

16. Wash and rinse the resident's face, ears, and neck well. Use towel to dry.

17. Expose far arm. Protect bed with bath towel placed underneath arm. Wash, rinse, and dry arm and hand. Repeat for other arm. Be sure axillae (armpits) are clean and dry. Apply deodorant and powder if requested or needed.

18. Wash each hand carefully. Rinse and dry. Push cuticle (base of fingernails) back gently with towel while wiping the fingers.

19. Clean under nails and shape with emery board. Be careful not to file nails too close. Do not cut nails if resident is diabetic. Inform the nurse if attention is needed.

20. Put bath towel over resident's chest and fold blanket to waist. Under towel, wash, rinse, and dry chest. Rinse and dry folds under breasts of female carefully to avoid irritating the skin. Powder lightly if necessary. Do not allow powder to cake.

21. Fold bath blanket down to pubic area. Wash, rinse, and dry abdomen. Fold bath blanket up to cover abdomen and chest. Slide towel out from under bath blanket.

22. Ask resident to flex knee if possible. Fold bath blanket up to expose thigh, leg, and foot. Protect bed with bath towel. Put bath basin on towel. Place resident's foot in basin. Wash and rinse leg and foot. When moving leg, support it properly.

23. Lift resident's leg and move basin to the other side of the bed. Dry leg and foot. Dry well between toes.

24. Repeat for other leg and foot. Take basin from bed before drying leg and foot.

25. Care for nails as necessary. Apply lotion to feet of patient with dry skin. File nails straight across. Do not round edges. Do not push back the cuticle because it is easily injured and infected.

26. Change water and check for correct temperature with bath thermometer. It may be necessary to change water before this point if it becomes cold.

27. Help resident to turn on side away from you and move toward the center of the bed. Place bath towel lengthwise next to patient's back. Wash, rinse, and dry neck, back, and buttocks. Use long, firm strokes when washing back.

28. A back rub is usually given at this time.

29. Help resident to turn on back.

30. Place a towel under the buttocks and upper legs. Place washcloth, soap, basin, and bath towel within convenient reach. Have person complete bath by washing genitalia. Assist if necessary. The geriatric health care provider must assume responsibility for the procedure if the patient has difficulty. People are often reluctant to acknowledge the need for help. If assisting a female, always wash from front to back, drying carefully. If assisting a male, be sure to carefully wash and dry penis, scrotum, and groin area.

31. Carry out range-of-motion exercises as ordered.

32. Cover pillow with towel and comb or brush hair. Oral hygiene is usually given at this time.

33. Discard towels and washcloth in laundry hamper.

34. Provide clean gown.

35. Clean and replace equipment according to facility policy.

36. Put clean washcloth and towels in bedside stand or hang according to policy.
37. Change the linen following occupied bed procedure. Discard soiled linen in laundry hamper.
38. Leave person in comfortable position. Place signal cord within reach. Replace furniture. Leave unit in order. Wash hands. Turn out ceiling light, if used.
39. Report completion of the tasks and any important observations to the nurse.

PROCEDURE 22

Giving a Back Rub

1. Wash hands and assemble the following equipment:

basin of water (105°F)	soap
	alcohol or lotion
bath towel	body powder

2. Tell the resident what you plan to do.
3. Screen the unit.
4. Place alcohol or lotion in basin of water to warm.
5. Turn the person on side with back toward you.
6. Expose and wash the back.
7. Pour a small amount of lotion into one hand. Apply to the skin and rub with a gentle but firm stroke. Give special attention to all bony prominences. Rubbing alcohol may also be used in some cases, if ordered by a physician.
8. Begin at the base of the spine and with long, soothing strokes rub up the center, around the shoulders, and down the sides of the back and buttocks. This procedure stimulates circulation over the bony prominences.

   a. Repeat this step four times, using the long, soothing upward stroke and a circular motion on the downstroke.

   b. Repeat, but on the downward stroke rub in a small, circular motion with the palm of the hand. Be sure to include area over coccyx.
   c. Repeat the long, soothing strokes to muscles for three to five minutes.
   d. Dry and apply powder.
   e. If pressure areas are noted, be sure to report to the nurse.
9. Straighten drawsheet.
10. Change the patient's gown if needed.
11. Replace equipment. Wash hands.

PROCEDURE 23

Giving a Partial Bath

Note: A partial bath is refreshing and assures cleaning of the hands, face, axillae, buttocks, and genitals. Many residents will be able to help with the process and should be encouraged to do so.

1. Wash hands and assemble the following equipment:

bed linen	alcohol or lotion,
bath blanket	powder
bath thermometer	equipment for oral
soap and soap dish	hygiene
washcloth	nail brush and
face towel	emery board
bath towel	brush, comb, and
gown	deodorant
laundry bag or	bedpan or urinal
hamper	and cover
bath basin with	paper towels or
water at 105°F	protector

2. Identify resident and explain what you plan to do.
3. Make sure windows and door are closed to prevent drafts.
4. Screen the unit.
5. Put towels and linen on chair in order of use. Place laundry hamper conveniently.

6. Offer bedpan or urinal. Empty and clean before proceeding with bath. Wash hands.
7. Elevate head rest, if permitted, to comfortable position.
8. Loosen top bedclothes. Remove and fold blanket and spread. Place bath blanket over top sheet and remove sheet by sliding it out from under the bath blanket.
9. Leave one pillow under the head. Place other pillow on chair.
10. Assist person to remove gown and place in laundry hamper.
11. Place paper towels or bed protector on overbed table.
12. Fill bath basin two-thirds full with water at 105°F and place on overbed table.
13. Push overbed table comfortably close.
14. Place towels, washcloth, and soap on overbed table within easy reach.
15. Instruct resident to wash as much as possible and say that you will return to complete the bath.
16. Place call bell within easy reach. Ask the person to signal when ready.
17. Wash hands and leave unit.
18. Wash hands and return to unit when patient signals.
19. Change the bath water. Complete bathing those areas the person couldn't reach. Make sure the face, hands, axillae, buttocks, back and genitals are washed and dried.
20. Give a back rub with lotion or alcohol and powder.
21. Assist the person in applying deodorant, powder, and a fresh gown.
22. Cover pillow with towel, and comb or brush hair. Assist with oral hygiene if needed.
23. Clean and replace equipment according to facility policy.
24. Put clean washcloth and towels in stand or hang according to facility policy.
25. Change linen following occupied bed procedure. Replace and discard soiled linen in laundry hamper.
26. Leave person in comfortable position with side rails up and bed in lowest horizontal position. Place signal cord within reach.
27. Replace furniture. Leave unit in order. Turn out ceiling light, if used.
28. Wash hands.
29. Report completion of task and any important observations to the nurse.

Oral Hygiene

The condition of the teeth affects the total health. Poor oral hygiene can result in loss of appetite and weight and be the focus of infection. Even if many teeth are missing, the remaining teeth should be cleaned regularly. Electric toothbrushes and waterpiks are relatively inexpensive. They do a good job when eyesight and hand manipulations are not dependable. Flossing should be a regular part of the regime.

Cavities should be given the same attention as they are in younger years. Regular dental checkups (four times a year) are essential. Unfortunately, neglect in early years leaves a large percentage of older people wearing dentures. Gum disease is the major reason that teeth are lost.

False teeth must be cleaned daily under running water with a brush especially made for this purpose. The older person should be cautioned to fill the washbowl half full of water so that if the teeth are dropped, there is less chance of breakage. Hot water and strong antiseptic solutions may injure dentures and should not be used. A place should be provided where they can safely be stored dry or in solution so they will not warp while out of the mouth. Denture wearers should routinely check their mouths and gums for signs of irritation. They should make periodic visits to the dentist to have the teeth checked and polished. Partial plates that are attached to the teeth on either side by small metal clips are removable. They should be given the same care as dentures. Be careful not to bend the clips. Lips should be inspected for excess dryness and fissures. These hygiene routines and observations are the responsibility of the health care provider when an individual is no longer able to do them.

Mouth care is important for the bed patient who is no longer able to maintain dentures in the mouth. A commercial mouthwash, a warm wash of saline and baking soda is refreshing if used before and after meals. Half-strength hydrogen peroxide can be used to removed dried secretions. Creams, petroleum jelly, or glycerin applied to the lips can prevent fissures from developing into deep sores and infections.

Eyes, ears, and nose should also be surveyed daily for any signs of irritation, redness, or excess dryness of the skin that could lead to breaks and fissures. Observations by staff members or self-observation by the patient should be part of routine care.

PROCEDURE 24

Brushing Teeth

1. Wash hands and assemble the following equipment:

toothbrush	paper bag
toothpaste or	bath towel
powder	drinking tube
mouthwash solution	tissues
in cup	cup of fresh water
emesis basin	

2. Identify resident and explain what you plan to do.
3. Screen the unit.
4. Raise back of bed so that the person may sit up if condition permits.
5. Place bath towel over gown and bed-covers.
6. Pour water over toothbrush and put toothpaste on brush. Insert toothbrush into the person's mouth with the bristles in a downward position. Turn toothbrush with bristles toward teeth and brush all tooth surfaces with an up-and-down motion.
7. Give resident water in cup to rinse mouth. Use straw if necessary. Turn the

head to one side with emesis basin near chin for return of fluid.
8. Repeat steps 6 and 7 as necessary. Offer mouthwash.
9. Remove basin. Wipe mouth and chin with tissue. Discard in paper bag.
10. Remove towel.
11. Rinse toothbrush with water.
12. Clean and replace equipment according to facility policy. Wash hands.

PROCEDURE 25

Assisting with Special Oral Hygiene

1. Wash hands and assemble the following equipment:

    mouthwash or solution in cup, or
    mixture of glycerin in lemon juice,
    or commercially prepared swabs
    bath towel
    paper bag
    applicators
    tissues
    tongue depressor
    lubricant for lips

2. Identify resident and explain what you plan to do.
3. Cover pillow with towel and turn the resident's head to one side. Place emesis basin under resident's chin.
4. Open mouth gently with tongue depressor.
5. Dip applicators into mouthwash solution or glycerin mixture. (In some cases, a physician may order hydrogen peroxide solution.)
6. Using moistened applicators, wipe gums, teeth, tongue, and inside of mouth.
7. Discard used applicators in paper bag.
8. Lubricate lips with cold cream or petroleum jelly.
9. Clean and replace equipment. Wash hands.

PROCEDURE 26

Assisting with Tooth Brushing

1. Wash hands and assemble the following equipment:

emesis basin	mouthwash (if
toothbrush	permitted)
toothpaste	hand towel
glass of cool water	bed protector

2. Identify resident and explain what you plan to do to help. Screen unit.
3. Elevate head of bed. Help person into a comfortable position.
4. Lower side rails and position overbed table across resident's lap.
5. Cover table with plastic protector.
6. Place emesis basin and glass of water on overbed table.
7. Place towel across patient's chest.
8. Be prepared to help as resident brushes teeth.
9. After resident has brushed teeth, push overbed table to foot of the bed. Remove towel, fold, and place on table. Help resident to assume a comfortable position and adjust bedding to leave the unit tidy.
10. Raise side rails.
11. Gather equipment. Clean and store according to facility policy. Discard soiled linen in proper receptacle.
12. Wash hands.
13. Report completion of task and your observations to the nurse.

PROCEDURE 27

Caring for Dentures

1. Wash hands and assemble the following equipment:

tissue	toothpaste or
emesis basin	powder
toothbrush or	gauze squares
denture brush	denture cup

2. Tell the resident what you plan to do.
3. Screen the unit.
4. Allow the person to clean dentures if able to do so. If not, present tissue and ask resident to remove dentures. Assist if necessary.
5. Place dentures in denture cup padded with gauze squares. Take to bathroom or utility room.
6. Put toothpaste or tooth powder on toothbrush. Place dentures in palm of hand and hold them under a gentle stream of warm water. Brush until all surfaces are clean.
   Note: Dentures may be soaked in a solution with a cleansing tablet before brushing, if necessary.
7. Rinse dentures thoroughly under cold running water. Rinse denture cup.
8. Place fresh gauze squares in denture cup. Place dentures in cup and take them to bedside.
9. Help resident to rinse mouth with mouthwash.
10. Use tissue or gauze to hand the wet dentures to resident. Insert if necessary.
11. Clean and replace equipment according to facility policy. Wash hands.
12. Store dentures in a denture cup inside the bedside stand when not in use. Some people prefer storing their dentures dry. Others prefer storing them in a special solution.

Facial Hair

Elderly women tend to have an increase in the growth and coarseness of the hairs on their chin and upper lip. This is distressing to many women who feel it defeminizes them. The hairs can be removed periodically with tweezers or, more permanently, professionally, with an electric needle. A mild bleach can also be used to lighten the hairs and make them less noticeable. Some women may require shaving. In some facilities, geriatric health care providers are not permitted to shave women residents. Be sure to check the policy of your facility and the preference of the resident.

Men need to shave or be shaved regularly, usually daily. It may be necessary to provide the equipment or to shave the older person. A rotary safety razor or electric razor is far safer then the straight razor that some elderly men are accustomed to using.

PROCEDURE 28

Shaving a Resident

1. Wash hands and assemble the following equipment:

electric shaver or   mirror
   safety razor   aftershave lotion or
shaving lather or   powder
   an electric pre-   basin of water
   shave lotion   (105°F)
face towel

2. Identify the resident and explain what you plan to do.
3. Screen unit.
4. Raise the head of the bed. Place equipment on overbed table.
5. Place face towel across resident's chest.
6. Moisten face and apply lather.
7. Starting in front of the ear, hold skin taut and bring razor down over cheek toward chin. Repeat until lather on cheek is removed and area has been shaved. Repeat on other cheek. Use firm, short strokes. Rinse razor frequently.
8. Lather neck areas and stroke up toward the chin in a similar manner.
9. Wash face and neck and dry thoroughly.
10. Apply aftershave lotion or powder if desired.
11. If the skin is nicked, apply pressure directly over the area and then an antiseptic. Report incident to nurse.
12. Clean and replace equipment. Wash hands.

Hand Care

Fingernails can be cleaned during the morning care period and should not be neglected. A soft brush and blunt-edged orangewood stick will clean the nails without causing injury. The hands can be soaked in warm water and the cuticles pushed back gently with a towel. Softening creams and olive oil soaks help to soften the cuticles. Fingernails should be cut and filed, following the contour of the fingertip. Care should be taken not to injure the corners. Improper cutting of fingernails and toenails is the biggest single cause of infections.

PROCEDURE 29

Giving Hand and Fingernail Care

Note: This procedure can be carried out independently or can be modified and incorporated with the bath procedure.

1. Wash hands and assemble the following equipment:

basin   plastic protector
soap   nail clippers
bath towel   nail file
lotion   orangewood stick

2. Identify resident and explain what you plan to do.
3. Screen unit.
4. Elevate head of bed, if permitted, and adjust overbed table in front of person. If allowed out of bed, help transfer to a chair and position overbed table waist high across lap.
5. Place plastic protector over the bedside table.
6. Fill basin with warm water approximately 105°F and place on overbed table.
7. Instruct person to put hands in basin and soak for approximately twenty minutes. Place towel over basin to help retain heat. Add warm water if necessary.

8. Wash hands. Push cuticles back gently with washcloth.
9. Lift hands out of basin and dry with towel.
10. Use nail clippers to cut fingernails straight across. Do not cut below tips of fingers. Keep nail clippings on protector to be discarded.
11. Shape and smooth fingernails with nail file.
12. Pour small amount of lotion in your palms and gently smooth on person's hands.
13. Empty basin of water. Gather equipment. Clean and store according to facility policy.
14. Return overbed table to foot of bed. If the person has been sitting up for the procedure, assist into bed.
15. Lower head of bed and make person comfortable. Leave call bell within easy reach. Make sure bed is in lowest position and side rails are up.
16. Leave unit tidy.
17. Wash hands.
18. Report completion of your task and any observations to the nurse.

Foot Care

Residents or those caring for them should be taught a basic routine of daily foot hygiene, figure 26-5. This should include careful washing and drying of the feet plus close inspection for any abnormalities. Lotions containing olive oil, lanolin, cocoa butter, or bland cream can be applied to dry, scaly skin. A light dusting of powder can be applied to perspiring feet. Do not apply cream or lotion between toes. The moisture will encourage microbial growth. Toenails should be kept trimmed and may require the services of a podiatrist. Toenails often grow thicker and have a tendency to become ingrown, figure 26-6. Small wisps of cotton under the nail can help redirect growth. Check facility policy concerning

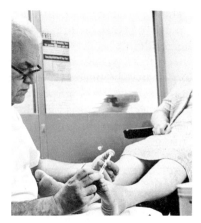

Figure 26-5 Aging feet require special care.

who can trim toe nails. Soak feet first or trim nails immediately after a tub bath.

Direct heat to lower extremities should be avoided. It increases cellular metabolism beyond that which aging circulation can maintain. Residents should be cautioned against self-care with commercial corn preparations, because severe trauma and infection may result.

Properly fitted shoes of a soft, pliant, porous texture, which are laced and have broad, low rubber heels, give the best support. The podia-

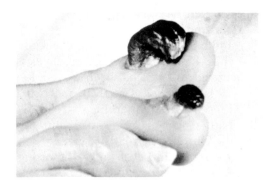

Figure 26-6 Toenail changes (Published from the *Journal of Practical Nursing*, October 1961, Practical Nursing II, with the permission of its publisher, the National Association of Practical Nurse Education and Service.)

trist may order well-fitting slippers that have cut-outs for painful conditions, and friction soles to prevent slipping, for some semiambulant patients.

PROCEDURE 30

Giving Foot and Toenail Care

1. Wash hands and assemble the following equipment:

wash basin	disposable bed
soap	protector
bathmat	bath towel/
lotion	washcloth
orangewood stick	

2. Identify resident and explain what you plan to do.
3. If resident is permitted, assist out of bed and into chair.
4. Place bathmat on floor in front of resident.
5. Fill basin with warm water (105°F). Put basin on bathmat.
6. Remove slippers and allow patient to place feet in water. Cover with bath towel to help retain heat.
7. Soak feet approximately twenty minutes. Add warm water as necessary. Lift feet from water while warm water is being added.
8. At end of soak period, wash feet with soap. Use washcloth to scrub roughened areas. Rinse and dry. Note any abnormalities such as corns, callouses, or nail irregularities.
9. Remove basin, covering feet with towel.
10. Use the orangewood stick to gently clean toenails. If nails are long and need to be cut, report this to the nurse. Do not undertake this task yourself.
11. Dry feet.
12. Pour lotion into palms of hands. Hold hands together to warm lotion and apply to feet.
13. Assist resident with slippers and to return to bed unless ambulatory.
14. Make resident comfortable.
15. Gather equipment, clean, and store according to facility policy. Leave unit tidy.
16. Wash hands.
17. Report completion of task and your observations to the nurse.

Hair Care

Hair care is important in maintaining personal appearance. Straggly, long, unclean hair makes anyone look unkempt. Hair should be brushed and arranged neatly. Consider the residents' preferences in hair styles to help maintain their individuality. Recognition of the relationship between neat appearance and high morale leads many care facilities to incorporate the services of a beautician and a barber into the basic cost of care. If they are not available, a family member or a volunteer can sometimes provide this service. The nurse is personally responsible for giving care or delegating the task to someone else.

An order is required for a shampoo to be given once or twice a month. An oil treatment will help correct the dryness of the hair before shampooing by lubricating the strands of hairs. A mild conditioning shampoo is best. A dryer will dry the hair quickly, decreasing the chance of chilling. The resident must be kept out of drafts while the hair is drying. Shampoos are most safely given in bed or, if the resident is seated, with use of a shampoo board.

PROCEDURE 31

Giving Daily Care of the Hair

1. Wash hands and assemble the following equipment:

towel	alcohol or petro-
comb and brush	leum jelly

2. Identify resident and ask resident to move to the side of the bed nearest you, or help sit in a chair if permitted.
3. Screen the unit.
4. Cover the pillow with a towel.
5. Part or section hair and comb with one hand between scalp and end of hair.
6. Brush carefully and thoroughly.
7. Have person turn so hair on the back of the head may be combed and brushed. If hair is snarled, apply alcohol to oily hair or petroleum jelly to dry hair as needed, working section by section. Unsnarl the hair beginning near the ends and working toward the scalp. Gum may be removed with ice.
8. Complete brushing and arrange attractively. Braid long hair to prevent repeated snarling.
9. Clean and replace equipment according to facility policy. Wash hands.
10. Report completion of task.

PROCEDURE 32

Giving a Bed Shampoo

1. Wash hands and assemble the following equipment and supplies:

   shampoo tray or plastic sheeting with the top and two sides rolled to drain

shampoo	large basin to collect used water
washcloths	hair dryer if available (portable)
three bath towels	
bath blanket	
basin of water (105°F)	small, empty pitcher or cup
safety pin	large pitcher of water (115°F) in case additional water is needed
two bed protectors	
waterproof covering for pillow	
hairbrush and comb	

2. Screen unit.
3. Identify resident and explain what you plan to do.

4. Place chair beside head of bed. Cover seat with bed protector. Place large, empty basin on chair.
5. Arrange on bedside stand within easy reach:

basin of water (105°F)	two bath towels
	shampoo
pitcher of water (115°)	empty pitcher
	washcloth

6. Replace top bedding with bath blanket.
7. Ask resident to move to side of bed nearest you.
8. Replace pillowcase with waterproof covering.
9. Cover head of bed with bed protector. Be sure to insert it well under the shoulders.
10. Loosen neck ties of gown.
11. Place towel under the person's head and shoulders. Brush hair free of tangles, working snarls out carefully.
12. Bring towel down around person's neck and shoulders and pin. Position pillow under shoulders so that head is tilted slightly backward.
13. Raise bed to high horizontal position.
14. Raise person's head and position shampoo tray so that drain is over the edge of bed directly above basin in chair.
15. Give person washcloth to cover eyes.
16. Recheck temperature of water in the basin. Using the small pitcher, pour a small amount of water over hair until thoroughly wet. Use one hand to direct the flow away from the face and ears.
17. Apply a small amount of shampoo, working up a lather. Work from scalp to hair ends.
18. Massage scalp with tips of fingers. Do not use fingernails.
19. Rinse thoroughly, pouring from hairline to hair tips. Direct flow into drain. Use water from pitcher if needed, but be sure to check temperature of water before use.
20. Repeat procedure a second time.
21. Lift person's head. Remove tray and bed

protector. Adjust pillow and slip a dry bath towel underneath head.

22. Place tray on basin and wrap hair in towel. Be sure to dry face, neck, and ears as needed.

23. Dry hair with towel. If available and not otherwise counterindicated, a portable hair dryer may be used to complete the drying. Brushing the hair as you blow it dry facilitates drying. Be sure to keep the dryer moving and not too close to the hair.

24. Comb hair appropriately. Remove protective pillow cover and replace with cloth cover.

25. Lower height of bed to comfortable working position.

26. Replace bedding and remove bath blanket. Help person into a comfortable position and lower bed to lowest horizontal position. Allow person to rest undisturbed. Length of procedure may tire patient.

27. Empty water from collection basin.

28. Clean equipment according to hospital policy and return to proper area.

29. Be sure unit is left in proper order. Wash your hands.

30. Record bed shampoo procedure and resident's reaction on chart.

Pressure Sores (Decubitus Ulcers or Dermal Ulcers)

Decubitus ulcers are sores that develop as a result of skin breakdown. They were previously called pressure sores, because unrelieved pressure contributes to their development. They are also known as *dermal ulcers*.

Decubitus ulcers are less apt to develop when geriatric health care providers actively work to prevent them. How much physical care is given to each patient depends upon the health care provider's role and function in a particular care unit. When being assisted in patient care by ancillary personnel, the nurse is still responsible for assuring that proper care is given. The prevention of decubiti is basic nursing care. The nurse must see that it is carried out properly, figure 26-7.

The average cost of treating decubitus ulcers runs into thousands of dollars annually and immeasurable misery for patients. An elderly person develops decubitus ulcers more quickly than a younger one does. There are several reasons for this, figure 26-8. The elderly are apt to be generally debilitated. When tissues are malnourished, decubiti develop much more rapidly. Circulation in old people is often less than adequate and the older person is generally less active.

Development of Decubiti

Decubiti develop when tissue is trapped between a surface such as a mattress or chair frame and a bony prominence such as the ankle or heel. Circulation is impeded by the pressure, which collapses the tiny blood vessels. The tissues quickly break down because the cells, lacking nourishment, can no longer live.

Even when patients are sitting in a wheelchair or in semi-Fowler's position in bed, shearing force slows the circulation to vulnerable points. *Shearing force* occurs as the weight of the torso and gravity tend to pull deep tissues such as muscle and bone in one direction while the skin held in place by linen tends to remain stationary. The result is a tension on blood vessels and a decrease in nourishment to the area. Try to limit the time in Fowler's position. Shearing force can also occur when patients dig their heels in as they are pulled to the head of the bed, when permitted to slump in the chair or bed, or when the head of the bed is too high. It is better not to elevate the head of the bed more than 30°. Encourage chairbound patients to push up from the chair every ten minutes.

The entire health care staff must watch carefully for signs that a decubitus ulcer may be developing. This observation is very important. The sites most likely to be involved are the anterior iliac crests, the hips, sacrum, scapulae, heels,

MOBILITY amount and control of body movement	**1. Immobile:** can't change position without help; dependent on others for movement	**2. Very limited:** offers minimal help in changing position; may have contractures, paralysis	**3. Slightly limited:** can control and move extremities, but still needs help changing position	**4. Full:** can control and move extremities at will; may need device, but can lift, turn, pull, balance, and sit up at will
ACTIVITY ability to walk	**1. Bedfast:** confined to bed	**2. Chairfast:** walks only to chair, with help, or confined to wheelchair	**3. Walks with help:** can walk with help of another, or with crutches, braces; possibly can't handle stairs	**4. Walks independently:** can rise from bed and walk without help; or with cane or walker can walk without help of another
NUTRITION quality of food intake	**1. Poor:** rarely eats complete meal; is dehydrated; has minimal fluid intake	**2. Fair:** occasionally refuses to eat, or leaves large portions of a meal; must be encouraged to take fluids	**3. Good:** eats some food from each basic food category every day; drinks 6-8 glasses of fluid a day; eats major portions of each meal, or is receiving tube feedings	
SKIN APPEARANCE observed skin characteristics	**SKIN TONE** degree of turgor and tension, determined by pinch at high-risk sites for pressure sores	**SKIN SENSATION** response to tactile stimuli	COMMENTS:	

Source: Davina J. Gosnell, RN, PhD, Copyright 1973 by the American Journal of Nursing Company. Reproduced with permission from *Nursing Research*, vol. 22, no. 1, January/February 1973.

Figure 26-7   Assessing a patient's potential for pressure sores

- Poor nutrition
- Immobilization
- Debilitation
- Poor circulation
- Edema
- Infection
- Aging
- Diminished reflexes
- Moisture/excessive dryness
- Prolonged pressure

Figure 26-8 Risk factors for decubiti formation

and shoulders, figure 26-9. Pressure areas can develop in different parts of the body, depending on position. For example, lying in a prone position could lead to the development of decubiti on the forehead or ear. A side-lying (Sims') position could lead to decubiti over the greater trochanter of the femur and the lateral maleolus

of the tibia. Improperly fitting braces, restraints, nasogastric tubes, oxygen tubes, and urinary catheters can also be sources of irritation, pressure, and breakdown.

Decubiti develop from friction burns as well. Skin surfaces should not be allowed to rub together. They will quickly break down, giving rise to ulcerations. This is especially true of moist surfaces, such as those between the legs and the buttocks and under breasts. The skin becomes macerated when in contact with urine, feces, and perspiration.

Signs of Tissue Breakdown

Tissue breakdown occurs in three stages. Nursing intervention at each stage can limit the process and prevent further damage.

In *Stage I*, the skin develops a redness or blue-gray discoloration over the pressure point. In darker-skinned people, the area may appear drier. If, after peripheral massage and relief of pressure, the blush has not subsided, it is probably the beginning of a decubitis. This first stage of redness is usually reversible if conscientious effort is made to alleviate the pressure. Refer to figure 26-10A.

In *Stage II*, the skin is reddened and there are blister-like lesions over the area, figure 26-10B. Sometimes the epidermis will be broken. The area around the breakdown site may also be reddened.

In *Stage III*, the process has advanced to deeper tissue breakdown, figure 26-10C. Ulceration may be so extensive that eventually the underlying bone may be visible. The figure shows the stages of breakdown and appropriate nursing care actions.

A constant assessment of the breakdown includes measuring the size of the area, figure 26-11, and of observing and evaluating the extent of healing. Frequently, photographs of the area are taken and are included in the chart as part of the documentation, figure 26-12. Documentation of progress is made weekly.

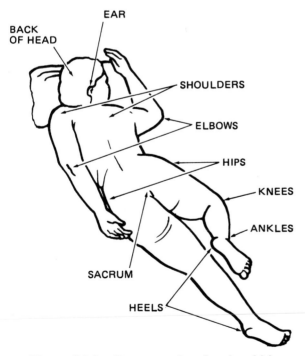

Figure 26-9 Common sites for decubiti

Stage   Nursing Care Actions
  I

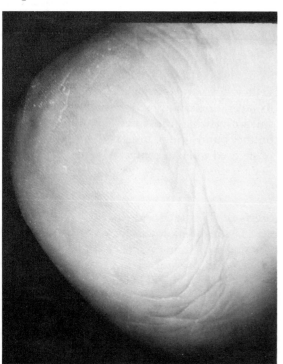

Remove pressure, gently massage around outside of affected area. Notify the nurse. Promote
adequate nutrition and fluids.

II

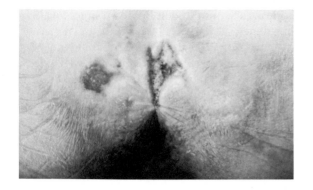

Gently massage outside broken area. Wash area
with a bacteriostatic agent. Keep breakdown area
clean and dry. Use mechanical aids as directed to
relieve pressure. Keep breakdown area covered
as ordered. Promote adequate nutrition and
fluids. Carry out treatments such as heart lamp,
as ordered. Notify the nurse of observations and
care.

Stage
III

Nursing Care Actions

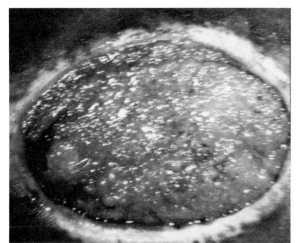

Continue care as for stage II. Apply debridgement ointments, pack and dress as ordered. Assist patient to whirlpool as ordered. Notify nurse of observations and care.

Figure 26-10   Decubitus formation and nursing actions
(Courtesy Emory University Hospital, Atlanta, GA.)

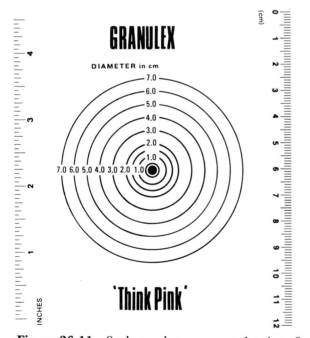

Figure 26-11   Scale used to measure the size of the area of breakdown. (Courtesy Don B. Hickam Inc.)

Prevention of Decubiti

In order to prevent decubiti, you must be alert to avoid those situations that contribute to their development. Nursing measures include encouraging proper nutrition and adequate fluids, keeping linens dry and free of wrinkles, and encouraging position changes. To prevent decubiti, position must be changed often, at least once every two hours, preferably once an hour. Research seems to indicate that the critical time for action is between one and two hours. It is not enough to help a patient out of bed and then allow the patient to remain sitting in a chair for the remainder of the day. Patients who must remain in bed require extra vigilance. This includes at least a minimum of position changes and regular range-of-motion exercises. Patients who can participate in their own skin care should be encouraged to do so even if their participation is only to the extent of explaining their needs to a health care provider.

Geriatric patients are often too weak or confused to make the necessary changes in position

DECUBITUS ULCER: To be assessed upon admission and every 7 days or PRN thereafter per Nursing Policy.

☐ DECUBITUS ULCER (SIZE, SITE, STAGE)

☐ PICTURE TAKEN BY:

USE DIAGRAMS TO SHOW SIZE, SITE, STAGE

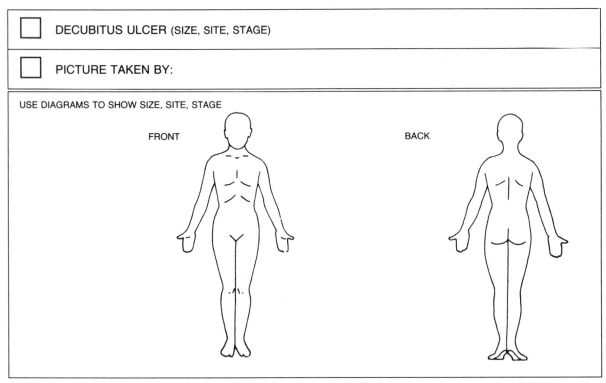

FRONT   BACK

Figure 26-12   Documentation of dermal ulcers is made on the patient's chart in words, pictures, and diagrams.

to relieve pressure. Many elderly patients tolerate the prone position with relative comfort, figure 26-13. But an individual turning regime needs to be developed that recognizes particular needs. Problems are often encountered when health care providers try to turn elderly patients regularly. Physical incapacities such as emphysema limit the positions that can be maintained. A paraplegic patient remains in position once aligned, when pillows are used for support. But confused elderly patients do not always remain quiet once positioned.

Health care providers need to recognize that changing a patient's position regularly in some geriatric units is difficult and time consuming but necessary. When staffing is short, health care providers may be frustrated in their attempts to

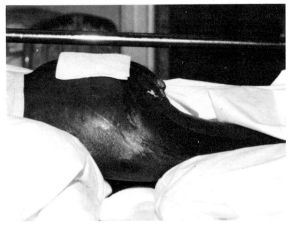

Figure 26-13   Bridging is a technique used to relieve pressure as the person is in the prone position.

give good nursing care when it is physically impossible. Fear of waking others in the unit when patients are uncooperative or resist and cry out makes some staff members reluctant to change patient's positions during the night. No excuse is being offered for failure to carry out turning assignments, merely an explanation of facts as they exist. It is important that all staff members appreciate the importance of turning so that a cooperative effort can be made.

Mechanical Aids

Nursing staffs must explore new ways of relieving pressure and be willing to try new techniques that offer promise. Over the past two decades, a great many mechanical devices have been developed in hopes of preventing or treating bedsores. These can be of great value, especially when used preventatively.

Pads   Sheepskin and artificial sheepskin pads provide a soft surface between patient and bottom bed linen, figure 26-14. They reduce friction and absorb moisture. However, they do not allow air to circulate, and pressure against them is constant. The artificial pads are in common usage. Incontinence is a problem unless an in-

dwelling catheter is in place. If an incontinence pad must be placed between the patient and the sheepskin pad, the advantage of the sheepskin is lost. Incontinence means frequent laundering, but indwelling catheters are avoided in the elderly unless there are no better alternatives. Although the sheepskin is helpful, it is not the total answer.

Padding can be used to relieve pressure, figure 26-15. Bridges can be formed with it to relieve pressure in specific areas. Highly inflated rings or cotton "doughnuts" are no longer used. They relieve pressure on the bony prominence in their center, but they create a ring of pressure themselves. Silicone gel pads, the consistency of fatty tissue, are another type of protective device. When they are placed under the patient, they conform to the body contours, distributing the body weight more evenly. Bed cradles can be used to keep the weight of the bedding off the patient's body, figure 26-16.

Mattresses   Various types of mattresses have been developed in hopes of decreasing pressure or at least equalizing it. Such mattresses include the alternating air pressure mattress, the water

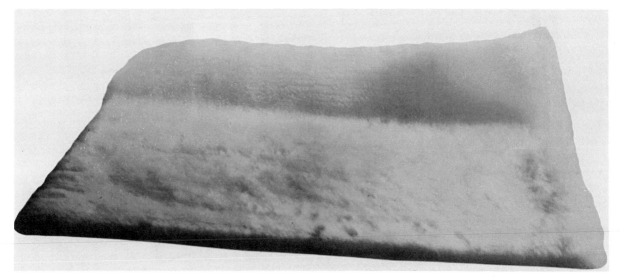

Figure 26-14   Sheepskin or artificial sheepskin pads are used to protect bony areas.

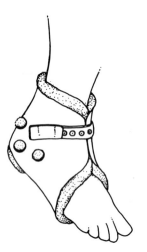

Figure 26-15 Specialized pads, such as the heel protector, also provide cushioning of bony prominences.

mattress or flotation unit, the egg crate mattress, and a unit that sends warm air through fine sand in the mattress. The weight of the patient's body is distributed so that pressure against the body is equalized. Shutting the unit off allows the patient's body to sink into a shallow well so that turning the patient and changing linens is easier.

Other mattresses have been developed for long-term use, such as the Mediscus™ low-air-loss therapy system, figure 26-17. Each system has the major focus of reducing the incidence of pressure areas that could lead to skin breakdown. These mattresses mold to the contours of the body, equalizing pressure over a wide area.

The alternating pressure mattress is similar in structure to the beach air mattress. It is motorized so that alternating cells are inflated for specific periods, figure 26-18. It is placed on a regu-

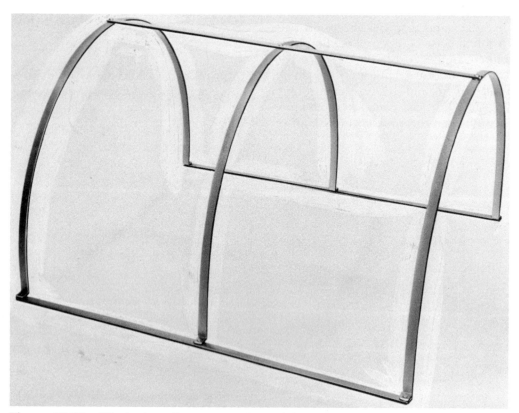

Figure 26-16 The bed cradle prevents the weight of the bedding from falling on the body. It must be padded so that no hard or rough edges touch the patient.

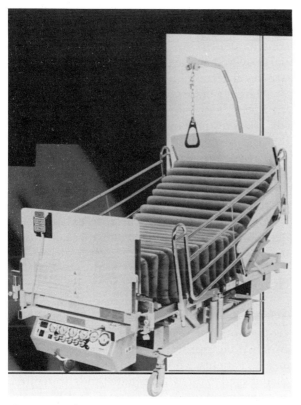

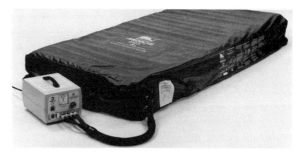

Figure 26-18B Auto-Matt™ mattress is a low-air-filled mattress that can maintain a constant below-capillary filling pressure or may automatically cycle different pressure every ten minutes. (Courtesy The Mediscus Group)

Figure 26-17 This low-air-loss therapy support system allows multiple position changes for the immobile patient. It has a patented air inlet/outlet valve creating an optimum environment to prevent pressure sores and to promote healing. (Courtesy The Mediscus Group)

lar mattress base and must be carefully monitored to make sure that the motor continues to function and the individual cells remain intact. One of the most common mattresses in use is the egg-crate mattress, figure 26-19. This has proved quite successful.

Flotation units, figure 26-20, have a waterproof mattress filled with water. The mattress is contained within a frame for stability. Most patients find the water bed quite comfortable. However, they require a gradual introduction to the feeling of weightlessness. Elderly patients on flotation mattresses must be watched carefully for signs of confusion and disorientation that might be brought on by the weightless feeling.

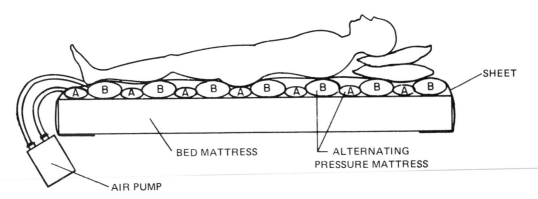

SECTIONS A AND B ALTERNATELY INFLATE EVERY 5 MINUTES

Figure 26-18A Air mattresses are used to relieve pressure on bony prominences.

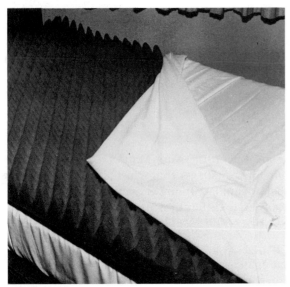

Figure 26-19 Egg crate mattress. (From Hegner & Caldwell, *Assisting in Long-Term Care,* copyright 1988 by Delmar Publishers Inc.)

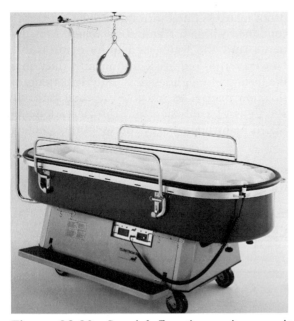

Figure 26-20 Special flotation units permit more even distribution of body weight, reducing the potential for tissue breakdown. (Courtesy Support Systems Inc.)

Body temperature has to be maintained. Range-of-motion exercises must be carried out conscientiously. Adequate fluid intake is essential to overcome the possibility of urine stasis and urinary infection.

The egg crate mattress is gaining in popularity. It evenly distributes the body weight over its surface and still allows air to circulate. Make sure that the pointed side of the crate faces the patient's body. Egg crate pads are also used to protect ankles, heels, and elbows.

These aids are only an adjunct to, not a substitute for, good nursing to prevent and care for decubitus ulcers. Much more experience is needed to completely evaluate these forms of therapy before they are generally available.

Nutrition

Breakdown occurs more readily and healing is delayed when the patient is poorly nourished. Proper nutrition may require tube feedings with enriched high-protein and high-vitamin supplements. Patients who are able to eat should be encouraged to do so. Adequate fluids are a must.

Serum albumin, hematocrit, and hemoglobin levels are important laboratory values in assessing nutritional status.

Treatment of Decubiti

If, in spite of all efforts, decubitus ulcers do develop, prompt attention is needed. Pressure areas must be relieved, using any of the aids available. If the area is reddened but not opened, the outer circumference is gently massaged to stimulate circulation. The patient should be placed on an egg crate mattress. The area can be covered by a porous skin barrier, such as a hydrocolloid dressing. The area must not be rubbed hard. Alcohol is not recommended because it has a drying and vasoconstrictive effect, making the skin more ischemic. A decrease in flow of blood to the skin must be avoided so the position must be changed at least every two hours. Heat lamps may be ordered. Do not permit plastic to come into contact with the skin.

Once the skin is broken, other measures

should be taken. The affected area can be washed with a bacteriostatic agent such as pHisohex™, CaraKlenz™, or Biolex™ wound cleanser. To inhibit infections, the wound is irrigated with hydrogen peroxide, Dakins solution (0.5 percent bleach), or acetic acid (0.25 percent vinegar). Antiseptic sprays have also proved of value in controlling infection. Antibiotic ointments are used if there is a low-grade infection and the area is protected with a dressing. Elase ointment, Biozyme ointment, or some other proteolytic preparation such as Santyl or Travase may be applied if local *debridement* (removal of dead tissue) is needed. Salt solutions, sugar and glycerin, Gelfoam sponges, and gold leaf are other materials sometimes applied directly to the lesion. Sugar and glycerin or Maalox are applied as a paste. These substances stimulate the development of healthy granulative tissue in the ulcer itself and decrease the toxicity of secondary invaders.

In some facilities, open lesions (Stage III) are packed loosely with gauze soaked in Carrington gel. The gel keeps the lesion moist, which promotes self-debridement and healing. The packing is kept moist by being covered with a hydrocolloid such as a thin sheet of Duoderm™ or Tegaderm®. The dressing must extend one inch beyond the wound edges and is held in place by a frame of either paper tape or silk tape, figure 26-21. The dressing must be changed every 3-5 days unless there is leakage.

Techniques that promote healing include exposure to ultraviolet radiation, air, and sunshine, and low concentrations of oxygen. These techniques have all demonstrated some value in the treatment of decubiti. Whirlpool therapy and ultrasonic sound promote circulation and help clean the lesion.

Sometimes it is necessary to surgically debride large lesions and to perform a graft to repair the lesion. Care must be taken in securing dressings. The elderly are more apt to be sensitive to regular tape. Cellophane tape, silk tape, paper tape, and elastoplast seem less irritating. The geriatric health care provider must remem-

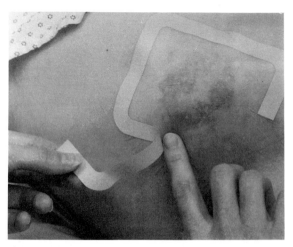

Figure 26-21   Special coverings protect areas of skin breakdown. (Courtesy 3M Health Care)

ber to loosen dressings with saline before removing them to avoid traumatizing the underlying tissue.

When more conservative methods fail to bring closure of ulcerations, debridement and skin grafting may be needed. Daily debridement is sometimes carried out for small areas and to prepare larger areas for grafting. In surgery, large decubiti are excised back to the healthy tissue and then closed with flap grafts, figure 26-22. It is essential that there be no pressure on the surgical area during healing. An effort must be made to increase the patient's appetite and improve overall condition. A high-protein diet will provide the nutrients necessary for tissue healing. It is believed that the negative nitrogen balance found in so many elderly people contributes to the formation of decubiti.

Remember that the elderly skin is very fragile. Skin tears (breaks in skin continuity) occur frequently in patients in extended care facilities. These are areas that must be protected. Bio-occlusive dressings such as Opsite or Duoderm™ can be used over these sites. These dressings can be seen through so that the condition of the lesion can be observed while the area is still protected.

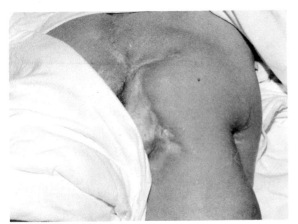

Figure 26-22 Areas of scarring following surgery (grafting) to close deep decubiti.

Summary

- As skin ages it becomes thinner, drier, less supple, more subject to injury, and less able to heal.
- Basic hygiene helps to protect the skin and its appendages.
- Any change in a skin lesion should be reported immediately.
- Decubitis ulcers begin as skin lesions and enlarge to involve deeper tissues.
- Decubiti are more easily prevented than cured.
- The elderly person, more susceptible to skin breakdown, must be protected by vigilant nursing care.
- A high-protein diet is important to provide the essential nutrients needed for healing.

Review Outline

   I. Behavioral Objectives

  II. Vocabulary

 III. The Integumentary System

      A. Structure
      B. Function

 IV. Senescent Changes

  V. Common Conditions

      A. Senile keratosis
      B. Basal cell epithelioma
      C. Leukoplakia
      D. Onychomysosis
      E. Pruritus
      F. Stasis dermatitis

 VI. Basic Care

      A. Skin
          1. Bathing
          2. Back rubs
      B. Oral hygiene
          1. Brushing teeth
          2. Special oral hygiene
          3. Denture care

        C.   Facial hair
        D.   Foot and toenail care
        E.   Hair care

VII.   Decubitus Ulcers

        A.   Contributing factors
        B.   Prevention
            1.   Mechanical aids
            2.   Pads and mattresses
        C.   Assessment
        D.   Treatment

Review

  I. Vocabulary

Word Search

Look at the word wheel. Identify five words from the vocabulary and write their definitions.

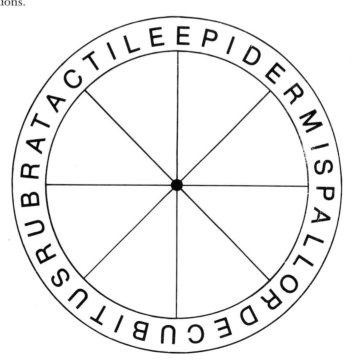

Definitions

    1. _____

    2. _____

    3. _____

    4. _____

    5. _____

II. Short Answers

1. Does the skin of an elderly person tend to be dry or oily, or neither?
2. What are the results of inadequate oral hygiene?
3. Why does a denture wearer still need to visit the dentist?
4. For safety, how should elderly people be positioned while having a shampoo?
5. Why is an elderly person more susceptible than a younger one to the development of decubitus ulcers?
6. Briefly describe the following:
    a. gel pad
    b. air mattress
    c. sheepskin
    d. water bed
    e. egg crate mattress
7. Why does shearing force tend to cause decubiti?
8. Why is it best not to use soap too freely on the elderly skin?
9. Why is lotion applied to the feet, but not between the toes?
10. Why are elderly people at great risk for the development of decubiti?

III. Clinical Situations

1. You notice an area of redness around a darkened skin lesion on a patient's skin. What do you do?
2. You have applied a dry sterile dressing over an open decubitus ulcer and need to secure it in place. What do you use?
3. Your patient's daughter asks why her father is not given a daily bed bath. What do you say?

CASE STUDY

Ralph Washington, an eighty-six-year-old male, had been a railroad worker for many years. He could tell many colorful stories about the days when the railroads were linking the oceans.

A year ago, he had fallen, breaking his left hip just below the greater trochanter. Unfortunately, he had been hurt when alone on the small farm in Georgia where he had been living since his retirement with another old friend. He had lain for two days before his friend found him and managed to get medical aid.

The fracture was compound. It healed poorly despite surgery and a prolonged period in traction.

On admission to the rehabilitation facility, a serious pressure area was noted over his sacrum, and his nutritional status seemed poor. His dark, leathery skin was in sharp contrast to the oozing, pink, draining ulceration on his back. Mr. Washington seemed depressed, with little interest in his future.

In the team conference, three immediate problems were identified:

1. Lack of motivation
2. Limited mobility
3. Decubitus ulcer

After discussion, it was determined that Juliette Potter, a geriatric health care provider, would be assigned, with a primary nurse, to Mr. Washington's care. Ms. Potter was chosen because her father worked for AMTRAK. It was hoped that the common tie with railroads might help Mr. Washington's depression and increase his motivation to become ambulatory again.

Range-of-motion exercises and special physiotherapy plans were instituted by the consulting physiotherapist.

The primary nurse outlined a routine of care to promote healing of the decubitus area. She also reviewed Mr. Washington's nutritional status with the dietitian. He was started on a high-protein diet with vitamin supplements.

The decubitus ulcer regime included:

1. Position on egg crate mattress
2. Position changes every hour
3. Area around decubitus to be washed with a bacteriostatic agent
4. Biozyme ointment for debridement
5. Exposure of area to low-level oxygen
6. Dry sterile dressings to be applied between treatments (secured with paper tape)

Mr. Washington responded both emotionally and physically to attentive nursing care. Although the decubitus began to respond, the area was too extensive to heal easily. Skin grafting became necessary.

Eventually, Mr. Washington was discharged to the Lakeview Rest Home, a short distance from the facility. He had become good friends with Ms. Potter, who promised to make frequent visits.

1. Name two major factors that limited Mr. Washington's healing power.
2. What three problems were identified?
3. List five techniques planned to heal the ulceration.

Unit 27
Musculoskeletal System Alterations

Objectives
After studying this unit, you should be able to:
- Name the parts of the musculoskeletal system and their functions.
- List the terms used to describe body movements.
- Describe senescent changes in bone, joints, and muscle.
- List the problems that result from sedentary living.
- Explain the hazards of immobility.
- Describe common musculoskeletal problems of the aged: osteoporosis, osteoarthritis, and rheumatoid arthritis.

Vocabulary
Learn the meaning and spelling of the following words or phrases.

abduction		
adduction		
alignment		
arthritis		
atrophy		
bunions	kyphosis	pannus
contract	lordosis	plantar flexion
crepitation	hallus valgus	podigeriatrics
dorsiflexion	Herberden's Nodes	rotation
extension	hypertrophy	sedentary
flatfoot	mobility	synovium
flexion	osteoporosis	tonus
hammertoes	palmar flexion	

Some elders are typical "pictures" of the pervasive effects of aging on the musculoskeletal system, figure 27-1. Muscles and bones shape and protect the body. As a person ages, however, body-shape changes and the body may be less protected. Muscles waste, bones thin, cartilage

434

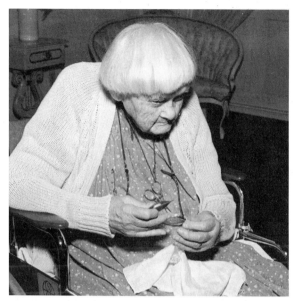

Figure 27-1 Postural changes become evident as the musculoskeletal system undergoes aging. Osteoporosis and loss of bone mass can cause marked changes.

compresses, and joints wear out. Senescent changes are listed in figure 27-2. When these changes occur, a person generally looks hunched over, potbellied, and frail. The elderly person may also walk more slowly and cautiously, and seem precariously balanced.

The most common physical problem among elders involves the musculoskeletal system. At least 80 percent of people sixty-five years and older have some problem in this system. Unfor-

---

- Loss of muscle tone and strength
- Increase in intramuscular fat
- Glycogen (energy) storage diminished
- Response to stimuli lessened
- Smooth muscle walls of organs lose strength
- Disks (pads) between vertebrae thin
- Rib cage more rigid
- Bone more porous and brittle

Figure 27-2 Senescent changes in the musculoskeletal system

tunately, many believe that all the changes they are experiencing are the result of aging and may delay seeking help. Some aches, pains, and fatigue are due to aging. Often, however, there is an underlying problem that can be diagnosed and treated to make an elder's life more comfortable and, above all, keep the older person mobile. Independence in activities of daily living is based on mobility (review B.A.D.L. and I.A.D.L. in Unit 11). Mobility is based on maintaining structure, functioning efficiently, and conserving energy.

Skeletal muscles stretch over joints. When these muscles are stimulated by nerves, they shorten *(contract)*, pulling two bones closer together. Many blood cells are also produced within the living bone tissue. When muscles, bones, or joints have been injured or fatigued, a period of rest and inactivity may be required for the part to heal. During this period, it is important that all other uninjured parts receive sufficient exercise.

Structure and Function

Bones

There are 206 bones in the body. Learn the name and general location of each bone. This is not as difficult as it may seem. Look at a skeleton, figure 27-3. You immediately see that if a line is drawn down the center, there are the same number and kinds of bones on each side. Already, the number of bones to be learned has been cut in half. Further examination shows that there are 12 ribs on each side, making a total of 24 bones, all called ribs.

Many structures within the body take their name from the name of the closest bone. The femoral artery runs close to the femur (the thigh bone). The radial artery that is used to take the pulse lies beside the radius (one of the lower arm bones). Bones are not all alike. Some are long, some short, some flat, and some irregular in shape.

Pay special attention to bones of the wrist, hip, and spine and to the long bones, especially those of the legs. The bones of the wrist, hip, and

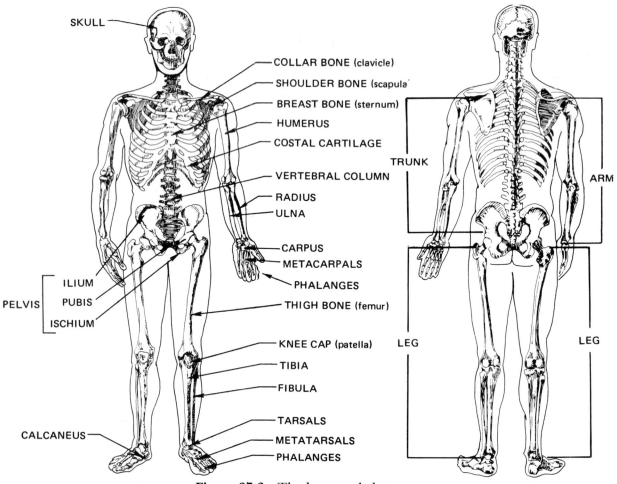

Figure 27-3   The human skeleton

spine are different from other bones. They are not as strong and lose more bone with aging. Older people are more at risk for fractures of these bones. The long bones maintain their strength by weight bearing. Therefore, it is essential for people to walk, to be mobile, even just to stand for periods of time, to keep the calcium in these bones.

Bones also serve a very protective purpose such as shielding the brain, heart, lungs, and kidneys. Muscles and joints help form our shapes and allow us to walk upright instead of slithering or oozing about.

Joints

Joints are points of possible movement. Several kinds of body movements are possible because not all joints are formed in the same way. The elbow joints and knee joints work like a door hinge, in that they bend in only one direction. The arm-shoulder and thigh-hip joints can move in a complete circle, like a ball and socket. The bones of the wrists, ankles, and spine have a more limited gliding type of motion. Bones are held together at the joints by bands of fibrous tissue called ligaments. Ligaments keep the bones of the joints in the proper relationships *(alignment).*

Muscles

There are more than 500 muscles in the body, and they work in groups. Skeletal muscles are attached to bones by tendons. They are called voluntary because the person can consciously control them. Other muscles, called involuntary or visceral muscles, form the walls of organs. These muscles operate without conscious control. An "automatic" center in the brain controls these muscles through special nerves.

Muscles receive their names in three ways: from their location, shape, or action. The major muscle groups responsible for an activity are easily located if the following points are remembered:

- Muscles can only shorten (contract) and lengthen (relax). Contraction occurs when nerves bring the message (stimulus) to the muscle cells. Although muscles relax when there is no stimulus, there is always a degree of *tonus.* Tonus is a normal state of partial muscle contraction which is maintained in healthy functioning muscles.
- Muscles have two points of attachment to the bone. As they stretch from one point (origin) to the other (insertion), they cross over one or more joints.
- As muscles contract they shorten, pulling their points of origin and insertion closer together. To bend the forearm at the elbow, the biceps muscle on the anterior upper arm, extending from the shoulder to below the elbow, contracts. At the same time the triceps muscle, which is attached to the posterior shoulder and to the arm below the elbow, relaxes. To straighten the arm at the elbow, the triceps contracts while the biceps stretches (relaxes).
- Muscles that are exercised increase in strength and size *(hypertrophy),* and those unused shrink and weaken *(atrophy).*

Muscles that are not exercised atrophy. In this country, *sedentary* (non-physically active) living has been identified as contributing to weakness in old age. Loss of muscle strength affects mobility and, in turn, the ability to carry out activities of daily living. Older women in particular tend to lose upper body strength from lack of exercise. For elders, atrophied muscles and an illness may mean prolonged time spent in extended care facilities or permanent long-term care.

Terms of Movement

Special terms are used to describe movements. You will hear these terms as you care for patients with orthopedic conditions, any long-term illness, and decreased mobility.

- *Flexion:* decreasing the angle between two bones
- *Extension:* increasing the angle between two bones
- *Rotation:* circular motion in a ball-and-socket joint
- *Abduction:* moving away from midline
- *Adduction:* moving toward midline
- *Plantar flexion:* pointing the toes and foot downward
- *Dorsiflexion:* pulling the toes and foot toward the knee; bending or cocking the wrist upward
- *Palmar flexion:* bending the wrist downward

Importance of Being Mobile

When a person is able to move about *(mobility),* either alone or with assistance, a vital first step has been taken in maintaining independence or in the rehabilitation process. Mobility, or lack of it, affects both physical functions and morale. The person who is able to be up and moving enjoys a degree of independence and a sense of well-being. That person is also able to participate in social occasions and other activities that contribute to overall adjustment.

All too often, a patient is considered mobile when able to walk across a room. True mobility means being able to negotiate stairs and bus steps and perform the usual activities associated with daily living. A person may be able to carry out many daily living activities and still be house-bound. Street curbs, bus steps, or stairs are often insurmountable obstacles. Many states are passing legislation to remove or reduce architectural barriers. For example, they are mandating building and sidewalk ramps.

Walking is probably the best exercise that the elderly person can engage in, because it exercises large muscle groups. Whenever possible, regular walking should be encouraged.

Ambulation

Wheelchairs, walkers, figure 27-4, canes, and crutches all aid mobility. Each appliance must be kept in good repair. Wheelchair supports should maintain proper alignment, figure 27-5, with the person's hips well back and the trunk supported. Pillows can be used to maintain the position.

Ambulation equipment must be fitted specifically to the individual. Check tips of walker legs, crutches, and canes for wear and fit. Be sure

adjustment holes are secure so there will be no slippage. Safety belts (gait belts) add a sense of security during ambulation, figure 27-6. They help the individual control the center of gravity. The health care provider should be alert and ready for a patient's loss of balance. To make the best use of body mechanics, stand close to the ambulating resident. Keep your knees slightly flexed and your spine erect, and maintain a broad base of support. Remember that successful ambulation requires strength and a sense of balance. Be ready to assist as needed. If a fall should start, maintain your own body mechanics. Ease the person to the floor, using your leg muscles as you go down into a squatting position. Try to keep your back straight. Do not leave, but call for help. Anyone who has fallen needs to be examined for injury before being moved.

When ambulating a person, do not hurry the process. Assist the resident to a sitting position and wait a few minutes before helping the resident into a standing position, figure 27-7. Remember that postural changes affect circula-

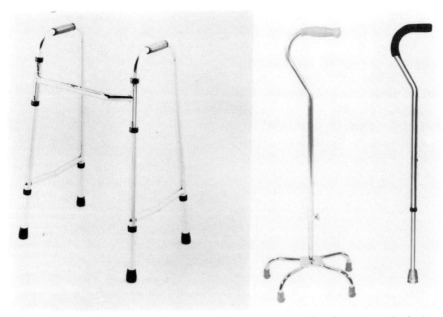

Figure 27-4 Walkers and canes add a measure of safety to ambulation. (Courtesy Invacare Corporation)

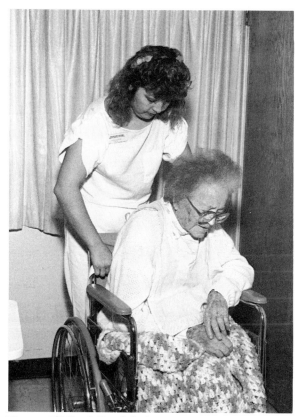

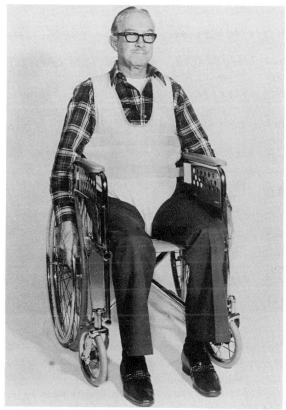

Figure 27-5 Wheelchair supports should maintain body alignment. The hips should be well back and the trunk supported.

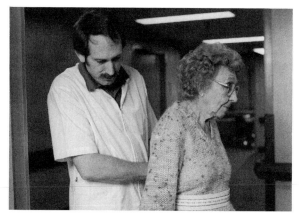

Figure 27-6 A gait belt helps patients control their center of gravity.

tion and too rapid movement may result in fainting and falls. Ambulate close to walls where guard rails can offer support. Do not allow patients to ambulate too ambitiously. Keep your expectations and those of the patient sensible, bearing in mind the person's physical condition and previous ambulatory experience. Too strenuous attempts can result in fatigue and discouragement. When ambulating in an open area, have chairs at spaced intervals for convenient resting if necessary.

Review procedures for ambulating patients with your instructor. Refer to figure 27-8 to review the beginning procedure and ending procedure actions.

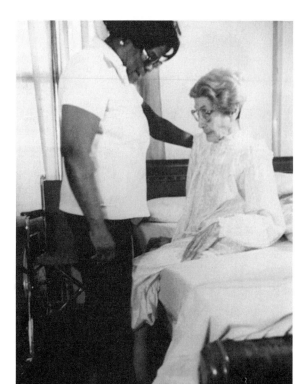

Figure 27-7 Always allow the resident to sit before attempting to stand.

PROCEDURE 33

Assisting a Person to Ambulate with Cane or Walker

1. Wash hands and assemble either of the following pieces of equipment:

   cane
   walker

2. Check appliance for worn areas or loose parts.
3. Identify resident and explain what you plan to do.
4. Lower bed to lowest horizontal position.
5. Raise head of bed and assist resident to a sitting position.

Beginning Procedure Actions

- Wash hands.
- Assemble all equipment needed.
- Knock on door and pause before entering resident's room.
- Politely ask visitors to leave. Tell them where they can wait.
- Identify the resident.
- Provide privacy by drawing curtains around bed and closing door.
- Explain what you will be doing and answer questions.
- Raise bed to comfortable working height.

Procedure Completion Actions

- Position resident comfortably.
- Leave signal cord, telephone, and fresh water where resident can reach them.
- Return bed to lowest horizontal position.
- Raise side rails, if required.
- Perform general safety check of resident and environment.
- Clean used equipment and return to proper storage, according to facility policy.
- Open privacy curtains.
- Wash hands.
- Tell visitors that they may reenter the room.
- Report completion of procedure.
- Document procedure following facility policy.

Figure 27-8 Beginning procedure actions and procedure completion actions.

6. Assist with robe and slippers. Swing resident's legs over edge of bed. Allow feet to rest on floor.
7. If necessary, apply a transfer belt around resident's waist.
8. Place cane or walker within easy reach.
9. Assist resident to standing position.
10. Have resident grasp walker or cane to maintain balance.

11. Walk beside resident, grasping transfer belt for additional support.
12. After ambulation, return resident to bed by reversing the procedure.
13. Leave resident in comfortable position with side rails up.
14. Wash hands.
15. Record on chart the date and time, procedure (ambulation with cane/walker), and the resident's reaction.

PROCEDURE 34

Lifting a Resident Using a Mechanical Lift

1. Wash hands.
2. Assemble equipment.
3. Obtain assistance from a co-worker.
4. Check slings and straps for frayed areas or poorly closing clasps.
5. Take mechanical lift to resident's bedside and screen unit.
6. Identify the resident.
7. Explain what you plan to do.
8. Place wheelchair or chair at a right angle to foot of bed, facing the head.
9. Lock the bed and roll resident toward you.
10. Position slings beneath the body behind shoulders and buttocks and upper thighs. Be sure the sling is smooth.
11. Roll resident back onto the sling and adjust position as necessary.
12. Attach suspension straps to sling. Check fasteners for security.
13. Position lift frame over bed with base legs in maximum open position and lock.
14. Elevate head of bed and bring person to a semisitting position.
15. Attach suspension straps to frame. Position resident's arms inside straps.
16. Secure restraint straps if needed.
17. While talking to the person, close the pressure value and pump the hydraulic mechanism.

18. Guide the lift away from the bed when the resident's buttocks are completely off the bed.
19. Position resident close to the chair or wheelchair (with wheels locked).
20. Slowly lower resident into chair or wheelchair. Pay particular attention to the position of the resident's feet.
21. Unhook the suspension straps and remove lift.
22. If the resident is to remain in the chair for a period of time, make resident comfortable and secure before leaving.
23. Wash hands.
24. Record the procedure on the resident's chart.
25. Readjust the resident's sitting position about every two hours.

PROCEDURE 35

Assisting a Person into a Chair or Wheelchair

1. Wash hands.
2. Identify the resident and explain what you plan to do and how you can be helped. Have slippers and robe close by.
3. Screen the unit.
4. Cover the chair or wheelchair with a cotton blanket or some other barrier.
5. Place chair or wheelchair near the head of bed facing the foot or head of the bed; lock the wheelchair and raise foot pedals. **Note:** Whenever possible, position chair or wheelchair securely against a wall or solid furniture to ensure that it will not slide backward.
6. Lock bed and elevate head. Lower the bed to lowest horizontal position.
7. Drape resident with a bath blanket and fanfold bedding to foot of bed.
8. Assist the resident to a sitting position by placing your arm (the one closest to the head of the bed) around shoulders. Place your other arm under the resident's

knees and pivot (rotate) the resident to-ward the side of the bed slowly and smoothly. Remain facing the resident to prevent a fall.

9. Help put on robe and slippers.
10. Still facing the resident, check to be sure he or she is ready to stand.
11. Have resident place feet on floor or foot-stool with both hands on your shoulders. Place your hands at the person's under-arms. Raise resident slightly and help to slide off edge of bed to a standing posi-tion. If using a footstool, have resident step to the floor.
12. Keeping hands in same position, help resident turn slowly until the person's back is toward the chair.
13. Have another person hold chair or move to side of resident, placing one foot be-hind front leg of chair. Lower resident gradually to a sitting position in chair, bending at your hips and knees. Keep your back straight. Arrange robe or blan-ket smoothly. If the resident is in a wheel-chair, place both feet on the footrests and lock the wheelchair securely.
14. Cover resident with bath blanket. Stay until you are sure there are no adverse side effects. Report anything unusual to supervising nurse.
15. Leave signal cord and drinking water in reach. Make sure bed and unit are tidy.
16. Wash hands and report completion of task to your supervisor.
17. Readjust the resident's position in the chair about every two hours.

PROCEDURE 36

Assisting a Person into Bed from a Chair or Wheelchair

1. Wash hands. Identify the resident and explain what you plan to do.

2. Screen unit for privacy.
3. Check to see that the bed is in the lowest horizontal position and that the wheels are locked. Raise head of bed, fanfold bedding to the foot, and raise opposite side rail.
4. Position chair or wheelchair at foot or head of the bed. Lock wheels of wheel-chair and lift foot pedals.
5. Have resident place feet flat on floor.
6. Remove bath blanket, fold, and return to bedside stand.
7. Stand in front of the resident. Keep your back straight and your base of support broad.
8. Place your hands on either side of the person's chest. Have resident place hands on your shoulders. Help resident to stand.
9. Pivot the resident toward the bed slowly and smoothly. Assist resident to sit on edge of bed.
10. Remove robe and slippers.
11. Place one arm around the resident's shoulders and one arm under the resi-dent's legs and swing the resident's legs onto the bed.
12. Lower head of bed and assist resident to move into center of bed.
13. Draw top bedding over person. Remake, if necessary.
14. Make resident comfortable with signal cord within reach.
15. Wash hands.
16. Report completion of assignment.

Hazards of Prolonged Immobility

Muscle tone is quickly lost when muscles are unused. This is especially true of the ankles, hips, shoulders, knees, and abdomen. Even vital ca-pacity is 10 percent less in the supine position. This, of course, further compromises any exist-ing respiratory condition.

Confinement with little activity predisposes to constipation, urinary retention and infection, renal calculi, metabolic disturbances, and development of decubitus ulcers. Circulation slows, and bones lose minerals. There is usually a decrease in weight because lagging appetite lowers food consumption. Mood may alter and morale suffer.

Inactivity causes serious muscle and joint problems. Stiffness develops into atrophy, loss of strength, contractures (figure 27-9), and permanent disability. Continuous lack of activity may ultimately lead to hypostatic pneumonia. When walking and active ambulation are not possible, range-of-motion (R.O.M.) exercises should be carried out for all joints, unless contraindicated, figure 27-10. Frequent position changes and attention to skin care are essential. Residents should be encouraged to move about on their own and care for themselves as much as they can. The bath is one of the best opportunities to carry out passive R.O.M. exercises and to encourage active R.O.M. exercises by the patients.

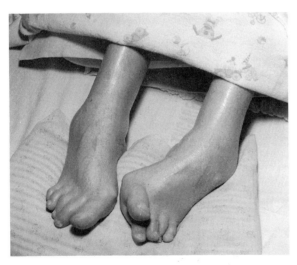

Figure 27-9 Contractures are a serious complication of immobility. (From Caldwell & Hegner, *Nursing Assistant, A Nursing Process Approach,* 5th Edition, copyright 1989 by Delmar Publishers Inc.)

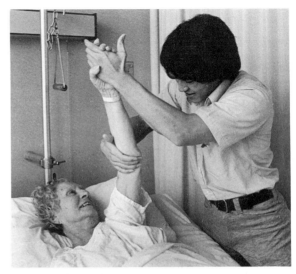

Figure 27-10 Range-of-motion-activities are essential to maintaining mobility.

The nurse will instruct you concerning the type of R.O.M. exercises to be performed. Be sure to ask before attempting to carry them out. Each exercise is usually performed three times. A joint should not be exercised to the point of pain, however. If pain or discomfort develops, stop the exercise and report the fact to the nurse. Always be gentle in handling the patient. Support the part above and below the joint being exercised. You may wish to review these procedures with your instructor.

PROCEDURE 37

Performing Range-of-Motion Exercises

1. Wash hands. Identify resident and explain what you plan to do and how you can be assisted.
2. Position person on back close to you.
3. Adjust the bath blanket to keep resident covered as much as possible.
4. Turn resident's head gently from side to side (rotation), figure 27-11.

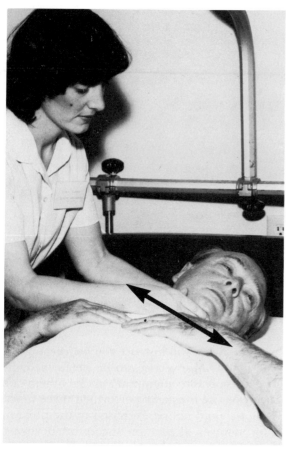

Figure 27-11 (From Caldwell & Hegner, *Nursing Assistant, A Nursing Process Approach,* copyright 1989 by Delmar Publishers Inc.)

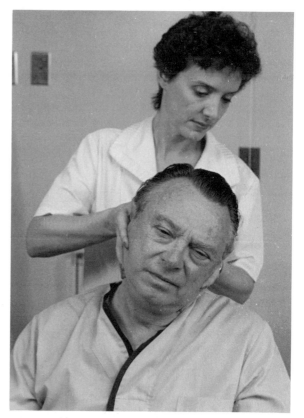

Figure 27-12 (From Caldwell & Hegner, *Nursing Assistant, A Nursing Process Approach,* copyright 1989 by Delmar Publishers Inc.)

5. Bend resident's head toward right shoulder and then left (lateral flexion), figure 27-12.
    Note: Although rotation and flexion are similar movements, the first resembles shaking the head. The second moves the head toward the shoulder.
6. Bring person's chin toward chest (flexion), figure 27-13.
7. Place pillow under person's shoulders and gently support head in a backward tilt (hyperextension). Return to straight position (extension). Adjust pillow under head and shoulders.

8. Supporting the elbow and wrist, exercise shoulder joint nearest you as follows:
    a. Bring entire arm out at right angle to body (abduction), figure 27-14.
    b. Return to position parallel to body (adduction).
9. With shoulder and arm in abduction (at right angle to the body), flex elbow and raise entire arm over head (shoulder flexion), figure 27-15.
10. With arm parallel to body, palm up, flex and extend elbow, figure 27-16.
11. Flex and extend wrist and each finger joint, figures 27-17 and 27-18.
12. Move each finger in turn away from the middle finger (abduction) and toward

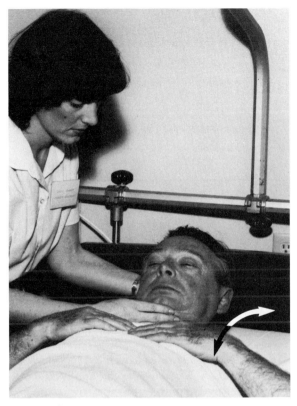

Figure 27-13 (From Caldwell & Hegner, *Nursing Assistant, A Nursing Process Approach,* copyright 1989 by Delmar Publishers Inc.)

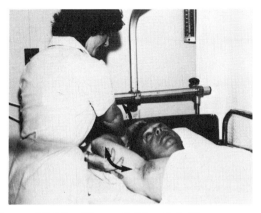

Figure 27-15 (From Caldwell & Hegner, *Nursing Assistant, A Nursing Process Approach,* copyright 1989 by Delmar Publishers Inc.)

the middle finger (adduction), figure 27-19.

13. Touch the thumb to each fingertip (opposition).
14. Turn palm down (pronation), then palm up (supination).
15. Point hand in supination toward thumb side (radial deviation), then toward little finger side (ulnar deviation).
16. Cover the resident's upper extremities and body. Expose only the leg being exercised. Face the foot of the bed.

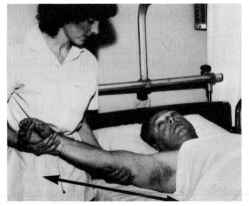

Figure 27-14 (From Caldwell & Hegner, *Nursing Assistant, A Nursing Process Approach,* copyright 1989 by Delmar Publishers Inc.)

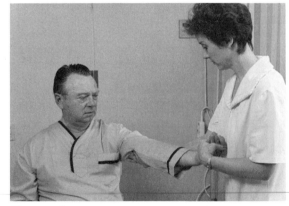

Figure 27-16 (From Caldwell & Hegner, *Nursing Assistant, A Nursing Process Approach,* copyright 1989 by Delmar Publishers Inc.)

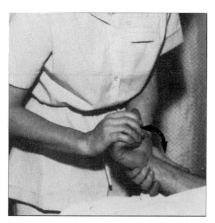

Figure 27-17 (From Caldwell & Hegner, *Nursing Assistant, A Nursing Process Approach*, copyright 1989 by Delmar Publishers Inc.)

17. Supporting knee and ankle, move entire leg away from body (abduction), figure 27-20, and toward body (adduction).

18. Turn to face bed. Supporting knee in bent position (flexion), raise knee toward pelvis (hip flexion), figure 27-21. Straighten knee (extension) as you lower leg to bed. With the resident in a side-lying position, leg closest to the bed bent for balance, support the upper leg under the knee and ankle and move the leg in a

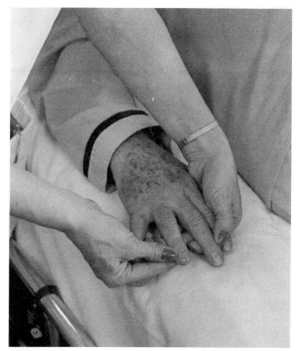

Figure 27-19 (From Caldwell & Hegner, *Nursing Assistant, A Nursing Process Approach*, copyright 1989 by Delmar Publishers Inc.)

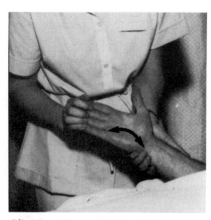

Figure 27-18 (From Caldwell & Hegner, *Nursing Assistant, A Nursing Process Approach*, copyright 1989 by Delmar Publishers Inc.)

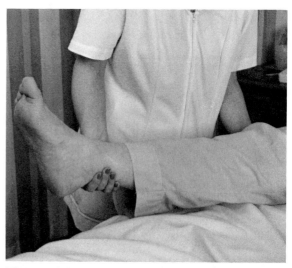

Figure 27-20 (From Caldwell & Hegner, *Nursing Assistant, A Nursing Process Approach*, copyright 1989 by Delmar Publishers Inc.)

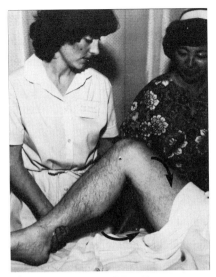

Figure 27-21   (From Caldwell & Hegner, *Nursing Assistant, A Nursing Process Approach,* copyright 1989 by Delmar Publishers Inc.)

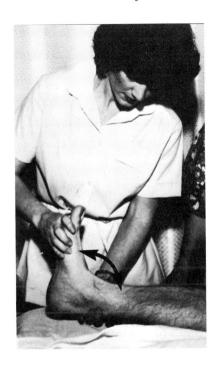

circular motion (rotation and hyperextension of the hip).

19. Place hand on ball of foot closest to toes while supporting ankle with other hand. Gently push the top of the foot toward the knee (dorsiflexion), figure 27-22. Still supporting the ankle, place hand on top of foot closest to toes and gently push down (plantar flexion), figure 27-23.

20. Turn to face foot of bed. Gently turn foot inward (inversion), figure 27-24, and downward (eversion), figure 27-25.

21. Place fingers over toes, bending toes (flexion) and straightening toes (extension).

22. Move each toe away from second toe (abduction) and then toward second toe (adduction), figure 27-26.

23. Cover leg with bath blanket. Raise side rail and move to the opposite side of the bed.

24. Move person close to you and repeat steps 7 to 12.

25. Wash hands.

26. Report completion of task.

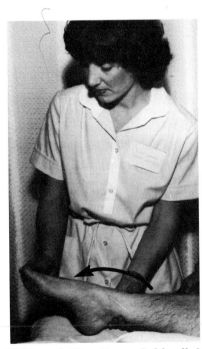

Figure 27-22 and 23   (From Caldwell & Hegner, *Nursing Assistant, A Nursing Process Approach,* copyright 1989 by Delmar Publishers Inc.)

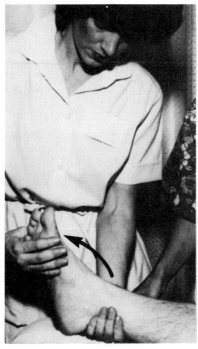

Figure 27-24 (From Caldwell & Hegner, *Nursing Assistant, A Nursing Process Approach*, copyright 1989 by Delmar Publishers Inc.)

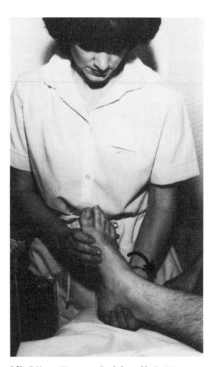

Figure 27-25 (From Caldwell & Hegner, *Nursing Assistant, A Nursing Process Approach*, copyright 1989 by Delmar Publishers Inc.)

Muscle tone can be maintained through a regular program of planned setting exercises When joints cannot, or should not, be moved because of pathology. In setting exercises, muscles are alternately contracted and relaxed for short periods without moving the joints. The nursing staff may be asked to help with these exercises and other special exercises that are planned by the doctor, nurse practitioner and physiotherapist, figure 27-27. Everyone must understand exactly the type and amount of exercise to be performed. They should also understand the extent of the nursing staff responsibility in seeing that the exercise is carried out.

Sometimes the strength of special muscle groups needs to be increased to prepare for certain activities. Operating a wheelchair or using a cane both require arm strength. In these cases, planned progressive resistive exercises are ordered. As the name implies, these exercises are

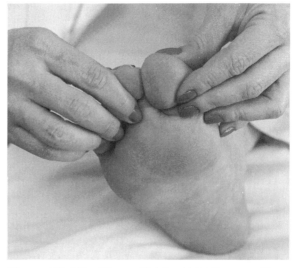

Figure 27-26 (From Caldwell & Hegner, *Nursing Assistant, A Nursing Process Approach*, copyright 1989 by Delmar Publishers Inc.)

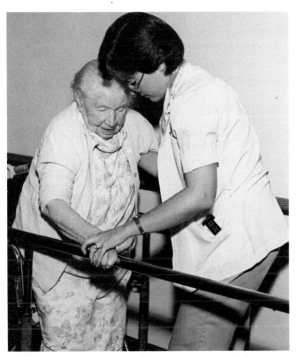

Figure 27-27 The physical therapist helps this patient to improve leg mobility.

planned so that increasing resistance is offered to the exercising muscle groups.

Alterations in Mobility

The musculoskeletal system changes with age. Muscle mass and response to stimuli generally decrease. Gaits become complex and motions awkward and limited as changes are made in posture to accommodate joint pathology. Elderly patients complain frequently of foot and leg cramps. Tremors make fine manipulations difficult, if not impossible. Superficially, reflexes become sluggish and less responsive, and perception of pain decreases. The ankle jerk reflex is lost or greatly diminished, and reflex reaction time is increased.

Both systemic and local conditions can interfere with a patient's mobility. Cardiovascular and respiratory problems, with their accompanying shortness of breath and discomfort, make move-

- Activity intolerance
- Alteration in comfort: Acute or chronic pain
- Alteration in nutrition: Less than or more than
- Diversional activity deficit
- Health maintenance deficit
- Impaired coping
- Impaired mobility
- Potential for injury
- Self-care deficit

Table 27-1 Nursing Diagnostic Categories Related to Musculoskeletal Problems

ment more difficult. Arthritic joints make movements painful. When joints become deformed, many movements that the healthy take for granted are impossible. Lowered general vitality and lack of incentive also hamper activity. Nursing diagnostic categories related to musculoskeletal problems are listed in table 27-1.

Alterations in mobility predispose the resident to falls. Falls are the leading cause of accidents in the elderly. The serious consequences of a fall for an elderly person cannot be overestimated. Among the consequences are physical injuries, especially fractures, loss of independence, and the hazards of immobility. An often-overlooked factor contributing to falls is the condition of the feet. Refer to table 27-2 for additional factors that contribute to falls.

Foot Problems

Musculoskeletal foot pathology is found in about 85 percent of the elderly, figure 27-28. It is the fourth most common cause of geriatric dis-

- Impaired balance, gait, mobility
- Impaired hearing and vision
- Impaired perception of health
- Impaired physical health
- Impaired mental status

Table 27-2 Disabilities Contributing to Falls

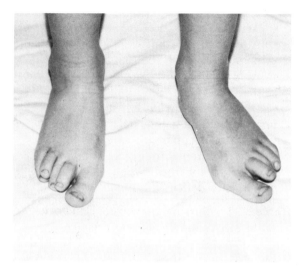

Figure 27-28   Flattened arches, bunions, overlapping toes, and thickened toenails are common to older persons.

comfort and is especially common among patients in long-term care facilities. Early diagnosis of infection has reduced the need for amputations and other surgery. Still, sore, aging feet continue to be one of the biggest problems in keeping the elderly ambulant.

Poor eyesight coupled with decreased coordination makes it difficult for the elderly to care for their own feet properly. *Podigeriatrics* is a specialty that deals with care of aging feet. Greater awareness of the need for foot care is demonstrated by the inclusion of podiatry services under Medicare. Some long-term care facilities have regular podiatry visits. Much still needs to be done to make these important services available to all long-term facilities and community centers.

The role of podiatry needs to be expanded if patients are to remain ambulant and well. "Keep them walking" programs conducted in community health centers focus on educating the public in foot care and hygiene. The aims of foot health programs include prevention, early diagnosis, maintenance, and rehabilitation. Foot conditions in the elderly are corrected slowly because of impaired circulation and retarded healing time.

Patients, or those caring for them, should be taught to carry out a basic routine of daily foot hygiene. This should include careful washing and drying of the feet and close inspection for any abnormalities. Olive oil, lanolin, cocoa butter, bland cream, or lotion can be applied to dry, scaly skin. A light dusting of powder can be applied to perspiring feet. Toenails should be kept trimmed and cut straight across.

Hose should be clean and properly fitted. Round garters increase the danger of circulatory impairment and should not be used. Properly fitted shoes of soft, pliant, porous material with broad, low, rubber heels give the best support. Well-fitted slippers that have cutouts for painful conditions and friction soles to prevent slipping may be ordered by the podiatrist for some residents.

Mechanical Deformities

Flatfoot is a fairly common condition caused by atrophy of the plantar muscles and consequent flattening of the arch. This causes unnatural areas of stress and discomfort. Although surgery is a corrective measure, the benefits for the elderly are questionable. Specially fitted shoes offer the best relief.

Bunions (hallus valgus) form when joints become misaligned because of basic weakness of the muscle structure and ill-fitting shoes. The tissues over the joints become tender, and the joints become deformed. Bunions can cause severe pain and inflammation when shoes are worn. Specially fitted shoes or cotton pads are prescribed to reduce pressure. In some cases, surgical removal of the bony overgrowth is necessary.

Hammertoes is a condition in which the toes are drawn into a tightly flexed position, causing deformity and pain. Corns often form on the tops of the curled toes from the pressure of footwear. It is possible to correct hammertoes surgically by shortening the proximal phalanx and releasing the contracture.

Corns and calluses occur in areas of pressure and friction. Pads or soft rings are used to reduce pressure. Nail files or emery boards may be used to reduce calluses. Residents must be cautioned against use of corn removal preparations. Treatment of these conditions should be directed by the podiatrist. Severe trauma and infection may result from mistreatment.

Thickened toenails that curve or become ingrown are also common. Soaking the nails prior to cutting them is helpful. The nails should be cut straight across, but left slightly longer than the toe. Wisps of cotton may be placed under the nail to encourage proper growth. It is recommended that only the podiatrist trim and cut the toenails.

Falls

Falls are not inevitable in elders. Geriatric health care providers have an important responsibility in identifying the factors that contribute to falls in their institution and in the elderly person's home. Contrary to popular belief, neither the environment nor medications are major factors in falls. The number of disabilities is. However, environmental hazards and polypharmacy in combination with disabilities create a major risk of falling. A study conducted in intermediate care facilities revealed that residents with three or fewer disabilities were frequent fallers. About one-third fell when they were acutely ill. Disabilities that contribute to falls are listed in table 27-2.

Fall risk assessment, figure 27-29, and fall prevention are the responsibility of all health care providers. Many long-term care facilities and geriatric physicians and nurses use a fall risk-assessment instrument to identify risks for residents and to plan individualized fall-prevention programs. Restraining residents in bed or in a chair as a general fall-prevention intervention creates problems of immobility. Assessments need to be done frequently. Changes should be made in the fall prevention plan as residents become less or more at risk for falls. Falls can make a resident fearful and less likely to move about, figure 27-30. This can create immobility problems and can result in a major catastrophe—fractures.

Risk Factors for Falls

- Age sixty-five or older
- Central nervous system depressants/hypnotics/analgesics/narcotics
- Confusion
- History of falls/previous fall in the hospital
- History of nocturia
- Incontinence/diarrhea/drugs that increase gastrointestinal mobility
- Organic brain syndrome
- Patients with impaired mobility/crutches/walker, etc.
- Postoperative twenty-four to forty-eight hours
- Use of diuretics
- Weakness related to disease process, tests, procedures

Figure 27-29 Patients whose assessment profiles include any combination of these risk factors must be considered at risk for falls and therefore need close observation.

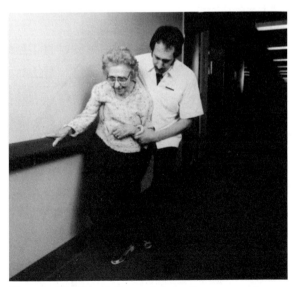

Figure 27-30 Falls and injuries can make an older person less likely to move about. (From Caldwell & Hegner, *Nursing Assistant, A Nursing Process Approach,* copyright 1989 by Delmar Publishers Inc.)

Fractures of the Femur

Osteoporosis, poor eyesight, difficulty in maintaining balance, and slow response to changes in body position are factors that make the elderly prone to falls and fractures. Fractures of the femoral neck of the left leg, figure 27-31, and of the intertrochanteric area are most common. In the past, treatment required traction and long periods of immobilization, with all its inherent dangers. Today, surgery is the treatment of choice because the elderly person can be mobilized quickly. Different types of surgical pins can be used. Figure 27-32 shows the surgical placement of two types of surgical pins to reduce and stabilize the fracture.

General Nursing Care

Before surgery, patients are frequently placed in Buck's extension or Russell traction, figure 27-33. This relieves muscle spasm and prevents further displacement of bone fragments. Patients in extended care facilities may be transferred to acute facilities for surgery. Russell traction may also be applied when surgery is contraindicated.

Preoperative routine includes maintaining traction and general supportive care. Patients should be provided with an overbed trapeze and encouraged to use it to maintain their upper body strength. Narcotics may be required for pain and sedatives for sleep, but they should be used wisely. The elderly patient tends to be highly sensitive to drugs. Side rails should be up for safety. The skin should be prepared carefully. Lacerations or abrasions of the skin cause the

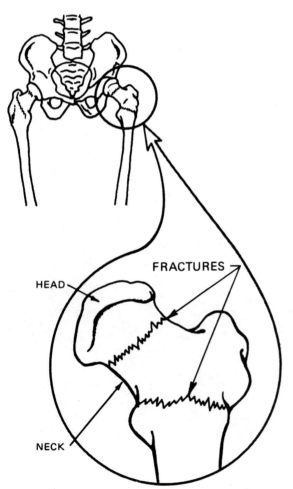

Figure 27-31 Common fracture sites of the femur head

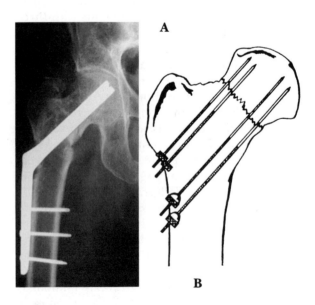

Figure 27-32 Fracture reduction with pin

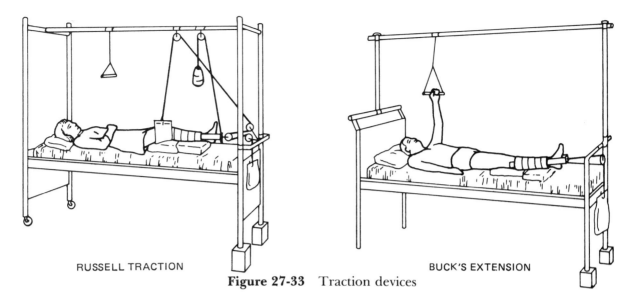

RUSSELL TRACTION   BUCK'S EXTENSION

Figure 27-33 Traction devices

surgery to be postponed because of the danger of infections. Special attention should be given to the heel of the foot. A small blanket folded and placed under the leg from thigh to ankle keeps pressure off the heel. A fracture bedpan is helpful both before and after surgery.

Postoperative Care

When certain internal fixation procedures using prosthetic devices are used to repair the fracture, immobilization following surgery is not usually needed. Minimal traction may be applied temporarily to help relieve muscle spasm. The patient can usually be gently rolled toward the nurse on either side. A pillow, placed lengthwise between the patient's legs, increases comfort during the moving procedure and prevents adduction that could cause dislocation of devices.

Deep breathing and other exercises are instituted to prevent pneumonia. With operative reduction of the fracture with internal fixation, the patient may begin weight bearing in a few days. If surgery is not possible, weight bearing could be prohibited for three to six months. The exact time depends on the type of fracture and the physician's preference. It also depends on the individual response and recovery of the resident.

Trochanter rolls can be used while the patient is in bed to control lateral rotation of the legs. In most instances, the patient should be encouraged to "toe in" to help control the tendency to lateral (external) rotation. Always check with the nurse first to determine whether the patient's hip can be positioned internally or externally.

The patient is allowed up in a chair by the first, second, or third postoperative day. He or she is encouraged to remain up for thirty-five to forty-five minutes, three times a day, to prevent complications of immobilization.

Following insertion of a hip prosthesis, an abduction pillow may be used or sandbags may be placed on either side of the affected leg to maintain the neutral rotation. The incisional line partly determines the exact position to be maintained. There must be no stress on the leg that would permit displacement of the prosthesis. Pillows can be used to maintain the position even while turning the patient to the unaffected side.

Initial ambulation may be in five days to six weeks. If the hip is very unstable, position may be maintained by an antirotation boot or either skin or skeletal traction. The extremity is placed in a Thomas splint with Pearson attachment, figure 27-34.

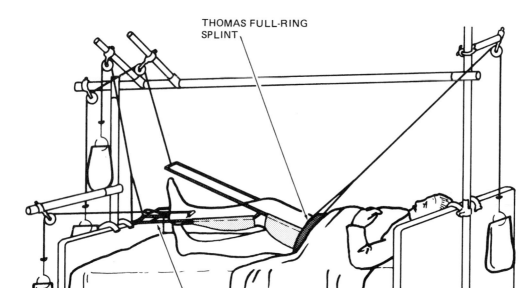

THOMAS FULL-RING
SPLINT

PEARSON ATTACHMENT

Figure 27-34   Thomas splint with Pearson attachment

Other Fractures

Small bone fractures of the wrist, arm, or leg may not require surgery or traction. They can be reduced (realigned) and maintained by splinting or casting.

Casting is done either by fiberglass casts that are lightweight and harden immediately or by wetting plaster of Paris rolls in water and wrapping them around the injured area. Sometimes the cast is then cut in half (bivalved) and held in place by straps. The casting material takes twenty-four to forty-eight hours to dry completely. It should be left uncovered. The part that is casted should be elevated to decrease swelling while drying takes place. No pressure should be applied to the cast. It should be handled only with the palms of the hand, not the fingertips. The cast edges may become rough as it dries. Once hardened, it may require some padding to prevent irritation of the tissues.

A trapeze bar helps the patient move in bed.

The casted area must be carefully positioned and supported each time the patient is moved. Be sure no bits of dried plaster are allowed to remain under the patient. They could lead to injury and decubiti.

The area beyond the cast should be checked carefully and frequently for changes in color, temperature, movement, and sensation. This could mean circulation impairment. Once the person is able to ambulate, an arm cast may be supported by straps or a sling. Patients with a leg cast may need a wheelchair or crutches for support.

Osteoporosis

Osteoporosis is a progressive bone-loss condition involving a defect in forming and maintaining bone tissue. Bone is lost faster than it is formed. The bones become brittle and porous, thus increasing the risk of fractures. Although the cause of osteoporosis is unknown, a number of factors are thought to contribute to it. Especially suspect are estrogen deficiencies, low levels of calcium in the circulatory system, and a sedentary life-style. Osteoporosis may also be seen in liver disease, hyperparathyroidism and hyperthyroidism (review the endocrine unit), alcoholism, and long-term use of steroid medications.

Being white, small, and female is another cluster of factors indicating that an individual may develop osteoporosis. It occurs in 30 to 80 percent of women over sixty-five years of age and is called postmenopausal osteoporosis. Because it is also found in older men and thought to be related to aging and inactivity, it is also called senile osteoporosis. Early diagnosis is made primarily through a person's history and by ruling out or excluding other possible causes. A definite diagnosis cannot be made with X rays until 30 to 50 percent of bone loss has occurred, when the disease is advanced. Unfortunately, the disease is mostly asymptomatic until the elder experiences severe pain as the result of a fracture in bones most affected by the disease (vertebrae, femur, and radius). Then the diagnosis is made. The increasing publicity about this condition among lay people, and the greater emphasis on dairy products and exercise throughout life, may help diagnosis and slow the progression of the disease among those who have it.

Signs and Symptoms

Some patients suffering from osteoporosis complain of aching pains, particularly in the back. Their skin may appear flaccid, dry, and atrophic. Frontal or cervical headaches are common. The major signs, however, are skeletal deformities. There may be *kyphosis* (dowager's hump or hunchback), decreased lower back curvature (reduced *lordosis*), and a loss of one to three inches in height. The major symptoms are fatigue, sudden severe pain, or chronic aching spine pain. Back pain is caused by a wedge fracture in the midback involving the thoracic or lumbar vertebrae. Usually an elder has bent to lift something and feels the severe pain because the brittle anterior part of the vertebra has snapped. Chronic spinal pain goes hand in hand with

fatigue. This kind of pain results from vertebrae collapsing on one another (collapse fractures). This pushes the ribs into a downward angle and reduces height.

Treatment

The primary goals of treatment for osteoporosis are to reduce bone loss, stimulate bone formation, and control pain so that the elder can participate in daily activities with a sense of well-being, despite disease. Treatment stresses mechanical stimulation by keeping the patient active. Adequate support must be provided by corsets or braces. Exercises to improve the musculature are prescribed. Supporting the patient in a weight-bearing position on an oscillating bed or tilt table is one means of increasing activity. Periods of weight-bearing are increased by walking or standing between parallel bars. Progressive resistive exercises are also used.

The diet should be adequate in protein and vitamin C, which is important to healthy connective tissues. It should include calcium and vitamin D in ordinary amounts. Excessive amounts of calcium should be avoided because they cannot be used by the bone. Therefore, they increase the tendency toward renal calculi. Calcium may also be deposited in muscles or joints, causing painful pathology in those areas. Good sources of calcium are ice cream and other daily products, sardines, and over-the-counter antacids such as Tums® which contain calcium carbonate. Usually 500 to 1,000 milligrams of calcium carbonate are given when a supplement is needed after menopause.

Dietary prescriptions must take into account that many of these patients have poor appetites and digestive disturbances. This includes a decrease in or lack of gastric hydrochloric acid.

Other measures for maintaining comfort and mobility include nonnarcotic analgesics, hot packs to aching areas, and gentle massage. The most beneficial treatment is activity and exercise. When an elderly resident cannot be out of bed, exercises in bed become of utmost importance. All geriatric health care providers must be very mindful that fractures in elders with severe bone loss are possible even with proper turning. Therefore, they must use extreme caution in turning and positioning these residents.

Arthritis

The term *arthritis* means joint inflammation. The number one crippler in the United States, arthritis strikes one family in five. Arthritis ranks second only to heart disease in causing permanent disability. Thirteen million Americans have some form of the disease. Because of the large number of people who are afflicted, arthritis is a natural focus for those who make money at the expense of others. Almost $300 million is spent yearly on arthritis remedies of no value. High-pressure advertising of diets, medications, devices, and spas tempt the suffering patient and family. The Arthritis Foundation engages in research and the dissemination of information about arthritis. It also provides various services directly to patients and their families.

Rheumatoid Arthritis

Rheumatoid arthritis was formerly called arthritis deformans because of its crippling effect. Although it may strike at any age, it usually first develops in those between thirty-five and forty-five. Its effects are carried into the senior years, leaving deformity and permanent damage. Onset may be late, the greatest incidence being after age sixty. It affects women two to three times as often as men.

The cause of rheumatoid arthritis is unknown. Heredity, hypersensitivity to foreign proteins, and autoimmune factors have been implicated. A rheumatoid factor usually composed of IgM globulin has been identified in 80 percent of the cases.

Pathological changes take place primarily in the joint lining (*synovium*). The synovial tissue becomes edematous and filled with inflammatory cells. It enlarges, forming a tissue called *pannus* that grows out over the articular cartilage. It gradually destroys the cartilage and invades the bone beneath. Wrists, feet, and the proximal in-

terphalangeal joints are most commonly involved. Usually more than one joint is affected, often symmetrically. Eventually, a fibrous ankylosing (fusion) of the joint occurs, with loss of motion. As the disease progresses, supporting ligaments are stretched and destroyed. Joint changes causes painful muscle spasms. The muscle spasms tend to "splint" the joints, holding them immobile. Because the flexor muscles are usually stronger, flexion contractures occur with varying degrees of deformity. The onset is usually insidious. But it may be abrupt, with polyarthritis, fever, and prostration.

Diagnosis is based on observation over a long time period. It also includes a serology indicating the presence of a rheumatoid factor and increased sedimentation rate, figure 27-35. X rays taken after a period of time reveal findings from soft tissue swelling to completely destroyed joints. Joint spaces are narrowed, indicating destruction of the cartilage. The synovial fluid may be studied as well.

Rheumatoid arthritis is characterized by periods of exacerbation (flare-ups) and remissions. There may be occasional flare-ups or a chronic progression. Periods of disease activity can be stimulated or exacerbated by stress, changes in diet or daily routines, and emotional problems.

Signs and Symptoms   The symptoms of rheumatoid arthritis include pain, heat, and swelling in

- Morning stiffness
- Joint tenderness or motion pain
- Joint swelling
- Symmetric joint swelling
- Subcutaneous nodules over bony prominences
- Rheumatoid arthritic X ray changes
- Positive tests for Rh factor
- Poor mucin precipitate from synovial fluid
- Characteristic cellular changes in the synovial membrane and nodules

Figure 27-35   Criteria for diagnosing rheumatoid arthritis (Courtesy American Rheumatism Association)

the joints and early morning stiffness. Systemically there may be fever, anemia, myositis, carditis, pneumonitis, and fatigue.

Treatment Early treatment gives the best results. Salicylates are used during the active periods to relieve inflammation and pain. Nonsteroidal anti-inflammatory agents, adrenocorticosteroids, anti-malarials, and gold salts are used in selected cases. Elderly patients being treated with these drugs should be observed carefully for adverse reactions.

Dry or moist heat gives comfort to many patients. Warm baths (104°F) or paraffin baths of 126° to 130°F are sometimes ordered. Periods of activity are alternated with periods of rest.

After the symptoms of pain, fatigue, and weakness subside, exercises may be started. During the active phase, it is important to continue range-of-motion exercises of all unaffected joints. Flexion contractures can be prevented by proper positioning, use of splints, and support of the patient. Flexion contractures of the hips can be prevented by making sure the patient spends part of each day on the abdomen.

If flexion contractures and joint deformities have occurred, specific orthopedic measures are needed. Gentle stretching via casts, splints, or manipulation may be tried. Surgical intervention may be required. Synovectomies, arthroplasty, and, in some cases, arthrodesis may be performed. Surgery should be performed when the disease is inactive.

Much of the treatment for the arthritic patient can be carried out on an outpatient basis or under visiting nurse supervision. A great deal of emotional support is required for both the patient and family. An effort must be made to involve patients physically and mentally in their progress. Self-help devices such as long shoehorns, grab bars, elastic shoelaces, and long pickup forceps, figure 27-36, can help the patient carry out activities of daily living. An overprotective or resentful family needs help in handling feelings positively. Rheumatoid arthritis is a chronic, progressive, disabling disease. The patient will need support for a long time.

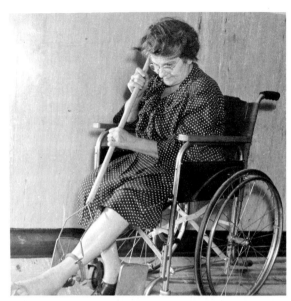

Figure 27-36 Special devices help arthritic patients remain independent.

Osteoarthritis

One of the most common forms of arthritis is osteoarthritis, also known as hypertrophic arthritis, degenerative or senescent arthritis, and osteoarthrosis. All joints undergo some degree of degeneration with age. Some symptoms are found in 97 percent of all people over sixty years of age. These patients are often overweight. The joints that are affected are those that receive the greatest trauma and strain, such as the knees and lumbar and cervical spine.

Osteoarthritis, for the most part, is not an inflammatory condition. There is usually no ankylosing of the joints. But there is destruction of the hyaline cartilage, figure 27-37. Each time the affected joint is moved, the friction against the joint surface results in further destruction until the subchondral bone is damaged. The most pronounced lesions develop in the greatest weight-bearing joints, and the knee is the joint most often affected. Initially, the cartilage becomes roughened and pitted. Additional stress stimulates the degenerative process, the joint loses its natural shape, movements become painful, and usual range of motion becomes limited.

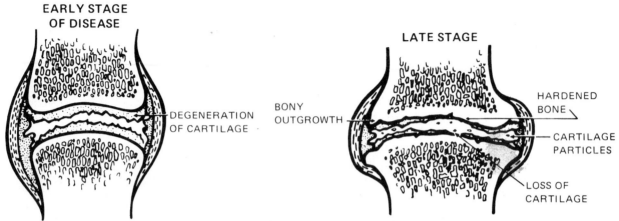

EARLY STAGE OF DISEASE

DEGENERATION OF CARTILAGE

LATE STAGE

BONY OUTGROWTH

HARDENED BONE

CARTILAGE PARTICLES

LOSS OF CARTILAGE

Figure 27-37   Osteoarthritis changes (Reprinted from *Osteoarthritis—A Handbook for Patients*, The Arthritis Foundation.)

X rays reveal thinning of the articular spaces resulting from loss of the cartilage. The subchondral bone becomes thickened. Bone spurs form near the point of attachment of the joint capsule and ligaments. Small pieces of cartilage come loose within the joint, adding to the destructive process. Osteoarthritis has been known to follow an episode of rheumatoid arthritis.

Symptoms   Pain and stiffness are the most common symptoms. Pain in the joints is aggravated by changes in temperature and humidity. Affected joints are tender and swollen. There is *crepitation* (a rubbing sound) when the joint is moved. Pain may be referred. For example, pain in the hips may be felt in the groin. Motion in affected joints is limited. Swelling of the distal interphalangeal joints, called *Herberden's Nodes*, is typical. There is a familial tendency toward the development of these nodes. Usually multiple, they may appear initially as early as forty years of age. They are usually painless. Nodes affecting the middle joint are called Bouchard's Nodes. Diagnosis of osteoarthritis is based on X rays and the presence of a normal sedimentation rate.

Treatment   The treatment of osteoarthritis includes nonsteroidal (nsaids) medication to relieve pain and reduce inflammation if it is present. Treatment also includes physiotherapy, light massage, and heat. At all times the staff must have a confident, positive, supporting attitude.

Salicylates are given for pain, and sometimes steroids are injected into the joint to reduce inflammation. These drugs cannot alter the disease progress, however.

Heat may be applied cautiously to the affected joints by means of an infrared light, usually twice daily for fifteen minutes. The light must be kept 30 inches away from the patient's skin to prevent burns. Heat may also be applied with warm baths, packs, and heated wax, figure 27-38. The joints, especially Herberden's Nodes, are massaged lightly for two minutes following a heat treatment. Exercise and limbering up can relieve joint stiffness and pain, figure 27-39. All too often, an elder reduces activity and then muscles waste and weaken. This leads to immobility and its attendant problems. Help elders learn that when joints are stiff and painful, activity will relieve these symptoms.

Physiotherapy must be carried on indefinitely, with range-of-motion exercises performed several times daily. Special exercises may be prescribed to build up muscular strength, and nursing care is directed toward preventing contractures. Patients should be provided with a firm mattress and bed board. Good posture in and out of bed should be encouraged. Support should be provided for a pendulous abdomen

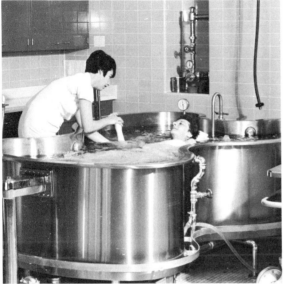
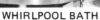

WHIRLPOOL BATH

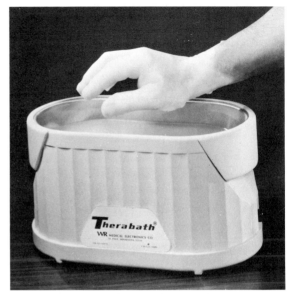

PARAFFIN BATH

Figure 27-38   Whirlpool and paraffin baths give temporary relief to the arthritis patient.

and breasts to improve posture. Mechanical stress on joint surfaces can be minimized by the use of crutches, canes, orthopedic collars, and arch supports. Gentle, intermittent, cervical traction is sometimes ordered to relieve muscle spasm. Weight puts more stress on the joints, so obesity must be reduced.

When all other treatments have not worked, orthopedic surgery is indicated for those in good mental and physical condition. Spinal fusion, total hip replacement, and total knee replacement have given many elders a new lease on mobility and well-being.

Summary

- Understanding the normal musculoskeletal system and the changes that occur with senescence provides a foundation for understanding the pathologies that can limit mobility.
- Mobility is important to a sense of well-being. It is a significant first step in rehabilitation.
- Many elderly people are not mobile because of foot discomfort and joint, muscle, and bone pathology.
- Arthritis, osteoporosis, and fractures are commonly seen among the older age group.
- Nursing care of the elderly with orthopedic disabilities attends to immediate needs and also provides support for long-term adjustment.

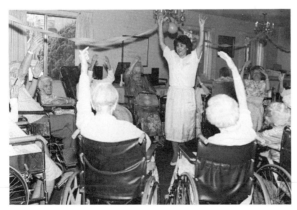

Figure 27-39   Even wheelchair-bound residents can participate in limbering-up exercises to music.

Review Outline

I. Behavioral Objectives

II. Vocabulary

III. Musculoskeletal System

    A. Structure

        1. Muscle
        2. Bones
        3. Joints
        4. Tendons/ligaments

    B. Function

    C. Types of movement

IV. Senescent Changes

V. Aids to Mobility

    A. Ambulation
    B. Wheelchairs
    C. Canes
    D. Walkers
    E. Mechanical lifts

VI. Hazards of Immobility

VII. Range-of-Motion Exercises

VIII. Alterations in Mobility

    A. Falls
    B. Foot problems
    C. Fractures
        1. Traction
        2. Surgery
    D. Osteoporosis
    E. Arthritis
        1. Rheumatoid arthritis
        2. Osteoarthritis

Review

I. Vocabulary

Write the definition of each of the following.

1. Alignment_____
2. Atrophy_____
3. Contract_____

4. Hypertrophy_____
5. Flexion_____
6. Abduction_____
7. Adduction_____
8. Arthritis_____
9. Mobility_____
10. Podigeriatrics_____

II. Short Answers

1. What is the best and least expensive form of exercise for the elderly?
2. What precaution must be taken for the patient who cannot ambulate freely?
3. What name is given to exercises that alternately contract and relax muscle groups without moving joints?
4. What are five musculoskeletal changes that take place with age?
5. What are the causes of flatfoot, bunions, and corns?
6. How should toenails be cared for?
7. What is the treatment for dry scaling feet?
8. What kinds of shoes are best for the elderly?
9. How is osteoporosis different from osteoarthritis?
10. What factors contribute to the development of osteoporosis?
11. What are three general methods of treatment used in both rheumatoid arthritis and osteoarthritis?
12. Why is careful preoperative care of the skin of a patient with a fractured hip important?
13. Why might a patient with a hip fracture be placed in traction preoperatively?
14. What nursing measures can be taken to add to the comfort and safety of the elderly person with a fractured hip?
15. What is the cause of rheumatoid arthritis, and how it is different from osteoarthritis?

III. Clinical Situations

1. The fingers of a resident with an arm cast look blue and feel cold. What do you do?
2. Your patient who has been ill with an upper respiratory infection is being ambulated for the first time. What do you do?
3. It is early morning and a resident complains of her fingers being stiff and painful. What can you do immediately to help?
4. You notice that a resident who had a hip pinning for a fracture lets his leg roll out laterally. How would you use a trochanter roll?
5. An elderly resident learned that her daughter and children were killed in a car accident. Her pain and disability from her rheumatoid arthritis worsened. Is there a connection? How can you help?

CASE STUDY

Mr. A.K. Jenner was a robust-looking man with a ruddy complexion and a quick smile. He was sixty-six. Until he started to rise and tried to walk, you would hardly be able to guess at his degree of disability.

For the thirty years before his retirement, he had worked as a mason and bricklayer. He had spent long hours on his knees, bending and stooping, creating what he laughingly called his "works of art." A skilled craftsman, his patios and fountain areas enhanced the landscape of the community.

In his late twenties, he had begun to notice twinges of pain in his right knee as he worked. The pain became increasingly severe in his thirties. Sometimes he used a small pad to kneel on. He also found himself favoring his right knee at times.

As the years passed, the twinges of pain that he first felt in his right knee he also felt in his left. Getting up in the morning was more difficult. He attributed the pain to "getting along in years" and started taking an aspirin compound for relief. Now, at sixty-six, his osteoarthritis was affecting not only his knees but his hips and ankles as well. He needed a cane for support and walked very little.

Over the years he had tried many advertised potions, spending by his own calculations hundreds of dollars for relief. On admission to the arthritis clinic, X rays revealed the thinning and pitting of articular cartilage characteristic of the disease process. Small pieces of cartilages had come loose within both knee joints, adding to the trauma and pain.

Mr. Jenner was advised to lose weight to reduce the stress on his weight-bearing joints. A program of physiotherapy, heat to the affected joints, and salicylates for pain were prescribed.

Currently, he is a possible candidate for arthroplasty of the right knee. If attention had been given to the pain and limitation earlier, some of the severe damage might have been prevented.

1. What factor probably produced the initial trauma to Mr. Jenner's knees?
2. Does osteoarthritis usually involve bilateral joints?
3. Why did both knees become involved?
4. What drug had been taken as an analgesic?
5. Why do arthritics tend to turn to quackery?
6. What effect did the osteoarthritis have on the articular cartilage?
7. What test helped to determine the diagnosis?
8. What three therapies were prescribed?

Unit 28
Gastrointestinal System Alterations

Objectives

After studying this unit, you should be able to:

- Locate the organs of the gastrointestinal system.
- Name the common pathologies affecting the senescent gastrointestinal tract.
- Demonstrate procedures for giving enemas.
- List the normal changes in the elimination pattern of solids as the body ages.
- Explain the purpose of bowel retraining.

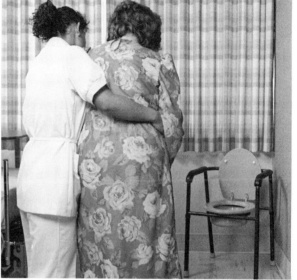

Vocabulary

Learn the meaning and spelling of the following words or phrases.

anabolic		
anabolism		
anus		
bile		
catabolic	dysphagia	masticated
catabolism	enzymes	metabolism
chyme	feces	ostomy
colon	flatus	peristalsis
colostomy	gallbladder	pylorus
constipation	gastritis	rectum
diarrhea	hernias	saliva
diverticulitis	herniorrhaphy	suppositories
diverticulosis	hydrochloric acid (HC1)	ulcers
dyspepsia	impaction	urgency

The gastrointestinal system is also called the G.I. or digestive tract. It extends from the mouth to the anus and is lined with mucous membrane. The organs of this system change food into simple forms able to pass through walls of the small intestine into the circulatory system. The circulatory system carries the nutrients to the body cells. Proteins are changed to amino acids, carbohydrates to simple sugars like glucose, and fats to fatty acids and glycerol. The changes are brought about by mechanical action and by chemicals called *enzymes*. The indigestible parts of food move through the intestines and are finally excreted from the body as feces. Many organs contribute to the digestive process and many disease conditions affect them. Each organ is affected in some way by the aging process.

Structure and Function

Mouth (Figure 28-1)

Food is *masticated* (chewed) by the teeth so that it can be swallowed and digested easily. Together, the teeth and tongue mix the food with *saliva*. Saliva is a fluid produced by the salivary glands that aids in digestion. The salivary glands produce several quarts of saliva daily. There are thirty-two adult teeth and with care they should last a lifetime. Tooth loss is not part of the natural aging process.

Stomach

After food has been chewed and swallowed, it passes through the pharynx and esophagus to the stomach, figure 28-2. To reach the stomach, the esophagus must pass through the posterior part of the diaphragm. The stomach is a hollow, muscular organ where food is mixed with and acted upon by gastric (stomach) enzymes. Food is

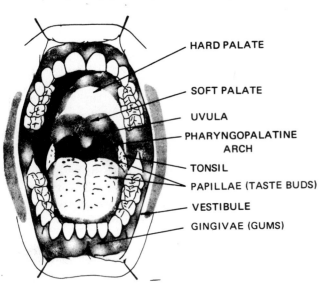

Figure 28-1   The normal anatomy of the mouth

HARD PALATE

SOFT PALATE

UVULA

PHARYNGOPALATINE ARCH

TONSIL

PAPILLAE (TASTE BUDS)

VESTIBULE

GINGIVAE (GUMS)

held within the stomach by sphincter muscles at either end while it is mixed with the digestive juices. The narrow, tapered end of the stomach is called the *pylorus*. The muscle guarding this exit point is called the pyloric sphincter. In addition to enzymes, the cells of the stomach lining produce *hydrochloric acid* (HCl). Hydrochloric acid helps to digest protein.

Intestines

When food leaves the stomach, it is in a semi-liquid form called *chyme*. Chyme enters the small intestine. There, any undigested nutrients are broken down by intestinal and pancreatic enzymes and bile from the liver.

The small intestine is about 20 feet long. It coils within the peritoneum. There are three main portions: the duodenum, the jejunum, and the ileum. The duodenum is about 12 inches long. It has an opening in the back to receive bile and pancreatic enzymes. Materials are moved through the intestines by rhythmic contractions of the involuntary muscles in the intestinal wall. These rhythmic contractions are called *peristalsis*. Most of the nutrients and food the body needs are absorbed into the bloodstream through the walls of the small intestine.

The small intestine is separated from the large intestine by the ileocecal valve. The large intestine is also called the *colon*. Names have been given to different portions of the large intestine: cecum, ascending colon, transverse colon, descending colon, sigmoid colon, rectum, and anus. The appendix extends from the cecum. Water is absorbed through the walls of the large intestine, changing wastes to a more solid form. In this way, the large intestine helps to maintain the water balance of the body. Peristalsis moves waste through the large intestine until it reaches the rectum. When a certain amount has been collected in the *rectum*, it is eliminated as *feces* (solid waste) through the *anus*.

Liver and Gallbladder

The liver is a large gland, located just beneath the right side of the diaphragm. It plays a major role in *metabolism*. Metabolism refers to all

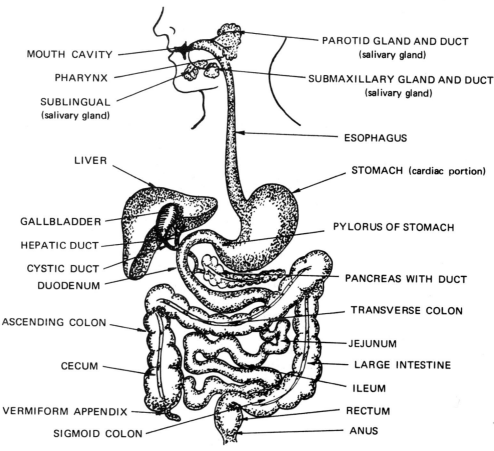

Figure 28-2 The digestive system

the chemical reactions that take place in the body. Some reactions are *catabolic*, breaking down complex compounds, which releases energy. Others are *anabolic* reactions in which complex compounds are synthesized by combining simple compounds. These reactions use energy.

The liver helps to control the sugar and the amount and kinds of proteins in the blood by changing and storing excess amounts. Two proteins necessary for blood clotting, prothrombin and fibrinogen, are produced by the liver. The liver also manufactures *bile*, which is used in the digestion of fats and the absorption of the fat-soluble vitamins A, D, E, and K. Bile is stored in the *gallbladder*, a small saclike organ on the under-side of the liver. When needed, bile is sent from the gallbladder to the duodenum. Bile gives feces their usual brown color.

Forty percent of Americans form gallstones by the age of eighty. Gallstones are hardened dehydrated bile that forms in the gallbladder or one of the bile ducts. The exact cause of gallstones is unknown.

Pancreas

This glandular organ extends from behind the stomach into the curve of the duodenum. It manufactures pancreatic juice, which is sent into the duodenum to aid in the digestion of foods. Special cells in the pancreas produce insulin.

Senescent Changes

The changes the digestive tract undergoes with age are related to a decrease in muscle tone and secretory ability, figure 28-3. Decreased muscle tone results in slower, less efficient peristalsis and elimination. Less blood flow slows absorption of nutrients. Nutrient utilization is also hampered by a decrease in levels of hydrochloric acid, and thickened saliva that fails to moisten and protect the mouth and tongue. It is also hampered by a less functional liver and diminished secretion of digestive enzymes in general. Less mucus is produced, so there is less protection of the lining of the tract.

Many older people develop an intolerance to lactose, or milk sugar. Therefore, milk and milk products are digested poorly. Fat absorption and absorption of fat-soluble vitamins is decreased. Minerals such as calcium and iron are utilized less efficiently. Also, the gag reflex is less active, leading to a greater likelihood of choking and aspirating food particles and saliva. Still, levels of enzymes remain adequate to maintain nutrition.

Liver function tests do not always show a deficiency. But flatulence (gas production), poor absorption of fat-soluble vitamins, and poor detoxification of drugs give clinical evidence of less functional ability. Decreased lubrication, loss of muscle tone, and less sensitivity to the urge to defecate increase the tendency to constipation. Fecal incontinence is associated with fecal impaction, loss of sphincter tone, confusion, and neurogenic changes.

Nursing diagnostic categories related to gastrointestinal problems are listed in table 28-1.

Frequently Encountered Conditions

Mouth Care

Older people often think that once they have dentures, they no longer have to make regular visits to the dentist. Those who have any natural teeth need to be checked for decay and can benefit from chloride treatments. Dentures need to be checked for irregularities or damaged edges. The mouth also should be checked for signs of irritation caused by ill-fitting dentures. Saliva normally keeps the mucous membranes moist and reduces microbial populations in the mouth. It lubricates dry foods, making them less traumatic to the mouth and tongue. Remember that the elderly do not have this full protection. Therefore, special and frequent mouth care and inspection is important. Further discussion of mouth care is found in Unit 26. Maintaining adequate fluids is also essential.

- Decreased number of taste buds
- Reduced digestive enzymes
- Thicker saliva
- More sensitive tongue
- Less efficient peristalsis
- Less effective gag reflex
- Poorer tolerance of some foods
- Slower absorption of nutrients
- Decreased chewing
- Ill fitting dentures
- Weaker muscular walls

Figure 28-3   Senescent changes in the digestive system

- Alteration in bowel elimination: Constipation, diarrhea, incontinence
- Alteration in comfort: Pain
- Alteration in nutrition: More than body requirements, less than body requirements
- Alteration in oral mucous membranes
- Fluid volume deficit
- Impaired skin integrity
- Impaired swallowing
- Knowledge deficit
- Potential for infection

Table 28-1   Nursing diagnostic categories related to gastrointestinal problems

Elimination Needs

Eliminating waste products regularly is one of the basic human needs. Being continent (able to control elimination) is important to everyone. You have specific responsibilities in helping continent elders to meet their elimination needs. You must be aware of the person's need to reach the proper facilities on time. Be observant so that you can be available to help the resident in your care to reach the toilet or commode. Answer call bells promptly for those who use a bedpan. Always note and chart the frequency and character of the excreta.

Normal feces should be soft, formed, and brown. Note bowel movements on the health record and report anything unusual. For example, infections and medications such as antibiotics can cause loose or watery stools. Iron can make the stool black. It can make stools loose in some patients, while constipating others. Hemorrhoids (piles) are varicose veins in the rectum. Hemorrhoids can sometimes bleed and can make the stool red or unusually dark.

Fecal Incontinence

Successful control of elimination is essential to a healthy and socially active life. Problems related to elimination are common among the elderly. The inability to predict when voiding or defecating will occur can cause embarrassment and a reluctance to participate in social engagements.

The reflex control of defecation is similar to that of urination, which is explained in Unit 29. Both forms of elimination are under reflex and voluntary control, figure 28-4.

Fecal incontinence is less common than urinary incontinence. It is also more easily controlled. Incontinence may be occasional or frequent. It may be a temporary condition or may require retraining. The elimination of loose, watery stools is called *diarrhea*. This may be caused by infection, intolerance to food, or fecal impaction.

You also have specific responsibilities in caring for the incontinent resident with diarrhea.

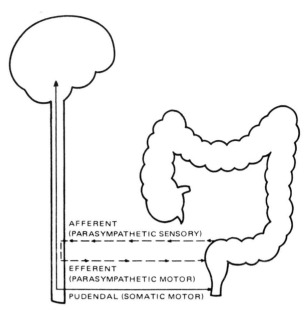

Figure 28-4 The defecation reflexes

Check the person frequently for soiling. Clean the resident as soon as evacuation occurs. Treat the care in a matter-of-fact manner, but be sensitive to the feelings of the patient. Use disposable gloves and be especially careful to wash your hands. If infection is present, it can be easily transferred to you from others on contaminated hands. Encourage a bland diet, if ordered. This kind of diet is easily digestible and has little bulk to irritate the colon. Report the frequency and character of the bowel movement to the nurse. Provide the patient with room deodorizers as needed to assure an odor-free environment. Fecal incontinence is most commonly caused by fecal *impaction*, the severest form of constipation. It may also be caused by inadequate hydrochloric acid (achlorhydria), diverticulosis, intolerance of certain foods, infections, and some medications such as antibiotics, which can cause diarrhea.

Constipation

Constipation (difficulty in evacuating bowels) is a common geriatric problem and can lead to the more serious problem of fecal impaction.

The cause of constipation is not always evident. However, improper diet, lack of exercise, inadequate fluids, anorexia, certain medications, and inaccessibility of the lavatory are contributing factors.

The person with the problem of constipation may not have any appetite and may complain of abdominal discomfort. The abdomen may be distended. Remember that the severest form of constipation is impaction.

You may assist the constipated patient by encouraging a high-roughage diet and as much activity as possible. Offer fluids frequently and help the resident to the bathroom, allowing adequate time for defecation. You may also need to administer bowel aids as ordered.

Impaction

An *impaction* results when the fecal mass becomes dehydrated from remaining in the bowel too long. This dehydrated mass acts as an irritant to the mucosa. Mucus production is increased, some of the outer fecal mass is dissolved by the mucus, and some liquid stool is formed and drains from the bowel. Absence of stool or the presence of diarrhea in the elderly should always be a warning of possible fecal impaction. Noting the frequency and character of bowel movements is an important nursing function. Fecal impaction is relatively common in the elderly, particularly in those whose activities are restricted. The presence of a fecal mass can be confirmed by a gloved digital examination. Some authorities believe that such an examination should be carried out two or three times weekly as a prophylactic measure.

In some facilities, geriatric health care providers are permitted to check for fecal impaction and report their findings so that an order for a bowel aid such as a suppository or enema can be ordered and given for relief. To check for fecal impaction, the patient must be in the Sims position and not sitting on the toilet. Be sure your facility permits you to perform this procedure before you undertake to do so. The mass may be felt by a lubricated, gloved finger gently inserted into the rectum.

Manual extraction of the mass is traumatic and should be avoided. A better technique is to give an oil enema to act as a lubricant, followed by a soapsuds enema. The soapsuds enema can be repeated daily until the colon is clear. Sometimes 50 ml of hydrogen peroxide may be administered to help break up the fecal matter, followed by a soapsuds enema. It is important to recognize that two or three bowel movements in a seven-day period may be adequate. Daily bowel movements are not necessary.

Retraining   The evaluation procedure and nursing assessment for bowel retraining are similar to those for bladder retraining—determination of bowel pattern and individual response to the problem. The first step after assessment is to recognize and treat any fecal impaction.

If difficulty in defecating is due to poor muscle tone, instruct the patient to take a deep breath and tighten the abdominal muscles as you gently massage the abdomen with a circular, downward motion. It may be helpful to exert gentle digital pressure with gloved fingers around the outside of the anus. Patients should be taught and encouraged to do this for themselves.

Regularity is the key to bowel retraining. Proper sitting helps considerably. The patient should be positioned comfortably and safely. Guard rails on either side of the toilet will increase the feeling of security. Privacy and an unhurried atmosphere are important. Something warm to drink may help to stimulate peristalsis.

Bowel Aids   Geriatric nursing assistants may give bowel aids such as oil-retention enemas, soapsuds enemas, and, in some facilities, lubricating suppositories. Each of these procedures requires a specific order. Sometimes bowel aids such as stool softeners and evacuants are needed to achieve a normal stool. These may be in the form of oral tablets, rectal suppositories, or contact laxatives, figure 28-5. Contact laxatives are preferred for the elderly because they are not absorbed and, therefore, create no toxicity problem. Action occurs in thirty to sixty minutes as they increase peristalsis of the large intestine.

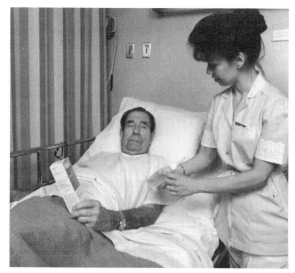

Figure 28-5 Bowel aids such as suppositories and enemas may be needed to restore regularity.

Care must be taken to place the contact laxative high against the bowel wall and to be sure it is not imbedded in the fecal mass. Enemas, another bowel aid, may be ordered. However, the use of all bowel aids is gradually diminished over the six- to eight-week retraining period.

Exercise and Diet A program of regular exercise commensurate with the person's general condition will stimulate circulation and improve intestinal muscle tone, figure 28-6. Keeping the elderly up and ambulant is important.

A basic diet rich in roughage and natural laxative foods, such as fruits, vegetables, and whole grain cereals and breads, makes a significant difference in bowel activity. Lemon juice and prune juice between meals is also helpful, figure 28-7. Some patients are given prune juice regularly with their medications. Others are routinely given juice nourishments twice a day. Routinely supervising dietary intake is important to the success of the bowel retraining program.

Continence is an essential step in the rehabilitative process. Too many care facilities do not have retraining programs. They rely heavily on laxatives, suppositories, enemas, and catheters for control.

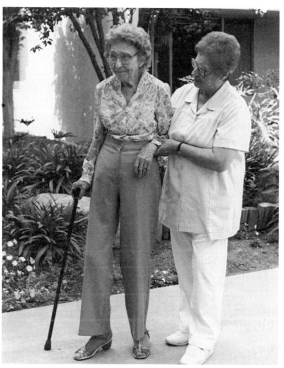

Figure 28-6 Regular exercise is essential for natural elimination patterns.

Hernias

Hernias occur when there is weakness in restraining muscle walls and a portion of an organ pushes through the weakened area. This may happen in the groin area (inguinal hernia). Hernias are also called ruptures. A surgical repair of the weakened wall is called a *herniorrhaphy*.

Hiatal hernias (protrusions of the upper stomach into the lower portion of the thorax through an enlarged esophageal opening in the diaphragm) become increasingly common after fifty years of age. They occur in 67 percent of those over sixty and are somewhat more common in women than in men. Signs and symptoms include *dysphagia* (difficulty swallowing), pain and pressure in the area of the lower sternum, and food trapped in the esophagus. The hiatal hernia is sometimes complicated by inflammation of the esophagus. Ulcerations and scarring occur as acid gastric juices flow upward.

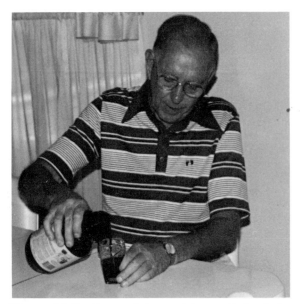

Figure 28-7   Prune juice and lemon juice help promote regularity.

Eating before retiring is inadvisable, because symptoms are more pronounced when lying down. Antacids and small, frequent, bland meals are recommended. Surgery to repair a hiatal hernia is rarely needed. But because obesity is a contributory factor, weight reduction is recommended. Elevating the bed slightly for sleep tends to reduce the incidence of reflux into the esophagus.

Diverticular Disease

Weakened areas in the wall of the intestinal tract due to decreased muscle tone result in the formation of small pouches called diverticula. A conservative estimate is that 30 to 50 percent of people over age sixty develop diverticula. A person with diverticula has *diverticulosis*. Hard food particles can become trapped in the pouches. This predisposes the person to infection and constipation. Inflamed diverticula cause *diverticulitis* in about 50 percent of the patients. Ulcerations sometimes develop, leading to bleeding. Low-residue or bland diets, weight reduction, and correction of constipation are usually sufficient to treat diverticulitis.

If diverticulitis does develop, it is usually signalled by pain. The patient in the acute phase should be given a low-residue diet. Adequate fluid and nourishment and spasmolytic agents also help reduce the bowel spasm. Transfusions may be needed. If conservative therapy and medication do not help, bowel resection surgery may be necessary.

Ulcers

Ulcerations of the stomach (peptic ulcers) and other parts of the tract are quite common. *Ulcers* are craterlike wounds formed as tissues break down. Some ulcers are stress induced, others drug induced. Still others form as a complication of diseases such as chronic pulmonary disease. The signs and symptoms—bleeding, *dyspepsia* (indigestion), and pain—are all related to erosion of the mucosa. Remember that signs and symptoms often may not be as pronounced in the elderly as they are in younger people. These ulcers are usually treated medically through bland diet, antacids, and correction of causal factors.

Gastritis

Gastritis means inflammation of the stomach and is frequently signalled by dyspepsia. Dyspepsia is fairly common among older people. Decreased vitality of the gastric mucosa means less tolerance to foods enjoyed previously. Eating foods that are too spicy, overeating, or overindulging in alcoholic beverages can lead to gastric distress. Small bland meals, antacids, and antispasmotics help. Reliance on excessive antacids can lead to electrolyte imbalance.

Malignancy

Malignancies (cancers) of the gastrointestinal tract are common. Carcinoma of the esophagus most often occurs between the ages of sixty and sixty-five. It is more frequently seen in women than in men. Malignancies of the stomach are most often developed somewhat later, between the ages of seventy-five and eight-five. Those of the esophagus and stomach demonstrate a poor prognosis.

Malignancies of the lower colon may be primary or metastatic. They affect both sexes with equal frequency. Symptoms depend on the location of the lesions. Diagnosis is confirmed by a G.I. series, sigmoidoscopy, and biopsy. Obstruction (blocking) of the passageway is sometimes the first major indication of a long-growing tumor. Indigestion, constipation, and changes in the shape or color of stool are signs and symptoms that may be overlooked.

Malignancies of the intestinal tract are usually treated surgically by removing the affected part. Making an artificial opening in the colon (*colostomy*) for the elimination of feces is common surgery for a malignancy of the bowel, especially among elderly men. The new opening is called an *ostomy* or stoma, figure 28-8. The ostomy may be temporary or permanent.

Different surgical techniques may be employed. For example, one part of the bowel may be removed and the remaining end brought through the wall, resulting in one stoma. When there is potential for reuniting the bowel in the future, both segments may be brought to the surface. This is called a double-barreled colostomy.

Because there is no sphincter around the stoma, voluntary control has been lost. There may be problems of leakage, odor, and irritation of the surrounding area. It is important to keep the area clean and dry. To collect the drainage, a disposable colostomy bag covers the stoma, figure 28-9. It may be held in place with a belt. If the ostomy is to be permanent, patients are taught to care for the colostomy themselves. You may be assigned to give stoma care.

A colostomy is traumatic at any age, but when it is added to the burden of age, it can be devastating. Patients fear that they will never have a normal life again. A retired person may have less incentive to gain control than a wage earner who must go back to work. The older person may feel there is no use in even trying.

In some major skilled care facilities, nurses with special training, called enterostomal nurses, care for the ostomy patient. They teach the new ostomy patient how to care for the stoma and do the irrigation. They also offer direct emotional support to both the patient and the family.

Skin protection is one of the major problems. This is especially true when the ostomy is high up in the intestines and the drainage is very wet.

There are many different appliances that are available for colostomy care. The skin around the stoma may be cleansed with a wound

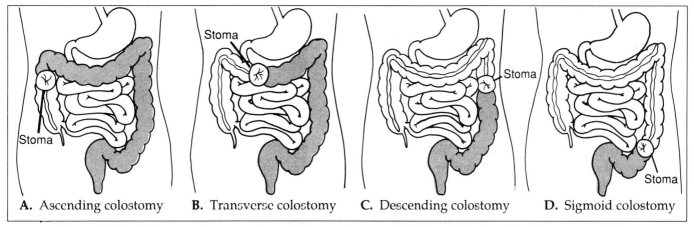

A. Ascending colostomy   **B.** Transverse colostomy   **C.** Descending colostomy   **D.** Sigmoid colostomy

Figure 28-8   Colostomy sites vary depending on the part of the bowel that needs to be removed. (From Caldwell & Hegner, *Nursing Assistant, A Nursing Process Approach,* copyright 1989 by Delmar Publishers Inc.)

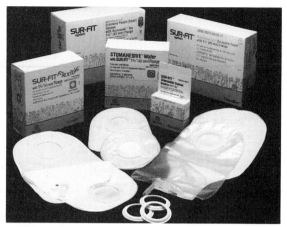

Figure 28-9 Various types of disposable drainage bags and accessories are available for the ostomy patient. (Photograph provided compliments of ConvaTec®, A Squibb Company)

cleanser such as Biolex.® A skin barrier is applied after the area is dried. There are skin barriers that can be cut to fit exactly the size of the ostomy, figure 28-10. Tegadem® or Duoderm® are skin

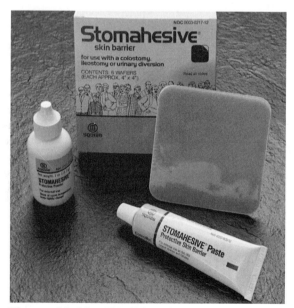

Figure 28-10 Flexible adhesive wafers help assure a secure fit around the ostomy. (Photograph provided compliments of ConvaTec®, A Squibb Company)

barriers that allow the health care provider to examine the skin around the stoma without removing the barrier. Adhesive wafers or gel pads to which the ostomy bag is attached can be used. The ostomy bag itself may be close ended or open ended for irrigation. Once regularity has been established, a small dressing is usually adequate to cover the stoma.

You may wish to review the procedures for caring for colostomies with your instructor. Figure 28-11 lists the beginning and ending procedure actions.

Beginning Procedure Actions

- Wash your hands.
- Assemble all equipment needed.
- Knock on door and pause before entering resident's room.
- Politely ask visitors to leave. Tell them where they can wait.
- Identify the resident.
- Provide privacy by drawing curtains around bed and closing door.
- Explain what you will be doing and answer questions.
- Raise bed to comfortable working height.

Procedure Completion Actions

- Position resident comfortably.
- Leave signal cord, telephone, and fresh water where resident can reach them.
- Return bed to lowest horizontal position.
- Raise side rails, if required.
- Perform general safety check of resident and environment.
- Clean used equipment and return to proper storage, according to facility policy.
- Open privacy curtains.
- Wash your hands.
- Tell visitors that they may reenter the room.
- Report completion of procedure.
- Document procedure following facility policy.

Figure 28-11 Beginning procedure actions and procedure completion actions

PROCEDURE 38

Caring for a Stoma

1. Wash hands and assemble the following equipment:

washcloth and towel	disposable colos-
basin of warm	tomy bag and
water	belt or adhesive
bed protector	disposable gloves
bath blanket	skin barrier, as
bedpan	directed
	toilet tissue

2. Take equipment to beside. Identify patient and explain what you plan to do.
3. Replace top bedding with the bath blanket.
4. Place bed protector under the person's hips.
5. Put on disposable gloves.
6. Remove the soiled disposable stoma bag and place in bedpan. Note amount and type of drainage.
7. Remove belt that holds stoma bag if used and save, if clean.
8. Gently clean area around stoma with toilet tissue to remove feces and drainage. Dispose of tissue in bedpan.
9. Wash area around stoma with soap and water.
10. Rinse thoroughly and dry.
11. If ordered, apply skin barrier around the stoma.
12. Position clean belt around person, if used or apply adhesive wafer or gel pad. Inspect area for irritation or breakdown.
13. Place clean ostomy bag over stoma and secure.
14. Remove bed protector. Check to be sure bottom bedding is not wet. Change if necessary.
15. Replace bath blanket with top bedding, making person comfortable.
16. Gather soiled equipment and dispose of according to facility policy.
17. Clean bedpan and basin and return to unit.
18. Wash hands.
19. Record on patient's chart the date and time, procedure (ostomy care), type and amount of drainage, signs of irritation, lotion applied (if any), and patient's reaction to the procedure.

Irrigation. A positive, unhurried attitude will help patients develop the necessary skill in handling irrigation equipment. A hurried approach is apt to make an elderly person feel defeated before beginning. Explain what is being done in simple terms. Let the patient help whenever possible. At first, the patient may be reluctant to even look at the stoma. Many register surprise that it is less unsightly than they imagined. Others have difficulty adjusting to the shock. Nevertheless, being able to look at the stoma is a vital first step in accepting the condition.

Gradually, the patient can learn to assume responsibility for self-irrigation. Figure 28-12 shows the irrigation equipment used and the patient positioned on the toilet for self-irrigation. Long irrigations may be exhausting to the older person. Offer assistance in any way that will help prevent fatigue. For example, preparing the equipment, figure 28-13, and cleaning it afterwards will not interfere with feelings of independence. But it will prevent the patient from becoming overtired. Equipment should be as simple as possible. Commercially produced plastic colostomy bags can be used to collect the drainage and can also be used for the irrigations. Use the patient's own equipment whenever possible.

PROCEDURE 39

Irrigating a Colostomy in the Bathroom

1. Wash hands and assemble the following equipment in the resident's bathroom:

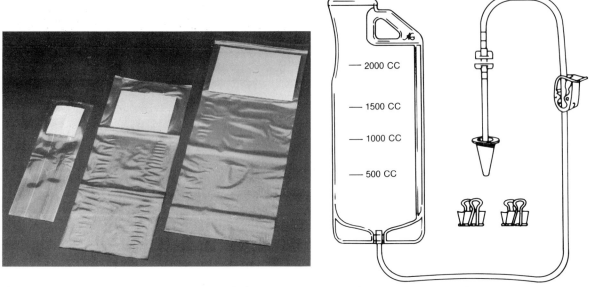

Figure 28-12A   Colostomy irrigation equipment (Courtesy of Mentor Corporation, Minneapolis, MN: Irrigation sleeve courtesy Bard Home Health Division, C.R. Bard, Inc.)

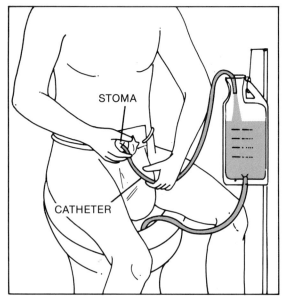

Figure 28-12B   Irrigating the colostomy in the bathroom

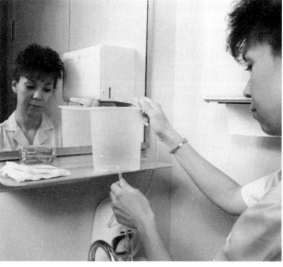

Figure 28-13   Assemble equipment before going to the bedside. (From Caldwell & Hegner, *Nursing Assistant, A Nursing Process Approach,* copyright 1989 by Delmar Publishers Inc.)

irrigating can,
tubing, and
clamp
connector and
catheter with cone
disposable gloves
lubricant
toilet tissue
washcloth and towel

disposable irrigating
apparatus
dressing for fresh
ostomy bag appli-
cation as needed
pole or some fixture
to support irri-
gating can

2. Identify resident and explain what you plan to do.
3. Assist resident into the bathroom.
4. Position resident on toilet and drape legs with towel.
5. Put on disposable gloves.
6. Remove disposable colostomy bag or dressing. Cleanse area of stoma with tissue and dispose of tissue in toilet.
7. Apply disposable irrigating sleeve by placing faceplate directly over the stoma. Secure with belt. Drop plastic drainage sheath between person's legs into toilet.
8. Attach catheter to connector and then to tubing. Attach tubing to irrigating container.
9. Fill container with solution as ordered, usually 1,000 to 2,000 ml of warm (100° F to 105°F) tap water or saline.
10. Allow a small amount of fluid to fill tubing and catheter to warm tubing and expel air.
11. Squeeze small amount of lubricant onto toilet tissue and apply to tip of catheter.
12. Gently insert catheter into stoma approximately 3 to 4 inches using a rotating motion. If cone tip is used, press against stoma to control return flow. If resistance is met, do not force but inform nurse.
13. Slowly allow approximately 500 ml of fluid to enter the ostomy by releasing clamp. Flexing the tube between your fingers will allow you to control the amount and speed of flow. Stop immediately if patient complains of discomfort.
14. Remove catheter and allow return to flow into toilet. Note character of return.

15. Repeat the procedure until returns are clear. This is a process that cannot be hurried and make take up to an hour. Be sure to check patient for fatigue. If patient becomes fatigued, return the patient to bed and use a bedpan to collect returns.
16. Detach irrigating bag from belt and dispose of according to hospital policy. You may reuse the sleeve. Wash and dry for reuse.
17. Clean area around stoma with warm, soapy water. Rinse and dry thoroughly.
18. Apply skin barrier as ordered.
19. Apply a small dressing or a clean ostomy bag and secure.
20. Remove gloves and dispose of them.
21. Assist person back to bed.
22. Clean equipment and replace according to facility policy.
23. Wash hands.
24. Record on patient's chart the date and time, procedure (colostomy irrigation), solution used, character and amount of returns, and patient's reaction to the procedure.

PROCEDURE 40

Irrigating an In-Bed Colostomy

1. Wash hands and assemble the following equipment:

bed protector/bath
blanket
toilet tissue
lubricant
basin
disposable gloves
solution as ordered
washcloth and towel
disposable irrigating
apparatus

irrigating can,
tubing, catheter
with cone,
and connector
emesis basin lined
with paper towels
dressing or fresh
ostomy bag
I.V. pole to hang
irrigating can

2. Identify resident and explain what you plan to do.

3. Replace top linen with bath blanket.
4. Position person close to edge of bed either sitting or in semi-Fowler's position.
5. Place protective bed covering in position.
6. Place bedpan on a chair beside bed.
7. Attach tubing, connector, and catheter to irrigating can. Clamp tubing.
8. Fill irrigating container with approximately 1,000 to 2,000 ml of solution at about 100°F to 105°F.
9. Allow a small amount of fluid to flow through tubing to expel air.
10. Hang container from I.V. standard near bed approximately 18 inches above stoma.
11. Place emesis basin on the bed with concave surface next to resident.
12. Remove dressing or disposable bag and place in emesis basin.
13. Clean gently around the stoma with toilet tissue and dispose of in emesis basin.
14. Apply disposable irrigation bag over stoma and place open end in bedpan so that return and drainage will flow into it.
15. Squeeze small amount of lubricant onto toilet tissue and apply to top of catheter.
16. Gently insert catheter cone approximately 3 to 4 inches into stoma, using a rotating motion. If cone tip is used, press against stoma to control return flow. If resistance is met, do not force but inform nurse.
17. Release clamp and slowly allow approximately 500 ml of fluid to enter the ostomy. Flexing the tube between your fingers will allow you to control the amount and speed of flow. Stop immediately if patient complains of discomfort.
18. Remove catheter and allow return to flow into bedpan. Note character of return.
19. Repeat procedure until returns are clear. The process cannot be hurried and may take up to an hour. Be sure to check the patient for fatigue. Stop procedure and allow patient to rest if fatigue occurs.
20. Detach irrigating bag from belt and dis-

pose of according to facility policy. You may reuse the sleeve. Wash and dry the sleeve for reuse.
21. Clean area around stoma with warm water. Rinse and dry thoroughly.
22. Apply skin barrier if needed.
23. Apply a small dressing or a clean bag and secure with belt.
24. Remove gloves and dispose of according to facility policy.
25. Clean equipment and replace according to facility policy.
26. Wash hands.
27. Report completion of procedure. Record observations.

Related Procedures

Enemas

An enema is the injection of fluid into the rectum in order to remove feces and *flatus* (gas) from the colon and rectum. Enemas are frequently ordered before tests and most kinds of surgery as well to relieve constipation. A soap solution, a salt solution, or tap water are the fluids usually ordered. These solutions are expelled a short time after they are given. *Urgency* is a term used to describe the need to defecate and empty the bowel.

Sometimes a small amount of oil is given to soften the feces. This is called an oil-retention enema. An enema of this type is usually followed by a soapsuds enema (S.S.E.) in about half an hour.

Disposable enema units contain a solution that draws fluid from the body to stimulate peristalsis. Usually 4 ounces of solution are administered. The solution contains sodium, which is not appropriate for all older people. Soapsuds and oil-retention enemas also come in disposable sets. Administration is simple, and the time spent preparing and cleaning the equipment is saved.

When possible, enemas should be given before the patient's bath or before breakfast. They should not be given within the hour following mealtime. An enema requires a doctor's order.

PROCEDURE 41

Giving a Soapsuds Enema

1. Wash hands and assemble equipment. Disposable enema equipment consisting of a plastic container, tubing, clamp, and lubricant is available commercially. Some units also contain a small amount of concentrated liquid soap.
   a. Connect tubing to solution container.
   b. Adjust clamp on tubing and snap shut.
   c. Fill container with warm water (105°F) to the 1,000-ml line.
   d. Open packet of liquid soap and put the soap in the water.
   e. Using the tip of the tubing, mix the solution gently so that no suds form.
   f. Run small amount of solution through tube to get rid of air and warm the tube.
2. Take the following equipment to bedside:

disposable enema unit	bedpan and cover towel
pack of lubricant	bath blanket
toilet tissue	bed protector
disposable gloves	

3. Identify resident and explain what you plan to do.
4. Place chair at foot of bed and cover with towel; place bedpan on it.
5. Cover the person with a bath blanket and fanfold linen to foot of bed.
6. Place bed protector under buttocks.
7. Help person to turn on left side and flex knees (Sims' position). Be sure opposite side rail is up.
8. Place container of solution on chair so tubing will reach person. Lubricate tip.
9. Adjust bath blanket to expose anal area.
10. Put on disposable gloves.
11. Expose anus by raising upper buttock.

12. Never force the tube. If tube cannot be inserted easily, get help. There may be a mass of feces (an impaction) blocking the bowel.
13. Open the clamp and raise container so that the fluid flows in slowly. Ask the person to take deep breaths to relax the abdomen. If person complains of cramping, clamp tube and wait. Then open the tubing to continue fluid flow.
14. When enough solution has been given, clamp the tubing.
15. Tell the person to hold breath while upper buttock is raised and tube is gently withdrawn.
16. Wrap tubing in paper towel. Put it in disposable container.
17. Place person on bedpan or assist to bathroom.
18. Raise head of bed to comfortable height.
19. Place toilet tissue and signal cord within reach of the person. If in bathroom, stay nearby.
20. Take tray to utility room. Rinse enema equipment thoroughly in cool water and then wash in warm, soapy water. Return it to bedside or discard according to hospital policy.
21. Remove disposable gloves and dispose of according to facility policy.
22. Remove bedpan or help person return to bed and observe contents. Cover bedpan. Remove bed protector.
23. Give the person soap, water, and a towel to wash hands.
24. Replace top bedding and remove bath blanket. Air the room. Leave room in order.
25. Clean and replace all other equipment used, according to facility policy.
26. Record on patient's chart the date and time; procedure (enema); type, amount, and temperature of solution; returns (color, consistency, unusual materials, flatus); and patient's reaction to the procedure.

PROCEDURE 42

Giving an Oil-Retention Enema

1. Wash hands and assemble the following equipment:

bedpan and cover	towel, soap, and
bed protector	basin with water
toilet tissue	prepackaged oil for
bath blanket	retention enema
disposable gloves	

2. Identify resident and explain what you plan to do. Say that it will be necessary to hold the solution at least 20 minutes.
3. Place chair at foot of bed. Cover with towel and place bedpan on it.
4. Cover person with bath blanket and fan-fold linen to foot of bed.
5. Place bed protector under buttocks.
6. Help the person assume the Sims' position.
7. Open the prepackaged oil-retention enema.
8. Put on disposable gloves.
9. Expose the anus. Remove cap from enema and insert the prelubricated tip into anus as the patient takes a deep breath.
10. Squeeze container until all the solution has entered the rectum.
11. Remove container and place in package box to be discarded.
12. Encourage the person to remain on side.
13. Check every 5 minutes until fluid has been retained for 20 minutes.
14. Position resident on bedpan or assist to bathroom.
15. If patient is on the bedpan, raise head of bed to comfortable height.
16. Place toilet tissue and signal cord within easy reach of the person. If in bathroom, stay nearby.
17. Dispose of expendable material according to facility policy.
18. Remove bedpan or help person return to bed. Observe contents of bedpan or toilet. Cover pan and dispose of or flush toilet.
19. Remove gloves and dispose of according to facility policy.
20. Give the resident soap, water, and towel to wash and dry hands.
21. Replace top bedding and remove bath blanket and bed protector. Dispose of according to facility policy.
22. Wash hands and record on patient's chart the date and time, procedure (oil-retention enema), returns, and patient's reaction to the procedure.

Insertion of Suppositories

Suppositories are given to stimulate bowel evacuation or to instill medications. Medicinal suppositories must be inserted by the nurse. Geriatric health care providers who have been trained may be asked to insert suppositories that soften the stool and promote elimination. These suppositories should be inserted 2 inches against the bowel wall.

PROCEDURE 43

Inserting a Suppository

1. Wash hands and assemble the following equipment:

suppository, as	gloves
ordered	bedpan and cover
lubricant	if needed
toilet tissue	

2. Identify resident and explain what you plan to do.
3. Help person assume the left Sims' position.
4. Expose buttocks only.
5. Put on gloves and unwrap suppository.
6. With left hand, separate the buttocks, exposing the anus.
7. Apply a small amount of lubricant to anus and insert the suppository. Suppository must be inserted deeply enough to enter the rectum beyond the sphincter (approximately 2 inches).
8. Encourage person to take deep breaths

and relax until the need to defecate is experienced, approximately 5 to 15 minutes.

9. Remove gloves and dispose of according to facility policy.
10. Adjust the bedding, helping person assume a comfortable position.
11. Place call bell near person's hand, but check every 5 minutes.
12. Assist patient to bathroom or position on bedpan.
13. Record time of insertion, type of suppository, and results.

PROCEDURE 44

Checking for Fecal Impaction

Note: Check the facility policy to be sure that this procedure is within the scope of your responsibilities.

1. Wash hands.
2. Assemble the following equipment:

   disposable gloves   toilet tissue
   lubricant   basin of warm water
   protective pad   washcloth and towel
   bath blanket

3. Identify the resident.
4. Explain what you plan to do.
5. Draw curtains for privacy.
6. Raise bed to comfortable working height.
7. Lower side rail on the side where you will be working.
8. Ask resident to raise hips. Assist as necessary.
9. Place bed protector under hips.
10. Turn resident to lay on side, facing away from you.
11. Cover resident with bath blanket.
12. Fanfold top bedclothes to foot of bed.
13. Put disposable glove on your dominant hand.
14. Ask resident to take a deep breath and bear down as you insert lubricated finger into rectum. **Note:** Rectum should feel soft and pliable.

15. You may feel no feces or you may feel a soft stool, a large solid mass, or multiple hard formations.
16. Withdraw finger. **Note:** If a spontaneous bowel movement occurs, note amount and character.
17. Wash resident's buttocks with warm water and dry.
18. Assist resident onto back.
19. Ask resident to raise hips. Assist as necessary. Remove bed protector.
20. Remove disposable glove.
21. Fold bed protector from outside to inside and place on chair.
22. Pull top bed covers over resident.
23. Remove bath blanket and fold and place in bedside stand, or in other proper storage area.
24. Make resident comfortable.
25. Raise side rail.
26. Place call bell where resident can reach it.
27. Empty basin and dry. Return to bedside stand.
28. Put towel and washcloth in laundry hamper.
29. Dispose of protector and glove according to facility policy.
30. Wash hands.
31. Report completion of procedure and record observations.

Collecting a Stool Specimen

Tests are sometimes performed on the feces that can reveal information about the gastrointestinal tract. Collect the specimen using proper technique. Be sure it is labeled correctly, stored properly, and reaches the laboratory promptly.

PROCEDURE 45

Collecting a Stool Specimen

1. Wash hands and assemble the following equipment:

   bedpan and cover
   disposable gloves

specimen container and cover
label including: resident's full name,
room number, date and time of collection, doctor's name, examination
to be performed, and other information as requested
toilet tissue
tongue blades

2. Put on disposable gloves.
3. Collect stool from daily bowel movement. Take covered pan to utility room. Offer wash water to patient.
4. Use tongue blades to remove specimen from bedpan and place in specimen container.
5. Wash hands. Do not contaminate the outside of the container.
6. Remove disposable gloves and dispose of according to facility policy.
7. Cover container and attach completed label. Make sure cover is on container tightly. Label the container appropriately.
8. Clean and replace equipment according to facility policy.
9. Promptly deliver specimen as directed.
10. Record procedure on resident's chart.

Summary

- The digestive tract breaks down food into simple substances that can be used by the body cells to carry on their work.
- Bowel problems are common among the elderly.
- Bowel problems in the elderly include constipation, impaction, and diarrhea.
- Through consistant retraining and the use of bowel aids and diet, it is often possible to help patients become continent of feces once again.
- Skin care is a significant part of the nursing care of all incontinent patients.
- Enemas are frequently ordered before tests and most kinds of surgery and to relieve constipation.
- Other procedures you may be assigned include inserting rectal suppositories, irrigating ostomies, collecting stool specimens, and checking for fecal impaction.

Review Outline

I. Behavioral Objectives

II. Vocabulary

III. The Gastrointestinal System
  A. Structure
  B. Function

IV. Senescent Changes

V. Conditions Related to the Tract
  A. Denture problems
  B. Elimination needs
    1. Fecal incontinence
    2. Constipation
    3. Impaction
  C. Bowel aids
    1. Exercise
    2. Diet
    3. Laxatives
    4. Suppositories
    5. Enemas

D.   Hernias
E.   Ulcers
F.   Gastritis
G.   Diverticular disease
H.   Malignancies

VI. Colostomies

A.   Types
B.   Stoma care
C.   Irrigations

Review

I. Vocabulary

Match the words in the left column with their meanings in the right column.

1.   Urgency   a.   To chew
2.   Rectum   b.   Dehydration
3.   Dyspepsia   c.   Chemical reactions that take place in the body.
4.   Suppository   d.   Strong urge to defecate
5.   Colostomy   e.   Indigestion
6.   Metabolism   f.   Difficulty swallowing
7.   Herniorrhaphy   g.   Severest form of constipation
8.   Dysphagia   h.   Terminal length of colon
9.   Impaction   i.   Medication inserted in the rectum
10. Masticate   j.   Repair of a weakened area in a body wall
                        k.   Artificial opening in colon for the
                             purpose of elimination

II. Name the organs shown in figure 28-14.

1.   _____
2.   _____
3.   _____
4.   _____
5.   _____
6.   _____
7.   _____
8.   _____
9.   _____
10. _____

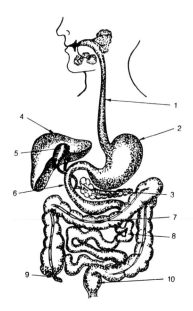

III. True or False

1. Digestion is the process by which complex foods are changed into simple forms.
2. Food is moved along the gastrointestinal tract by rhythmic contractions called urgency.
3. An elderly person having a small amount of diarrhea should be checked for fecal impaction.
4. Diminished liver function can result in poor fat digestion and inability to absorb fat-soluble vitamins.
5. An oil-retention enema is given to harden the stool.
6. Oil-retention enemas are usually followed by S.S.E.
7. It is important to irrigate a colostomy quickly to avoid fatiguing the patient.
8. The person is best positioned for fecal elimination sitting with feet flat on the floor.
9. Guard rails on either side of the toilet add to the security of the resident.
10. Two factors that encourage proper elimination are proper diet and adequate exercise.

IV. Clinical Situations

1. You have an order to give an S.S.E. and the resident has just finished breakfast. What do you do?
2. The resident complains of cramping while you are giving an enema. What do you do?

CASE STUDY

Jessie Yates was a difficult patient. At least that is what the entire staff of Wheelsboro Convalescent Hospital believed.

She was a diminutive person, barely 5 feet tall but full of spunk and energy. She was anemic and received daily nutrients with iron. Her ninety-one years had been lived to the fullest. As a former social worker, she was perhaps the best informed of all the residents about all the other residents. She was hard of hearing and sometimes mixed up facts. She created problems by repeating these inaccurate facts and giving unsolicited advice.

Besides this, she was forgetful and tended to be cranky. Perhaps this is why her crankiness and lack of appetite over a four-day period were not considered significant.

During exercise hour, the geriatric health care provider missed her and commented that her lack of participation *was* unusual. The assistant went to locate Mrs. Yates and found her in her room, sitting by the window. She told the assistant her stomach was upset and she seemed to have a small amount of diarrhea.

The assistant reported the situation and the team leader talked with Mrs. Yates. She told the assistant to give Mrs. Yates a soapsuds enema because she suspected that the resident was constipated. When the assistant attempted the carry out the procedure, she met resistance to the rectal tube. She withdrew the tube and notified the team leader.

The team leader confirmed a fecal mass by digital examination and ordered an oil-retention enema, according to facility policy. An oil-retention enema followed by a soapsuds enema proved successful in relieving the impaction.

The team leader called a staff conference later that day and discussed the following points:

1. Careful noting of the character and frequency of bowel movements is an important nursing responsibility.
2. Diarrhea in the elderly is often a sign of fecal impaction and should be reported immediately.
3. The elderly are at risk for constipation and impaction because of poor appetites, lack of fluid intake, inactivity, and loss of muscle tone.
4. The elderly can become dependent on bowel aids. Although helpful, they should be avoided by simple nursing awareness.
5. All resident should have bowel movements recorded. Fluids and activity should be promoted.

All staff members realized the importance of what had been discussed.

1. How was the fecal impaction determined?
2. List four clues that might have made the staff aware of an impending problem.
3. What senescent bowel change contributed to the develpment of constipation?
4. Why did the assistant discontinue the first soapsuds enema?
5. Why was an oil retention enema given before the S.S.E.?
6. Can you think of a reason that the early signs might have been missed?
7. It is necessary to have a bowel movement every day?

Unit 29
Urinary System Alterations

Objectives
After studying this unit, you should be able to:
- Name and locate the parts of the urinary system.
- Describe the function of the urinary system.
- Review the characteristics of the aging urinary system.
- List the normal changes in the elimination pattern as the body ages.
- Explain the purpose of bladder retraining.
- Give proper nursing care to a patient who is incontinent.

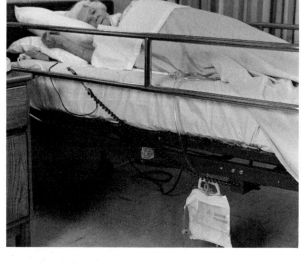

Vocabulary
Learn the meaning and spelling of the following words or phrases.

concentration	incontinence	rectocele
cystocele	micturating cystogram	renal calculi
cystometrogram	micturate	retention
cystoscopy	nephron	uremia
hemodialysis	nocturia	void

The urinary system is sometimes referred to as the excretory system. The organs of this system produce urine (liquid waste), which is excreted from the body. The urinary system also helps to control the vital water and electrolyte balance of the body. Inability to secrete urine by the kidneys is known as suppression. Inability to excrete urine that has been produced is called *retention*. Urine with few dissolved substances is more dilute. Urine with many dissolved substances is more concentrated.

Structure and Function

Kidneys
The two bean-shaped kidneys are located behind the peritoneum, the membrane that lines the ventral cavity. The kidneys are held in place by capsules of fat. The outer portion of the kidney is called the cortex, figure 29-1. Urine is produced in this area. The middle area (medulla) is a series of tubes that drain the urine toward the pelvis of the kidney.

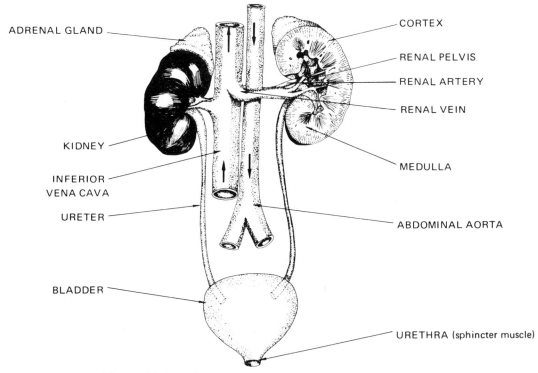

ADRENAL GLAND

CORTEX

RENAL PELVIS

RENAL ARTERY

RENAL VEIN

KIDNEY

INFERIOR
VENA CAVA

MEDULLA

URETER

ABDOMINAL AORTA

BLADDER

URETHRA (sphincter muscle)

Figure 29-1 The normal anatomy of the urinary system

Ureters

The two ureters extend from the pelvises of the kidneys to the urinary bladder. The ureters are approximately 10 to 12 inches long and 1/4 inch wide. They act as passageways for the urine.

Urinary Bladder

The urinary bladder, within the pelvic cavity, is a reservoir for urine until it is expelled from the body. The muscular walls of the bladder are able to contract and force the urine out. The bladder can be controlled voluntarily, but it can empty involuntarily as well. Before being toilet trained, children automatically empty their bladders as the smooth muscle walls contract and the muscles that guard the opening relax. The urge to urinate (*micturate* or *void*) occurs when there is 200 to 300 ml of urine in the bladder. However, the bladder is capable of holding much more.

Urethra

The urethra in the female is about 1 1/2 inches long. In the male it is about 8 inches long. Surrounding the neck of the male bladder is a doughnut-shaped gland called the prostate, which normally functions in reproduction. The urethra passes through its center. The opening of the urethra to the outside is called the external urinary meatus. The meatus is guarded by a round sphincter muscle that relaxes to release the urine.

Urine Production

The renal arteries carry blood to each kidney. Their many branches pass through the medulla to the cortex. In the cortex the blood vessels branch to form balls of capillaries called glomeruli. There are approximately one million glomeruli in each kidney. The blood vessels merge to leave the kidney as the renal vein.

Each glomerulus is surrounded by a blind tube, the end of which resembles a cup. This cup is called Bowman's capsule. Extending from Bowman's capsule is a tube that twists and coils within the cortex and then extends down into the medulla of the kidney. Blood vessels extend from the glomerulus and wrap themselves around the coiled tubules. This entire structure is called a *nephron*, figure 29-2. Waste products in large amounts of water are passed from the glomerulus to Bowman's capsule. The filtering ability of the kidneys depends in large measure on an adequate flow of blood to the kidneys.

All the water needed to filter waste products cannot be permanently lost from the body. Much of it is absorbed back into the bloodstream as the branches of the glomerulus encircle the twisted tubule in the cortex. Concentrating urine to conserve water and solids is an important function of the kidneys. Much of this *concentration* of urine goes on at night. The final product of the filtration and reabsorption processes is called urine. The urine is drained into the pelvis of the kidney. From there, it flows to the ureters and then to the urinary bladder. People drink less during the night or sleeping hours. Therefore, urine is normally more concentrated and darker than usual when first voided in the morning.

Waste products excreted in urine include urea, creatinine, uric acid, and various salts. The average urine output is 1,500 to 2,400 ml every twenty-four hours. Hormones influence how much urine is produced.

Elimination

The normal act of voiding is brought about through the integrated action of the internal sphincter, external sphincter, and the muscle

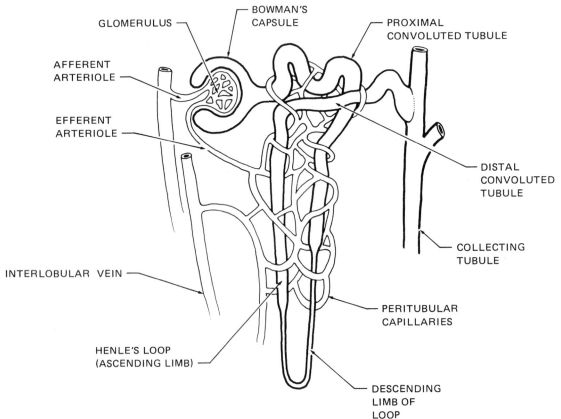

Figure 29-2   The functional unit of the kidney that produces urine is the nephron.

mass of the bladder wall. As the bladder fills, the muscle fibers stretch. This stimulates autonomic nerve fibers embedded within, figure 29-3. The sensation is carried to the spinal cord for reflex action and to the cerebral cortex for awareness.

Autonomic nerve impulses allow the muscle mass of the bladder to relax and fill. The stretching stimulus of the bladder wall gradually becomes stronger as urine accumulates. Unless impulses from the cerebral cortex intervene and cause inhibition, a reflex reaction at the cord level occurs. Reflex impulses cause the sphincters to relax and the bladder wall to contract, and urine is expelled.

Messages from the cerebral cortex may either initiate or inhibit this activity. When cerebral control is lost, as it is in a stroke, emptying of the bladder will occur automatically. Loss of voluntary control may result in premature, frequent emptying of the bladder, or *incontinence*. Continuous catheter drainage causes the bladder muscle to lose tone. This makes continence even more difficult to achieve after the catheter has been removed.

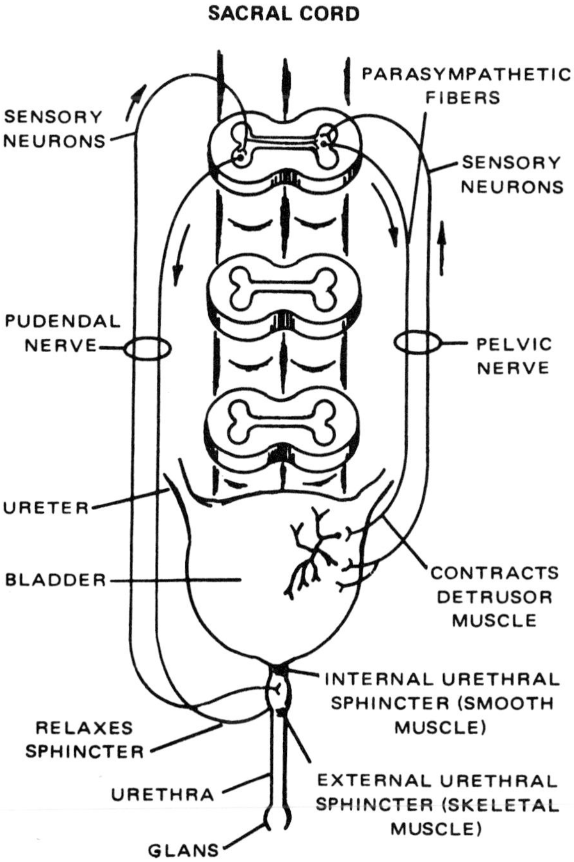

Senescent Changes

* Kidneys decrease in size
* Scars replace renal cells
* Renal concentration is poorer, with nocturia
* Bladder emptying becomes less efficient
* Filtration ability is reduced

Figure 29-4   Senescent changes in the urinary system

As a person grows older, the relaxation of perineal structures and the enlargement of the prostate gland form mechanical barriers to urine elimination. There is a tendency for urine to be retained and bladder stones to form. Under these conditions, bladder infections become more common. The bladder muscle loses tone, and bladder capacity decreases. The older person is less aware of the need to void or defecate, because the sensations of a full bladder or rectum have diminished. The ability of the kidneys to concentrate urine at night decreases. As a result, frequency and *nocturia* (voiding often during the night) are encountered more often.

Refer to table 29-1 for the nursing diagnostic categories related to problems of elimination.

* Alteration in urinary elimination: Incontinence, retention
* Altered sexual patterns
* Anxiety
* Impaired skin integrity

Table 29-1   Nursing diagnostic categories related to problems in urinary elimination

Figure 29-3   The voiding reflexes (From *Dynamic Anatomy and Physiology* by Langley, et al., copyright 1969, McGraw-Hill Book Company)

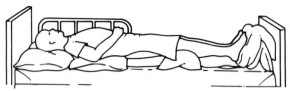

Figure 29-5 The bedpan should be padded and the body supported with pillows.

Positioning for Elimination

Proper positioning makes elimination easier. Remaining in the supine position for a long period of time predisposes to both infections and bladder stones because of incomplete bladder emptying. In this position, it is much more difficult to relax the external sphincter and perineal muscles to initiate elimination.

Sitting upright, with knees and hips flexed and feet flat for support, is the best position. A bedside commode may be used. The patient may also sit on a bedpan on the edge of the bed with the feet resting on a footstool. The height of the regular toilet seat may be raised for maximum comfort, safety, and support. A height of 20 inches is usually the most satisfactory. Men find it easier to void in the standing position, but they may require support. When patients must remain in bed, the bedpan should be padded and the body supported with pillows, figure 29-5. Use of an orthopedic bedpan may provide additional comfort.

Refer to figure 29-6 to review the beginning procedure actions and the procedure completion actions.

Beginning Procedure Actions

- Wash hands.
- Assemble all equipment needed.
- Knock on door and pause before entering resident's room.
- Politely ask visitors to leave. Tell them where they can wait.

- Identify the resident.
- Provide privacy by drawing curtains around bed and closing door.
- Explain what you will be doing and answer questions.
- Raise bed to comfortable working height.

Procedure Completion Actions

- Position resident comfortably.
- Leave signal cord, telephone, and fresh water where resident can reach them.
- Return bed to lowest horizontal position.
- Raise side rails, if required.
- Perform general safety check of resident and environment.
- Clean used equipment and return to proper storage, according to facility policy.
- Open privacy curtains.
- Wash hands.
- Tell visitors that they may reenter the room.
- Report completion of procedure.
- Document procedure following facility policy.

Figure 29-6 Beginning procedure actions and procedure completion actions

PROCEDURE 46

Giving a Bedpan

Note: Check the policy of your facility regarding the use of disposable gloves during this procedure.

1. Wash hands and assemble the following equipment:

bedpan and cover	soap
toilet tissue	washcloth
basin of warm water	towel

2. Identify the person and explain what you plan to do.
3. Screen the unit.
4. Lower the head of the bed.

5. Take the bedpan and tissue from the bedside stand and place the bedpan on the bedside chair. Never place it on the side stand or overbed table. Put tissue on the bedside stand within easy reach of the patient. Put the remainder of the articles on the bedside table.

6. Place bedpan cover at the foot of the bed between the mattress and springs. The bedpan may be warmed by running hot water into it and emptying it. In hot weather, talcum powder may be used on the bedpan to prevent the patient's skin from sticking to it. Plastic bedpans may be comfortable without warming.

7. Fold top bedcovers back at a right angle and raise the patient's gown. Pad the bedpan with a folded towel if the person is thin or has a pressure sore.

8. Ask the person to flex knees and rest weight on heels if able.

9. Help the person to raise buttocks by putting one hand under the small of the back and lifting gently and slowly with one hand. With the other hand, place the bedpan under the person's hips. If the person is unable to raise the buttocks, two people may be needed to lift, or the pan may be placed by rolling the patient to one side, positioning the bedpan against the buttocks, and rolling the person back on it. Alternatively, if a trapeze is in place over the bed, the assistant may place the bedpan as the person lifts up using the trapeze. The person's buttocks should rest on the rounded shelf of the bedpan. The narrow end should face the foot of bed.

10. Replace top bedcovers. Raise the head of the bed to a comfortable height.

11. Make sure the signal cord is within easy reach. Leave the person alone unless contraindicated.

12. Answer the call signal immediately. Fill the basin with warm water and get soap, washcloth, and towel. Lower the head of the bed.

13. Ask the person to flex knees and rest weight on heels. Place one hand under the small of the back and lift gently to help raise the buttocks off bedpan. Take the bedpan with the other hand. Cover it and place it on the chair. If the person is unable to raise the buttocks, two people may be needed to lift. Otherwise, roll the person off the pan to the side and remove the pan. Lift and move it carefully. Hold the pan firmly with one hand. Many people have difficulty cleaning themselves adequately after using the bedpan. You may need to clean and dry the person yourself.

14. Assist the person to a clean area of the bed, if necessary. Discard tissue in bedpan unless specimen is to be collected. Cover the bedpan again and place on chair. Cleanse person with warm water and soap if necessary.

15. Replace bedclothes. Encourage the person to wash hands and freshen up after the procedure. Change linen or protective pads as necessary.

16. Take the bedpan to the bathroom or utility room and observe contents. Measure, if required.

17. Empty bedpan. Rinse with cold water and disinfectant, rinse, dry, and cover the bedpan.

18. Put bedpan inside the bedside table. Clean and replace other articles.

19. Wash hands. Leave unit in order.

20. Report any unusual observations to your supervisor and chart according to facility policy.

PROCEDURE 47

Giving a Urinal

Note: Check the policy of your facility regarding the use of disposable gloves during this procedure.

1. Wash hands and assemble the following equipment:

urinal and cover	soap
basin of warm	washcloth
water	towel

2. Identify the person and explain what you plan to do.
3. Screen the unit for privacy.
4. Lift the bedcovers and place the urinal under the covers so the patient can grasp the handle.
5. Make sure the signal cord is within easy reach. Leave the person alone if possible.
6. Answer the signal immediately. Fill a basin with warm water and lay out the soap, washcloth, and towel so the patient can wash and dry hands.
7. Ask the person to hand the urinal to you. Cover it and rearrange bedclothes if necessary.
8. Take the urinal to the bedroom or utility room and observe the contents. Measure, if required. Do not empty urinal if anything unusual (such as blood) is observed, but save contents for your supervisor's inspection.
9. Empty the urinal. Rinse with cold water and clean with warm, soapy water. Rinse, dry, and cover urinal.
10. Place urinal inside bedside table. Clean and replace other articles. Leave person comfortable and unit tidy.
11. Wash hands.
12. Report any unusual observations to supervisor, and chart according to facility policy.

PROCEDURE 48

Assisting with a Bedside Commode

Note: Check the policy of your facility regarding the use of disposable gloves during this procedure.

1. Wash hands and assemble the following equipment:

portable commode	washcloth and soap
basin of warm	toilet tissue
water	towel

2. Identify person and explain what you plan to do.
3. Draw curtains for privacy.
4. Place tissue on bedside table within reach.
5. Position commode beside bed, facing head. Lock wheels and remove cover. Be sure receptacle is in place under seat.
6. Lower side rails and bed to lowest horizontal position.
7. Assist person to sitting position. Swing person's legs over edge of bed.
8. Put patient's slippers on and help patient to stand.
9. Have person place hands on your shoulders.
10. Support patient under the arms, pivot person to the right, and lower to commode.
11. Leave call bell and tissue within reach.
12. When signalled, return promptly. Draw warm water in basin and bring to bedside along with soap, towel, and washcloth.
13. Assist person to stand.
14. Cleanse anus or perineum if person is unable.
15. Allow person to wash and dry hands.
16. Help person return to bed. Adjust bedding and pillows for comfort.
17. Put cover on commode.
18. Remove receptacle. Cover with bedpan cover.
19. Take to bathroom. Note contents and measure if required.
20. Empty and clean according to facility policy. Return commode. Clean remainder of articles and return to their place.
21. Put commode in proper place (probably in the corner of the room).
22. Wash hands.

23. Report completion of task. Indicate any unusual observations. Record on appropriate record form.

Urinary Retention and Incontinence

Incontinence and retention are two equally serious problems involving the urinary system. It is estimated that one of every ten patients receiving home care is plagued by one or the other of these problems. The situation is three times more common in institutions. It is twice as common in women as in men.

Incontinence and retention have many causes. Included are psychological withdrawal with loss of interest in surroundings, lack of awareness of the need to eliminate, and organic changes affecting the process of elimination. Medications such as diuretics produce larger volumes of urine. Other medications such as tranquilizers and sedatives may promote incontinence at night. These drugs depress the nerve sensations that signal the need to void. Control can be achieved in some cases by simply increasing the mental stimulation and social involvement of the patient. Getting a patient up and dressed may be sufficient to promote control.

Some incontinence may be due to difficulty in getting to the toilet or unfastening clothing in time. Geriatric health care providers can assist by planning activities that take toileting time into consideration. They can also be available to routinely assist with toileting, manage fluid intake, and encourage Velcro fasteners on clothing. For example, encouraging fluids during the day, limiting the amount of fluids after 8 P.M., and keeping a call bell close at hand can often solve the incontinence problem.

Urinary retention most often results from poor bladder tone or incomplete emptying because of mechanical obstructions. Enlargement of the male prostate and relaxation of female perineal structures act as mechanical obstructions.

Urinary incontinence may be due to one or a combination of causes. Any interruption of cerebral control will lead to incontinence. This would include a stroke, brain damage that destroys the control centers or pathways, or cerebral clouding and decreased awareness due to general cerebral degeneration or aphasia. Incontinence may also be related to a fecal impaction. The impaction acts as a mechanical obstruction by compressing the urethra. This causes urine to be retained. The incontinence is actually overflow. Perhaps the most common reason for incontinence is infection. Inflammation irritates sensory nerve endings in the bladder, causing mucosa and bladder contractions to increase and leading to incontinence.

Incontinence in elderly women may be stress induced. Sneezing, laughing, and coughing may cause the woman to expel a small amount of urine. Two approaches may be helpful. Exercises to improve the strength of pelvic floor musculature can be learned and practiced, or cystoceles (herniations of the bladder wall into the vagina) or rectoceles (herniations of the rectum into the vagina) can be repaired surgically.

Incontinence may be temporary, lasting only a few days, as during a period of illness. Attention to the underlying causes and the temporary use of incontinence pads or adult disposable diapers may be all that is needed. When adult diapers are required, be sensitive to the patient's emotional response. Diapers connote babies, dependence, and failure of self-control. Treat the application as a routine but temporary measure to assure better skin protection. Choose less demeaning terms such as incontinence pants, skin protection pads, or undergarments when speaking of them. Emphasize the temporary need (if true) and the patient's increased comfort.

These disposable undergarments will make your task easier, because the bedding will be protected. Do not forget to change the pads frequently and to give good skin care, however. The area should be washed and dried at each changing. Urine left on the skin will promote rapid breakdown. Every effort should be made to help the patient become ambulant as soon as possible, with little reference to the temporary incontinence. You can do much to give emotional support and reassurance to the patient. Incontinence may continue even though the patient is ambulant and making progress in other areas of rehabilitation. This is a more difficult but still not impossible form of incontinence to treat. Catheterization should be considered only as a last resort.

Diagnosis

Diagnostic procedures include *cystoscopy* (visualization of the bladder), and *micturating cystogram* (X rays taken before and during *micturition*). They also include *cystometrogram* (a record made by filling the bladder slowly to note its capacity and uninhibited bladder contractions).

After the diagnostic tests have been completed, a program of bladder retraining may be found advisable. The purpose of retraining is to achieve a pattern of nearly normal filling and emptying of the bladder. The first step is to determine the present incontinence pattern. An incontinence chart covering a period of seventy-two hours is helpful. It shows the times and amounts of urine and feces and any drugs or bowel aids that have been used. The patient's emotional reaction is observed carefully.

Urinalysis is the most common laboratory test made in the hospital. The specimen is usually taken when the patient first voids in the morning. When a urine specimen is needed that is free of contamination from organisms found in areas near the urinary meatus, it is collected either by inserting a sterile tube (catheter) or by collecting a midstream specimen. For the latter, the area is cleansed and the person is instructed to void. After the flow is started, the container is moved into position to catch the urine. This is the best way to obtain any urine specimen. If a twenty-four-hour urine specimen is ordered, all urine excreted in a twenty-four-hour period is collected and saved in a large, carefully labeled container. The container is usually surrounded by ice or kept in a refrigerator. The person is asked to

void, and this first urine is discarded so that the bladder is empty when the test begins. All other urine is saved, including that voided as the test time ends. No toilet tissue should be allowed to enter the specimen. If you or the person forgets to save a specimen during the test period, report this fact immediately to the nurse.

PROCEDURE 49

Collecting a Routine Urine Specimen

Note: Check the policy of your facility regarding the use of disposable gloves during this procedure.

1. Wash hands and assemble the following equipment:

    disposable gloves
    bedpan or urinal and cover
    container and cover for specimen
    graduate
    laboratory requisition slip, properly filled out
    label, including patient's full name, room number, hospital number, date and time of collection, doctor's name, examination to be done, and other information as requested

2. Identify person and explain what you plan to do. Tell person not to discard toilet tissue in the pan with the urine. Provide paper towels or a small plastic sack in which to place the soiled tissue.
3. Screen the unit. Offer bedpan or urinal.
4. After person has voided, take pan to utility room. Offer wash water to patient.
5. Put on disposable gloves if they are to be used. Pour specimen from the bedpan into the graduate, figure 29-7. Note the amount if intake and output are to be recorded.
6. Pour about 120 ml into the specimen container.
7. Remove disposable gloves and dispose of them according to facility policy. Wash

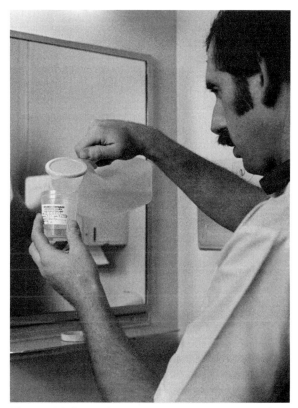

Figure 29-7   Urine specimens must be carefully obtained and sent to the laboratory.

hands. Do not contaminate outside of container.

8.   Cover container. Attach completed label and requisition slip to container.

9.   Clean and replace equipment according to facility policy.

10.   Take or send specimen to appropriate area.

11.   Record procedure on the chart.

PROCEDURE 50

Collecting a Clean-Catch (Midstream) Urine Specimen

1.   Wash hands and assemble the following equipment:

disposable gloves
sterile urine specimen container
gauze squares or cotton
antiseptic solution
label for container with resident's full name, room number, date and the time of collection, physician's name, type of specimen/test to be performed, and any other information requested

2.   Identify the person and explain what you plan to do.

3.   Put on disposable gloves. Wash the person's genital area or have the person do so.

For the female:

a.   Using the gauze or cotton and the antiseptic solution, cleanse the outer folds of the vulva (the folds are also called labia or lips) with a front-to-back motion.

b.   Discard the gauze/cotton.

c.   Cleanse the inner folds of the vulva with another piece of gauze and antiseptic solution, again with a front-to-back motion. Discard gauze/cotton.

d.   Finally, cleanse the middle, innermost area (meatus or urinary opening) in the same manner. Discard gauze/cotton.

For the male:

a.   Using the gauze or cotton and the antiseptic solution, cleanse the tip of the penis from the urinary meatus (opening) down, using a circular motion.

b.   Discard the gauze/cotton.

4.   Instruct the person to void, allowing the first part of the urine stream to escape. Then, catch the urine stream that follows in the sterile specimen container. Allow the last portion of the urine stream to escape. **Note:** If intake and output are being monitored or if the amount of urine passed must be measured, catch the first and last part of the urine in a bedpan or urinal.

5. Place the sterile cap on the urine container immediately to avoid contaminating the urine specimen.
6. Allow the person to wash hands.
7. With the cap securely tightened, wash the outside of the specimen container.
8. Remove gloves and dispose of them according to facility policy. Wash hands.
9. Label the container as instructed and attach requisition slip for appropriate test.
10. Clean and replace all equipment according to facility policy.
11. Take or send specimen to appropriate area immediately.
12. Record procedure on the chart.

PROCEDURE 51

Collecting a Fresh Fractional Urine Sample

1. About one hour before testing is to be done, wash hands and assemble the following equipment:

   disposable gloves
   two specimen containers
   urinal or bedpan
   testing materials if urine testing is to be performed (Clinitest, Acetest, Ketostix, or Testape)
   small plastic bag for used toilet tissue

2. Identify the person and explain what you plan to do. Tell the person that two samples will be taken, an initial sample now and a smaller sample in about one hour.
3. Screen unit. Put on disposable gloves and offer bedpan or urinal (assist person to the commode if permitted).
4. Encourage person to empty bladder.
5. Do not permit tissue to be placed in receptacle. Place in plastic bag and discard.
6. Take receptacle to bathroom or utility room.
7. Pour sample into one specimen container. Test this sample in case resident fails to void second specimen.

8. Note the test results but do not officially record them.
9. Clean equipment according to facility policy and return to proper area. Measure and record urine if person is on I & O.
10. Remove and dispose of gloves according to facility policy. Wash hands.
11. Offer wash water for the person to wash hands.
12. If permitted, encourage the person to drink water. Be sure to record intake on intake/output sheet.
13. Tell person when you will return for the second sample. Return to the unit at the proper time.
14. Wash hands. Identify person and explain what you plan to do.
15. Repeat steps 3 to 11.
16. Report and record findings of the second testing.

PROCEDURE 52

Collecting a 24-Hour Urine Specimen

1. Wash hands and assemble the following equipment:

   disposable gloves
   twenty-four-hour specimen container
   label and sign for person's bed
   label for the container with the person's name, room number, test ordered, type of specimen, date, and physician's name

2. Identify the person and explain what you plan to do. Emphasize the necessity for saving all urine passed.
3. Allow the resident to void. Put on gloves and assist with the bedpan/urinal as needed. Measure the amount of urine passed if the person's I & O is being monitored.

4. Discard the urine specimen. Note the date and time of voiding. This time will mark the start of the twenty-four-hour collection period.
5. Remove gloves and dispose of them according to facility policy. Place a sign on the person's bed to alert other health care team members that a twenty-four-hour urine specimen is being collected (sign may read "Save all urine—24-hour specimen").
6. From this time on, all urine is voided into the specimen container for a period of twenty-four hours. The container is refrigerated when not in use. Check facility policy regarding handling of the specimen container. If any urine is discarded accidentally, the test must be discontinued and started again for another twenty-four hours.
7. At the end of the twenty-four-hour period, ask the person to void one last time. Put on disposable gloves and add this urine to the specimen container. Remove gloves and dispose of them according to facility policy.
8. Remove sign from bed. Check label for accuracy and completeness and attach appropriate requisition slip.
9. Clean and replace all equipment used according to facility policy.
10. Wash hands.
11. Take or send specimen to appropriate area immediately.
12. Record the procedure on person's chart.

Nursing Assessment

A nursing assessment is an essential part of the retraining regime. During the assessment the nurse tries to determine the patient's previous habits and feelings about the present illness. It is sometimes necessary to gather information from the family. You can help by closely observing and accurately reporting your findings to the nurse. This information is added to the medical diagnosis and an analysis of the incontinence pattern is made. A retraining program is then planned.

Although the professional nurse usually makes the nursing assessment, all staff members must participate in keeping the incontinence record up to date.

Retraining

Western society views incontinence as totally undesirable in an adult. In fact, it is barely tolerated in the young, as shown by the pride many mothers take in the early toilet training of their children. It is not surprising that mature people who are incontinent suffer shame or embarrassment and feel hopeless or despondent. Families may be reluctant to accept responsibility for care of the incontinent at home. Feelings of disgust or annoyance are quickly communicated to the patient. Family members may so resent the problems of an incontinent adult that they refuse to give care at all. Incontinence may be the factor that determines whether a person can remain at home or must be institutionalized.

Cultural mores influence the attitude of the nursing staff as well. Too often nurses view incontinence with resignation, as an inevitable condition of advanced age. But the patient with elimination problems represents a challenge to enlightened geriatric health care providers who understand that control can often be achieved. This type of staff conveys a feeling of hope to the patient. Positive acceptance helps the patient recognize that, with patience, retraining is possible.

The first step in retraining is to enlist the patient's cooperation. Not all patients are able to cooperate to the same degree, but they should be given the opportunity to participate. An hourly incontinence record is kept for at least forty-eight hours. Intake and output are measured, and times are noted. Nursing assessments consider patient awareness, cooperation, and medications or related treatments. From this record a continence training program is developed. The second step is to provide the patient with the opportunity to void, figure 29-8. Nocturnal incontinence can be helped by making sure that a urinal is kept at the bedside in an easily accessible

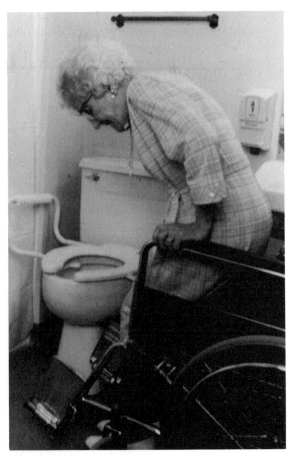

Figure 29-8 The toileting facility must be easily available when retraining for continence.

spot or by taking the patient to the bathroom. It can also be helped by offering the bedpan at midnight. When the incontinence record shows a specific time that incontinence occurs, the patient should be awakened routinely one hour before that time.

Some authorities advocate control of fluids as an aid to continence. Fluids are forced during daytime hours and restricted at night. Others believe that limitation of fluids is inadvisable because of the danger to the elderly of dehydration, increased confusion, and even *uremia*. Uremia (accumulation of urea in the blood) develops as the kidneys fail.

Drugs are sometimes used to achieve bladder control. When decreased bladder capacity is the problem, anticholinergic drugs may be given. These drugs block transmission of motor impulses to the bladder. Such drugs diminish the frequency of uninhibited bladder contractions and thus increase the capacity of the bladder. Two such drugs, propantheline and orphenadrine, are usually prescribed on a 7- to 10-day trial basis. They are not effective for all patients.

Voiding

Voiding may occur as often as every 1 to 1½ hours in the early training stages. Gradually, however, as intake and voiding opportunities are planned, the intervals become greater. During the weeks of retraining, the importance of emotional support cannot be overemphasized. The nursing staff must all present a confident attitude. They must help to assure the patient that new habits can be established with diligence, patience, and time. Retraining usually takes from six to eight weeks of continuous effort. Successes should be praised and lapses accepted as a natural part of the training process. The attitudes and reactions of the nurse and staff members must be consistently positive.

When difficulty initiating the flow is encountered, attention to position, a glass of water to drink, or a measured amount of water poured over the perineum may act as a stimulus. Helping the patient to lean forward, gently stroking the inner thigh, or tickling the side of the urinary meatus with a wisp of cotton can be tried. Patients should be encouraged to bear down at the end of voiding to completely empty the bladder. Slight pressure over the abdomen at this time aids the process.

Intractable Incontinence

When retraining is not successful, means must be found to protect the skin against breakdown from constant contact with the urine. This problem is more simply solved for men than it is for women through the use of external drainage appliances.

For men, urosheaths and condoms attached to drainage tubing and collection bags are quite convenient and effective, figure 29-9. Care should be taken to remove the urosheaths or condoms every twenty-four hours. The penis should be carefully washed and dried and observed for signs of irritation. A thin film of tincture of benzoin should be applied to the penis and the condom or urosheath placed in position. Tape is used to secure the sheath so that circulation is not impeded. Some urosheaths are packaged with special sponge tape. Portable urinals are sometimes used by patients, but they usually present problems with odor and skin irritations. The sheath, when applied properly, is a better approach to a difficult situation.

You have the following responsibilities when patients have urinary drainage, whether through a condom, urosheath, or catheter.

• Make sure tubes are in good position and unblocked.

• Measure output carefully. Note color and anything unusual.
• Keep the end of the drainage tubing above the urine in the bag.
• Do not permit the drainage bag to touch the floor. Connect it to the bed frame, not to the side rail.
• Always keep the bag below the patient's hip.
• Keep the drainage tubes coiled smoothly in the bed so that there is a direct drop to the drainage bag.

Activity should be planned on twenty-four-hour basis. Adequate fluid intake (3,000 ml daily) is essential. Infection tends to make urine alkaline. A patient may develop kidney stones because of this. Therefore, an acid-ash diet is ordered to make the urine more acid (lower the pH), figure 29-10. Activity, adequate fluid intake, and diet help decrease the incidence of stone formation and bladder infections. There is an ever present danger that resistant strains of

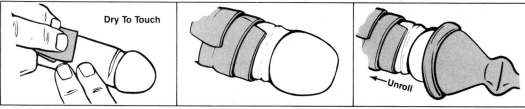

1   PREPARATION   Wipe the penis completely with Shield Skin to increase holding power of the liner and provide added skin protection. Let this dressing dry completely to a smooth, non-tacky surface (about 30 seconds). Make sure the penis is completely dry and free of all moisture before applying the Uro-San Plus liner.

2   APPLYING THE LINER   Starting at the head of the penis, wrap the water-proof stretchable double-sided adhesive foam liner gently around the penis in an overlapping fashion. Wrap it snug but not tight. Continue to spiral wrap the liner back toward the base of the penis. The liner should wrap around the penis one full turn or more. (Do not wear gloves, as the liner will stick to them.)

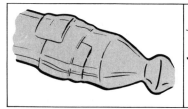

3   ROLLING ON SHEATH   Place the cone end of the rolled up sheath next to the head of the penis. Unroll the sheath over the outside of the foam liner and all the way up the length of the penis. Make sure the funnel is not touching head of penis.

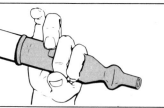

4   SEALING IN PLACE   Squeeze the sheath all around to seal the sheath and liner in place. The liner has now formed a water-tight and non-constricting barrier against urine. The free end of the catheter is then attached to a urine collection bag.

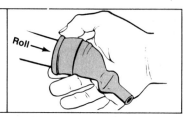

5   REMOVAL IS QUICK AND EASY.   Grasp the end of the sheath at the base of the penis. Roll it forward gently. Liner and sheath roll right off together.

Figure 29-9   A urosheath connected to a drainage bag is placed over the penis to protect the skin of the incontinent male. (Courtesy of Mentor Corporation, Minneapolis, MN)

microorganisms may develop. Therefore, broad-spectrum antibiotics may be employed to combat the infections that do occur.

External drainage is not feasible for the female with intractable urinary incontinence. Catheterization may be the final answer. The insertion of a catheter is a sterile procedure, usually performed by the nurse or physician. Do not try to perform the procedure until you have been taught and have practiced under supervision, and until you have gained proficiency.

Indwelling catheters should be employed only when all other measures have failed and skin breakdown is probable or present. Prolonged use of indwelling catheters causes the bladder to lose muscle tone and normal capacity. As a preventative measure, the catheter may be clamped at intervals during the day. An order is required to clamp the catheter. Be sure the clamp is left on only for the specific amount of time ordered.

Only those who have been properly taught and supervised and who have legal authorization may carry out advanced procedures such as catheterization.

Catheter Techniques The smallest catheter possible, usually size 14 to 16, should be used for the elderly person. A french-type catheter will be used for simple catheterization, such as for a urine specimen. A Foley (indwelling) catheter will be used when the catheter is to be attached

for continuous drainage, figure 29-11. To relieve pressure, the catheter must be taped to the inner thigh of the female and in an upward position for a male patient, figure 29-12. The upward position decreases the pressure on the penoscrotal junction.

Three areas of possible contamination include the entrance to the urethra, connections between the catheter and drainage tube, and the end of the drainage tube, figure 29-13. Special attention should be given to these areas. The urinary meatus must be kept clean and free of secretions. The area around the meatus should be washed daily with a solution specified by the hospital. This is called indwelling catheter care. Any signs of irritation or urinary discomfort should be reported.

PROCEDURE 53

Routine Drainage Check

1. Wash hands.
2. Identify the resident.
3. Explain what you plan to do.
4. Close the privacy curtains.
5. Raise bedding to observe tubing. Do not expose the resident.
6. Check position of catheter and meatus.
7. Keep drainage tube coiled smoothly on bed so there is a direct drop to collection bag, figure 29-14.

Acid-Ash Foods	Alkaline-Ash Foods
Cranberries	Vegetables
Prunes	Milk
Meat	Citrus fruits
Eggs	
Fish	
Plums	
Poultry	

Figure 29-10   An acid-ash diet helps to prevent the formation of kidney stones. Acid urine also inhibits bacterial growth.

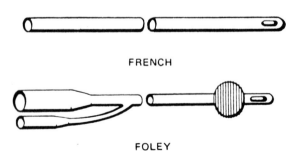

FRENCH

FOLEY

Figure 29-11   Two types of catheters used to drain urine

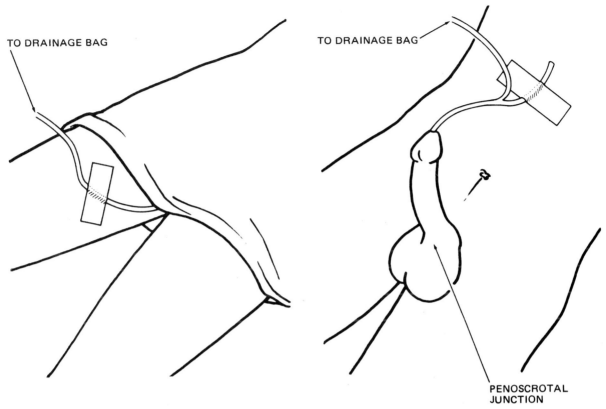

TO DRAINAGE BAG

TO DRAINAGE BAG

PENOSCROTAL
JUNCTION

Figure 29-12   To relieve pressure, the indwelling catheter is taped to the inner thigh of the female and to the abdomen of the male patient.

8. Adjust collection bag level below resident's hips.
9. Keep end of drainage tube above urine level in bag.
10. Attach drainage tube to bed frame.
11. Note color, character, and flow of urine.
12. Measure urine using proper technique.
13. Wash hands.
14. Report completion of procedure.
15. Record your observations.

Indwelling catheter care may be performed during the routine morning care, as part of perineal care, or as a separate procedure. Safe techniques must be used when the catheter is irrigated. It is better not to introduce anything into the catheter unless there is evidence that the catheter is not draining freely.

PROCEDURE 54

Disconnecting a Catheter

Note: It is preferable never to disconnect the drainage setup, but it may be necessary. If sterile caps and plugs are available, they should be used. If not, the disconnected ends must be protected with sterile gauze sponges.

1. Wash hands.
2. Identify resident.
3. Explain what you are going to do.
4. Put on disposable gloves.
5. Clamp the catheter.
6. Disinfect the area to be disconnected.
7. Disconnect the catheter and drainage

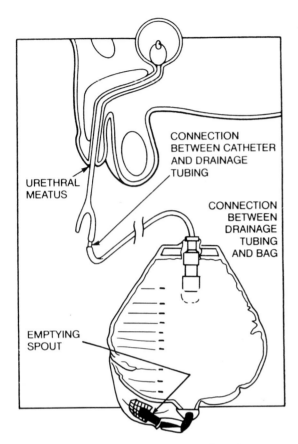

Figure 29-13 Special care must be taken to protect the possible sites of contamination in the closed urinary drainage system. (From Caldwell & Hegner, *Nursing Assistant, A Nursing Process Approach*, copyright 1989 by Delmar Publishers Inc.)

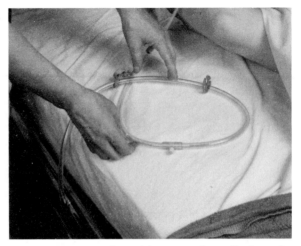

Figure 29-14 The tubing must be coiled on the bed with a direct drop to the collection bag. (From Caldwell & Hegner, *Nursing Assistant, A Nursing Process Approach*, copyright 1989 by Delmar Publishers Inc.)

connected tube in the bed or on the floor, do not reconnect it, but report the situation at once.

Skin Care Regular, routine cleansing of the skin of any incontinent patient must be meticulous if breakdown is to be avoided. Heat lamps, carefully used, and a fine dusting of zinc oxide powder help to heal excoriated areas. You may wish to review with your instructor the procedures related to the urinary system.

PROCEDURE 55

Replacing a Urinary Condom

1. Wash hands and assemble the following equipment:

basin of warm water	gloves
	plastic bag
washcloth	tincture of benzoin
towel	condom with drain-
bed protector/bath	age tip
blanket	paper towels

tubing. Do not put them down or allow them to touch anything.

8. Insert a sterile plug in the end of the catheter.
9. Place a sterile cap over the exposed end of the drainage tube, figure 29-15.
10. Secure the drainage tube to the bed so that it will not touch the floor.
11. Remove gloves and dispose of them according to facility policy.
12. Wash hands.
13. Reverse the procedure to reconnect the catheter. If you find an unprotected, dis-

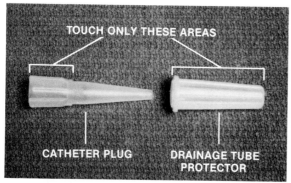

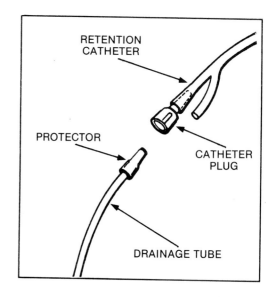

Figure 29-15 Left: Sterile catheter plug and protective cap. Right: Plug and protective cap in place. (From Caldwell & Hegner, *Nursing Assistant, A Nursing Process Approach,* copyright 1989 by Delmar Publishers Inc.)

2. Identify person and explain what you plan to do.
3. Screen unit and elevate bed to comfortable working height. Arrange equipment on overbed table.
4. Lower side rail closest to you.
5. Cover person with bath blanket and fanfold bedding to foot of bed. Place bed protector under patient's hips.
6. Adjust bath blanket to expose genitals only.
7. Put on gloves.
8. Remove present sheath by rolling toward tip of penis. Place in plastic bag if disposable. Place on paper towels to be washed and dried if reusable.
9. Wash and dry penis carefully. Observe for signs of irritation.
10. Check to see whether condom has "ready stick" surfaces. If not, a thin spray of tincture of benzoin may be applied to the penis. Do not spray on head of penis.
11. Apply fresh condom and drainage tip to penis by rolling it toward base of penis. If the person is uncircumcised, be sure that the foreskin remains in good position.
12. Reconnect drainage system.
13. Remove gloves.

14. Adjust bedding and remove bath blanket. Fold bath blanket and leave in bedside stand.
15. Lower bed and raise side rail. Make patient comfortable, call bell at hand. Leave unit tidy.
16. Clean and replace equipment and disposables according to hospital policy.
17. Wash hands.
18. Report completion of task to nurse. Record on patient's chart the date and time, procedure (urinary condom replaced), and any observations you have made.

PROCEDURE 56

Giving Indwelling Catheter Care

1. Wash hands and assemble the following equipment:

disposable gloves	daily catheter care
bed protector	kit
bath blanket	antiseptic solution
plastic bag for	sterile applicators
disposables	tape

2. Identify person and explain what you plan to do. Screen unit.

3. Raise bed to working height and lower side rail closest to you. Be sure opposite side rail is up and secure. Position patient on back, legs separated and knees bent, if permitted.

4. Cover person with bath blanket and fanfold bedding to foot of bed.

5. Position bath blanket so that only genitals are exposed.

6. Ask person to raise hips, and place bed protector underneath.

7. Arrange catheter care kit and plastic bag on overbed table. Open kit.

8. Put on gloves and draw drape back.

9. For the male:
    a. Gently grasp penis and draw foreskin back.
    b. Dipping a fresh applicator in antiseptic solution for each stroke, cleanse the glans from meatus toward shaft for approximately 4 inches.
    c. Place each applicator into disposable plastic bag after use.
   For the female:
    a. Separate the labia.
    b. Using a fresh applicator dipped in antiseptic solution for each stroke, cleanse from front to back.
    c. Place each used applicator after one stroke in plastic bag.

10. Remove gloves and place in plastic bag.

11. Check catheter to be sure it is taped properly. Retape and adjust for slack, if needed.

12. Check to be sure tubing is coiled on bed and hangs straight down into drainage container. Check level of urine in container. End of tubing should not be below urine level. Empty bag and measure if necessary.

13. Replace bedding and remove bath blanket.

14. Fold bath blanket and leave in bedside stand for reuse.

15. Help person to assume a comfortable position, call bell within easy reach.

16. Lower bed and raise and secure side rail. Leave unit tidy.

17. Dispose of equipment according to facility policy.

18. Wash hands and report completion of task. Record on patient's chart the date and time, procedure (catheter care), antiseptic solution used, and any observations you have made.

PROCEDURE 57

Emptying a Urinary Drainage Unit

Note: Check the policy of your facility regarding the use of disposable gloves during this procedure.

1. Wash hands and assemble the following equipment:

   disposable gloves
   graduate
   sterile cap or sterile 4 x 4

2. Identify person and explain what you plan to do.

3. Put on gloves.

4. If drainage bag has an opening in the bottom, place a graduate under it and allow the urine to drain, figure 29-16.

5. If there is no opening, the tube must be removed before emptying. Protect the end of the drainage tube with a sterile cap or a sterile gauze sponge.

6. Empty urine and measure it.

7. Remove protective cover from the end of the tube and reinsert it in the bag. Be careful not to hit the sides of the bag.

8. Remove gloves and dispose of them according to facility policy.

9. Wash hands.

10. Record output according to facility policy.

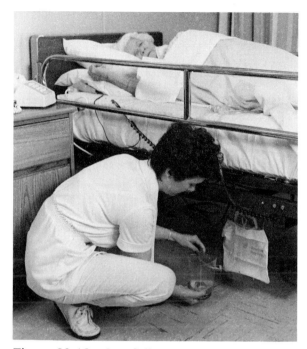

Figure 29-16 Carefully open the tubing in the drainage bag and allow urine to drain into the container or graduate. (From Hegner & Caldwell, *Assisting in Long-Term Care,* copyright 1988 by Delmar Publishers Inc.)

PROCEDURE 58

Inserting Indwelling Catheter to Female Patient

Note: Only those who have been properly taught and supervised and have legal authorization may carry out the following advanced procedures.

1. Wash hands and assemble the following equipment:

    bath blanket
    sterile catheterization tray
    gloves, if not included with tray
    emesis basin lined with paper towels
    spotlight

2. Take equipment to bedside and identify the patient.
3. Explain what you plan to do.
4. Draw curtains for privacy.
5. Drape and help patient assume the dorsal recumbent position.
6. Position spotlight to illuminate the perineum.
7. Wash and dry hands.
8. Place disposable tray between patient's legs and emesis basin lined with paper towels near the foot of the bed.
9. Remove cover carefully so as not to contaminate the contents. Remember, the contents are sterile.
10. Put on sterile gloves.
11. Protecting gloved hands, ask patient to lift hips; slip protective towel underneath.
12. Place inner sterile tray and contents on sterile drape.
13. Open lubricant, squeezing some onto sterile drape.
14. Fill syringe (if not prefilled) with sterile solution.
15. Remove cover of specimen jar if specimen is to be taken.
16. Open package of premoistened cotton balls. Make sure all equipment that requires two hands is ready before proceeding to the next step.
17. With one hand, gently separate the labia, moving upward to expose the vestibule and meatus. This hand is now contaminated and must not be used to handle sterile supplies.
18. With the other hand, pick up cotton balls, forming a pad between gloved fingers and patient's body. Stroke from top of vestibule downward once on one side and drop on paper towels. Taking a second cotton ball, repeat on opposite side of vestibule and drop the cotton ball. Bring the third moist cotton ball directly down

over the meatus and drop it in a similar fashion. Remember to maintain the separation of the labia.

19. Pick up the catheter and lubricate about 1½ inches of the tip.

20. Gently insert the catheter about 2½ to 3 inches into the meatus at a slight downward angle (no more than 4 inches should ever be inserted). Urine will run into the closed drainage system. Do not force if resistance is met. In this case, discontinue and report to nurse. If the catheter touches any area other than the meatus, it is considered contaminated and must be discarded. You must then begin again with a new sterile setup. *Be careful.*

21. Using the syringe provided, fit tip into balloon channel and inflate the catheter balloon with 5 ml of sterile water.

22. Gently test the stability of the catheter.

23. Remove gloves.

24. Tape catheter to side of patient's leg, allowing some play in length.

25. Suspend drainage bag below level of patient's pelvis by attaching to bed frame. Wind excess tubing in a circle on the bed, securing with a pin. Never attach to side rails.

26. Place all used equipment into tray and dispose of according to hospital policy.

27. Reposition patient and remove drapes.

28. Leave unit in good order.

29. Return light to utility room.

30. Record procedure and amount and color of urine obtained.

PROCEDURE 59

Inserting Indwelling Catheter to Male Patient

1-5. Same as for female patient.

6. Position light to shine on penis.

7. Wash and dry hands.

8. Open sterile tray on overbed table.

9. Put on sterile gloves.

10. Place sterile protective sheet over person's legs.

11. Arrange equipment by placing inner sterile tray and contents on sterile drape.

12. Open lubricant, squeezing some onto sterile drape.

13. Fill syringe (if not prefilled) with appropriate amount of sterile solution.

14. Remove cover of specimen jar if specimen is to be obtained.

15. Open package of premoistened cotton balls. Make sure all equipment that requires two hands is ready before proceeding to the next step.

16. With one hand, gently grasp penis, retracting foreskin. Position penis at about a 60° to 90° angle to the body.

17. Cleanse the exposed area using one cotton ball for each stroke from tip toward shaft, and drop cotton ball on paper towels.

18. Lubricate about 1½ inches of the catheter tip.

19. Insert the catheter about 6 to 8 inches with a slight rotating motion. Lower the penis slightly after about 5 inches have been inserted.

20. Using the syringe provided, inflate the catheter balloon with proper amount of sterile solution.

21. Gently test the stability of the catheter.

22. Remove gloves and secure catheter to side of patient's leg with tape, allowing some play in length.

23. Suspend drainage bag below level of patient's pelvis by attaching to bed frame. Wind excess tubing in a circle on the bed, securing with a pin. Do not attach to bed rail.

24. Place all used equipment on tray and dispose of according to hospital policy.

25. Reposition patient and remove drapes.

26. Leave unit in good order.

27. Return light to utility room.

28. Record procedure and amount and color of urine obtained.

PROCEDURE 60

Inserting a Urethral Catheter

1-13. Same as for inserting indwelling catheter for female patient.

14. Place urine container on the sterile bed protector close to the vulva, but not touching it.

15. Pick up the catheter in the right hand, gently curling it around hand so that end is close to open box.

16. Lubricate tip of catheter and insert about 2½ to 3 inches into meatus using a gentle rotating motion.

17. As urine begins to flow, direct stream of urine into container.

18. Hold catheter in place until urine stops flowing. Do not remove more than 1,000 ml at one time. If a sample is needed, allow a small amount of urine to flow and then direct stream into specimen bottle.

19. Pinch off catheter, remove, and place in tray. Dry perineal area.

20. Remove gloves and drapes and place in tray.

21. Reposition patient for comfort and safety.

22. Dispose of equipment according to hospital policy, leaving unit in good order.

23. Record procedure and amount and color of urine obtained. Be sure to report to the nurse if the urine excretion could have exceeded 1,000 ml.

Other Conditions

Renal Calculi

Just as stones sometimes form in the gallbladder, stones may also form in the kidney and along the urinary tract. Kidney stones *(renal calculi)* can cause obstruction when they become lodged in the ureters. Many renal calculi are passed in the urine. Forcing fluids encourages increased output. All urine must be strained and inspected for stones before it is discarded. There may be no sign of developing renal obstruction by calculi until actual blockage occurs. Then there is sudden intense pain (renal colic).

When it is impossible for the patient to pass the stones, surgery may be necessary. Sometimes during cystoscopy, the stones may be crushed so that they can then be passed in the urine. Otherwise, the stones must be removed through a surgical incision. A new technique has been developed that fragments the stones with ultrasonic waves while the patient is submerged in a tub of water. But this is not suitable for all patients.

Prostate Problems

From 60 to 70 percent of all men over fifty suffer from hypertrophy (enlargement) of the prostate gland, and 20 percent require some form of surgery. An enlarged prostate puts pressure on the urethra, causing urinary retention. The older man may have had difficulty initiating the urine stream or experienced dribbling at the end of voiding for some time before seeking medical attention. Removal of all or part of the prostate gland will relieve the obstruction.

The incidence of cancer of the prostate, usually an adenocarcinoma, increases with age. It is the main cause of death in men over seventy-five. The tumor begins in the posterior lobe and may not produce signs and symptoms until the cancer is advanced. The condition is sometimes picked up on a routine physical. Cancer of the prostate is usually treated with radiation, surgery (prostatectomy), and hormonal therapy.

Various surgical approaches are used to remove all or part of the prostate gland to relieve the retention. These procedures are performed even in men over age ninety. When only enough of the gland is removed from inside the urethra to permit urine to pass, the operation is called a transurethral prostatectomy (T.U.R.P.). The gland may also be removed through surgical incisions in the perineum (perineal prostatectomy) or through an incision right over the bladder (suprapubic prostatectomy).

A Foley (indwelling) catheter is always in place following prostate surgery. In addition, a suprapubic drain through the surgical incision or a perineal drain may be present. Be careful that the tubes do not become kinked, stressed, or dislodged when positioning the patient. Carefully note the amount and color of the drainage from all areas. Any sudden increase in bright redness or the appearance of clots that seem to block the tube must be reported at once. If dressings become wet with urinary drainage, report it to your team leader who will reinforce them. At times, it will be necessary to irrigate (wash out) the drainage tubes. This is a sterile procedure that will be carried out by the nurse or doctor unless you have been specifically trained for it and it is within your job description.

Men often fear that they will not be able to have sexual intercourse after a prostatectomy, but loss of the prostate gland does not necessarily mean a loss of libido or ejaculatory ability. Be sure to refer these questions to your team leader, who can provide the patient with accurate information.

Rectocele and Cystocele

Rectoceles and cystoceles usually occur, in females, at the same time. The conditions are due to a weakening of the muscles in the walls between the vagina and bladder *(cystocele)* and between the vagina and rectum *(rectocele)*. Frequent pregnancies and general loss of muscle tone with aging contribute to the development of both conditions. Cystoceles cause urinary incontinence. This may be associated with stress such as coughing or laughing and can be embarrassing. Rectoceles cause constipation and hemorrhoid development. Rectoceles, once formed, have little tendency to get worse, but cystoceles do.

Many women accept the urinary problems associated with cystoceles as inevitable after childbirth and may be reluctant to seek medical attention because they believe nothing can be done. Today, however, a surgical procedure called colporrhaphy can be performed to tighten the vaginal walls. This procedure can be done under local anesthesia with minimal stress or complications to the older woman. *Pessaries*, used

in the past, have not proven as effective. Following surgery, ice packs, heat lamps, Sitz baths, and sterile vaginal douches (irrigations) may be ordered. Pain and type and amount of drainage should be reported. Returning from surgery, the patient will probably have a urinary catheter in place. Since there is no nerve involvement, perineal exercises are helpful. Patients should be instructed to alternately start and stop the stream of urine and to contract gluteal, perineal, and abdominal muscle groups.

Renal Failure

Renal failure may be chronic or acute. Older patients usually suffer from chronic renal failure.

Chronic failure is associated with advanced renal insufficiency following other chronic conditions such as nephrosis or arteriosclerosis. Specific signs and symptoms become apparent as the kidneys fail and waste products accumulate in the blood. These include:

- Edema
- Hypertension
- Anuria or oliguria
- Acidosis and electrolyte imbalance
- Headache, nausea, and unpleasant taste
- Twitching, muscle spasms, and convulsions
- Uremia

In later stages, poor appetite and electrolyte imbalance lead to malnutrition, generalized tissue wasting, and a yellow skin discoloration. In terminal stages, there may be itching from the crystallization of urea in the sweat on the skin, called uremic frost. Ultimately, as the kidney fails, symptoms become systemic and include generalized edema, increased blood pressure, and eventual metabolic acidosis.

Acute failure may be temporary and respond to hemodialysis, figure 29-17, with the kidneys eventually resuming independent functioning. In chronic failure, unless a compatible transplant can be found, survival is not possible. Transplants of compatible kidneys have been performed for many years. The problem is to find a suitable donor.

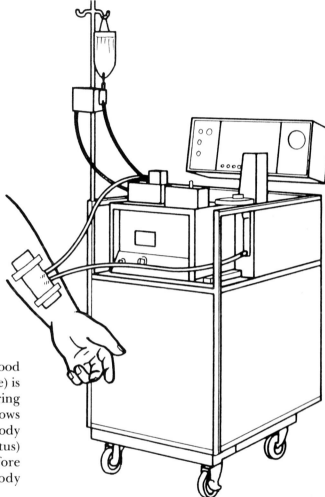

Figure 29-17 *Hemodialysis* (separation of blood components by passing through a membrane) is a life-preserving treatment for patients suffering either acute or chronic renal failure. Blood flows through a cannula (tube) from the patient's body into a membrane package (dialysis apparatus) that allows separation of waste products before the blood is returned to the patient's body through another cannula.

Summary

- Bladder problems are common in elderly persons.
- The most common bladder problems are incontinence and retention.
- Inability to control elimination has psychological as well as physical aspects. It often creates impossible situations for both patient and family.
- Through consistent retraining, it is often possible to help patients become continent of urine once again.
- Conditions involving the pelvic structures, such as prostatic hypertrophy, rectoceles, and cystoceles, contribute to elimination problems.
- Surgical approaches are commonly used to correct these conditions.
- Skin care is a significant part of the nursing care of all incontinent patients.
- Catheter care is a process that must be carried out meticulously.

Review Outline

   I. Behavioral Objectives

  II. Vocabulary

 III. Urinary System

     A. Structure
     B. Function

  IV. Senescent Changes

   V. Positioning for Elimination

     A. On bedpan
     B. On commode

  VI. Elimination Problems

     A. Retention
     B. Incontinence
        1. Cause
        2. Diagnostic techniques
        3. Urinalysis
        4. Retraining
        5. Intractability

 VII. Urinalysis
     A. Specimen collection

VIII. Urine Specimen Collection

  IX. Urinary Catheters

     A. Purpose
     B. Care
     C. Insertion

   X. Urinary Drainage

  XI. Catheterization

     A. Types
     B. Techniques
     C. Authorization

 XII. Other Related Conditions

     A. Renal calculi
     B. Prostate problems
     C. Rectocele
     D. Cystocele
     E. Renal failure

Review

I. Vocabulary

Word Puzzle

Circle the words that are defined in the puzzle.

1. Renal stones
2. The ability to control voiding
3. A four-letter word meaning to urinate
4. Weakened anterior vaginal wall
5. Accumulation of urea in the blood
6. Excessive urination at night
7. Weakened wall between rectum and vagina
8. Another term for urine elimination

```
A   E   N   N   O   C   T   U   R   I   A   B   P   A
G   F   K   M   D   N   C   L   E   O   F   I   H   J
E   D   O   C   Y   S   T   O   C   E   L   E   R   B
I   N   K   A   L   C   I   M   T   E   O   E   K   N
H   C   I   L   G   K   A   S   O   F   C   T   L   C
A   L   O   C   R   E   Q   C   C   N   J   P   F   O
M   J   U   U   M   O   B   H   E   R   M   G   E   J
B   I   R   L   F   P   K   N   L   S   C   T   D   R
L   N   E   I   N   H   I   M   E   H   I   V   S   F
P   T   M   I   C   T   U   R   I   T   I   O   N   N
D   L   I   S   N   M   F   A   J   H   I   L   K   O
Q   E   A   O   J   B   N   C   E   O   K   D   L   D
F   Q   C   M   A   O   K   P   I   G   S   C   J   I
J   N   B   L   K   N   D   H   Q   B   M   A   N   G
I   G   O   E   I   C   L   P   J   F   O   C   K   E
```

II. Anatomy

Identify the structures indicated in figure 29-18.

1. _____
2. _____
3. _____
4. _____
5. _____

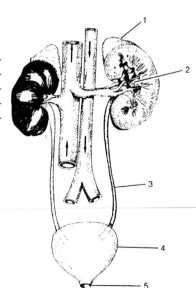

III. True or False

    1. Two equally important problems related to elimination are incontinence and micturition.
    2. Incontinence of urine is twice as common among men as it is among women.
    3. Typical elderly reactions to incontinence are shame and embarrassment.
    4. The bladder of the elderly patient tends to lose muscle tone and capacity.
    5. Urination is under both voluntary and involuntary control.
    6. The purpose of bladder retraining is to achieve a pattern of filling and emptying that is as nearly normal as possible.
    7. Anticholinergic drugs block motor impulses to the bladder, causing a decrease in bladder contractions and capacity.
    8. When collecting a 24-hour urine specimen the last specimen is discarded.
    9. Incontinence is easily accepted by most adults.
    10. Frequent urination is to be expected early in a retraining period.

IV. Select the one best answer.
    1. Changes in the aging urinary system include

        a. increased kidney size.
        b. improved vascular pathways.
        c. increased reabsorption.
        d. less efficient elimination.
    2. Your patient has difficulty starting the urine stream. You might try
        a. turning the person to the left side.
        b. assisting the person to sit very straight.
        c. supporting the person as he or she leans forward.
        d. encouraging the person to hold his or her breath and relax the abdominal muscles.
    3. For a female, the best position for elimination is
        a. sitting upright with knees and hips flexed.
        b. standing.
        c. on a low toilet.
        d. on a bedpan in the supine position.
    4. In a male, a major cause of urinary retention is
        a. unwillingness to cooperate.
        b. mechanical obstruction.
        c. cystocele.
        d. presence of an indwelling catheter.
    5. When collecting a fresh fractional urine sample, it is best to
        a. save the first complete sample in case the second is lost.
        b. collect three samples.
        c. stay with the patient for a short time after taking the sample.
        d. withhold fluids for one hour before and after the test.

V. Clinical Situations

    1. Your charge nurse tells you to put adult disposable diapers on a temporarily incontinent patient. What do you do?
    2. Your male patient has difficulty voiding in bed and cannot walk very well. What do you do?

CASE STUDY

Adele Berenstein, age eighty-seven, sat defiantly staring out of the window. She was in a wheelchair. She said to the young woman before her, "I'm not a child and I refuse to be treated as one. You certainly may not put one of those paper diapers on me."

Ms. Berenstein, a former history professor and very much a women's rights activist, had suffered a small stroke that had left her partially paralyzed on her left side. Her speech was unaffected and she had made excellent progress until she developed the flu. Now, lack of urinary continence was a major problem for her. She was embarrassed over her loss of control and indignant at the suggestion that she be put into diapers like a child. The geriatric health care provider could hear her still mumbling under her breath as she left the room to report to her supervisor.

A team conference was called and plans made to help Ms. Berenstein regain bladder control. The first step was to offer protection for the skin, so the nurse respectfully explained to Ms. Berenstein that the pads were not diapers but skin protection pads and were only to be used temporarily to prevent possible skin breakdown. She assured Ms. Berenstein that she would gain control again. The staff was cautioned not to refer to the pads as anything other than skin protection pads when making application and to do so in a routine manner.

The second step in the retraining program was to carry out diagnostic procedures, so Ms. Berenstein was scheduled for a cystoscopy, micturating cystogram, and cystometrogram. These were performed during a temporary hospitalization after which she returned to the facility.

After the laboratory tests were evaluated, it was determined that a bladder infection was complicating the picture. The patient was put on a sulfa compound to correct that aspect of the problem. Sometimes, bladder infections alone can cause frequency and incontinence.

Because the incontinence persisted, step three of the program was instituted. An incontinence record detailing the pattern of incontinence was compiled for seventy-two hours. All members of the staff participated in its formulation. The patient was greatly upset each time she was incontinent and was almost hostile to the staff when they came to change the linen and pads.

The staff recognized that this was a defense mechanism to hide embarrassment. They calmly changed the linen with little comment. Enlisting Ms. Berenstein's cooperation was difficult until the charge nurse found that if the incontinence was referred to as a "mishap," the patient was able to respond more positively. Obviously, loss of bladder control was not in keeping with Ms. Berenstein's self-image. All staff members were made aware of this approach. As they followed through, they found a great change in the patient's willingness to cooperate.

The incontinence record showed that one period of incontinence most often occurred about 1 A.M. Fluids were forced during the day and ambulation encouraged. After dinner, fluids were limited but not withheld. Ms. Berenstein was encouraged to empty her bladder before retiring for the night.

At midnight each night, the night staff moved the commode close to the bed. They awakened Ms. Berenstein and helped her transfer to the commode. They positioned her slippered feet flat on the floor and provided her with privacy. This same technique was followed one hour before each time of incontinence indicated by the record. The staff maintained a positive attitude, which was quickly transferred to the patient. Each time a "mishap" occurred, little fuss was made, and each dry period was accepted as normal.

Ms. Berenstein's sharp mind soon became involved. She recognized that there was a pattern to her incontinence and that retraining would be most successful if she cooperated. She had a friend bring her a small wristwatch with an alarm. She set the alarm one hour before her "mishap" times. It was found that a major part of the incontinence problem was difficulty in reaching the facilities in time. In a relatively short time (3½ weeks), Ms. Berenstein was continent, much to her relief and peace of mind.

1. Why was Ms. Berenstein upset over the incontinence pads?

2. What characteristics of the patient's personality might you deduce from this incident?
3. How did the staff handle the problem?
4. What term was used to describe incontinence pads in a more acceptable way?
5. What three tests were done in the hospital to determine adequacy of urinary function?
6. Why was Ms. Berenstein put on a sulfa compound?
7. What is an incontinence record?
8. What was found to be a major cause of the resident's incontinence?

Unit 30
Reproductive System Alterations

Objectives

After studying this unit, you should be able to:

- Name the location and functions of the male and female reproductive organs.
- Describe common senescent problems of the reproductive organs.
- Identify sexually transmitted diseases.
- Prepare and give a nonsterile vaginal douche.

Vocabulary

Learn the meaning and spelling of the following words or phrases.

acquired immune deficiency syndrome (A.I.D.S.)
A.I.D.S. related complex (A.R.C.)
chancre
chlamydial organisms
communicable
contagious
ejaculation
erection
germs
gonorrhea
human immune virus (H.I.V.)
incubation period
infectious
irrigate
Kaposi's sarcoma
lesion

mammary glands
mastectomy
masturbation
moniliasis
nongonorrheal
  urethritis (N.G.U.)
normal flora
orchiectomy
pneumocystis carinii
  pneumonia
procidentia

prolapse
pruritis
sexually transmitted
  diseases (S.T.D.)
signs or symptoms
syphilis
transurethral prostatec-
  tomy (T.U.R.P.)
vaginitis
venereal
yeast

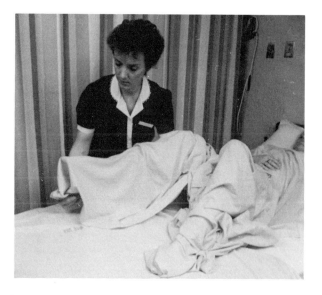

Reproductive Tract

Both the male and female organs of reproduction have dual functions. They produce the hormones responsible for masculine and feminine characteristics. They also produce the living cells (sperm and ovum) that unite to form a baby.

The female also houses the new baby until birth. The female breasts (*mammary glands*) produce milk after delivery to nourish the newborn. In the male, the urethra is a passageway for both urine and sperm. Conditions affecting the urethra in the male may result in both urinary and reproductive problems. Disease conditions that affect the reproductive organs have tremendous psychological effects on older patients.

Male Organs: Structure and Function

The male organs include the penis, the two testes (gonads) in the scrotum, and accessory structures, figure 30-1. The testes produce sperm and masculine hormones throughout life. Leading from each testes is a tube. The first part of the tube (epididymis) is coiled on top of the testes. The next part (the vas deferens) passes with the nerves and blood vessels into the pelvis. The vas deferens passes behind the urinary bladder to the seminal vesicle. This pouch stores the sperm and adds nutrients to the seminal fluid. A small tube (ejaculatory duct) leads from the seminal vesicles, entering the urethra just below the bladder. Urine and seminal fluid (sperm and other secretions) do not mix. The acidity of the urine would cause the sperm to become inactive.

Surrounding the male urethra, just below the bladder, is the prostate gland. It secretes a fluid that increases the ability of the sperm to move in the seminal fluid. Enlargement of the prostate gland may prevent urine from passing through the urethra. This is a fairly common occurrence in older men. Partial removal of this gland does not necessarily render the man impotent (unable to have an erection).

The penis is composed of special tissue that can become filled with blood, causing an *erection.* The organ becomes enlarged and stiffened so that it may enter the vagina to deposit seminal fluid. The movement of the seminal fluid through the tube system to the outside is called *ejaculation.* The fluid is referred to as the ejaculate. Loose-fitting skin called the prepuce or foreskin covers the penis. The section of foreskin that covers the penis tip (glans) is often removed by a surgical procedure called circumcision shortly after birth.

Female Organs: Structure and Function

The female internal organs include the ovaries, fallopian tubes (oviducts), uterus, and vagi-

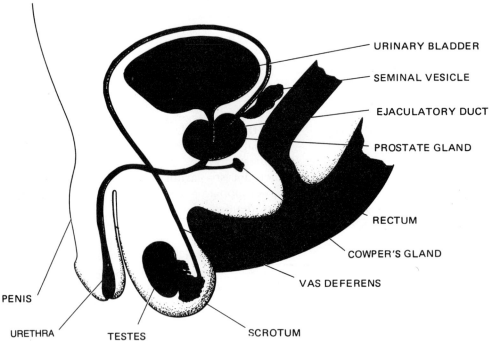

Figure 30-1   Male reproductive organs

URINARY BLADDER

SEMINAL VESICLE

EJACULATORY DUCT

PROSTATE GLAND

RECTUM

COWPER'S GLAND

VAS DEFERENS

PENIS

URETHRA

TESTES

SCROTUM

na, figure 30-2. The external genitals include the vulva, which is made up of two liplike structures, the labia majora and labia minora, figure 30-3. The labia majora are covered with hair and padded with fat. The labia minora are hairless and the edges gently meet when the legs are together. When the labia are separated, other external structures may be seen: the clitoris, the urinary meatus, and the vaginal opening. The clitoris is similar in structure to the male penis but it is mostly sheltered by a hood of tissue. It is a sensitive erotic area.

Ovaries and Oviducts   The ovaries are two small glands on either side of the uterus at the ends of the oviducts in the pelvis. They produce two female hormones, estrogen and progesterone, and egg cells. The eggs are contained in small sacs called follicles. From the onset of puberty at nine to seventeen years until menopause at fifty to fifty-five, a follicle matures and releases an egg about once each month. The egg makes its way into one of the 4-inch oviducts. This process is called ovulation. The cells of the follicles that are left produce progesterone. This hormone causes changes within the uterus to prepare it for pregnancy in case the egg is fertilized.

Uterus   The uterus is a hollow, pear-shaped organ. Its walls are made of smooth involuntary muscles, and it is lined with a tissue called endometrium. Each month, under the influence of estrogen and progesterone, the lining builds up

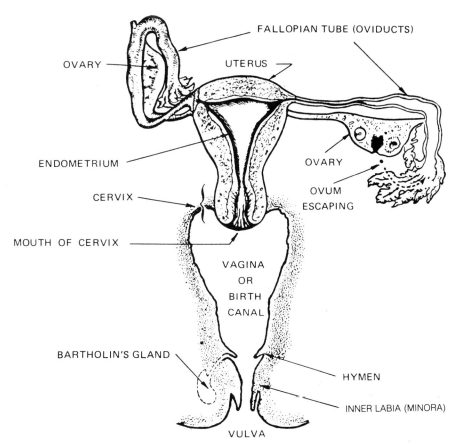

Figure 30-2   Internal female reproductive organs

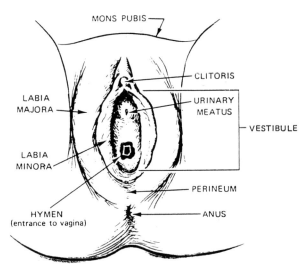

Figure 30-3 External female reproductive organs

in anticipation of pregnancy. When pregnancy doesn't occur, the endometrium is shed. This is called menstruation. The uterus has three main parts: the fundus, the body, and the cervix. The body and the fundus can stretch to hold a baby and much fluid. The cervix extends into the vagina. During labor, it opens up to allow the baby to be delivered through the birth canal.

Vagina The vagina is between the urinary bladder and the rectum. Its muscular walls are capable of stretching and are lined with mucous membrane. Two glands (Bartholin's glands) are found on either side of the external vaginal opening. The vagina is the female organ of copulation and the passageway for menses and delivery of the baby.

Menstruation and Ovulation Menstruation is the loss of an unneeded part of the endometrium. It occurs for approximately three to five days each month. At the end of each menstrual period, another egg begins to mature in a follicle in one of the ovaries. As the follicle and its egg grow, they produce the hormone estrogen. It causes the endometrium to begin developing new blood vessels and tissues.

Ovulation takes place about twelve to four-

teen days after the first day of the last menstrual period. When ovulation occurs, the follicle secretes the hormone progesterone. Progesterone causes the endometrium to become somewhat thickened, soft, and sticky in preparation for pregnancy. Sperm are capable of traveling from the vagina, through the uterus, to the oviduct. If the egg unites with a sperm in the oviduct, it begins to divide into many cells. It then journeys to the uterus where it grows and develops into a baby. If the egg does not meet a sperm as it passes through the oviduct, it is expelled from the body. It is too small to be seen.

If pregnancy does not occur after ovulation, the production of progesterone is slowed down about twelve days later. Shortly thereafter, the unneeded, newly built-up portion of the endometrium is shed as menstrual flow. The processes of ovulation and menstruation are known as the menstrual cycle. Terms used in discussing menstruation include dysmenorrhea (painful menstruation), amenorrhea (without menstruation), and menorrhagia (excessive bleeding).

Breasts The breasts are two modified sweat glands located on the anterior chest wall. They develop at puberty, but they do not produce milk until pregnancy. Ducts from the glandular cells drain into a central duct that opens into the nipple. Surrounding the nipple is slightly darker tissue called the areola. The size of the breasts is due to the amount of fat between the ducts.

Senescent Changes

With aging, the following changes take place in the reproductive system. For men, there will be the following:

- Slower sexual response
- Delayed ejaculation
- Decrease in the number of sperm (but the number is still adequate for reproduction)
- Gradual decrease in testosterone levels.

For women, the changes due to aging include the following:

- Decrease in estrogen levels
- Thinning of tissue of the vulva and vaginal walls and a decrease in lubrication of the vagina (because of this, elderly women more prone to vaginal infections)
- Weakening of breast tissues and muscles (sagging of breasts)

Impotence

True impotence in older men is usually more psychological than physiological. Some diseases such as diabetes can contribute to the inability of the male to achieve an erection. This is also true of certain surgical procedures and drugs such as tranquilizers, sedatives, and anti-hypertensives. There are implants that can help men achieve erections. These implants are soft, hollow tubes that can fill with fluid housed in the abdomen. When pressure is applied to the abdomen, fluid moves forward into the tube, making the penis firm and coitus easier.

Older men with erection problems, and their partners, can still enjoy manual and oral stimulation, thus providing each other with pleasure and satisfying the need for intimacy. The need for more direct stimulation can be helped by using a vibrator.

There are some health problems that might interfere with sexual activity. These include systemic illnesses such as cardiac illness, hypertension, atherosclerosis, arthritis, muscle and bone weakness, diabetes mellitus, and hearing and sight problems. Conditions that affect the reproductive organs themselves include senile vaginitis, uterine prolapse, cystoceles, rectoceles, and Peyronies disease. Even people with these health problems can be helped if they so desire and if there are willing, mature, knowledgeable health care providers to offer help. Some adjustments may be made following a heart attack or hip replacement that make sexual intercourse less stressful. Positions in which the recovering patient is more passive cause less stress and discomfort.

Table 30-1 lists the diagnostic categories related to problems of the reproductive system.

- Alterations in patterns of urinary elimination
- Altered sexual patterns
- Anxiety
- Chronic pain
- Impaired social interactions
- Potential for infection
- Self-concept disturbance

Table 30-1 Diagnostic categories related to problems of the reproductive system

Depression and organic brain changes may alter the individual's perception of sexual need and expression. The depressed person may become too introverted to be interested. Those with organic brain changes may not be fully aware of their actions.

If an older resident makes sexual advances to you, be firm but gentle in rejecting these advances. Calmly let the person know that the behavior is not appropriate or acceptable. Even if you feel irritated, do not show anger.

Use diversion techniques if you observe a person making unwelcome advances toward another in your care. Gently but firmly intervene and engage the sexually aroused person in some other activity. You may wish to ask another health care provider to help you by physically assisting the unwilling partner to another location while you are occupied in the diversion activity.

When opportunities for sexual interactions are limited, many men and women derive satisfaction through self-stimulation (*masturbation*). This is not wrong, immoral, or abnormal. It can bring pleasure and continued comfort to the later years.

Benign Prostatic Hyperplasia

Benign hyperplasia of the prostate is an enlargement of the prostate gland without tumor development. It causes narrowing of the urethra that passes through the center of the prostate gland, causing urinary retention. It is a noncancerous condition. The man with prostatic hyperplasia has difficulty starting the stream of urine and emptying the bladder completely.

Various surgical approaches are used to remove all or part of the prostate gland (prostatectomy) to relive the retention. *Transurethral prostatectomy (T.U.R.P.)* removes only enough of the gland from inside the urethra to permit urine to pass. This is commonly performed on the elderly male. In perineal prostatectomy, the entire gland is removed through a surgical incision in the perineum. In suprapubic prostatectomy, an incision is made just above the pubis, and part of the gland is removed.

Male patients are very apt to be disturbed by the necessity for prostate surgery. Men often fear that they will not be able to have sexual intercourse after a prostatectomy and that their very manhood is threatened.

In addition to routine postoperative care, the prostatectomy patient will have a Foley catheter in place following the surgery. He may have a suprapubic drain through the suprapubic incision or a perineal drain in the perineal incision.

As a geriatric health care provider, you must be careful to be sure that the tubes do not become twisted, stressed, or dislodged when positioning the patient. Carefully note the amount and color of drainage from all areas. Report at once any sudden increase in bright redness, the appearance of clots that seem to block the tube, or urinary drainage on the dressings. Be patient and understanding of the patient's emotional stress. Refer questions of possible sexual limitations to your supervisor so that the patient can be provided with accurate information.

At times it will be necessary to *irrigate* (wash out) the drainage tubes. This is a sterile procedure that will be carried out by the nurse or physician.

Cancer of the Testes

This cancer is more common today. It may require the removal of the testicles. *Orchiectomy* is a procedure performed when there is testicular malignancy. Early diagnosis can ensure early treatment, and an orchiectomy can be avoided.

Testicular self-examination is an important way to locate lumps or changes in the testes. This procedure should be performed at least once each month. It is best done during a warm shower so that the scrotum will be relaxed. Each testis should be palpated with soapy fingers.

Peyronies Disease

This is a painful bending of the penis resulting from fibrous scarring usually associated with inflammation, figure 30-4. The condition makes insertion of the erect penis difficult and uncomfortable. Some cases can be helped by injections of corticosteroids, but others require surgery to release the contracture.

Procidentia

Procedentia refers to *prolapse* (drop) of the uterus downward into the vagina. It usually occurs in older women who have had children and received injury such as tearing or excessive

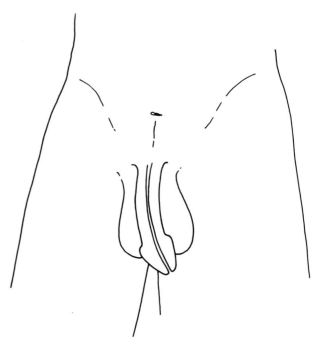

Figure 30-4 The patient with Peyronies disease experiences a painful deviation of the penis during erection.

stretching to the birth canal during delivery. The effects of these injuries are not evident until aging takes place and supportive structures are less efficient.

Older women suffering from partial or complete procidentia complain of pulling sensations in their lower abdomen. They frequently experience incontinence and incomplete emptying of the bladder. Incomplete emptying of the bladder can predispose to urinary infection. A mass may be felt in the vagina. The procidentia is corrected with surgery that may or may not include removal of the cervix. Postoperative care is similar to that following colporrhaphy. Patients should be checked carefully after any vaginal surgery for signs of excessive bleeding or foul discharge.

Vaginitis

Inflammation of the vagina, or *vaginitis*, can occur throughout a female's lifetime. In the older woman, the atrophic less secretory vaginal walls offer less protection against microbial invasions and irritation. Secretions are less acidic and lower acid levels encourage microbial growth. This condition is known as senile vaginitis. All these factors contribute to a greater incidence of infections, which tend to become chronic and difficult to cure.

The irritation and inflammation can result in bleeding and the formation of adhesions (scarring) around the urinary and vaginal openings. Senile vaginitis responds well to estrogen therapy, vaginal suppositories, and douches with mild acid solutions. Douches are irrigations used to wash the vaginal canal. They should not be given too often and never without an order. Too-frequent douching can decrease the vaginal lubrication even more. Cleanliness is important and Sitz baths may be ordered.

Pruritus Vulvae and Ani

Older women often suffer from itching (*pruritus*) around the anus and vulva. Many factors contribute to this discomfort: lower hormone levels, moisture and incontinence, local irritation, and rubbing. Continued irritation can

lead to tissue breakdown and superimposed infection.

Treatment involves a search for underlying causes and control of any infection that may be present. Soap should be avoided because it can increase the irritation. Creams and soothing colloidal baths and compresses can increase comfort. Keeping the area clean and free of excessive drainage is done by careful routine perineal care.

Perineal care is a simple procedure that greatly adds to the comfort of many patients. The technique reduces odor and provides an opportunity to closely inspect the patient for abnormalities. Daily attention to the perineum is also given in conjunction with indwelling catheter care.

Nongonorrheal Urethritis (N.G.U.)

Vaginitis may also be infections, caused by a variety of infectious organisms (pathogens or germs). Some of these organisms are part of the *normal flora* (usual microbial population) of the vaginal tract. *Chlamydia* are microorganisms which commonly cause vaginal infections. When there is evidence of vaginitis, the vaginal secretions may be checked for gonorrhea. If the results are negative, the patient is treated with antibiotics and the condition is labeled as *nongonorrheal urethritis (N.G.U.)* or nonspecific urethritis (N.S.U.). This indicates that the exact cause was not identified.

Moniliasis (Yeast Vulvovaginitis)

Yeast organisms that are part of the normal flora of the female vaginal tract often cause an infection (*moniliasis* or *yeast vulvovaginitis*). The *yeast*, which is a fungus (*Candida albicans*), causes a watery vaginal discharge. The vulva and vagina are inflamed, and itching can be intense. Douches are not usually given for this condition. However, special drugs and creams are prescribed to relieve the itching and combat the infection.

Carcinoma of the Female Tract

After menopause, any bleeding from the vagina must be reported immediately. Such bleeding is frequently due to a malignancy in the reproductive tract.

Cancer of certain parts of the older female's reproductive tract is fairly common. Malignant lesions of the vulva are frequently preceded by the development of white, shiny patches (leukoplakia) of the labia, clitoris, and vestibule. The condition is usually treated by a radical excision of the vulva.

Malignancies of the vagina are not common, but cervical, endometrial, and ovarian cancers are. These malignancies may spread before they can be diagnosed. When diagnosed early, they are best treated by surgery and radiation, depending upon the age and general condition of the patient.

Cancer of the female breast is most often seen in older women. Its incidence increases rapidly after menopause. Women who have fibrocystic disease are also at greater risk. Paget's disease is a malignancy that affects the breasts of older women. This is an invasive form, and the prognosis is less than favorable.

All women should examine their breasts regularly and report any lumps, irregularity of contour, skin dimpling, or bleeding from the nipples. Early investigation through mammography, thermography, or other diagnostic methods offers the best hope for curative therapy.

Mastectomy (excision of the breast), radiation, chemotherapy, and hormal therapy are used in combination, depending upon the type of malignancy and the health and age of the woman. Malignancies in older people are often associated with anemias that leave the individual weakened and less able to cope with other physical stresses.

Breast Surgery A simple mastectomy means removal of the breast tissue. A radical mastectomy includes the breast tissue, underlying muscles, and the glands in the axillary area. A lumpectomy removes the abnormal tissue and only a small amount of the breast tissue. Lumpectomies are more often the current technique of choice. A mastectomy requires a great psychological adjustment by the patient. Because a large amount of blood may be lost during a mastectomy, transfusions may be ordered. Pressure dressings must be checked frequently for signs of excess bleeding. The bed linen should also be checked because blood may drain to the back of the dressing. Circulation to the arm may be lessened. Therefore, swelling and numbness should be reported immediately. Walking may be difficult because the patient feels unbalanced. Be ready to offer support.

Breast surgery or surgery on the other sex organs can threaten a woman's feeling of femininity. Many excellent breast prostheses are available for the mastectomy patient. There are also support groups to aid in the psychological adjustment. After recuperation and counseling, surgery to implant a breast prosthesis may be an option for some mastectomy patients.

You may wish to review procedures related to the reproductive system with your instructor.

Sexually Transmitted Diseases

Older persons are subject to the same types of *sexually transmitted diseases (S.T.D.s)* as younger persons are. *Venereal* (sexually) transmitted diseases are *infectious* (caused by microorganisms), *communicable* (transmittable), and, in some instances, *contagious* (easily spread from person to person). In general, they are caused by disease-producing microbes that do not live for long outside the warm, moist membranes and tissues of the body.

There are a number of different agents that cause venereal diseases. The most important diseases are gonorrhea, syphilis, herpes genitalia, and trichomoniasis, which is caused by a protozoan. At present, the incidence of *A.I.D.S., (acquired immune deficiency syndrome)*, caused by the human immune virus, is not as common among the elderly as it is among younger people, but more cases are being diagnosed. *Human immune virus (H.I.V.)* infection is a sexually transmitted disease that greatly concerns the public and health care providers.

Gonorrhea *Gonorrhea* is an infectious disease caused by a small bacterium, *Neisseria gonorrhea.*

It affects the mucous membranes of the reproductive tract of both men and women, causing an acute inflammation. Males usually have a greenish-yellow discharge and pain and burning upon urination. Females often will have no *signs or symptoms* (indications) at all until an abscess of inflammation develops in the pelvis. It takes two to six days after contact with the organisms for the disease process to begin. This is called the *incubation period.*

The secretions are infectious and can be transferred directly to other mucous membranes such as the eyes if precautions are not taken during care. The condition is cured with antibiotics.

Syphilis   *Syphilis* is another sexually transmitted disease that has been known for centuries. It is primarily transmitted by direct sexual contact with the *lesion* (sore) that develops when the organisms enter the skin or mucous membranes. It is caused by a bacterium called *Treponema pallidum.* This disease has an unusually long incubation period of up to ninety days between exposure and the development of the *chancre* or lesion.

Characteristically, this disease may pass through two and, in some cases, three stages. *Stage one* is the development of the chancre. This lesion is painless and appears at the point of contact. If it is deep in the female vagina, it may not be noticed. Without any treatment, the chancre disappears.

Stage two appears two to eight weeks later. By this time, the organisms have moved deep into the body. The person may have a variety of signs and symptoms that should include sore throat, hair loss (alopecia), rash, canker sores, fever, and malaise (general worn-out feeling). Kissing or biting during this stage could transmit the disease.

Stage three may occur next. Not all persons initially infected with the organisms progress to the third stage. Those who do, develop noninfectious lesions in the bones, nervous tissue, and cardiovascular system. They may become blind, demented, or paralyzed. Some patients develop weakened areas in the walls of blood vessels (aneurysms) or lesions that weaken other tissues and bones. Evidence of third-stage syphilis (tertiary syphilis) may not show up for many years after the original contact.

Trichomonas Vaginitis   Trichomonas vaginitis is caused by a parasitic microbe, the *Trichomonar vaginalis.* In females the infection causes a large amount of white, foul-smelling vaginal discharge (leukorrhea) and itching.

The organisms may infect the mate's reproductive tract without signs or symptoms. The disease can be treated with medication, but both sex partners must be treated to prevent reinfection.

Genital Herpes   Genital herpes *Herpes simplex II)* is an infectious disease caused by the herpes simplex virus. The person who has herpes develops red blisterlike sores on the reproductive organs. The sores are associated with a burning sensation. The fluid in the blisters is infectious.

A person infected with the virus may have only one episode or may have repeated attacks. Usually, subsequent attacks are less severe. Drugs can reduce discomfort and communicability, but there is no cure at present.

Venereal Warts   This sexually transmitted disease is caused by a virus. Lesions develop on the genitals and can be found on both skin and mucous membranes.

The warts (lesions) are cauliflower shaped, raised, and dark. They can be numerous and tend to spread. They may cause discomfort during intercourse and may bleed if dislodged. Venereal warts can be removed with chemicals and surgery, but they often reoccur.

A.I.D.S.   A.I.D.S. is a viral disease that is transmitted primarily through direct contact with the bodily secretions of an infected person. There is a greater incidence of the disease among intravenous drug users, homosexual males, hemophiliacs, sex partners of infected persons, and babies of mothers who are infected. The virus can be transmitted blood-to-blood through transfusions of infected blood, needle sharing among drug users, and unsterile instruments used for ear piercing or tattooing.

The virus can also be transmitted from an infected sexual partner through vaginal or anal intercourse. It can also be transmitted from infected mothers to their infants during pregnancy, the birth process, or nursing.

There is currently *no evidence* that the disease is transmitted through kissing, touching, hugging, or eating at the same table with an infected person. Toilet seats and insect bites are not modes of transmission.

The A.I.D.S. virus has many variants, but does not live long outside the body. It is affected by common chemicals. Its action in the body is to depress the immune system of the infected person. The person is then more susceptible to a large variety of infections.

Two common complications of A.I.D.S. are *pneumocystis carinii pneumonia* (a serious lung infection) and *Kaposi's sarcoma* (a serious malignancy that affects many body organs). The brain may be damaged by the virus, leading to dementia. Other opportunistic infections are commonly seen. The presence of pneumocystis carinii pneumonia and Kaposi's sarcoma are diagnostic for A.I.D.S. Not everyone who comes in contact with the disease becomes infected.

There is usually an initial period between contact with the organisms and the onset of the signs and symptoms. No indications are usually seen during the first six months to one year. The incubation period may be sixteen years or more, but 25 to 50 percent of people show evidence of disease within five to ten years of antibody development (becoming sero positive).

A.I.D.S. related complex (ARC) is an early step in the progression of A.I.D.S. The person with A.R.C. demonstrates a positive blood test for A.I.D.S. antibodies, has a suppressed immune response, and suffers chronic illness. The person with A.R.C. may experience signs and symptoms that include fatigue or listlessness or loss of 10percent of body weight. The person may have a recurrent fever of 100°F with drenching night sweats, swollen lymph nodes, and diarrhea. Of the people with A.R.C., 25 to 35 percent develop A.I.D.S. within five years of the onset of A.R.C.

There is no specific treatment for A.I.D.S. at the present time. No vaccine has been developed to prevent the infection from developing. Much effort is being directed in this area, however. An A.I.D.S. blood test has been developed that detects A.I.D.S. antibodies (chemicals produced by the infected person in reaction to the virus) in the blood so that the blood supply given to patients who need transfusions can be checked. A similar test is available to detect the presence of the A.I.D.S. antibodies in a person's own blood. The presence of the antibodies indicates exposure to the organisms, but it does not indicate the specific course that the disease will take. Therapy is directed toward treating each opportunistic infection vigorously as it arises.

The incidence of A.I.D.S. among hospital workers not otherwise exposed is very low. It is, however, a disease that can be transmitted to anyone who has direct blood-to-secretion contact with bodily fluids such as blood or semen that are infected with H.I.V.

Nursing Precautions

Any infection can be transmitted directly into the bloodstream of another through open cuts or small breaks in the skin or mucous membranes. Precautions to be followed in caring for patients with infections such as S.T.D.s, which are easily transmittable, include gloving, proper handwashing, careful handling of any sharp equipment such as needles and razor blades, and, where appropriate, complete isolation technique including gowns and masks.

Refer to figure 30-5 for a review of the beginning procedure actions and the procedure completion actions.

Beginning Procedure Actions

- Wash hands.
- Assemble all equipment needed.
- Knock on door and pause before entering resident's room.

- Politely ask visitors to leave. Tell them where they can wait.
- Identify the resident.
- Provide privacy by drawing curtains around bed and closing door.
- Explain what you will be doing and answer questions.
- Raise bed to comfortable working height.

Procedure Completion Actions

- Position resident comfortably.
- Leave signal cord, telephone, and fresh water where resident can reach them.
- Return bed to lowest horizontal position.
- Raise side rails, if required.
- Perform general safety check of resident and environment.
- Clean used equipment and return to proper storage, according to facility policy.
- Open privacy curtains.
- Wash hands.
- Tell visitors that they may reenter the room.
- Report completion of procedure.
- Document procedure following facility policy.

Figure 30-5 Beginning procedure actions and procedure completion actions

---

PROCEDURE 61

Giving a Nonsterile Vaginal Douche

1. Wash hands. Assemble disposable douche and bring to bedside the following:

    irrigation standard
    disposable gloves
    small cup with cotton balls and
       disinfectant
    toilet tissue
    bed protector
    bedpan and cover
    bath blanket
    paper bag

2. Pour a small amount of the specified disinfecting solution over the cotton balls in the cup.
3. Close clamp on tubing. Leave protector on sterile tip.
4. Measure water in douche container. Temperature should be about 105°F. Add powder or solution as ordered.
5. Identify person and explain what you plan to do.
6. Assemble all equipment conveniently at bedside and screen unit.
7. Remove the perineal pad, if in place, from front to back and discard in paper bag.
8. Give bedpan and ask person to void.
9. Drape the person with bath blanket. Fanfold top bedding to foot of bed.
10. Assist the person into the dorsal recumbent position.
11. Place bed protector beneath the person's buttocks.
12. Place bedpan under person.
13. Wash hands. Put on gloves for your protection.
14. Cleanse perineum. Use one cotton ball and disinfectant for each stroke. Cleanse from vulva toward anus. Cleanse labia minora first, exposing with thumb and forefinger. Give special attention to folds. Discard cotton balls in emesis basin.
15. Open clamp to expel air. Remove protector from sterile tip.
16. Allow small amount of solution to flow over inner thigh and then over vulva. Do not touch vulva with nozzle.
17. Allow solution to continue to flow and insert nozzle slowly and gently into the vagina with an upward and backward movement for about 3 inches.
18. Rotate nozzle from side to side as solution flows.
19. When all solution has been given, remove nozzle slowly and clamp tubing.

20. Have the person turn on side. Dry buttocks with tissue.
21. Remove douche bag from standard and place on paper towels.
22. Dry perineum with tissue. Discard tissue in bedpan.
23. Cover bedpan and place on chair.
24. Have person turn on side. Dry buttocks with tissue.
25. Place clean pad over vulva from front to back.
26. Remove bed protector and bath blanket. Replace with top bedding.
27. Make the person comfortable and leave unit in order.
28. Observe contents of bedpan. Note character and amount of discharge if any.
29. Clean and return equipment according to facility policy.
30. Record on chart the date and time; procedure (vaginal irrigation); type, amount, and temperature of solution; your observations; and the patient's reaction.

PROCEDURE 62

Giving Routine Perineal Care to a Female

1. Wash hands and assemble the following equipment:

bath blanket	ordered solution (if
bedpan and cover	other than water)
graduate pitcher	plastic bag to dis-
cotton balls	pose of used
disposable gloves	cotton balls
bed protector or	perineal pad and
bath towel	belt, if needed

2. Identify person and explain what you plan to do.
3. Fill pitcher with warm water (or ordered solution) at approximately 100°F and take to bedside.
4. Screen unit.
5. Lower side rail and position bed protector (or towel) under person's buttocks.
6. Fanfold spread to foot of bed.
7. Cover person with bath blanket and fanfold sheet to foot of bed.
8. Position person on bedpan.
9. Put on disposable gloves.
10. Have person flex and separate knees.
11. Draw bath blanket upward to expose perineal area only.
12. Unfasten perineal pad if in use. Touch only the outside. Note amount and color of discharge. Fold with the insides together and place in plastic bag.
13. Holding pitcher of water approximately 5 inches above the pubis, allow all the water to flow downward over vulva and into the bedpan.
14. Dry vulva using cotton balls in the following manner:

    a. Use each cotton ball once only and dispose of into plastic bag.
    b. Bring one or more cotton balls down one side of vulva from pubis to perineum until dry.
    c. Repeat on opposite side of vulva. Remember, use each cotton ball only once and discard.
    d. Dry area over center of vulva.

15. Remove and dispose of disposable gloves.
16. Ask person to raise hips and carefully remove bedpan. Cover and place on chair.
17. Apply perineal pad if needed and secure to belt. Never touch fingers to inside of pad. Apply from front to back, then fasten belt.
18. Remove bath towel or disposable pad and dispose of according to facility policy.
19. Draw sheet and spread up over person and remove bath blanket.
20. Fold bath blanket and store in bedside stand.

21. Make person comfortable and leave unit tidy.
22. Clean equipment and discard disposables according to facility policy.
23. Wash hands.
24. Report completion of task and observations to the nurse.

Summary

- A knowledge of the normal male and female reproductive anatomy and physiology is important for the geriatric health care provider who wishes to understand the related nursing care.

- Although changes take place in the reproductive tract with aging, there are no normal senescent changes that preclude sexual activity throughout life.
- Sexual behavior is part of human nature influenced by cultural expectations.
- Pathologies affecting the reproductive tract of older men and women include inflammations, tumor development, and decreased ability to carry out coitus.
- Diseases transmitted sexually are referred to as S.T.D.s. They can affect the elderly as well as the young.
- Any therapy involving the reproductive organs can have both physical and psychological effects.

Review Outline

   I. Behavioral Objectives

  II. Vocabulary

 III. Reproductive System

     A. Structure
     B. Function
        1. Male
        2. Female

  IV. Senescent Changes

   V. Problems of the Reproductive System

     A. Male
        1. Impotence
        2. Benign prostatic hyperplasia
        3. Cancer of the testes
        4. Peyronies disease
     B. Female
        1. Procidentia
        2. Vaginitis
        3. Pruritus
        4. Nongonorrheal urethritis
        5. Carcinoma of the system

VI. Sexually Transmitted Diseases

    A.   Gonorrhea
    B.   H.I.V.
    C.   Syphilis
    D.   Trichomonas vaginitis
    E.   Genital herpes
    F.   Venereal warts

Review

I. Vocabulary

Complete the pattern with the names of six sexually transmitted diseases you learned in this unit.

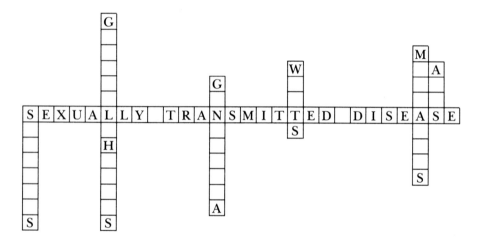

II. Anatomy

Label the figures.

Figure 30-6

1. _____
2. _____
3. _____
4. _____
5. _____

Figure 30-7

1. _____
2. _____
3. _____
4. _____
5. _____

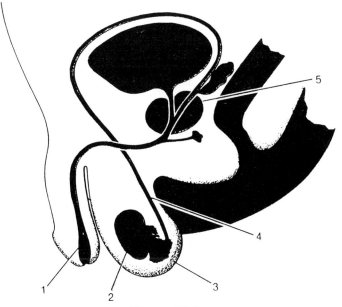

Figure 30-6

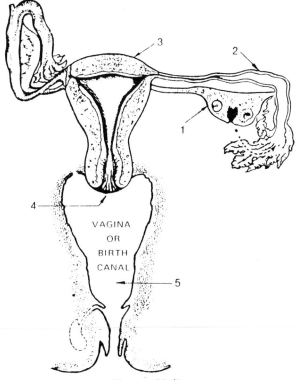

VAGINA
OR
BIRTH
CANAL

Figure 30-7

III. True or False

1.   The female and male gonads are known as the ovaries and testes.
2.   Another name for the female womb is the uterus.
3.   A female sex organ closely resembling the male penis is the vagina.
4.   The male and female organs of copulation are the penis and labia minora.
5.   The menstrual cycle prepares the female uterus for pregnancy approximately once a month.
6.   The primary lesion of syphilis is called a chancre.
7.   The temperature of a douche solution is about 90°F.
8.   When an elderly man suffers from benign prostatic hyperplasia, a surgical procedure called T.U.R.P. is often performed.
9.   Contagious diseases are easily transmitted infectious diseases.
10. Germs (pathogens) cause infectious diseases.

IV. Short Answers

1.   List the ways that males and females change sexually with aging.
2.   What are the phases of coitus?
3.   List five things to remember when giving an older woman a nonsterile vaginal douche.

V. Clinical Situations

1.   You notice an area of dimpling in the breast of an elderly patient as you are bathing her. What do you do?
2.   You are giving perineal care to a newly admitted resident and notice a large amount of frothy, white vaginal discharge. What do you do?

CASE STUDY

Breakwater Home is a sheltered facility that provides board and care for mostly ambulatory older people who need some assistance in carrying out their activities of daily living. It is located in a rural setting with wide, rolling lawns and large oak trees.

Bettina Heinz, seventy-nine, had been a resident for two years when Albert Moore joined the "family," as the residents call themselves. Bettina had entered the United States forty years ago as a domestic worker from Germany. She hade been brought to this country by a socially prominent family. Over the years she had worked for several wealthy families in New York, first as a housekeeper and then as chief cook. She had never married

but had always been a great favorite of the children in the households where she worked.

She had frequently had a dog or cat as a pet. Since her admission to Breakwater, she had "adopted" a stray black-and-white cat she called "One Eye." She loved to sit and stroke its fur, and the cat in turn would be quiet and content on her lap for hours.

When Bettina was forty-two she developed cancer in her right breast and a radical mastectomy was performed. She is very self-conscious about the scar and tries to shield it from view as she is assisted in dressing and undressing. She suffers from arthritis in her hips, hands, and spine, and she frequently uses a wheelchair to get around.

Albert Moore, a widower of twenty years, is a tall stately gentlemen of eight-seven. A former certified public accountant, his attention to detail still prevails as can be noted in his grooming. His shock of pure white hair is always in place and his clothing neat and well pressed. He has suffered a stroke and now requires some help in maintaining himself. He is ambulatory with the aid of a walker, has a hearing aid, and enjoys the wide open area of the Breakwater facility. His daughter had invited him to make his home with her family in the city, but he declined. He prefers to remain with his "friends" in the country setting. His daughter and grandchildren visit frequently, but he finds the children tiring and seems relieved when they leave.

Albert and Bettina were a somewhat unlikely couple, he with his rather precise English and she with her deep German accent, but a couple they became nonetheless. They spent hours in the yard, he on a bench and she in a wheelchair, talking and just enjoying each other's company.

Sometimes the younger geriatric health care providers would laugh and make joking remarks to each other about the couple. In a moment of frankness, Bettina confided her sexual interest in Albert Moore to a geriatric health care provider. She told the assistant that she thought Mr. Moore was interested in her "that way" also but she was afraid his daughter might not approve. Besides, there were always other people around. She said she knew it might be difficult because of her arthritis. Besides, he might find her body ugly. But she expressed a desire to "make love" once before she died.

The health care provider reported the information to the supervisor, who had a private conference with Miss Heinz and Mr. Moore. The nurse then arranged a private room in which Miss Heinz and Mr. Moore could be alone. She made a sign that was hung on the outside of the door to ensure their privacy.

1. Why did the younger health care providers make fun of Miss Heinz and Mr. Moore? Do you share their attitude?
2. Should the geriatric health care provider have repeated the information to the supervisor?
3. What if there had been no Mr. Moore? Were there ways to increase Miss Heinz's sensual satisfaction without involving another person?
4. Why did Miss Heinz need extra emotional support?
5. Should the supervisor have made provision for the two residents to have privacy? Should the supervisor have contacted the daughter before assisting the couple to be alone?

Unit 31
Basic Skills

Objectives

After studying this unit, you should be able to:

- List some basic skills carried out by geriatric health care providers.
- Demonstrate proficiency in carrying out basic nursing skills.
- Relate specific nursing care principles to nursing care procedures.
- List steps in common to all patient procedures.

Vocabulary

Learn the meaning and spelling of the following words or phrases.

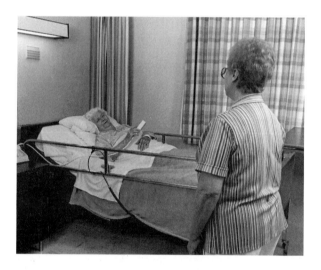

bradycardia		
diastolic		
diathermy	metric system	sphygmomanometer
dyspnea	mitered corner	stethoscope
electronic	occupied	systolic
enteric	probe	tachycardia
exudate	prostheses	unoccupied
hypertension	pulse pressure	vasoconstriction
hypotension	rules	vasodilation

The nursing skills needed to care for older people are usually taught in basic nursing programs. These skills are then adapted to the geriatric setting. Today, geriatric health care providers may be prepared to function specifically in extended care facilities. Therefore, they may not need some of the skills related to the acutely ill. Still, some fundamental procedures must be mastered by all who wish to function as geriatric health care providers.

This unit may be used to introduce or to review these concepts. Experienced geriatric nursing assistants may be competent in these procedures, whereas new health care providers must learn and practice the skills.

All procedures that involve patient care have some elements in common. These are referred to as procedure reminders and include beginning procedure actions and procedure completion actions. They are identified in figure 31-1. These actions are an integral part of every patient care procedure. Students should practice them often enough to make them a habit.

Beds and Bedmaking

Patients in extended care facilities do not spend as much time in bed as they would in an acute care facility, but proper bedmaking is still

Beginning Procedure Actions

- Wash hands.
- Assemble all equipment needed.
- Knock on door and pause before entering resident's room.
- Politely ask visitors to leave. Tell them where they can wait.
- Identify the resident.
- Provide privacy by drawing curtains around bed and closing door.
- Explain what you will be doing and answer questions.
- Raise bed to comfortable working height.

Procedure Completion Actions

- Position resident comfortably.
- Leave signal cord, telephone, and fresh water where resident can reach them.
- Return bed to lowest horizontal position.
- Raise side rails, if required.
- Perform general safety check of resident and environment.
- Clean used equipment and return to proper storage, according to facility policy.
- Open privacy curtains.
- Wash hands.
- Tell visitors that they may re-enter the room.
- Report completion of procedure.
- Document procedure following facility policy.

Figure 31-1 Beginning procedure actions and procedure completion actions

important. Beds may be made with occupants out of them (*unoccupied*) or in them (*occupied*). Linens are usually changed two to three times a week. But whenever they are soiled, they should be changed at once. Pillowcases are usually changed every day. If a supplemental drawsheet is used, it should also be changed daily.

The Hospital Bed

Before attempting to make the bed, be sure you know how to operate it. Not all beds are operated in the same way. Some are electrically controlled; others operate by the turning of cranks. The height of most beds may be raised so that there is less strain for those giving care. All beds break in the middle so that the head may be raised. This permits the patient to be supported in a sitting position. Side rails, which keep the patient from falling, may be attached to the bed or may be separate from it. They may extend the full length of the bed or only part way. Before you leave any patient, check to make sure the rails are raised and securely attached.

Beds should always be left in the lowest horizontal position when side rails are down, figure 31-2. Side rails should be up at night, because patients may become disoriented in dim light and unfamiliar surroundings. If restraints are being used, be sure that they are never tied to the side rails and that tubes such as I.V. lines or catheters are always free of the side rails. Raising and lowering the side rails could put undue stress on them.

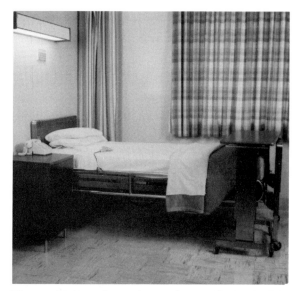

Figure 31-2 Always leave the resident's bed in the lowest horizontal position when side rails are down. (From Caldwell & Hegner, *Nursing Assistant, A Nursing Process Approach,* copyright 1989 by Delmar Publishers Inc.)

PROCEDURE 63

Making the Unoccupied Bed

1. Wash hands and assemble the following equipment:

pillowcases	cotton drawsheet or
spread	half sheet
blankets, as	mattress pad and
needed	cover
2 large sheets	
(90″ × 108″)	

    Hospital mattresses that are treated with plastic do not require a moisture-proof sheet or cotton half sheet (drawsheet). In selected cases, the half sheet is used as a lifter to assist in moving the patient or simply to keep the bottom sheet clean. Some hospitals use fitted bottom sheets. If so, substitute a fitted sheet for one of the large sheets.

2. Lock bed wheels so the bed will not roll, and place chair at the side of the bed.
3. Arrange linen on chair in order in which it is to be used.
4. Position mattress to head of bed by grasping handles on mattress side.
5. Place mattress cover on mattress and adjust it smoothly for corners. Work entirely from one side of the bed until that side is completed. Then go to the other side of the bed. This conserves time and energy.
6. Place and unfold bottom sheet, smooth side up with wide hem at the top, and center fold at the center of the bed, figure 31-3.
7. Tuck 12 to 18 inches of sheet smoothly over the top of the mattress.
8. Make a *mitered corner* (triangular), figure 31-4. The square corner, preferred by some facilities, is made in a similar way.
9. Tuck in the sheet on one side, keeping it straight, working from the head to the foot of the bed. Or adjust fitted sheet over the head and bottom ends of mat-

tress (see figures for proper and improper placement).

10. If used, place the plastic drawsheet and half sheet with upper edge about 14 inches from head of mattress and tuck under one side.
11. Unfold the top sheet and place wrong side up, hem even with the upper edge of the mattress, and center fold in the center of the bed.
12. Spread the blanket over the top sheet and foot of mattress. Keep blanket centered.
13. Tuck top sheet and blanket under mattress at the foot of the bed as far as the center only and make a mitered corner.
14. Place spread with top hem even with head of mattress. Unfold to foot of bed.
15. Tuck spread under mattress at the foot of bed and make mitered corner.
16. Go to other side of the bed. Fanfold the top covers to the center of the bed in order to work with lower sheets and pad.
17. Tuck bottom sheet under head of mattress and make mitered corner. Working from top to bottom, smooth out all wrinkles and tighten sheet as much as possible to provide comfort. Or adjust fitted bottom sheet smoothly and securely around mattress corners.
18. Grasp protective drawsheet, if used, and cotton drawsheet in the center. Tuck these sheets under the mattress.
19. Tuck in top sheet and blanket at foot of bed and make mitered corner.
20. Fold top sheet back over blanket, making an 8-inch cuff.
21. Tuck in spread at foot of bed and make a mitered corner. Bring top of spread to head of mattress.
22. Insert pillow in case.

    a. Place hands in the clean case, freeing the corners.
    b. Grasp the center of the end seam with hand outside the case and turn case back over hand.
    c. Grasp the pillow through the case at

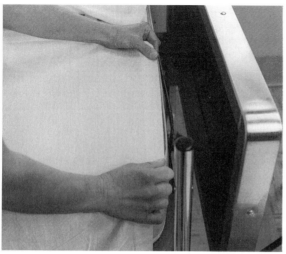 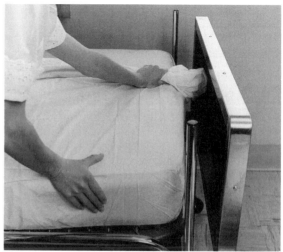

Figure 31-3 Making the unoccupied bed. A. Place flat bottom sheet even with the end of the mattress at the foot of the bed. B. If a fitted bottom sheet is used, fit it properly and smoothly around one corner. (From Caldwell & Hegner, *Nursing Assistant, A Nursing Process Approach,* copyright 1989 by Delmar Publishers Inc.)

the center of one end and pull the case over the pillow.

   d.   Adjust the corners of the pillow to fit in the corners of the case.

23. Place pillow at head of bed with open end away from the door.

24. Lower bed to lowest horizontal position.

25. Replace bedside table parallel to bed. Place chair in assigned location. Place overbed table over the foot of the bed opposite the chair. Place signal cord or call panel within easy reach of the patient.

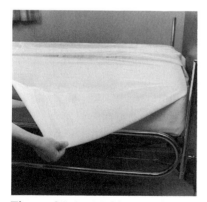 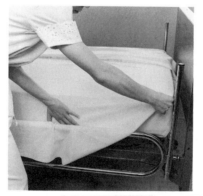 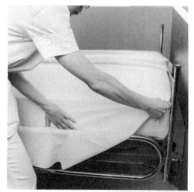

Figure 31-4 Making a mitered corner. A. To make a mitered corner, pick up sheet hanging at side of bed, about 12 inches from the bed, forming a triangle. B. Bring the fold down and begin to tuck under the mattress. C. Complete tucking in the corner and smooth. (From Caldwell & Hegner, *Nursing Assistant, A Nursing Process Approach,* copyright 1989 by Delmar Publishers Inc.)

PROCEDURE 64

Making the Occupied Bed

1. Wash hands and assemble the following equipment:

   cotton drawsheet or turning sheet for selected patients
   2 large sheets (or fitted bottom sheet)
   2 pillowcases
   laundry hamper

2. Identify the patient and explain what you plan to do.
3. Place bedside chair at the foot of the bed.
4. Arrange linen on chair in the order in which it is to be used.
5. Screen the unit for privacy.
6. Bed should be flat with wheels locked unless otherwise indicated. Raise to working horizontal height.
7. Loosen the bedclothes on all sides by lifting the edge of the mattress with one hand and drawing bedclothes out with the other. Never shake the linen; this spreads germs. Adjust mattress to head of bed. Have patient bend knees, grasp bed head frame with hands, and pull on frame as you draw mattress to the top, or have another person help from the opposite side.
8. Remove top covers except for top sheet, one at a time. Fold to bottom and pick up in center. Place over the back of chair.
9. Place the clean sheet over top sheet. Have the patient hold the top edge of the clean sheet if able. If not, tuck the sheet beneath the patient's shoulder.
10. Slide the soiled top sheet out, from top to bottom. Discard in hamper.
11. Ask the patient to roll toward you and assist if necessary. Move one pillow with the patient and remove the other pillow. Pull up the side rail.
12. Go to the other side of the bed. Fanfold the cotton drawsheet, if used, and bottom sheet close to the patient.
13. Straighten out mattress pad. Place a clean bottom sheet on the bed so that the narrow hem comes to the edge of the mattress at the foot and the lengthwise center fold of the sheet is at the center of the bed.
14. Tuck top of sheet under the head of the mattress.
15. Make a mitered corner.
16. Tuck side of sheet under mattress, working toward the foot of the bed.
17. Position fresh turning sheet. If drawsheet is used, position and tuck it under the mattress.
18. Ask patient to roll toward you and assist as needed. Move the pillow with the patient. Raise side rails.
19. Go to the other side of the bed. Remove the soiled linen by rolling the edges inward and place in hamper. Keep soiled linen away from your uniform.
20. Complete the bed as an unoccupied bed. Make toe pleats in top sheet and blanket so that pressure is not exerted on the toes. There are several methods of making toe pleats. One is to make a mitered corner but before making the final tuck to grasp the linen and make a 3-inch fold toward the foot of the bed. Then complete the mitered corner. Some patients prefer not to have the blanket, topsheet, or spread tucked in.
21. Turn patient on back. Place clean case on pillow not being used. Replace pillow. Change other pillowcase.
22. Adjust bed position for the patient's comfort. Be sure side rails are up and secure. Lower bed to lowest horizontal height.
23. Place signal cord within patient's reach. Replace bedside table and chair. Remove hamper. Wash hands.
24. Let the nurse know you have completed the task.

Admission, Transfer, and Discharge

Admission to a care facility is a period full of anxiety and uncertainty, figure 31-5. Often people view admission to a long-term facility as the final separation from society. The event may closely follow loss of a spouse or home or a period of serious illness. Independence has been eroded. People fear they will be abandoned and never see familiar surroundings again. A few people, frail and no longer able to care for themselves, feel a measure of comfort. Most, however, will require a period of adjustment before settling into their new residence. This is also a trying time for those accompanying the new admission. Feel-

ings of guilt and sadness may be strong. They, too, will need support and understanding. Courtesy and an unhurried approach are important in helping new residents to relax. Anything done to make them feel welcome helps reduce the stress.

During admission, the resident's belongings are listed, identified, and put away. Valuables should be placed in the facility safe or listed and sent home with the family. If the resident insists on keeping valuables, inform the nurse. Assist in arranging personal articles as the new resident wishes. Explain regulations, such as times of meals and when visits are permitted. Try to make residents feel that they still have some control and choice. Remember, this will become their home and they need to feel secure. Additional procedures related to admission will be carried out at this time. These include weighing, measuring, and determining vital signs. Each of these findings must be reported and recorded appropriately.

Residents are weighed and measured when they are admitted. They may be weighed at intervals thereafter. The initial weight serves as a baseline for assessment. Disease is often related to body weight. Changes in body weight indicate general health. Drug dosages are sometimes determined according to the resident's weight. Weights are recorded in pounds or kilograms, and height is recorded in feet and inches or centimeters. Refer to figures 31-6 and 31-7 for conversions.

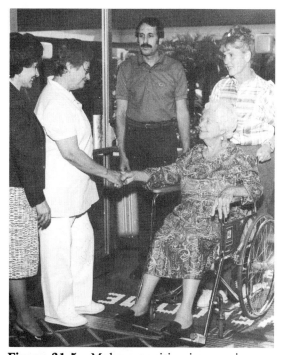

Figure 31-5 Make a positive impression on the new resident and her family by making them feel welcome. (From Hegner & Caldwell, *Assisting in Long-Term Care,* copyright 1988 by Delmar Publishers Inc.)

---

1 kilogram = 2.2 pounds
12 inches = 1 foot
2.5 centimeters = 1 inch
To convert kilograms to pounds, multiply by 2.2.
To convert pounds to kilograms, divide by 2.2.
To convert feet to inches, multiply by 12.
To convert inches to feet, divide by 12.

Figure 31-6 Conversion chart for weight. Some facilities record weights in kilograms while others record weights in pounds.

1 foot is equal to 12 inches.

- To convert from feet to inches, multiply the number of feet by 12.
  Example: 6 feet × 12 = 72 inches
- To convert from inches to feet, divide the number of inches by 12.
  Example: 72 inches ÷ 12 = 6 feet

1 inch equals 2.5 centimeters

- To convert from inches to centimeters, multiply inches by 2.5
  Example: 6 inches × 2.5 = 15 centimeters
- To convert from centimeters to inches, divide centimeters by 2.5.
  Example: 15 centimeters ÷ 2.5 = 6 inches

MULTIPLES OF 12

12 × 1 = 12	12 × 7 = 84
12 × 2 = 24	12 × 8 = 96
12 × 3 = 36	12 × 9 = 108
12 × 4 = 48	12 × 10 = 120
12 × 5 = 60	12 × 11 = 132
12 × 6 = 72	12 × 12 = 144

Figure 31-7 Some facilities measure height in feet and inches. Other facilities measure height in centimeters.

Transfer to an acute hospital or other facility is handled as a discharge if the resident is to be absent for an extended period, and the record is closed, figure 31-8. A return at a later time is treated as a new admission.

Observations

Carefully observe the new resident. Note any limitations such as hearing difficulties or the need for glasses or other *prostheses* (artificial parts). Try to determine the resident's ability to communicate and degree of reality orientation. As mentioned previously, observing means more than just looking. To observe properly, you must use all your senses. Note anything unusual and then record and report these findings to the nurse. Observations at this time serve as a baseline for future comparisons, figure 31-9.

Certain patient conditions make some observations particularly significant. For example, attention to the skin color and respirations of a patient with pneumonia is particularly important. Body language sometimes reveals a lot. A patient in pain tends to be somewhat protective of the painful area. Tears may be indicative of depression. Be alert to body language. Make sure your own sends a message of welcome and confidence.

If it is necessary to ask visitors to leave during the admission procedure, do so kindly. Visitors will be anxious to see the resident settled and comfortable. Show them where they may wait. Let them know approximately how long they will have to wait and the availability of coffee and smoking areas. Your courtesy will go a long way toward establishing peace of mind for them and their loved one.

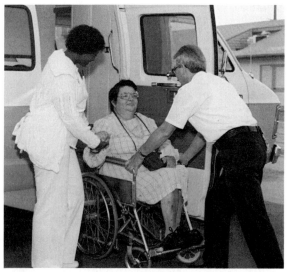

Figure 31-8 Transfer to a new facility can be a very stressful experience unless you sensitively lend support. (From Hegner & Caldwell, *Assisting in Long-Term Care,* copyright 1988 by Delmar Publishers Inc.)

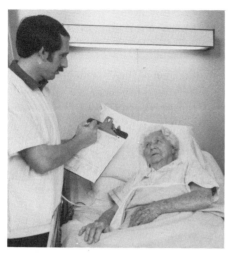

Figure 31-9 Think of each body system as you make and record your observations. (From Hegner & Caldwell, *Assisting in Long-Term Care,* copyright 1988 by Delmar Publishers Inc.)

PROCEDURE 65

Admitting a Resident

1. Wash hands and assemble the following equipment:

pad and pencil	equipment for
patient's record	taking tempera-
stethoscope	ture
blood pressure cuff	watch with second
equipment for	band
urine specimen	

2. Prepare the unit for the patient by making sure that all necessary equipment and furniture are in their proper places. Check the unit for adequate lighting and provide ventilation.

3. Identify the new resident by asking his or her name and by checking the identification. Introduce yourself and take the patient and family to the unit. Do not rush. Be courteous and helpful.

4. Ask the new resident to be seated or assist into bed from the stretcher. Ask the family to go to the lounge or lobby while you carry out the admission procedure. Introduce the resident to others in the room. Explain the signal system and the standard regulations. Insofar as it is permitted, explain what will happen in the next hour.

5. Screen the unit.

6. Care for clothing and personal articles according to facility policy.

7. Valuables or jewelry that have not been left at the office should be listed. Ask the resident to sign the list if possible; this protects the facility. The relatives should also sign the list and take the valuables home, or you should put them in the safe.

8. Check the patient's weight and height.

9. If ordered, help patient get undressed and into bed. Adjust side rails if ordered. Otherwise, residents are encouraged to stay up and in their own clothes as much as possible.

10. Take temperature, pulse, respiration, and blood pressure. Record.

11. Clean and replace equipment according to facility policy.

12. Record information according to facility policy on the patient's chart.

PROCEDURE 66

Weighing and Measuring a Resident

1. Escort the patient to the scale, if ambulatory. If not, use a portable scale, wheelchair scale, or overbed scale.

2. Place a paper towel on the platform of the scale.

3. Be sure the weights are at the extreme left and the balance bar hangs free. The lower bar indicates weights in large (50-pound) increments. The upper bar indi-

cates smaller increments. Even-numbered pounds are marked with numbers. Long lines between even numbers indicate the odd numbers. Each small line indicates one-quarter of a pound.

4. Help the patient remove shoes and step onto the scale platform. Stand close for support. The balance bar will rise to the top of the bar guide.
5. Move the large weight to the closest estimated weight.
6. Move the small weight to the right until the balance bar hangs free halfway between the upper and lower bar guide.
7. Add the two figures and record the total weight in pounds or kilograms according to facility policy. For example, if

Large weight   150 pounds
Small weight   8 pounds
    Total   158 pounds
or 158 ÷ 2.2 = 71.8 kilograms

8. While the patient stands on the platform, raise the height bar until it rests levelly on the top of the patient's head.
9. Make the reading at the movable point of the ruler. Record this information in inches, feet and inches, or centimeters, according to facility policy. (There are 12 inches to 1 foot, and 2.5 centimeters to 1 inch.) For example, a height of 62 inches might be recorded as 62 inches, 5 feet 2 inches (62 ÷ 12 = 5 feet 2 inches), or 155 centimeters (62 inches × 2.5).
10. Help the patient step off the scale and put on shoes.
11. Enter the height and weight in the appropriate place on the patient's record.

Vital Signs

Temperature, pulse, respiratory rate, and blood pressure are referred to as the patient's vital signs. They must be measured accurately, because they tell a great deal about the patient's condition. Never tell the resident the results.

This is the responsibility of the physician or professional nurse. Vital signs are always taken on admission and at other times as ordered.

Equipment for Vital Signs

Clinical thermometers are used to take the patient's temperature. A watch with a second hand is used to count the pulse and respiratory rate. Both a *stethoscope* (an instrument used to hear body sounds) and blood pressure cuff (*sphygmomanometer*) are needed to determine the blood pressure. Each vital sign will be discussed separately, although they are usually taken together.

Temperature

Temperature is the balance between the heat that is produced by the body and the heat that is lost. Normal body temperature is 98.6°F or 37°C. To take oral temperatures, wait fifteen minutes after a patient has smoked or drunk cold or hot fluids.

There are three methods of taking the temperature. They are:

- Oral—most common. This method should not be used if there is any difficulty breathing or closing the lips around the thermometer.
- Rectal—most accurate. Rectal temperature registers one degree higher than oral. A rectal temperature should not be taken when there is rectal bleeding or the resident is uncooperative or has diarrhea.
- Axillary or groin—least accurate. This method is used only when the patient's condition does not permit the use of oral or rectal thermometers. Axillary temperatures register one degree below oral temperature.

Clinical Thermometers Three types of glass clinical thermometers are in general use. They are the oral, security, and rectal thermometers, figure 31-10. The thermometers differ mainly in the size and shape of the bulb (the end that is inserted into the patient). When only the security

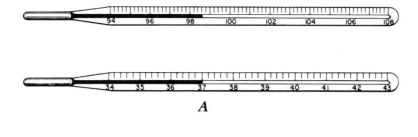

A

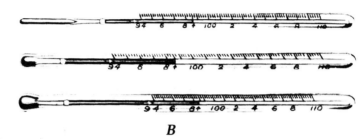

B

Figure 31-10   Fahrenheit and Celsius thermometer scales. B. Clinical thermometers—from top to bottom: oral, security, and rectal. (From Hegner & Caldwell, *Assisting in Long-Term Care,* copyright 1988 by Delmar Publishers Inc.)

or stubby type is in use, the rectal thermometers are marked with a red dot at the end of the stem.

Other Types of Thermometers

Electronic Thermometers   The electronic (battery operated) thermometer is used in many facilities, figure 31-11. One unit can serve many residents by simply changing the disposable sheath that fits over the probe.

- The electronic thermometer is battery operated. It registers the temperature on the viewer in a few seconds.
- The portion called the *probe* is inserted into the resident.
- The probes are colored red for rectal use and blue for oral use.
- The probe is covered by a plastic sheath before use. The plastic sheath stays on during use. It is discarded after use.

Plastic or Paper Thermometers   Plastic or paper thermometers are used in some facilities, figure 31-12. They are used once and discarded. They have dots on them. The dots are treated to change color from brown to blue, according to the resident's temperature.

Reading the Thermometer   Mercury (the solid color line) in the bulb of the thermometer rises in the hollow center of the stem. To read the thermometer, hold it at eye level, figure 31-13. Look along the sharper edge between the numbers and lines to find the solid column of mercury. Temperature may be measured in degrees Celsius or Fahrenheit and converted from one to the other. Starting with 94°F (34°C), each long line indicates a one-degree elevation in temperature. Only every other degree is marked with a number. In between each long line are four shorter lines. Each shorter line equals two-tenths (2/10 or 0.2) of a degree. The thermometer is "read" at

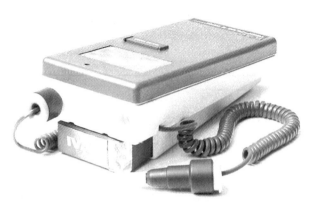

Figure 31-11 An electronic thermometer (From Caldwell & Hegner, *Nursing Assistant, A Nursing Process Approach,* copyright 1989 by Delmar Publishers Inc.)

the point where the mercury ends, figure 31-14. If it falls between two lines, read it to the closest line. If it falls exactly halfway between, read to the next higher line.

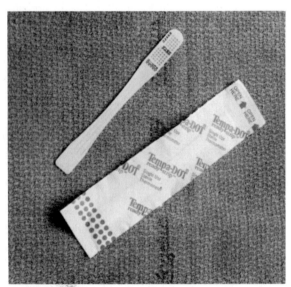

Figure 31-12 A plastic thermometer (From Caldwell & Hegner, *Nursing Assistant, A Nursing Process Approach,* copyright 1989 by Delmar Publishers Inc.)

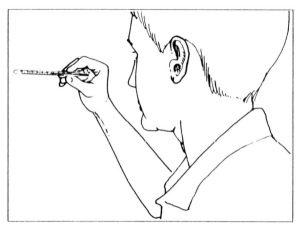

Figure 31-13 Read the thermometer by holding it at eye level. Locate the column of mercury and read to the closest line. (From Caldwell & Hegner, *Nursing Assistant, A Nursing Process Approach,* copyright 1989 by Delmar Publishers Inc.)

PROCEDURE 67

Taking Oral Temperature
(Glass Thermometer)

1. Wash hands and assemble the following equipment on a tray:

    pad and pencil
    container for used thermometers
    container with clean thermometers

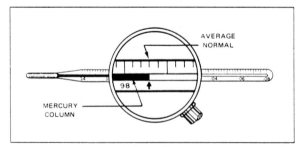

Figure 31-14 Each long line represents one degree difference. Each short line represents 0.2 of one degree difference. (From Caldwell & Hegner, *Nursing Assistant, A Nursing Process Approach,* copyright 1989 by Delmar Publishers Inc.)

watch with second hand
container for soiled tissues
container with tissues

2. Identify patient and explain what you plan to do.

3. Have patient rest in comfortable position in bed or chair.

4. Remove thermometer from container by holding stem end. Wipe with tissue and check to be sure the thermometer is intact. Read mercury column. It should register below 96°F. If necessary, shake down. To shake down, move away from table or other hard objects. Grasp stem tightly between thumb and fingers and shake with downward motion until mercury falls below 96°F.

5. Insert bulb end of thermometer under patient's tongue, toward side of mouth. Tell patient to hold thermometer gently with lips closed for 3 minutes.

6. Remove thermometer, holding by stem. Use tissue to wipe from stem end toward bulb end.

7. Discard tissue in proper container.

8. Read thermometer and record on pad.

9. Place thermometer in container for used thermometers. If thermometer is to be reused for this patient, be sure to wash it in cold water and soap, rinse and dry it. Return it to the individual disinfectant-filled holder.

10. Clean and replace equipment according to policy.

11. Record the temperature on the resident's chart. Report any unusual variation in reading immediately to supervising nurse.

PROCEDURE 68

Taking Rectal Temperature

1. Wash hands and assemble equipment as for oral temperature. Add lubricant. Use rectal thermometer with rounded bulb.

2. Identify patient and explain what you plan to do.

3. Screen unit.

4. Lower backrest of bed. Ask patient to turn on side. Assist, if necessary.

5. Place small amount of lubricant on tissues.

6. Remove thermometer from container by holding stem end and read mercury column. Be sure it registers below 96°F. Check condition of thermometer.

7. Apply small amount of lubricant to bulb with tissue.

8. Fold the top bedclothes back to expose anal area.

9. Separate buttocks with one hand. Insert the thermometer gently into rectum 1½ inches. Hold in place. Replace bedclothes as soon as thermometer is inserted.

10. Thermometer should remain in place for 2 minutes.

11. Complete procedure as for oral temperature, steps 6 to12.

12. Record an "R" beside temperature reading; for example, 98°FR.

PROCEDURE 69

Taking Axillary or Groin Temperature

1. Wash hands and assemble equipment as for oral temperature. The procedure for taking temperature in the groin or axilla (underarm) is basically the same as for taking temperatures in the mouth or rectum.

2. Identify patient and explain what you plan to do.

3. Wipe the area dry, and place the thermometer. The patient should hold arm close to body if axillary site is used. Thermometer must be in the fold against the body if groin site is used. The thermometer is left in place for 10 minutes.

4. In recording, place "AX" after axillary temperature; for example, 98°F AX. For a groin temperature, use the abbreviation "GR": 98°FGR.

Pulse and Respiration

The pulse and respiration of the patient are usually counted during the same procedure. Because breathing is partly under voluntary control, patients may alter their breathing pattern without meaning to do so when they realize that their breathing is being monitored. To avoid this, count respirations immediately following the pulse count, while seeming to continue counting the pulse.

The Pulse Pulse is the pressure of the blood against the wall of an artery as the heart alternately beats (contracts) and rests (relaxes). It is more easily felt in arteries fairly close to the skin surface that can be gently squeezed against a bone by the finger. The pulse rate and its character provide a good indication of how the cardiovascular system is able to meet body needs.

You will usually take the pulse over the radial artery (at the base of the thumb), figure 31-15. The age, sex, size, and condition of the patient may influence the pulse rate (speed), rhythm (regularity), and volume (fullness). Rate and character (rhythm and volume) should be noted when taking the pulse.

The heart rate is usually the same as the pulse rate, but sometimes all the heartbeats are not strong enough to be transmitted along the radial artery. This is true in some forms of heart disease. If a pulse deficit (difference between the heart and pulse rates) is suspected, it may be necessary to determine the heart rate with a stethoscope and compare it to the pulse rate. This is referred to as the apical pulse, figure 31-16.

An unusually fast heartbeat is called *tachycardia*. An unusually slow heartbeat is called *bradycardia*. Both extremes—pulse rates under 60 or over 100—should be reported immediately.

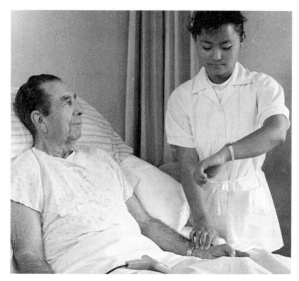

Figure 31-15 Count the pulse for one full minute. (From Hegner & Caldwell, *Assisting in Long-Term Care*, copyright 1988 by Delmar Publishers Inc.)

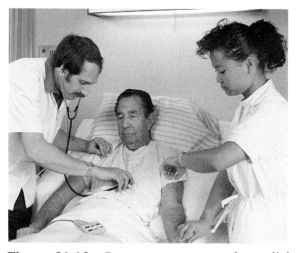

Figure 31-16 One person counts the radial pulse while another counts the apical pulse. The two rates should be the same. (From Hegner & Caldwell, *Assisting in Long-Term Care*, copyright 1988 by Delmar Publishers Inc.)

Respiration The main function of respiration is to supply the body cells with oxygen and to rid the body of excess carbon dioxide. When respirations are inefficient, carbon dioxide accumulates in the bloodstream. This makes the skin dusky, bluish, or cyanotic.

There are two parts to each respiration: one inspiration (inhalation) followed by one expiration (exhalation). *Dyspnea* is difficult or labored breathing. A period of no respirations is known as apnea. Periods of dyspnea followed by apnea are called Cheyne-Stokes respirations. At times fluid (mucus) will collect in the air passages, giving rise to a characteristic "bubbling" type of respiration called *rales*. Rales are common in the dying patient.

The character of respirations must be noted as well as the rate. Respirations are described as normal, shallow, deep, labored, or difficult. Rate is determined by counting the rise and fall of the chest for 1 minute, using a watch equipped with a second hand. One rise and one fall equal one respiration. The normal rate for adults is fourteen to eighteen respirations per minute. If the rate is more than twenty-five per minute, it is said to be accelerated and should be reported.

PROCEDURE 70

Counting the Pulse

1. Wash hands and go to bedside. Identify patient and explain what you plan to do.
2. Place patient in a comfortable position, with arm resting across chest, palm of hand down.
3. Locate the pulse on the thumb side of the wrist with the tips of your first three fingers. Do not use your thumb because it contains a pulse that may be confused with the patient's pulse.
4. When a pulse is felt, exert slight pressure. Using second hand of watch, count for 1 minute. It is the practice in some hospitals to count for one-half minute and multiply

by 2, but counting for 1 minute is preferred.
5. Record the rate and character of the pulse.

PROCEDURE 71

Counting Respirations

1. When the pulse rate has been counted, leave your fingers on the radial pulse and start counting the number of times the chest rises and falls during 1 minute.
2. Note depth and regularity of respirations.
3. Record the time, rate, depth, and regularity of respirations.

Blood Pressure

Blood pressure is the fourth vital sign. The *systolic* pressure is the greatest force exerted on the walls of the artery by the blood as the heart contracts. The *diastolic* pressure is the least force exerted as the heart relaxes. Blood pressure is measured by means of a sphygmomanometer and a stethoscope. *Pulse pressure* is the difference between systolic and diastolic readings.

Blood pressure depends upon the volume (amount) of blood in the circulatory system, the force of the heartbeat, and the condition of the arteries. Arteries that have lost their elasticity (stretch) give more resistance. Therefore, the pressure is greater. Blood pressure is also increased by exercise, eating, stimulants, and emotional disturbance. It is decreased by fasting (not eating), rest, depressants (drugs that slow down body functions), and hemorrhage (loss of blood). In resting adults, any reading between 60 and 90 diastolic is considered normal. Blood pressure rises slightly with age. High blood pressure (greater than 140/90) is called *hypertension*. Low blood pressure (below 100/70) is called *hypotension*. Hypertension can lead to a stroke. Hypotension can lead to shock. In either case, unusual or changed findings must be reported.

Equipment The sphygmomanometer consists of a cuff with a rubber bladder inside and two tubes. One tube is connected to a pressure control bulb and the other to a pressure gauge. The gauge may be a round dial or a column of mercury, figure 31-17. Both are marked with numbers. Be sure to use a cuff of the proper size. Cuffs that are too wide or too narrow will give inaccurate readings.

The gauges are marked with a series of large lines at 10-mm (millimeter) intervals. In between the large lines are shorter lines. Each indicates 2 mm. For example, the small line above 80 mm marks 82 mm. The small line below 80 mm marks 78 mm. The gauge should be at eye level when reading it. The mercury column gauge must not be tilted. The top of the mercury column is the reading.

PROCEDURE 72

Determining Blood Pressure

1. Wash hands and collect the following equipment:

   sphygmomanometer
   stethoscope (clean earpieces with antiseptic solution)

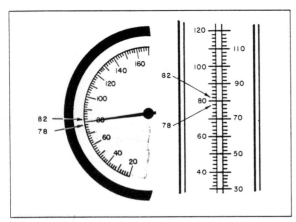

Figure 31-17 Two common sphygmomanometer gauges: aneroid (left) and mercury gravity (right). (From Caldwell & Hegner, *Nursing Assistant, A Nursing Process Approach*, copyright 1988 by Delmar Publishers Inc.)

2. Identify patient and explain what you plan to do.
3. Place the patient's arm palm upward and support it on bed or table. The same arm should be used for all readings.
4. Roll patient's sleeve up about 5 inches above elbow. Be sure it is not tight on the arm.
5. Apply the cuff above the elbow and directly over the brachial artery. The brachial artery is on the inside of the arm just above the elbow.
6. Wrap the rest of the armband smoothly around the arm. Tuck the ends under a fold, hook, or simply press if Velcro is used to secure. Be sure cuff is secure but not too tight.
7. Place stethoscope earpieces in ears. Locate the brachial artery with the fingers. Place stethoscope head directly over the artery.
8. Close valve attached to hand pump (air bulb) and inflate cuff until indicator registers 20 mm above where pulse ceases to be heard.
9. Open valve of pump and let air escape slowly until the first sound is heard.
10. At this first sound, note reading on manometer, figure 31-18. This is the systolic pressure.
11. Continue to release the air pressure slowly until there is an abrupt change in the sound from very loud to soft. The reading at which this change is heard is the diastolic pressure. (In some hospitals the last sound heard is taken as diastolic pressure.) If a repeat procedure is necessary, completely deflate the cuff, wait 1 minutes, and begin again.
12. Remove cuff, expel air, and replace apparatus. Clean earpieces of stethoscope with antiseptic solution.
13. Record time and blood pressure. The blood pressure is recorded as an inverted fraction. For example, in 120/80, 120 is the systolic pressure and 80 is the diastolic pressure. Remember, the pulse pres-

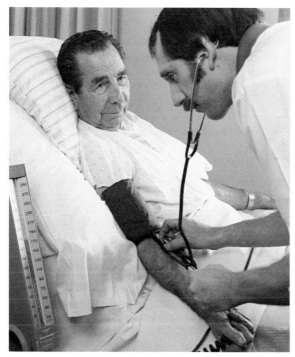

Figure 31-18 As you listen, note the level of the mercury column when you hear the first regular beat and the point at which the sound becomes muffled. (From Hegner & Caldwell, *Assisting in Long-Term Care,* copyright 1988 by Delmar Publishers Inc.)

sure is the difference between the systolic and diastolic pressures. In this example, it is 40.

Intake and Output

An accurate recording of intake and output (I & O) is basic to the care of many patients. A knowledge of measurement is essential in performing this procedure. Most of the scientific work in the United States is done with the *metric system.* Medical facilities generally use the metric system to measure fluids.

The containers used in hospitals for measuring fluids such as urine are marked in metric units. Cubic centimeters (cc) or milliliters (ml) are the units of fluid measurement in the metric system, figure 31-19. One cubic centimeter

U.S. Customary Units	Metric Units
1 minim	0.06 milliliter (ml)
16 minims	1 ml
1 ounce	30 ml
1 pint	500 ml
1 quart	1000 ml (1 liter)
2.2 pounds	1 kilogram
1 inch	2.5 centimeters (cm)
1 foot	30 cm

Figure 31-19 Comparison of U.S. customary and metric measurements. (From Caldwell & Hegner, *Nursing Assistant, A Nursing Process Approach,* copyright 1989 by Delmar Publishers Inc.)

equals one milliliter. There are approximately fifteen drops of fluid in one milliliter. For the purposes of general measurement, a drop is approximately a minim.

Food containers used in facilities are fairly standardized as to volume, or amount of fluid they hold, figure 31-20. Many facilities have a printed record on the top of I & O sheets as a reminder. Learn the fluid content of the containers used at your facility.

Coffee/tea cup, 8 oz	240 ml
Water carafe, 16 oz	480 ml
Foam cup, 8 oz	240 ml
Water glass, 8 oz	240 ml
Soup bowl, 6 oz	180 ml
Jello, 1 serving	120 ml
Ice chips, full 4 oz glass	120 ml

Figure 31-20 Approximate liquid amounts of common containers and servings (30 ml equals one ounce).

PROCEDURE 73

Recording Intake

1. Wash hands and assemble the following equipment:

   intake and output record at bedside
   pen
   graduated pitcher

2. Identify the patient and explain what you plan to do. Explain that the patient can help by recording the amount of fluid he or she takes by mouth.

3. Record intake on the I & O record at the bedside. How it is taken should also be recorded. Intake includes the amount of liquid taken with meals. This includes anything liquid at room temperature such as ice cream or jello, water and other liquids taken between meals, and all other fluids given by mouth, intravenously, or by tube feeding.

4. Copy information onto the chart from the bedside I & O record according to hospital policy. Remember, I & O are recorded in milliliters (ml). Total is recorded at the end of each shift and at the end of twenty-four hours.

PROCEDURE 74

Recording Output

1. Save urine specimen if one has been ordered and take it to utility room or resident's bathroom.

2. Pour urine from bedpan or urinal into graduate. Measure amount, figure 31-21.

3. Record amount immediately under output column on bedside I & O record. All liquid output should be recorded. Output includes urine, vomitus, drainage from wound or stomach, liquid stool, blood loss, and perspiration.

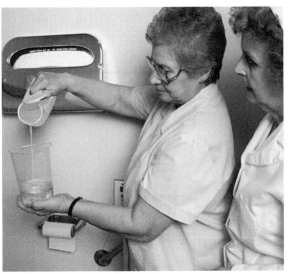

Figure 31-21 Urine can be poured into a graduate for measuring or into a specimen container to go to the lab before discarding the remainder. Do not spill the urine on your hands or over the container. (From Hegner & Caldwell, *Assisting in Long-Term Care,* (copyright 1988 by Delmar Publishers Inc.)

4. Empty urine into bedpan hopper. If specimen is accidentally lost, estimate amount and make notation that it is an estimate.

5. Rinse graduate with cold water. Clean according to facility policy.

6. Clean bedpan or urinal and return to proper place according to facility policy.

7. Wash hands.

8. Copy information onto chart from I & O record according to facility policy. Perspiration and blood loss may be described as little, moderate, or excessive.

Collecting Specimens

Samples of body fluids, such as urine, are frequently collected and tested. This may occur during the admission procedure or any time during the resident's stay. Because body fluids may be infectious, some facilities now require those collecting and handling any body fluids (excretions or secretions) to wear disposable gloves while doing so. Acute care facilities such as hospitals often have strict regulations about the use of barriers such as disposable gloves. Each health care provide must know and follow the procedures recommended by the facility.

For this reason, when carrying out any procedure involving body fluids such as genital secretions, urine, or sputum, check your facility policy regarding the use of disposable gloves. The same precautions should be followed when handling *exudate* (drainage) from infections or *excreta* (intestinal) discharge. Whether or not gloves are used, avoid exposure to the fluids or discharge and always wash your hands carefully.

Hot and Cold Applications

Hot or cold applications may be ordered. These treatments are used to relieve pain, combat local infection, check bleeding (hemorrhage), and reduce body temperature.

Local applications of hot and cold are made with ice bags or hot water bags applied to a small area of the body. Standard ice bags are being replaced in many areas by the electronically operated Aquamatic K-Pad, figure 31-22. K-Pads are available in many shapes and sizes. They can be used to apply dry heat and, by using an attachment, for cooling. Prepackaged, single-use units for the application of hot and cold are now available. A single blow to the surface activates the contents, providing a controlled temperature.

General treatments of hot and cold consist of special baths such as alcohol sponge baths. The alcohol sponge bath is used to reduce an elevated temperature. Thermal mattresses (hypothermia blankets) are also widely used for this purpose. Hot and cold applications are used only on written orders of the doctor.

Types of Heat and Cold

There are two kinds of heat and cold: dry and moist. Dry heat is produced by the use of hot

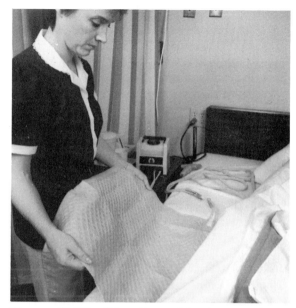

Figure 31-22 The disposable Aquamatic K-Pad® and control unit maintain an even temperature. (From Caldwell & Hegner, *Nursing Assistant, A Nursing Process Approach,* copyright 1989 by Delmar Publishers Inc.)

water bags, electric heating pads, and heat lamps. Dry cold is provided by ice bags, ice caps, and ice collars. Moist hot and cold applications are more penetrating than dry types. Wet compresses, soaks, and packs provide moist heat or cold depending on the temperature of the moisture. Moisture intensifies the application of heat, so extra care must be taken.

Body Response

Cold causes blood vessels to constrict or become smaller *(vasoconstriction)*. Intense cold numbs the sensation of pain. It also slows all life processes, including inflammation. Therefore, it reduces inflammation and itching. Heat *(diathermy)* has the opposite effect. It makes blood vessels larger *(vasodilation)* and increases the blood supply to the area. The additional blood supply promotes healing and can be soothing.

Cautions

Extreme care is mandatory when cold or hot applications are used on the aged, especially if the patient is uncooperative or unconscious. An electric heating pad must not be used with moist dressings unless a rubber cover is placed over the pad. If the wires should become damp, a short circuit would result. The patient must not lie on the pad; severe burns can result. Sensitivity to heat varies, so patients receiving heat treatments must be checked frequently.

Heat cradles are sometimes used to stimulate circulation in the legs and feet. A bed cradle is equipped with ordinary 25-watt light bulbs, placed 3 feet from the area to be treated to provide continuous dry heat. The bulbs are hung under the top of the cradle and encased in wire frames to avoid contact with the patient. The length of treatment is always specified. Other lamp treatments, such as infrared and ultraviolet, are given by experts because of the danger involved with their penetrating heat.

PROCEDURE 75

Applying Ice Bag

1. Wash hands and assemble the following equipment in the utility room:

   ice bag or collar
   spoon or similar utensil
   cover (usually muslin)
   ice cubes or crushed ice
   paper towels

2. If ice cubes are used, rinse them in water to remove sharp edges.
3. Fill ice bag half full, using ice scoop or large spoon. Avoid making ice bags too heavy.
4. Expel air by resting ice bag on table in horizontal position with top in place but not screwed on. Squeeze the bag until air has been removed.
5. Fasten top securely.
6. Test for leakage.

7. Wipe dry with paper towels.
8. Place muslin cover on ice bag. Never permit rubber or plastic to touch patient's skin.
9. Take equipment to bedside on tray.
10. Identify resident and explain what you plan to do.
11. Apply ice bag to the affected part with metal away from patient.
12. Refill bag before all ice is melted.
13. Record the procedure on the patient's chart.
14. Check skin area with each application. Report to supervising nurse immediately if skin is discolored or white or if patient reports that skin is numb.
15. When ice bag is removed after use, wash with soap and water, drain, and screw top on. Leave air in ice bag to prevent sides from sticking together.
16. If a reusable cold pack is used, wash thoroughly with soap and water and return it to the refrigerator. Discard a disposable pack.

PROCEDURE 76

Applying Hot Water Bag

1. Wash hands and assemble the following equipment in the utility room:

hot water bag	cover
container for hot	thermometer
water	paper towels

2. Fill container with water and test for correct temperature, which should be approximately 115°F unless otherwise ordered.
3. Fill hot water bag one-third to one-half full to avoid unnecessary weight.
4. Expel air by placing hot water bag horizontally on flat surface, holding neck of bag upright until water reaches neck. Close the top when all air has been expelled.

5. Wipe bag dry with paper towels and turn upside down to check for leakage.
6. Place cover on hot water bag so that resident's skin does not come in contact with rubber or plastic.
7. Take equipment to bedside on tray. Identify resident and explain what you plan to do.
8. Apply hot water bag to the affected area as ordered. Never allow patient to lie on the hot water bag.
9. Check the patient's condition at intervals.
10. Clean and replace equipment according to policy. Place cover in laundry hamper.
11. Repeat procedure as necessary. Check condition of skin with each reapplication. Report any unusual observations immediately to supervising nurse.
12. Record the procedure on the resident's chart.

PROCEDURE 77

Applying Aquamatic K-Pad

1. Wash hands and assemble the following equipment:

    K-Pad and control unit
    covering for pad
    distilled water

2. Identify resident and explain what you plan to do.
3. Place the control unit on the bedside stand.
4. Remove the cover and fill the unit with distilled water to the fill line.
5. Screw the cover in place and loosen it one-quarter turn.
6. Cover the pad and place it on the patient. Be sure that the tubing is coiled on the bed to facilitate the flow. Do not allow it to hang below the level of the bed.
7. Turn on the unit. The temperature, usually 95° to 100°F, is set by a key that is removed after setting.

8. Record the procedure on the resident's chart.

PROCEDURE 78

Giving Cooling Bath (Alcohol Sponge Bath)

1. Wash hands and assemble the following equipment:

2 bath towels	5 covered ice bags,
2 bath blankets	filled
1 washcloth	covered, filled hot
basin of tap water	water bottle
(ice cubes if	alcohol (70%)
ordered)	

2. Identify resident and explain what you plan to do.
3. Screen unit for privacy and to prevent drafts.
4. Take the patient's temperature.
5. Cover the patient with a bath blanket. Remove gown. Fanfold top bedding to foot of bed.
6. Position bath blanket under the patient.
7. Add alcohol to water. The temperature should be about 70°F.
8. Apply ice bag to head.
9. Apply hot water bag to feet, groin, and axilla.
10. Sponge with washcloth. Expose only one area at a time. Cover and allow to air dry. Sponge strokes should be in direction of heart. Continue procedure for approximately 20 minutes.
11. Bathe entire body. Avoid the eyes and genitals.
12. Replace gown and top bedding. Remove bath blankets and discard.
13. Clean equipment according to hospital policy.
14. Take vital signs 10 minutes after sponge bath. Procedure may be repeated if temperature is still elevated.

15. Report and record cooling bath, vital signs at beginning and termination of procedure, and resident's response.

Documentation

Most of your observations will be recorded, figure 31-23, either by you or by the person to whom you report. Your observations must be accurate.

Keeping the patient's chart or legal record may or may not be part of your responsibility. If charting is your responsibility, follow these guidelines:

- Chart on the proper form and resident chart.
- Use the correct color of ink.
- Be objective, brief, and legible; spell accurately.
- Date each entry.
- Never erase an entry. If an entry is in error, draw a single line through it, print "error," and initial.
- Sign each entry with your first initial, last name, and job title.

Remember, the resident's record is a legal and confidential document.

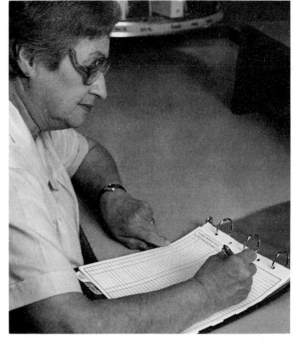

Figure 31-23 Make sure your observations and actions are documented carefully.

Summary

- Skills basic to nursing care are outlined and explained in this unit. Everyone giving care must be proficient in these skills.

- These skills include care of the environment; bedmaking; taking vital signs; admitting, discharging, and transferring residents; and making and recording observations.
- Exact procedures may differ from facility to facility and may need to be adjusted to meet varying resident conditions, but the principles remain constant.

Review Outline

    I. Behavioral Objectives

   II. Vocabulary

 III. Procedure Reminders

     A. Carried out in relation to each procedure
     B. Beginning procedure actions
     C. Procedure completion actions

IV. Special Basic Procedures

    A   Beds and bedmaking
        1. Types of beds
        2. The unoccupied bed
        3. The occupied bed
    B.   Admitting a resident
    C.   Discharging or transferring a resident
    D.   Weighing and measuring a resident
    E.   Vital signs
        1. Temperature determination
        2. Pulse counting
        3. Respiration counting
        4. Blood pressure determination
    F.   Measuring intake and output
    G.   Hot and cold applications
        1. Types of heat and cold
        2. Body responses
        3. Cautions
            a. Icebags
            b. Aquamatic K-Pads
            c. Cooling sponge bath
    H.   Collecting specimens
    I.   Documentation

Review

I. Vocabulary

Locate the terms that are defined by placing a circle around them.

```
A  N  O  X  R  A  L  E  S  O  J  Q  T  D  Q  U  F  N  K  V  A
L  Q  E  T  W  U  R  P  V  B  V  D  S  D  S  I  W  C  P  Z  O
I  B  D  G  S  T  S  F  M  F  S  M  H  T  T  R  M  Z  V  D  T
K  W  Q  T  U  O  H  K  U  S  E  E  O  Y  E  R  A  S  X  G  E
P  E  P  S  G  C  P  B  Y  A  Q  C  R  T  T  N  Q  E  S  U  O
D  S  R  C  S  L  U  Y  H  T  G  L  E  W  H  J  G  L  M  O  C
L  A  O  T  W  A  E  T  D  L  P  M  Y  S  O  S  C  I  X  I  W
H  R  T  F  X  Y  J  V  O  K  O  V  B  F  S  V  O  W  R  T  K
N  U  H  Y  P  E  R  T  E  N  S  I  O  N  C  D  U  E  O  J  P
M  I  E  X  D  M  I  N  A  J  A  S  I  P  O  S  T  R  A  B  Y
Y  O  S  B  T  G  V  M  P  E  R  C  L  K  P  N  F  E  P  L  E
C  R  I  H  Y  P  O  T  E  N  S  I  O  N  E  P  S  X  T  G  M
U  P  S  Q  P  M  R  A  Y  F  N  C  Q  K  U  I  N  U  A  V  H
R  A  M  L  G  T  I  R  M  D  L  L  Y  F  W  C  T  D  R  T  C
N  O  X  Y  Y  G  T  T  A  C  H  Y  C  A  R  D  I  A  Q  L  S
J  Y  H  Z  O  U  B  W  E  Q  N  N  R  O  X  J  Y  T  X  F  P
S  P  K  T  E  P  K  L  T  R  A  N  S  F  E  R  S  E  Y  W  K
S  M  W  B  E  Q  I  Y  C  R  Z  F  X  T  L  W  M  H  F  N  C
```

1. Instrument used to measure blood pressure
2. Instrument used to hear body sounds
3. Elevated blood pressure
4. Procedure when a resident moves from one facility to another
5. Solid body wastes
6. Triangular corner made with bed linen
7. Rapid pulse rate
8. Low blood pressure
9. Pertaining to the intestinal tract
10. Drainage or discharge
11. Artificial part
12. Moist respiration sounds

II. True or False

1. In an extended care facility, linens are usually changed once a week.
2. Pillowcases are changed every day in extended care facilities.
3. All beds used for nursing care break in the middle so patients may sit up.
4. I.V. lines or catheters should be attached to side rails.
5. Making a bed with a person in it is known as making an occupied bed.
6. One side of a bed is made at a time.
7. A rectal thermometer may safely be used in the same resident's mouth.
8. If the mercury falls between two lines, it should be read at the next lowest number.
9. A person whose height is 62 inches might also be described as being 6 feet 2 inches.
10. The equipment needed to determine blood pressure is the sphygmomanometer and the stethoscope.

III. Short Answers

1. Explain how a resident's weight of 160 pounds is expressed in kilograms.
2. Explain how you may use your senses in making observations of the resident.

IV. Clinical Situations

1. You are admitting a resident and she insists on keeping a ring with a very large stone on her finger. What do you do?
2. The resident has just been given a cooling bath to reduce his temperature. How long should you wait before taking the temperature?
3. Make the conversions from U.S. customary units to metric units or metric units to U.S. customary units as indicated.

U.S. Customary Units	Metric Units
a. 32 minims	_____
b. 3 ounces	_____
c. _____	2,000 ml
d. _____	165 centimeters
e. 160 pounds	_____
f. _____	79 kilograms

4.   Total the input and output for the following record.

7:30 A.M.	urine	500 ml
8:00 A.M.	grape juice	90 ml
	milk	120 ml
9:30 A.M.	water	180 ml
	coffee	120 ml
	soup	180 ml
1:00 P.M.	urine	500 ml
1:15 P.M.	water	90 ml
3:00 P.M.	orange juice	120 ml
3:15 P.M.	vomitus	120 ml
4:20 P.M.	tea	120 ml
	milk	60 ml
5:30 P.M.	urine	400 ml
6:00 P.M.	water	150 ml
9:00 P.M.	ginger ale	150 ml
9:30 P.M.	urine	300 ml
10:00 P.M.	water	90 ml

Glossary

INTRODUCTION

A glossary is a tool for understanding. The Spanish language translation of glossary terms was carried out by a Central American, Chilean, and North American translation team organized by World Education, Inc. The most difficult part of the team's work was to accurately translate English-language acronyms—the many abbreviations in English that have themselves become words. Wherever it makes sense to Spanish-speakers, an English language acronym such as AIDS is translated with a Spanish-language acronym such as SIDA. Unfortunately, only a few of the English-language acronyms also have widely used acronyms in Spanish.

Since so many of the English-language acronyms and abbreviations in this glossary do not have an acronym form in Spanish that is widely recognizable to Spanish-speakers, the team has provided a literal translation. For example, the English-language acronym CVP (central venous pressure) is translated as presión venosa central rather than as PVC.

Introducción

Un glosario es un instrumento para una mejor comprensión. La traducción al Castellano fué llevada a cabo por un equipo de traductores de Centro-América, Chile y Norte-América organizados por World Education, Inc. La parte más dificil del trabajo ha sido la traducción precisa de las siglas en Inglés—siglas en Inglés, significativas a hispano-parlantes, como AIDS, fueron directamente traducidas al Castellano como SIDA. Desafortunadamente solo algunas siglas en Inglés tienen su correspondiente en Castellano. Puesto que muchas de las siglas y abreviaciones en Inglés en éste glosario no tienen equivalente, el equipo ha optado por una traducción literal de aquellas. Por ejemplo, las siglas en Inglés CVP (central venous pressure) fueron traducidas como "presión venosa central" en lugar de PVC.

A.A.R.P. (Asociación Americana de personas jubiladas) — American Association of Retired Persons

abduction (abducción) — movement away from midline or center

abuse (abuso) — to maltreat or abuse

acceptance (aceptación) — state of grieving when a person with a terminal diagnosis comes to terms with the inevitable

achlorhydria (aclorhidria) — lack of hydrochloric acid

acidosis (acidosis) — pathologic condition resulting from accumulation of acid or depletion of the alkaline reserve in the blood and body tissues

activities of daily living (actividades de la vida diaria) — the activities that help patients fulfill their basic human needs

adduction (aducción) — movement toward midline or center

A.D.E.A. (leyes en contra de la discriminación por edad) — Age/Discrimination in Employment Act

A.D.L. (actividades de la vida diaria) — activities of daily living

agar (agar) — gelatinous substance sometimes used to increase intestinal bulk

aged (envejecido) — old; usually refers to those over seventy-five years of age

ageing (envejecimiento) — natural, progressive process that begins at birth

ageism (discriminación basada en la edad) — discrimination based on age

aiding and abetting (ayudar y encubrir) — observing someone committing a crime, and not reporting it

A.I.D.S. (SIDA) — acquired immune deficiency syndrome; viral infection that suppresses the immune system, leaving the patient vulnerable to opportunistic infections that often cause death

air compressor (compresor de aire) — machine used to deliver aerosol medication and moisture

aldosterone (aldosterona) — electrolyte-regulating hormone of the adrenal cortex

alert (alerta) — mentally responsive

alignment (alineación) — proper position

ambivalence (ambivalencia) — opposing feelings being experienced at the same time, for example wanting to be independent and still wanting to feel taken care of

anabolism (anabolismo) — process by which the body converts nutritional substances into living matter

anemia (anemia) — deficiency of quality or quantity of red blood cells

anesthesia (anestesia) — loss of feeling or sensation

aneurysm (aneurisma) — blood-filled sac formed by dilatation of the walls of a blood vessel, usually an artery

anger (enojo) — state of grieving when a patient is no longer able to deny awareness of a terminal diagnosis and exhibits feelings of frustration

A.N.S. (SNA, sistema nervioso autónomo) — autonomic nervous system; portion of nervous system that controls visceral activity

anus (ano) — outlet of the rectum lying in the fold between the nates

aphasia (afasia) — language impairment

A.R.C. (complejo relacionado al SIDA) — AIDS-related complex

arteriosclerosis (arterosclerosis) — narrowing of the blood vessels that can result in subsequent tissue hypoxia

artery (arteria) — vessel through which the blood passes away from the heart to various parts of the body

arthritis (artritis) — joint inflammation

ascites (ascitis) — fluid accumulation in the abdomen

aspiration (aspirar) — drawing of foreign material into the respiratory tract

assault (asalto/agresión) — attempt or threaten to do violence to another

assessment (evaluación) — judgment about information related to a problem

asthenia (astenia) — weakness

asthma (asma) — chronic respiratory disease characterized by bronchospasms and excessive mucus production

ataractic (ataractic) — drug that has a tranquilizing effect

atherosclerosis (aterosclerosis) — hardening of the inner coat of blood vessels

atrium (cavidad/cámara) — chamber on either side of the heart

atrophy (atrofia) — shrinking or wasting away of tissues

autoclave (autoclave) — machine that steam sterilizes articles

autoimmune reactions (reacciones de autoinmunidad) — destructive reactions against the body's own healthy cells

B.A.D.L. (actividades básicas de la vida diaria) — basic (personal) activities of daily living

bargaining (negociar/concertar) — state of grieving when a patient with a terminal diagnosis attempts to find ways to prolong his or her life

bath itch (salpullido) — condition that affects the less oily, elderly skin; characterized by tiny, red eruptions and itching

battery (agresión) — unlawful attack on another person

bile (bilis) — secretion of the liver which aids in digesting fats

bisexuality (bisexualidad) — desiring sexual intimacy with both sexes

bradycardia (bradicardia) — unusually slow heartbeat

call bell (timbre) — signal device

capillary (capilar) — hairlike blood vessel

carbohydrate (carbohidrato) — energy food used by the body to produce heat; essential nutrient

carbonic anhydrase inhibitors (inhibidores de la anhidridaza carbónica) — drugs used to decrease production of the aqueous fluid by the carbonic anhydrate enzyme

cardiac cycle (ciclo cardiaco) — all the (mechanical and electrical) events that occur between one heart contraction and the next

catabolism (catabolismo) — opposite of anabolism; process by which complex substances are broken into simpler substances

cataract (catarata) — opacity of the lens resulting in loss of vision

celibacy (celibato) — abstaining from sexual intercourse

cellulose (celulosa) — carbohydrate foods that supply the body with roughage

census (censo) — survey taken every ten years to gather information about the population

cerebrospinal fluid (fluido cerebroespinal) — blood filtrate that acts as a hydrostatic cushion and tissue fluid for the central nervous system

chancre (chancro) — primary lesion of syphilis

chart (archivo) — record of information concerning a patient

chemical restraint (restricción química) — the use of drugs to control the behavior or actions of a person

chlamydia (clamidia) — organism that causes infections of the reproductive system

choroid (coroides) — vascular (nutritive) layer of the eye

chronic bronchitis (bronquitis crónica) — condition in which there is excessive mucus secretion in the bronchi

chyme (quimo) — semiliquid form of food as it leaves the stomach

claudication (claudicación) — increased pain in the legs with exercise associated with peripheral vascular disease

client (cliente) — another term for patient

climacteric (climaterio) — menopause or "change of life"

clinical nurse specialist (enfermera especialista) — advanced nurse practitioner who has further education and clinical preparation in the care of elders, sick and well

C.N.S. (sistema nervioso central) — central nervous system; consists of the brain and spinal cord

cochlea (cóclea) — portion of the inner ear that receives and then transmits sound waves to the brain

coitus (coito) — genital sexual union between male and female

cold (catarro/resfriado) — acute and highly contagious viral infection of the upper respiratory tract

colon (colon) — another name for the large intestine

colostomy (colostomía) — artificial opening in the abdomen for the purpose of evacuation

coma (coma) — state of profound unconsciousness from which the patient cannot be aroused, even by powerful stimuli

comatose (comatoso/a) — in a coma; unconscious

communicable (transmisible) — transmissible from person to person, such as from an infectious disease

communication (comunicación) — passage of a message from a sender to a receiver

compensation (compensación) — defense mechanism in which abilities in one area are used to make up for disabilities in another

concentration (concentración) — increase in the amount of dissolved substances in a liquid

condominiums (condominio) — privately owned apartments in which all residents share the cost of the upkeep of communal areas

cones (conos) — photo receptor cells of the retina; receptors for daylight and color vision

confidential (confidencial) — keeping what is said or written to oneself

confidentiality (confidencialidad) — maintaining privacy

confusion (confusión) — disturbed orientation concerning time, place, or person; sometimes accompanied by disoriented consciousness

congregate (congregar) — to group

conjunctiva (conjuntiva) — membrane that lines the eyelids and covers the eye

constipation (constipación) — a condition in which the solid wastes are too hard to pass easily

constrict (estrechar/apretar) — to make narrow by squeezing

contagious (contagioso) — disease that is easily and directly communicable from person to person

contaminated (contaminado) — unclean; carrying germs

contractures (contracturas) — permanent contractions of a muscle due to spasm or paralysis

convalescent home (casa para convalescientes) — a long-term care facility

C.O.P.D. (enfermedad pulmonar obstructiva crónica) — chronic obstructive pulmonary disease

cordotomy (cordotomía) — destruction of a nerve tract to relieve intractable pain

cor pulmonale (mal cardio-pulmonar) — serious cardiac condition resulting from pulmonary involvement

cortex (corteza) — outer portion of the cerebrum and cerebellum, kidneys, or adrenal glands

crepitation (crepitación) — dry, crackling sound or sensation, such as that produced by the grating of the ends of a fractured bone

criterion (criterio/norma) — standard against which actions may be measured

cryoprobe (criosonda) — instrument used in cryosurgery

cryosurgery (criocirugía) — destruction of tissue by the application of extreme cold

cunnilingus (cunilingüo) — oral sexual stimulation

C.V.A. (accidente cerebrovascular) — cerebrovascular accident

C.V.P. (presión venosa central) — central venous pressure; blood pressure in the large central veins

cyanosis (cianosis) — bluish skin discoloration from lack of oxygen

cyclopedic (ciclopedic) — drug that paralyzes the ciliary structure of the eye

cystocele (cistocele) — bladder hernia

cystometrogram (cistograma) — record made by filling the bladder slowly to rate its capacity and to measure uninhibited bladder contractions

cystoscopy (cistoscopía) — visualization of the bladder

day center (centro de servicios para ancianos) — place where elders may go to receive various services

debridement (desbridamiento) — removal of all devitalized tissue

decaliter (decalitro) — 10 liters (2.64 gallons)

decompensation (descompensación) — inability of the heart to maintain adequate circulation

decubitus (decúbito) — pressure sore

decubitus ulcer (úlcera decúbita) — bedsore or pressure sore

defamation (difamación) — act of casting aspersions on the good name or reputation of a person

defecation (defecar) — bowel movement

defense mechanism (mecanismo de defensa) — technique used to protect self-esteem

delirium (delirio) — mental condition in which the patient's speech is incoherent and illusions, delusions, and hallucinations are experienced

delusion (delirio) — false belief

dementia (demensia) — progressive mental deterioration due to organic disease of the brain

demographics (demográfico) — information of a statistical nature

denial (negación/rechazo) — a defense mechanism in which reality is rejected

density (densidad) — the compactness of a substance

depression (depresión) — feelings of sadness; one of the stages of grieving

dermal ulcer (úlceras dérmicas) — decubitus ulcer or bedsore

dermatitis (dermatitis) — inflammation of the skin

developmental tasks (tareas/estados del desarrollo) — stages to be mastered in the development of the personality

diagnostic category (diagnóstico) — patient problem

dialysis (diálisis) — separating substances by passing them through a membrane

diaphoresis (diaforesis) — profuse sweating

diarrhea (diarrea) — loose, watery stool

diastolic (diastólico) — relaxation phase of the cardiac cycle; blood pressure reading taken when pressure is lowest, between contractions

diathermy (diatermia) — extreme heat

digiti flexis (flexión dactilar) — hammertoes, a condition in which toes are drawn into a tightly flexed position

dilate (dilatar) — to get bigger, as in capillaries

dilemma (dilema) — situation involving choice between equally unsatisfactory choices

directive (tipo de testamento/mandato) — type of living will

disability (incapacidad) — physical or mental restriction or disadvantage

disorder, psychological (trastorno psicológico) — formerly called neurosis

disorientation (desorientación) — loss of recognition of time, place or person

displacement (desplazamiento/sustitución) — defense mechanism in which an emotion is shifted from its real cause to some more acceptable one

disposable (desechable) — not reusable

diuretics (diuréticos) — drugs that increase urine output

diverticulitis (diverticulitis) — inflammation of diverticuli, small blind pouches that form in the lining and wall of the colon

D.K.A. (diabetes acetoacidosica) — diabetic ketoacidosis

dorsiflexion (flexión dorsal) — toes pointed toward the knee

D.R.G. (diagnóstico de grupos) — diagnosis related grouping

dyspareunia (dispareunia) — painful intercourse

dyspepsia (dispepsia) — indigestion

dysphagia (disfagia) — difficulty in swallowing

dyspnea (disnea) — difficult or labored breathing

ectropion (ectropión) — eversion of an eyelid

edema (edema) — excessive accumulation of fluid in tissues

ejaculate (eyacular) — forcefully expelling the semen

ejaculation (eyaculación) — forcible, sudden expulsion of semen from the male urethra

electrocoagulation (electrocoagulación) — process by which unhealthy tissues are destroyed through high-frequency electrical impulses

elimination (eliminación) — discharge from the body of indigestible materials and of waste products of body metabolism; excretion

empathy (empatía) — being able to put oneself in another's place

enteric (entérico) — pertaining to the alimentary canal; intestinal

entropion (entropión) — inversion of an eyelid

enzymes (enzimas) — organic catalysts produced by living cells but capable of acting independently of the cells that produce them

epidermis (epidermis) — top layer of skin

erection (erección) — process of becoming upright and turgid

E.R.I.P. (Plan incentivo de jubilación prematura) — Early Retirement Incentive Plan

E.R.I.S.A. (Ley de Seguridad de Salario para Empleados Jubilados) — Employee Retirement Income Security Act

erotic (erótico) — sexual

erythrocyte (eritrocito) — red blood cell

ethics (ética) — rules of moral or responsible conduct

eustachian tube (trompa de Eustaquio) — one of two small tubes leading from the nasopharynx to the middle ear; carries air to equalize pressure on either side of the tympanic membrane (eardrum)

euthanasia (eutanasia) — easy death; mercy killing

evaluation (evaluación) — comparison of a situation against an accepted standard

expiration (expirar) — expulsion of air or other vapor from the lungs

extended care facility (establecimiento para cuidado a largo plazo) — long-term care facility

extension (extensión) — two ends of any jointed part moving away from each other; to increase the angle between two bones

exteroceptor (exteroceptor) — sense organ such as the eye that receives stimuli from outside the body

extremism (extremismo) — quality or state of being extreme; radicalism

false imprisonment (encarcelamiento ilegal) — unlawfully restraining another

fat (lipidos/grasa) — energy food used by the body to produce heat; essential nutrient

feces (heces) — stool eliminated from the bowel

fibers (nerve) (fibras nerviosas) — axons or dendrites of the neuron

F.I.C.A. (Ley de Contribuciones al Seguro Social Federal) — Federal Insurance Contributions Act (Social Security Tax)

flatus (flatus/flatulencia) — gas or air in the stomach or intestine

flexion (flexión) — decreasing the angle between two bones

flow rate (razón o tasa de flujo, flujo) — rate at which a fluid moves

fomites (fomes/fomites) — objects that contain germs

forced fluids (alimentación forzada de líquidos) — encouraging the patient to take as much fluid as possible

Foster Grandparents (Abuelos Adoptivos) — federal program that recruits, trains, and employs persons over sixty years of age to work with neglected, deprived, and mentally retarded children

gallbladder (vesícula biliar) — small, saclike organ on the underside of the liver

gastritis (gastritis) — inflammation of the stomach

gastrostomy tube (tubo gastrastómico) — tube inserted through the abdominal wall directly into the stomach

gavage (alimentación por sonda) — tube feeding

gay men (homosexual) — homosexual males

genitals (genitales) — sexual organs

geriatric care technician (técnico de cuidado geriatra) — geriatric nursing assistant; one who assists, under supervision, in the care of the elderly

geriatrician (geriatra) — specialist concerned with old age and its diseases

geriatrics (geriatría) — care of the elderly

geri chair (silla geriatra para ancianos) — chair with a table or tray affixed

germs (gérmenes) — organisms capable of causing infection

gerontology (gerontología) — study of the aging process

glaucoma (glaucoma) — increased intraocular pressure that ultimately results in loss of vision

gonorrhea (gonorrea) — sexually transmitted disease (infection) caused by a bacterium

gossip (chisme) — to talk about patients or coworkers

Gray panthers (Panteras Grises, movimiento de reformas para proteger a los ancianos) — movement for urgent reforms needed to protect the elderly

gustatory (gustativo) — pertaining to the sense of taste

hallucination (alucinación) — idea or perception not based on reality

hallux valgus (hallux valgus/juanete) — bunion

health care provider (trabajadores al servicio de la salud) — one who assists in the health care of the elderly

heloma (heloma/callosidad) — corns

hemiparalysis (hemiparálisis) — paralysis of one side of the body

hemiparesis (hemiparesis) — paralysis affecting one side of the body

hemiplegia (hemiplegia) — paralysis of one side of the body

hemodialysis (hemodiálisis) — removal of certain elements from the blood by diffusion through a membrane

hemoptysis (hemóptisis) — expectoration of blood

Heberden's Nodes (Nódulos de Haberden) — swelling of distal nodes of interphalangeal joints

hernia (hernia) — protrusion of an organ or part of an organ through the wall of the cavity that normally contains it

herniation (herniación) — protrusion of an organ out of its normal location

herniorrhaphy (herniotomía/quelotomía) — surgical operation for hernia

heterosexual (heterosexual) — male or female who prefers sexual intimacy with the opposite sex

H.H.N.C. (coma hiperglicémica hiperosmolar no cetósica) — hyperglycemic, hyperosmolar, nonketotic coma

H.I.V. (Virus de inmunodeficiencia) — human immune virus; cause of A.I.D.S.

home health services (servicios de salud a domicilio) — help provided to the chronically homebound and to convalescents in their homes after an acute hospitalization

homophobia (homofobia) — irrational fear of homosexuals

homosexual (homosexual) — male or female who prefers sexual interaction with members of his or her own sex

hospice (hospicio) — special facility that provides care for the terminally ill

hydrochloric acid (ácido clorhídrico) — an aqueous solution of 35 to 38 percent hydrogen chloride (HCl)

hygiene (higiene) — system of rules designed to promote health

hyperalimentation (hiperalimentación) — technique of providing nutrition directly into a large vein

hyperchlorhydria (hiperclorhidria) — excessive amount of hydrochloric acid in the stomach

hyperglycemia (hiperglicemia) — excessive levels of sugar in the blood

hyperkalemia (hiperalcalemia) — excessive levels of potassium in the blood

hyperopia (hiperopía) — farsightedness

hypertension (hipertensión) — high blood pressure

hypertrophy (hipertrofia) — increase in size of an organ or structure that does not involve tumor formation

hypochlorhydria (hipoclorhidria) — abnormally low level of hydrochloric acid in the stomach

hypochondriasis (hipocondriasis) — abnormal concern about one's health

hypoglycemia (hipoglicemia) — abnormally low level of sugar in the blood

hypokalemia (hipoalcalemia) — abnormally low level of potassium in the blood

hyponatremia (hiponatremia) — abnormally low level of sodium in the blood

hypoproteinemia (hipoproteinemia) — abnormally low level of protein in the blood

hypotension (hipotensión) — low blood pressure

hypothermia (hipotermia) — below normal body temperature

hypoxia (hipoxia) — lack of adequate oxygen supply

I.A.D.L. (actividades instrumentales de la vida diaria) — instrumental activities of daily living (social and household activities)

I & O (entrada y salida) — intake and output

illusion (ilusión) — mental impression derived from misinterpreting an actual sensory stimulus

I.M. (intramuscular) — intramuscular

impaction (impactarse) — condition of being tightly wedged, for example, the feces in the bowel

implementation (implementación) — to put into action

incest (incesto) — culturally prohibited sexual activity between close relatives

incident (incidente) — occurrence

incontinence (incontinencia) — inability to resist the urge to defecate or urinate

indurated (endurecer) — hardened

induration (endurecimiento) — hardness; process of hardening

infectious (infeccioso) — capable of causing infection

insomnia (insomnio) — sleeplessness

inspection (inspección) — gaining information through the sense of sight

inspiration (inhalar) — drawing of air into the lungs

insulin (insulina) — active antidiabetic agent secreted by the islets of Langerhans in the pancreas

intercourse (relaciones sexuales) — interchange or communication between individuals; coitus

interpersonal relationships (relaciones interpersonales) — interactions between people

intertrigo (intértrigo) — skin irritation caused by friction between two moist, adjacent skin surfaces

intervention (intervención) — action performed for the patient

intimacy (intimidad) — close relationship characterized by love and affection

intravenous infusion (infusión intravenosa) — nourishment given through a sterile tube into the veins; also the injection of a solution, such as medication, to secure an immediate result

I.R.A. (cuenta individual para jubilados) — Individual Retirement Account; tax-deferred savings plan to encourage the accumulation of income for retirement

iridencleisis (iridencleisis) — surgery in which the iris is cut and inverted to form a wick into the subconjunctival space to promote drainage

ischemia (isquemia) — deficient blood supply to body tissues

isolation (aislar) — place where patients with easily transmitted diseases are kept separate from other patients

isolation technique (técnica de aislamiento, cuarentena) — name given to the method of caring for patients with easily transmitted diseases

jaundice (ictericia) — yellowing of the skin due to obstruction of the flow of bile

joint mouse (fragmentos de cartílago entre articulaciones) — loose cartilage in a joint

kardex (kardex) — carrier in which nursing care plans are kept

Keogh plan (Plan Keogh) — tax-deferred savings plan for the self-employed

keratitis (queratitis) — corneal infection

keratosis (queratosis) — roughened, scaly, wart-like lesions

ketosis (cetosis) — diabetic coma

kyphosis (cifosis) — hunchback

laxative (laxante) — a medicine that loosens the bowel contents and encourages evacuation

leisure (desocupación/ocio) — free time

lentigines (lentigines/pecas) — elevated yellow or brown spots on exposed skin; sometimes referred to as "liver spots"

lesbian (lesbiana) — homosexual female

lesion (lesión) — any damage to a tissue

lethargic (letárgico) — being stuperous or in coma resulting from disease or hypnosis

leukocyte (leucocito) — white blood cell

liable (confiable, propenso) — responsible

libel (calumnia y difamación) — written defamatory statement

libido (líbido) — instinctual energy or drive, often used with special reference to the motive power of the sex drive

life-care facility (establecimiento de cuidado de ancianos) — apartments that offer services, health care, and recreational facilities for the elderly

lipodystrophy (lipidodistrofia) — abnormal changes in the subcutaneous fat as the result of repeated insulin injections

living will (documento en el que el signatario instruye descontinuar tratamiento médico en caso de enfermedad incurable) — will written by a terminally ill patient expressing the wish that no extraordinary means be employed to prolong life

lordosis (lordosis) — abnormally increased concavity in the curvature of the lumbar spine

lover (amante) — sexual partner

lumen (lúz) — cavity or channel within a tube or tubular organ

macula (mácula) — part of the retina that is slightly lateral to and below the optic disc

malignancy (maligno) — cancerous condition that, if left untreated, leads to death

malpractice (negligencia o incompetencia profesional) — improper care by a health care professional, or care given without proper training

mammary (mamario) — pertaining to the breast

masochism (masoquismo) — self-punishment

mastectomy (masectomía) — removal of a breast

masticate (masticar) — to chew food with the teeth in preparation for swallowing

masturbation (masturbación) — sexual gratification by self-manipulation of the genitals

Medicaid (Seguro de Salud Estatal) — state program of medical insurance for the needy

Medicare (Seguro de Salud Federal para Ancianos) — federal program of health insurance to assist those over sixty-five with hospital and medical costs

meninges (meninges) — membranes that surround the brain and spinal cord

menopause (menopausia) — climacteric or "change of life"; the time that a female is no longer able to conceive children

metabolism (metabolismo) — sum total of the physical and chemical processes taking place among the ions, atoms, and molecules of the body

metric system (sistema métrico) — system of measurement based on multiples of ten, generally used to measure fluids

micturating cystogram (cistograma urinario) — X rays taken before and during urination

micturition (micción, emisión de orina) — urination

mineral (mineral) — substance that builds body tissues and regulates body fluids; essential nutrient

minority (minoría) — less than half of the total number

miotic (miótico, miósis) — drug that constricts the pupil of the eye

mitered corner (dobléz de las sabanas en las esquinas de las camas) — one type of corner used in making a hospital bed

mobility (mobilidad) — ability to move about

moniliasis (moniliasis) — infection by yeast organisms

morbidity (patología) — sickness

mortality (mortalidad) — state of being mortal or having to die; death

multi-infarct (infarto múltiple) — multiple strokes

myocardium (miocardio) — heart muscle

myth (mito) — popular belief or tradition; false notion

narcosis (narcosis) — stuporous state

nasoenteric tube (tubo nasalentérico) — tube inserted in the nose and extending into the intestines

nasogastric tube (tubo nasal-gástrico) — tube inserted in the nose and extending into the stomach

N.C.O.A. (Congreso Nacional de la Vejez) — National Council on Aging; a nonprofit, nongovernmental agency concerned with problems of ageing

necrosis (necrósis) — tissue death

negligence (negligencia) — failure to give the care that can reasonably be expected

nephron (nefrona) — functional unit of the kidney

neuron (neurona) — nerve cell

neurotransmitters (neurotransmisores) — chemicals that make transmission of the nerve impulse possible between neurons

N.G.U. (Uretritis por causas no identificadas) — urethritis of unidentified cause

N.I.D.D.M. (diabetes mellitus independiente de insulina) — noninsulin dependent diabetes mellitus

nocturia (nocturia) — excessive urination at night

normal flora (flora normal) — usual populations of organisms living on a particular body surface

nosocomial (perteneciente a hospital o nosocomio) — pertaining to a hospital or infirmary

N.R.T.A. (Asociación Nacional de Maestros Jubilados) — National Retired Teachers Association

nurse practitioner (enfermera o practicante) — professional nurse who has advanced education and clinical preparation in managing commonly occurring physical and emotional health problems of elderly people

nursing care plan (plan de tratamiento) — written, detailed program of the care to be given to a specific patient

nursing diagnosis (diagnóstico médico) — statement of the specific emotional, psychological, and physical needs of the patient

nursing process (proceso médico) — method used to determine the needs of the patient and the nursing activities to meet those needs

nursing technician (asistente de enfermería) — nursing assistant

nutrient (nutriente) — food that supplies heat and energy, builds and repairs body tissues, and regulates body functions

nutrition (nutrición) — the process by which the body uses food for growth and repair and to maintain health

obesity (obesidad) — condition of being overweight

objective (objetivo) — information collected through the senses

O.D. (ojo derecho) — right eye

oncology (oncología) — study of tumors

Operation REASON (operación REASON, programa de empleo y cuidado médico) — Responding to Elderly's Abilities and Sickness Otherwise Neglected; employment and health care program

orgasm (orgasmo) — climax of sexual excitement

orthopnea (ortopnea) — condition in which one can breathe only in an erect position

orthostatic hypotension (hipotensión hortoestática) — drop in blood pressure due to a sudden change in position

O.S. (ojo izquierdo) — left eye

osmotic agents (agentes osmóticos) — drugs that increase the water-drawing power of plasma

ossicles (osículos, huesecillos (del oído interno)) — three small bones in each ear that transmit sound waves from the outer ear to the inner ear

osteoporosis (osteoporosis) — systemic disease relating to a defect in the formation and maintenance of bone tissue

palliative (paliativo) — something that relieves symptoms without curing the disease

pallor (palidez) — less skin color than normal

palmar flexion (flexión palmar) — bending of the wrist downward

palpate (palpitación) — to examine using the sense of touch

pannus (pannus, pligue de la membrana sinovial) — gray, cloudy, vascular membrane associated with rheumatoid arthritis

paralysis (parálisis) — loss or impairment of the ability to move parts of the body

paranoia (paranoia) — state in which one has delusions of persecution

paraphrenia (parafrenia) — diagnosis of schizophrenia that develops after age forty-five

parasympathetic (parasimpático) — pertaining to one section of the autonomic nervous system that controls visceral activity

paroxysmal (paroxismal) — characterized by episodes of abrupt onset and termination

pathogenic organisms (organismo patógeno) — germs or disease-producing organisms

patient (paciente) — person who needs health care

patient rights (derechos del paciente) — list of standards, treatment, and care to which a patient is entitled

P.A.W.P. (presión arterio-pulmonar) — pulmonary arterial wedge pressure

pension (pensión) — retirement income or fund

perceptual processes (procesos perceptuales) — means of interpreting sensory information

peridontal (periodontal) — pertaining to the teeth

peristalsis (peristático) — progressive, wavelike movement that occurs involuntarily in hollow tubes of the body, especially in the digestive system

pes planus (pie plano) — flatfoot

pessary (pesario) — appliance inserted into the vagina to support the uterus

phenomenon (fenómeno) — a fact or event known through the senses rather than through thought or intuition

phlebotomy (flebotomía) — incision of a vein to withdraw blood

phlegm (flema) — mucus

pinna (pabellón de la oreja) — outer portion of the ear that is attached to the head

pitting edema (edema depresible) — condition in which tissue remains indented when pressure is applied to edematous areas

plantar flexion (flexión plantar) — pointing of the toes downward

plasma (plasma) — liquid portion of the blood

podiatrist (podiatra) — physician who specializes in care of the feet

podigeriatrics (podigeriatra) — medical specialty that deals with ageing feet

polydipsia (polidipsia) — excessive thirst

polyphagia (polifagia) — excessive ingestion of food

polyuria (poliuria) — excessive excretion of urine

potency (potencia) — power; especially the ability of the male to perform coitus

prefix (prefijo) — common beginning of words

presbyopia (prebiopia, presbicia) — impaired near vision resulting from changes in the eye's lens with age

p.r.n. (como sea necesario) — as needed

problem-solving technique (técnica de solución de problemas) — systematic manner used in identifying patient needs, determining appropriate goals or outcomes, planning the activities to achieve the outcomes, implementing the plan, and evaluating the outcomes for effectiveness

procidentia (procidencia, prolapso) — falling down, or state of prolapse, especially prolapse of the uterus

procreation (procreación) — act of begetting or generating life

projection (proyección) — defense mechanism in which responsibility for one's own actions is placed elsewhere

prolapse (prolapso) — falling down, or downward displacement, of an organ; to drop out of position

proprioception (propiocepción) — reception of internal stimuli

protein (proteína) — basic material of every body cell; essential nutrient

protocol (protocolo) — written statement of actions to be followed in a specific set of circumstances

pruritus (prurito) — itching

psychosis (psicosis) — major emotional disorder with derangement of the personality and loss of contact with reality, often with delusions, hallucinations, or illusions

psychosocial (psicosocial) — psychological and social

psychotic (psicótico) — out of touch with reality

pulmonary emphysema (enfisema pulmonar) — chronic lung disorder in which the terminal bronchioles become plugged with mucus and lung elasticity is lost

pulse pressure (presión diferencial) — difference between systolic and diastolic blood pressures

P.V.D. (mal vascular periférico) — peripheral vascular disease

pylorus (píloro) — narrow, tapered end of the stomach opening into the duodenum

pyorrhea (piorrea) — peridontitis

rales (estertor) — bubbling type of respiration caused by fluid that collects in the air passages

rationalization (racionalización) — defense mechanism in which a logical explanation is given to cover one's less logical feelings

reaction (reacción) — opposite action or counteraction; response

reality orientation (orientación a la realidad) — technique of assisting patients to become more aware of their surroundings or environment

rectocele (rectocele) — protrusion of the posterior vaginal wall

rectum (recto) — lower part of the large intestine, about 5 inches long, between the sigmoid flexure and the anal canal

refraction (refracción) — bending of light rays to focus on the area of most acute vision reception

rehabilitation (rehabilitación) — maximum possible restoration of function

resident (residente) — patient in a long-term care facility

rest home (hogar de descanso) — long-term care facility

retention (retensión) — inability to excrete urine

retina (retina) — nervous tissue layer of the eye containing photoreceptor neurons

retinopathy (retinopatía) — noninflammatory disease of the eye

retirement (jubilación) — time after leaving employment

rods (bastones) — photoreceptor cells of the retina for night vision

R.S.V.P. (Programa de Jubilados Voluntarios) — Retired Senior Volunteer Program

rubra (rubor) — unusual redness or flushing of the skin

saliva (saliva) — the first digestive secretion; emitted from the salivary glands into the mouth

schizophrenia (esquizofrenia) — chronic mental disorder characterized by the inability to distinguish fantasy from reality; often accompanied by hallucinations and delusions

sclera (esclerótica) — fibrous outer protective coat of the eye; "white of the eye"

S.C.O.R.E. (Cuerpo de Servicio de Ejecutivos Jubilados) — Service Corps of Retired Executives

S.C.S.E.P. (Programa Comunal para Empleo de Ancianos) — Senior Community Service Employment Program

S.D.A.T. (demencia senil) — senile dementia (Alzheimer's disease)

sedative (sedante) — agent that calms nervousness, irritability, and excitement

sedentary (sedentario) — pertaining to a sitting or inactive posture

seizure (convulsión) — sudden attack

senescence (senectud) — growing old

senile (senil) — affected with the infirmities of age

senile keratoses (queratosis senil) — roughened, scaly, slightly elevated, wartlike lesions thought to be related to sunburn damage in fair-skinned individuals

senior citizen center (centro de ancianos) — place where older people get together for socialization, recreation, learning, exercise, and health care (such as testing or innoculations)

sensuality (sensualidad) — experiencing through the senses

septum (septum, tabique) — wall or partition dividing a body cavity or space

shearing force (fuerzas de corte) — damaging pressure that occurs as the weight of the torso and gravity tend to pull deep tissues such as muscle and bone in one direction while the skin tends to remain stationary

signs and symptoms (señales y síntomas) — objective and subjective indications of disease

skilled nursing facility (establecimiento de cuidado avanzado) — long-term care facility

sleep apnea (apnea nocturna) — stoppage of breathing during sleep

Social Security (Seguro Social Federal para los retirados o incapacitados) — Old Age, Survivors, and Disability Insurance

society (sociedad) — structured group of people with common interests and goals

somnifacients (somnífero) — drugs that induce sleep

sphygmomanometer (baumanómetro) — instrument for determining arterial pressure; blood pressure gauge

spouse (cónyuge) — married man or woman

S.S.I. (suplemento social de renta) — Supplemental Security Income

standard (patrón, norma) — level of quality or quantity or value

standard (columna, pilar) — pole used to hang treatment fluids

S.T.D. (enfermedad sexualmente transmitida) — sexually transmitted disease

stereotype (estereotipo) — characteristic assigned to entire groups of people

steroids (esteroides) — complex compounds that improve the protective function of tissues; cholesterol is the main building block of steroid hormones in the body

stethoscope (estetoscopio) — instrument used in auscultation to convey to the ear the sounds produced in the body

stoma (estoma) — artificial, mouthlike opening

stuporous (asombrado, pasmado) — being in a state of near unconsciousness; a state of lethargy and immobility with diminished responsiveness to stimulation

subjective (subjetivo) — known only to the individual

substance abuse (drogadicción) — inappropriate use of drugs

suffix (sufijo) — common ending of words

suppository (supositorio) — device used to help the bowels eliminate feces

sympathetic (simpático) — portion of the nervous system that prepares the body for emergency situations through control of the viscera

sympathy (simpatía) — sharing similar feelings with another

synovium (membrana sinovial) — joint lining

syphilis (sífilis) — sexually transmitted disease caused by a spirochete

systolic (sistólico) — blood pressure reading taken when pressure is greatest, during contractions; refers to the contraction phase of the cardiac cycle

tachycardia (taquicardia) — unusually fast heartbeat

tact (tacto, delicadeza) — sensitivity in the treatment of others

tactile (táctil) — relating to the sense of touch

terminal (final, terminal) — final or fatal condition

theories (teorías) — unproven ideas; logical attempts to explain that which is not understood

therapeutic (terapeútico) — pertaining to results obtained from treatment; healing agent

therapeutic communication (comunicación terapeútica) — communication with a designed purpose

thrombocyte (trombocito) — platelet produced in the bone; important in blood clotting

thyroxine (tiroxina) — hormone of the thyroid gland that contains iodine

tic douloureaux (neurálgia del trigémino) — trigeminal neuralgia

tonography (tonografía) — recording of change in intraocular pressure due to sustained pressure on the eyeball

tonometry (tonometría) — measurement of tension or intraocular pressure

tonus (tono) — normal state of firmness; normal state of slight contracture of all skeletal muscles

toxicity (toxicidad) — quality of exerting deleterious effects on an organism or tissue

tranquilizers (tranquilizantes, calmantes) — any of a group of compounds that calm or quiet an anxious person without causing drowsiness

trephination (trepanación) — surgical procedure in which a small circle of tissue is removed, chiefly from the skull, cornea, or sclera

trigeminal neuralgia (neurálgia del trigémino) — bouts of severe pain felt following the path of the trigeminal nerve

trochanter roll (rodillo trocanter) — rolled towel or bath blanket placed against the lateral thigh to maintain proper alignment

tunica intima (túnica íntima, capa endotelial) — inner coat of an artery

turgor (skin) (turgor, turgencia) — having normal firmness or tone

T.U.R.P. (escición transuretral prostática) — transurethral prostatic resection

tyloma (callosidad) — calluses

ulcers (úlceras) — open sores caused by blood stoppage and broken skin

uremia (uremia) — presence of increased urea, a waste product, in the blood

urgency (urgencia) — need to urinate or defecate

vaginitis (vaginitis) — inflammation of the vagina

validation therapy (terapia de auto-estima) — interactions that reinforce the patient's self-esteem

vasodilators (vasodilatadores) — nerve or agent that causes blood vessels to dilate

venereal (venéreo, venérea) — encouraged by intercourse

ventilation (ventilación) — process of supplying with fresh air

ventilator (ventilador) — machine used to assist the delivery of oxygen or medication into the lungs

ventricle (ventrículo) — small cavity or chamber, as in the brain or heart

vertigo (vértigo) — dizziness

viscera (víscera) — organs

V.I.S.T.A. (Voluntarios al Servicio de Estados Unidos de Norteamérica) — Volunteers in Service to America

visual accommodation (acomodación visual) — adjustment of the eye to see objects at various distances

vital capacity (capacidad vital) — volume of air a person can forcibly expire from the lungs after a maximal inspiration

vitamin (vitamina) — substance that regulates body processes; essential nutrient

void (vaciar) — to release urine from the bladder

volunteerism (voluntariado) — contribution of time to help others

vomitus (vómito) — matter ejected from the stomach through the mouth

withdrawal (mecanismo de retracción) — defense mechanism in which one absents oneself mentally and/or physically from a situation that is too threatening

withhold (ayuno, abstención alimenticia) — order whereby a patient is not to be served food

yeast (levadura) — microorganism that can sometimes cause infection

Index

family reaction to, 23
Sight, loss of, 50, 331–32
Signal lights, 194
Skilled care facilities, 78, 124
Skin. *See also* Integumentary system.
    aging of, 52–53
    care of, 406–8
    structure of, 404–6
Slander, 171–72
Social Security benefits, 4, 89–91
Socialization, 118–20
Soporifics, 253–54
Spinal cord, structure of, 281–82
Spleen, function of, 361
Sputum specimen, collection of, 391
Stereotypes, about aging, 6–10
Sterile packages, opening of, 204–5
Sterilization, of equipment, 204
Steroids, 256
Stockings, elasticized, 373
Stoma, care of, 386–87, 473
Stool specimen, collection of, 479–80
Stress, 21–23, 38–39
Stroke. *See* Cerebrovascular accident.
Substance abuse, 39
Suicide, prevention of, 312
Suppositories, insertion of, 478–79
Syphilis, 521

T
Technician, health care, geriatric, 131, 135–39. *See also*
        Nursing assistant and Health workers.
Teeth, brushing of, 412–14
Temperature, taking of, 539–42
Terminal illness, 263–74
Terminology, medical, 160–62
Testes, cancer of, 518
Theft, 171
Thermometers, types of, 538–40
Thymus, 53–54
Thyroid, 53, 343
T.I.A.s. *See* Transient ischemic attacks.
Tic douloureux, 286–88
Tinnitus, 255, 256
Tipping, 158
Toenails, 52, 416–17, 451
Tonography, 329
Tourniquets, rotation of, 368–69
Tracheostomy, care of, 386–87
Transient ischemic attacks (T.I.A.s), 292. *See also*
        Cerebrovascular accident.

dementia and, 313
Tremors, 288–89
Trichomoniasis, 521
Trigeminal nerve, 286–88
Tuberculosis, 387–88

U
Ulcers, decubitus, development of, 419–23
        prevention of, 423–28
        treatment of, 428–29
    peptic, 470
Unemployment, of older workers, 104–5
Universal Precautions, 201, 203
Urethritis, nongonorrheal, 519
Urinal, procedure for, 489–90
Urinalysis, 492
Urinary system, alterations in, 241, 484–507
        nursing diagnoses for, 487
    senescent changes in, 487
    structure of, 484–85
Urine, drainage unit for, emptying of, 502–503
    elimination of, 486–87
    incontinence of, 491–92, 495–98
    production of, 485–86
    retention of, 491–92
    specimen, collection of, 492–95
    testing of, 351–54
Urosheaths, 497–98
Uterus, anatomy of, 515–16

V
Vaginitis, 519
Vascular disease, 372–77
Vasodilators, 252
Venereal disease, 520–22
Venereal warts, 521
Vertigo, 50
Vital signs, 538–45
Vitamin(s), 214, 253
Voiding, techniques for, 496
Volunteerism, 112, 121–22

W
Walking, as exercise, 438
Warts, venereal, 521
Watch record, neurosurgical, 284–85
Water, changing of, 225
    diet and, 214–15
Weighing, procedure for, 537–38
Wheelchair, assisting with, 441–42
Workers, health. *See* Health Workers.